Management of Treatment-Resistant Major Psychiatric Disorders

Management of Treatment-Resistant Major Psychiatric Disorders

EDITED BY

Charles B. Nemeroff, MD, PhD

Leonard M. Miller Professor and Chairman
Department of Psychiatry and Behavioral Sciences
University of Miami Miller School of Medicine
Miami, FL

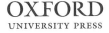

OXFORD
UNIVERSITY PRESS

OXFORD
UNIVERSITY PRESS

Oxford University Press is a department of the University of Oxford.
It furthers the University's objective of excellence in research,
scholarship, and education by publishing worldwide.

Oxford   New York
Auckland   Cape Town   Dar es Salaam   Hong Kong   Karachi
Kuala Lumpur   Madrid   Melbourne   Mexico City   Nairobi
New Delhi   Shanghai   Taipei   Toronto

With offices in
Argentina   Austria   Brazil   Chile   Czech Republic   France   Greece
Guatemala   Hungary   Italy   Japan   Poland   Portugal   Singapore
South Korea   Switzerland   Thailand   Turkey   Ukraine   Vietnam

Published in the United States of America by Oxford University Press
198 Madison Avenue, New York, NY 10016, United States of America
www.oup.com

Oxford is a registered trademark of Oxford University Press in the UK
and in certain other countries

Library of Congress Cataloging-in-Publication Data
  Management of treatment-resistant major psychiatric disorders / edited
by Charles B. Nemeroff. — 1st ed.
    p.; cm.
  Includes bibliographical references.
  ISBN 978-0-19-973998-1 (hardcover)
  I. Nemeroff, Charles B.
  [DNLM: 1. Mental Disorders—therapy. 2. Drug Resistance.
3. Treatment Outcome. WM 400]
  616.89—dc23   2012000394

9 8 7 6 5 4 3 2 1
Printed in the United States of America on acid-free paper

To my patients, who have taught me so much,

and

To my wife, Gayle, and children (Gigi, Ross, Amanda, and Michael),
who have taught me even more

Contents

Preface

The need for a summary on the management of treatment-resistant psychiatric disorders became evident to me over the last several years when interacting with busy practitioners and academics at various continuing medical education programs and professional meetings. From these discussions, the seed for this book was sown. The toll of treatment-resistant disorders on patients and their families in terms of suffering and economic cost is staggering. The cost to society in terms of loss of life from suicide, increased drug and alcohol abuse, loss of productivity, and increases in overall health care costs is almost unfathomable. The magnitude of the problem is generally greater than appreciated by most practitioners. A very large number of our patients with major psychiatric disorders do not achieve remission, certainly not with monotherapy, either pharmacologically or psychotherapeutically. Although many patients with these disorders are treated by non–mental health professionals, generally family practitioners and internists, those who do not respond to initial therapies are referred to psychiatrists, and this treatment population comprises a large percentage of most psychiatrists' practices.

The goal of this book is to assemble many of the leaders in the psychiatric treatment field to summarize the evidence for management of patients with the major mood, anxiety, and psychotic disorders who fail their initial treatment. The chapter authors are well known to many of the readers because of their manifold contributions to the literature. With the exception of the chapter on generalized anxiety disorders (GAD), the chapters are all written by authors based in the United States. This might be viewed as a shortcoming by some because of the frequent references to the United States Food and Drug Administration (FDA), but space constraints precluded consideration of regulatory agency approval in different countries worldwide. The GAD chapter is of special interest not only because of its wealth of knowledge but because of its uniquely European focus. The chapters are remarkably up to date and the publication delay has been truly minimal, undoubtedly due to the diligent efforts of David D'Addona and Craig Panner of Oxford University Press. They have been truly a pleasure to work with. Together we believe this book will be a welcome addition to the busy practitioner's library.

Contributors

Jacob S. Ballon, MD
Department of Psychiatry
College of Physicians and Surgeons
Columbia University; and
New York State Psychiatric Institute
New York, NY

Kathleen T. Brady, MD, PhD
Department of Psychiatry
Clinical Neuroscience Division
Clinical and Translational Research
South Carolina Clinical and Translational
   Research Institute; and
Medical University of South Carolina
Charleston, SC

Eric Bui, MD, PhD
Department of Psychiatry
Massachusetts General Hospital
Boston, MA

Kevin Ryan Connolly, MD
VISN 4 MIRECC
Philadelphia Veterans Affairs Medical
   Center; and
Department of Psychiatry
Perelman School of Medicine
University of Pennsylvania
Philadelphia, PA

Karl Doghramji, MD
Department of Psychiatry and Human
   Behavior; and
The Jefferson Sleep Disorders Center
Thomas Jefferson University
Philadelphia, PA

Darin D. Dougherty, MD
Department of Psychiatry
Massachusetts General Hospital
Boston, MA

Mark A. Frye, MD
Department of Psychiatry and Psychology
Mayo Clinic
Rochester, MN

Glen O. Gabbard, MD
Department of Psychiatry
Baylor College of Medicine
Houston, TX

Priya Gopalan, MD
Department of Psychiatry
Western Psychiatric Institute and Clinic
Pittsburgh, PA

Emily Grenesko-Stevens
Department of Psychiatry
University of California-San Diego
La Jolla, CA

Paul E. Holtzheimer, MD
Department of Psychiatry
Dartmouth-Hitchcock Medical Center
Lebanon, NH

Robert Hudak, MD
Department of Psychiatry
Western Psychiatric Institute and Clinic
Pittsburgh, PA

Walter H. Kaye, MD
Department of Psychiatry
University of California-San Diego
La Jolla, CA

Jeffrey A. Lieberman, MD
Department of Psychiatry
Columbia University College of Physicians
    and Surgeons; and
New York State Psychiatric Institute; and
New York Presbyterian Hospital-Columbia
    University Medical Center
New York, NY

Kerry-Ann Louw, MB ChB
Department of Psychiatry and Mental Health
University of Cape Town
Cape Town, South Africa

R. Bruce Lydiard, MD, PhD
Ralph H. Johnson VA Medical Center and
    Department of Psychiatry and Behavioral
    Sciences
Medical University of South Carolina
Charleston, SC

Enrica Marzola, MD
Department of Neuroscience
Section of Psychiatry
University of Turin
Turin, Italy

Charles B. Nemeroff, MD, PhD
Department of Psychiatry and Behavioral
    Sciences
University of Miami Miller School of Medicine
Miami, FL

**David J. Nutt, DM, FRCP, FRCPsych,
FMedSci**
Edmond J Safra Chair
Neuropsychopharmacology Unit
Imperial College London
London, United Kingdom

Victoria Osman-Hicks
Academic Unit of Psychiatry
University of Bristol
Bristol, UK

Mark H. Pollack, MD
Department of Psychiatry
Rush University Medical Center
Chicago, IL

John Potokar, MD, MRCPsych
Academic Unit of Psychiatry
University of Bristol
Bristol, UK

Charles F. Reynolds III, MD
Western Psychiatric Institute and Clinic
University of Pittsburgh School of
    Medicine
Pittsburgh, PA

Patricio Riva Posse, MD
Department of Psychiatry and Behavioral
    Sciences
Emory University
Atlanta, GA

Dan J. Stein, FRCPC, PhD
Department of Psychiatry and Mental
    Health
University of Cape Town
Cape Town, South Africa

Michael E. Thase, MD
Department of Psychiatry
Perelman School of Medicine
University of Pennsylvania
Philadelphia Veterans Affairs Medical
    Center
Philadelphia, PA

Mary Ellen Trunko, MD
Department of Psychiatry
University of California-San Diego
La Jolla, CA

Karen Dineen Wagner, MD, PhD
Department of Psychiatry
The University of Texas Medical
    Branch
Galveston, TX

Management of Treatment-Resistant Major Psychiatric Disorders

The Problem of Treatment-Resistant Psychiatric Disorders

Patricio Riva Posse and Charles B. Nemeroff

Introduction

Mental disorders occur in all cultures and at all stages of life. They are associated with poverty, marginalization, social disadvantage, violent conflicts, and other major disasters, and they are the most prominent causes of deliberate self-harm, the 10–20 million suicide attempts, and the 1 million completed suicides every year worldwide (Churchill, 2010). Unfortunately, in most parts of the world, mental health and mental disorders are not considered as important as physical health. Instead, they have been largely ignored or neglected. Partly as a result, the world is suffering from an increasing burden of mental disorders and a widening "treatment gap." According to a World Health Organization (WHO) report, in 2001 approximately 450 million people suffered from a mental or behavioral disorder, yet only a small minority of them received even the most basic treatment. In developing countries, most individuals with severe mental disorders are left to cope as best they can with depression, dementia, schizophrenia, and substance dependence. Globally, many are victimized for their illness and become the targets of stigma and discrimination (WHO, 2001). The rate of outpatient treatment for depression in the United States has been increasing in the past 20 years, but it is still below the population prevalence estimates. In 1987, 0.73% of the population was receiving treatment, increasing to 2.37% in 1998 and 2.88% in 2007 (Marcus & Olfson, 2010). This is still below the community prevalence estimates of 6.6% to 7.1% for major depressive disorder prevalence in 1 year (Compton, Conway, Stinson, & Grant, 2006). In addition to the scores of patients who remain untreated, there is another group of patients who are not improving despite receiving medical care. There is also evidence that patients receiving psychiatric treatment are not receiving the optimal care they should, for example, being underdosed in the antipsychotic regimen in psychotic depression (Rasmussen et al., 2006). It seems that inadequate treatment is often the norm rather than the exception in the treatment of mental illness. For example, in one study only 33% of

801 patients with chronic depression had ever had a prior adequate trial of antidepressant medication (Kocsis et al., 2008).

New advances in pharmacotherapy have had a remarkable impact on the course and outcome of psychiatric disorders. However, studies consistently demonstrate that a significant proportion of patients who receive drug treatments achieve minimal or no improvement in their symptoms. In the last decades of psychopharmacological research, the response rates of medication for depression have overall remained stable (Holtzheimer & Mayberg, 2011).

A treatment-resistant psychiatric disorder refers to the occurrence of an inadequate response following adequate therapy among patients suffering from a defined psychiatric disorder. For example, when considering depression, this could mean that adequate antidepressant treatment does not result in an adequate response in a unipolar depressed patient (Dickerson et al., 2006). This "inadequate" response is a relative term in that patients' responses range from complete remission, to moderate improvement, to absolute nonresponse. There are some psychiatric disorders that generally show a better response to currently available treatments than others.

There are no universally accepted definitions of what defines treatment resistance for all of the individual psychiatric disorders. In medicine there is a clear distinction between chronicity and refractoriness. Most cases of diabetes and essential hypertension are, although chronic disorders, highly treatment responsive. Patients can often remain on stable doses of the same medications during their entire lives, for example, the same doses of hypoglycemic agents or antihypertensives (Elkis, 2007). In contrast, after receiving multiple trials of various pharmacological agents at adequate doses for a substantial amount of time, some patients remain severely ill with little or no symptomatic or functional improvement. There are also patients for whom treatments that had worked earlier in the course of their illness become ineffective.

Magnitude of the Problem

The Global Burden of Disease report revealed the worldwide impact of mental illness (WHO, 2008). Severe depression and active psychosis are in the same range of severity (i.e., highest level of disability) as quadriplegia and terminal cancer. WHO ranks the disability caused by these illnesses as severe as blindness or Down syndrome. Depression was identified in the WHO report as the leading global cause of years of health lost to disease in both men and women. Unipolar depression makes a large contribution to the worldwide burden of disease. It is the eighth leading cause of loss of health in low-income countries and the primary cause of loss of health in middle- and high-income countries. In 2004 depression was the third most prevalent cause of moderate and severe disability in the world (after hearing loss and refractive errors), with the additional fact that it was the most common in individuals under 60 in both low- and middle-income as well as high-income countries. It was overall the leading cause of disability in high-income countries. In addition to depression, alcohol dependence, bipolar disorder, schizophrenia, dementias, panic disorder, and drug dependence are all in the top 20 causes of disability. In the year 2000, depression was already the fourth leading contributor to the global burden of disease in terms of "disability adjusted life years"; it is projected to become the second leading contributor by the year 2020 (second only to heart disease)—indeed, it has already reached second place in the age category 15–44 years and is expected to reach first place by 2030 (WHO, 2008).

The purpose of this chapter is to introduce the discussion of the problem of treatment-resistant psychiatric disorders and to focus on treatment-resistant psychiatric disorders as a public health problem. Treatment resistance is understood differently across separate disorders. Many times treatment resistance is used interchangeably with "difficult-to-treat" disorders. Some disorders are inherently more difficult to treat than others, for example, schizophrenia compared to specific phobias. Some treatments are incomplete (i.e., the paucity of options to treat cognitive and negative symptomatology in schizophrenia), and other disorders seem less impairing than others but may show little response to current available treatments (i.e., certain anxiety disorders).

What Is Treatment Resistance?

If we define treatment resistance by lack of response to adequate treatments, this prompts several questions: What is adequate treatment? How many lines/steps of approved treatments render an individual "treatment resistant"? Do patients become treatment resistant? Do medicines generate treatment resistance, similar to antibiotic exposure generating resistant strains? Depressed patients tend to have less chance of achieving remission with increasing cumulative episodes (Holtzheimer & Mayberg, 2010). Patients in the third step of treatment of major depressive disorder in STAR*D exhibited only a 13.7% remission rate, compared to the 36.8% in the first step (Rush et al., 2006). There has also been confusion in recent years between the terms "treatment resistant" and "treatment refractory." The latter term has come to imply an inability to respond to any treatment and as such is generally avoided in this chapter and the volume in general. We do not believe that there is sufficient data to suggest that any patient with a psychiatric disorder cannot respond to any currently available or novel treatments developed in the future.

It is also important to define treatment goals, in order to understand treatment resistance as an inability to attain them. The past few years have seen a rise in the "recovery models" for different psychiatric disorders, an issue that had been largely overlooked previously (Warner, 2009). Does symptom remission mean functional remission (Wingo, Baldessarini, Holtzheimer, & Harvey, 2010)? There is a significant difference between syndromal recovery (no longer fulfilling *DSM-IV* episode criteria) and functional recovery (regaining baseline vocational and residential status). For example, in bipolar disorder, functional recovery is 2.6 times less likely than syndromal recovery (Tohen et al., 2000). In schizophrenia, recovery is defined as a 2-year duration of (1) remission of symptoms, (2) engagement in productive activity such as work or school, (3) independent management of day-to-day needs, (4) cordial family relations, (5) recreational activities, and (6) satisfying peer relationships (Liberman, 2008). In most psychiatric disorders, including schizophrenia (Andreasen et al., 2005), major depression (Nierenberg & Wright, 1999), and anxiety disorders (Ninan, 2001), the goal is recovery and full remission of symptoms.

The recovery model in psychosis also takes into consideration the multiple clinical features of schizophrenia, including disability in everyday functioning (social functioning, everyday living skills, productive activities, and independence in living), cognitive impairments, various comorbidities (substance abuse, medical illness, and medication side effects), and other symptoms, including depression and anxiety, that are not part of the formal diagnostic criteria for this illness (Harvey & Bellack, 2009).

The National Comorbidity Survey Replication (NCS-R) results show 12-month *DSM-IV* disorders to be highly prevalent in the United States. Although over one third of cases are mild, the prevalence of moderate and serious cases is substantial (14% of the population). Although anxiety disorders are by far the most common mental disorders, they are often considered less serious than other classes of disorders, though the disability associated with them is often quite severe and comorbidity is the rule, not the exception. Mood disorders are the next most common and have the greatest severity. The NCS-R did not include schizophrenia or nonaffective psychosis in the survey (Kessler, Chiu, Demler, Merikangas, & Walters, 2005).

The US lifetime prevalence of major depressive disorder is 16.6%. For bipolar I and II disorders it has been estimated to be 3.7%–3.9%. The overall lifetime prevalence rate of mood disorders is therefore 20.8%. There are almost twice as many women affected as men (Kessler, Berglund et al., 2005). The incidence of depression is growing worldwide and by 2030 it is predicted to be the primary cause of years lost to disability (WHO, 2008). This incidence has been steadily growing (Murray & Lopez, 1997). Between 10% and 30% of depressed patients will not remit and stay well while receiving adequate therapy (Nierenberg & Amsterdam, 1990). The results of STAR*D revealed that 33% of patients failed to achieve remission despite multiple treatment steps, and that relapse occurred in about 50% of patients in less than a year (Rush et al., 2006). After adequate first-line treatment with citalopram, approximately 70% of patients remain symptomatic (Trivedi et al., 2006). Antidepressant medications are effective in the treatment of major depressive disorder, but only 25%–45% of patients experience remission after one antidepressant monotherapy trial (Nierenberg et al., 2006). Patients with recurrent episodes are more likely to exhibit a longer latency to respond to the next phase of treatment.

The impact (in terms of duration of episodes and quality of life) of depressive episodes in bipolar patients is substantially worse than the impact of manic episodes (Calabrese, Hirschfeld, Frye, & Reed, 2004; Judd et al., 2002). Unfortunately, far less research attention has been paid to the treatment of bipolar depression as compared to acute mania or unipolar depression (Gijsman, Geddes, Rendell, Nolen, & Goodwin, 2004; McEvoy et al., 2005).

Evidence is increasing that for most patients, mood disorders are chronic relapsing illnesses. Attention is therefore shifting from acute treatment strategies to evaluation of relapse prevention (Kellner et al., 2006).

In schizophrenia, depending on the definition, between 30% and 60% of patients are considered treatment resistant (Solanki, Singh, & Munshi, 2009). How do we define treatment resistance in schizophrenia? Given that schizophrenia is a chronic disease and that close to 90% of patients develop social or occupational dysfunction, precisely defining its treatment resistance is a challenge. Some authors propose the failure to respond to a certain number of medications (Kane, Honigfeld, Singer, & Meltzer, 1988) or the number of acute or chronic hospitalizations (Conley & Kelly, 2001), though it is generally agreed that the latter does not constitute, by itself, the sole criterion to define treatment resistance

(Brenner et al., 1990). The initial trials of clozapine (Multicenter Clozapine Trial) had inclusion criteria that were (1) at least three periods of treatment in the preceding 5 years (from at least two different drug classes) at dosages equivalent to or greater than 1000 mg/d of chlorpromazine for a period of 6 weeks, each without significant symptomatic relief, and (2) no period of good functioning within the preceding 5 years (Kane et al., 1988). Before starting clozapine, patients were treated for 6 weeks with haloperidol (10–60 mg/d) and exhibited a less than 20% reduction in Brief Psychiatry Rating Scale (BPRS) scores or were intolerant to the drug. Given that doses greater than or equal to 400 mg/d of chlorpromazine block 80%–90% of dopamine D2/D3 receptors, and that higher doses produce no direct therapeutic benefit, now the standard accepted dose of chlorpromazine is 400–600 mg (Barnes & McEvedy, 1996). "Treatment-resistant" schizophrenia is used interchangeably in different trials when considering patient's eligibility for clozapine (Juarez-Reyes et al., 1995), and by this standard about 43% of patients fulfill the criteria.

"Response" is a relative term in schizophrenia and many patients will continue to suffer from low-level symptoms even after response to a medication is seen. Typically, "response" for a treatment-resistant patient was defined by Kane et al. as a ≥20% decrease in total BPRS score (18-item scale) and a final score of ≤36 (Kane et al., 1988), obviously not close to any reasonable definition of remission. Because some patients who exhibit very high levels initially may exhibit significant reductions in BPRS scores but never reach an end point score of 36 or less, modified response criteria are often used. These usually include a 20% reduction on the total BPRS score and either a final score of 36 or a decrease on another dimensional measure such as the Clinical Global Impression (Guy, 1970) or the Bunney-Hamburg Global Psychosis Rating Scale (Bunney & Hamburg, 1963), usually to a score equivalent of mild psychosis (Conley & Kelly, 2001; Pickar et al., 1992). Partial response to clozapine was defined as a 20% reduction in the total BPRS score. When switching from first-generation antipsychotics, only 9% of patients who were nonresponders to one drug exhibited a response to higher doses of the same drug or another first-generation drug (Kinon et al., 1993).

Some authors propose the term "incomplete recovery" to describe this particular subtype of schizophrenia (Pantelis & Lambert, 2003). They emphasize the potential of improved therapeutic outcomes with more advanced pharmacological options, and the term reduces the stigma implied in treatment resistance because some consider the term to imply lack of collaboration by the patient.

Anxiety disorders are highly prevalent both in men and women (Ansseau et al., 2004). Generalized anxiety disorder affects 3%–5% of the general population in the United States and is twice as prevalent among women than men (Kessler, Chiu, et al., 2005). Anxiety disorders tend to be chronic and the rate of remission is low. Remission rates vary between 0.30 and 0.60 at 5-year follow-up (Yonkers, Bruce, Dyck, & Keller, 2003). The likelihood of remission of generalized anxiety disorder is 15% after 1 year and 25% after 2 years (Yonkers, Warshaw, Massion, & Keller, 1996). Over 8 years, only 38% of women and 32% of men experienced a complete remission of social phobia, according to a longitudinal study conducted by the Harvard-Brown Anxiety Research Program (Yonkers, Dyck, & Keller, 2001). Relapse is frequent and characteristic of many anxiety disorders. Generalized anxiety disorder is typically a chronic disorder with a waxing and waning course (Wittchen, 2002), and patients who do not achieve a full symptomatic remission have higher chances of relapse (Yonkers, Dyck, Warshaw, & Keller, 2000).

Obsessive-compulsive disorder exhibits several differences with the other anxiety disorders. It is the only anxiety disorder that has a similar prevalence in men and women (Karno, Golding, Sorenson, & Burnam, 1988). It is recognized as an inherently difficult-to-treat disorder and most of the trials accept a 25%–35% reduction in the symptoms as a measure of response to the treatment (Goodman, Ward, Kablinger, & Murphy, 2000). Between 40% and 60% of patients fail to respond to first-line pharmacological or psychotherapeutic treatments (Mancebo et al., 2006). When considering a patient with obsessive-compulsive disorder to be treatment resistant, the question of adequate trials of medications that include high enough doses (often the maximum recommended dose) for long enough periods of time (10–12 weeks) is important (American Academy of Child and Adolescent Psychiatry [AACAP], 1998). It is also critical for optimal management for the patients to have a meaningful trial of behavioral therapy, usually exposure and relapse prevention (Albert, Bergesio, Pessina, Maina, & Bogetto, 2002; Foa & Kozak, 1996).

Factors Contributing to Treatment Resistance

As summarized in Table 1.1, there are multiple factors that contribute to treatment resistance (Bystritsky, 2006). Without intending to oversimplify this complex issue, we can divide these factors into those related to the pathophysiology; factors related to the environment, such as stressors; factors related to patients; and factors related to clinicians, who for a variety of reasons often use ineffective therapeutic options.

Comorbidity between different psychiatric disorders renders each individual disorder more difficult to treat. In a survey from the Systematic Treatment Enhancement Program for Bipolar Disorder (STEP-BD), patients with bipolar disorder had a high degree of comorbidity with anxiety disorders, with a lifetime prevalence of >50% (Simon et al., 2004). Bipolar patients with a comorbid anxiety syndrome had several poor prognosis indicators, including a younger age at onset, decreased likelihood of recovery, poorer role functioning and quality of life, less time euthymic, and greater likelihood of suicide attempts, with an odds ratio for history of suicide attempts of 2.45 (95% CI = 1.4–4.2).

The coexistence of Axis I disorders such as major depression with substance use disorders confers a greater overall severity and worse health-related outcomes, including increased risk of suicide (Nunes & Levin, 2004). This is particularly worrisome in patients with bipolar I disorder (Tondo et al., 1999).

Comorbidity among psychiatric disorders is very common, not only with Axis I but also with Axis II disorders. The relationship between personality and depression is complex and multifactorial, and it includes at least three different processes: predisposition, complication, and coaggregation. "Predisposition" refers to the tendency for people with selected pathologic personality traits, for example, neuroticism or excessive interpersonal dependence, to be at greater risk for depression. "Complication" refers to the development or exaggeration of personality traits as a consequence of the primary disorder. "Coaggregation" describes how related vulnerabilities are simultaneously expressed in the same individual. For example, patients with borderline personality disorder have a higher co-occurrence of

TABLE 1.1 Outline of Reasons for Poor Response to Treatment of Psychiatric Disorders

Pathology related
- Exact underlying pathophysiology unknown
- Multiple neurotransmitters' participation and interaction
- Complex receptor and feedback structure of every single transmitter system
- Diagnosis-dimensional approach
- Genetics of disorders is overlapping and unclear what is inherited
- Current biological treatments are empirical and have limitations

Environment related
- Severe acute or long-term persistent stressors
- Childhood stressors, early life trauma
- Life cycles
- Cost of and access to available treatments, including new drugs, therapeutic approaches (e.g., electroconvulsive therapy, repetitive transcranial magnetic stimulation, deep brain stimulation), or evidence-based psychotherapy

Patient related
- Severity
- Medical comorbidity
- Psychiatric comorbidity
- Noncompliance
- Discordance between symptomatic remission and functional improvement
- Cultural factors

Clinician related
- Lack of knowledge in primary care
- Nonadherence to recommended treatment guidelines
- Lack of use of illness severity and rating scales to optimize available treatments
- Lack of recognition of subsyndromal states, without pursuing treatments to achieve remission
- Underdosing of adequate medications
- Inadequate polypharmacy

Source: Modified from Bystritsky (2006).

bipolar disorder (Gunderson et al., 2006). Depressed patients have an increased rate of personality disorders and more pathologic personality traits when compared with healthy controls (Thase, 1996). The presence of a personality disorder diagnosis negatively influences the chances of achieving remission in patients with anxiety disorders (Massion et al., 2002). Patients with borderline personality disorder are at a higher risk of developing substance use disorders as well (Walter et al., 2009).

Consequences of Treatment Resistance

Suicide

In the year 2020, suicide is expected to represent 2.4% of the global burden of disease, up from 1.8% in 1998, and it is among the 10 leading causes of death for all ages in most countries (WHO, 1999). It is estimated that by 2020, approximately 1.53 million people will die from suicide per year (Bertolote & Fleischmann, 2002). The same study group from the WHO reported that the majority (98%) of a series of cases of completed suicides had a diagnosis of at least one psychiatric disorder. Among all diagnoses, mood disorders accounted for 30.2%, followed by substance-use-related disorders (17.6%), schizophrenia (14.1%), and personality disorders (13.0%). Patients with treatment-resistant depression are more likely than not to report prominent suicidal ideation and hopelessness, indicating their increased risk for suicide (Papakostas et al., 2003). The implications of treatment resistance in psychiatric disorders on suicide risk are most relevant for mood, anxiety, and substance use disorders than in psychotic disorders, given that the risk in the former disorders is particularly increased at the beginning of the course of the illness (Pompili et al., 2011). Suicide prevention must focus not only on depression but also consider, especially in treatment-resistant disorders, the influence of substance use and anxiety disorders.

Increased Morbidity and Mortality

There is growing awareness within the medical community that patients with severe mental illness die earlier than the general population (Saha, Chant, & McGrath, 2007). The somatic health of patients with severe psychiatric illnesses is too often neglected adding to an already remarkable health disparity (Fleischhacker et al., 2008).

When schizophrenia is analyzed, data suggest that the mortality gap with the general population has increased from the 1970s to the present. The standardized mortality ratios increased from 1.84 in the 1970s to 2.98 in the 1980s to 3.2 in the 1990s. It may now be slowly decreasing from when it peaked in the mid-1990s, but it is still unacceptably high (Bushe, Taylor, & Haukka, 2010). The main causes of mortality in patients with schizophrenia are suicide, cancer, and cardiovascular disease, with evidence that cancer mortality rates are similar to cardiovascular mortality rates. It is estimated that 4.9% of patients with schizophrenia will die by suicide (Palmer, Pankratz, & Bostwick, 2005). The average life expectancy of the general population in the United Stated is 76 years (72 years in men, 80 years in women), whereas the corresponding figure is 61 years (57 years in men, 65 years in women) among patients with schizophrenia. Thus, patients with schizophrenia exhibit a 20% reduced life expectancy compared with the general population. Although patients with schizophrenia are 10 to 20 times more likely than the general population to commit suicide (Meltzer, 1998), more than two thirds of patients with schizophrenia, compared with approximately one half in the general population, die of coronary heart disease (CHD). The chief risk factors for this excess risk of death are cigarette smoking, obesity leading to dyslipidemia, insulin resistance and diabetes, and hypertension (Hennekens, Hennekens, Hollar, & Casey, 2005). Tobacco in particular seems to be an important factor in the increased mortality of individuals with mental illness. Persons with mental illness are almost twice as likely to be smokers (Lasser et al., 2000).

Medical Comorbidities

The preponderance of evidence suggests that depression, anxiety disorders, bipolar disorder, and schizophrenia are all important cardiac risk factors, and patients with these disorders are at significantly higher risk for cardiac morbidity and mortality than are their counterparts in the general population (Sowden & Huffman, 2009). Carney and Freedland (2009) have proposed that nonresponse to treatment of depression should be considered a cardiac risk marker in patients with coronary artery disease, in an effort to underscore the significance it has in the outcome of these patients. The reasons for this association are not yet very well understood, but an abnormal autonomic nervous system, increased inflamation, platelet and clotting cascade alterations, and decreased adherence to treatment as well as physical inactivity and smoking might be contributors (Carney, Freedland, Rich, & Jaffe, 1995). As many as 27% of patients with coronary artery disease have major depression, but a substantially larger number of cardiac patients have subsyndromal depressive symptoms. Patients with coronary artery disease and depression have a twofold to threefold increased risk of future cardiac events compared to patients without depression, independent of baseline cardiac dysfunction (Rudisch & Nemeroff, 2003).

Obesity continues to be an ongoing problem in the United States (Mokdad et al., 2001). There is increasing evidence associating severe mental illness and obesity (Keck & McElroy, 2003; Wirshing, 2004). Obesity is associated with a shorter life span, and the effect of obesity in decreasing life expectancy might be even greater in younger adults, one of the populations of interest in severe mental illness (Fontaine, Redden, Wang, Westfall, & Allison, 2003). Obese individuals are at an increased risk for a number of general medical conditions, including type 2 diabetes mellitus, cardiovascular disease (coronary artery disease, cerebrovascular disease, peripheral artery disease), dyslipidemia, hypertension, certain cancers (in men: esophagus, stomach, liver, pancreas, multiple myeloma, rectum, and gallbladder; in women: uterus, kidney, cervix, pancreas, breast, ovary, among others), gastrointestinal disease (gastroesophageal reflux disease, gastritis, gallbladder disease, steatohepatitis), kidney disease (kidney stones, chronic renal disease), endocrine changes (insulin resistance, disturbed menstrual cycles, altered cortisol metabolism), infertility (polycystic ovarian syndrome), sleep apnea, respiratory problems, and obstetrical risks (Caesarean section, neonatal mortality) (Bray & Wilson, 2008). In addition to its adverse effects on disease outcomes, weight gain also impairs physical functioning, reduces quality of life, and is associated with poor mental health. Obesity appears to shorten life span, especially in young adults (Fontaine et al., 2003). These psychological and mental health consequences of weight gain can become an added burden for patients with schizophrenia and other mental disorders (Kawachi, 1999). When analyzing US patients with schizophrenia who enrolled in the CATIE trial, males were 138% more likely to fulfill criteria for metabolic syndrome than a matched control epidemiological group from the National Health and Nutrition Examination Survey (NHANES) III, and females were 251% more likely than their counterparts (McEvoy et al., 2005).

Individuals with severe obesity have high rates of depression (Dixon, Dixon, & O'Brien, 2003). Sociodemographic, psychosocial, and genetic factors may render certain obese individuals more prone to depression or vice versa (Faith, Matz, & Jorge, 2002). Patients who consulted to an outpatient medical center for weight loss had significantly higher rates of depressive symptomatology and psychosocial disability than patients presenting for regular medical treatment (Goldstein, Goldsmith, Anger, & Leon, 1996). Obesity has also been shown to correlate with poor outcome in the treatment of bipolar I disorder (Fagiolini, Kupfer, Houck, Novick, & Frank, 2003).

Obesity and weight variations are also very important factors to consider when evaluating treatment options (Michelson et al., 1999; Stunkard, Fernstrom, Price, Frank, & Kupfer, 1990). Some authors propose that chronically mentally ill patients, who already suffer from unfavorable metabolic profiles, are in a particularly fragile position when placed on medications that have potential for worsening their general condition (Newcomer, 2007; Wieden & Newcomer, 2007).

Functional Impairment

Psychiatric disorders are within the top causes of functional impairment and disability in the world. In mood disorders, functional impairment appears to be related to the severity of the illness, which makes treatment-resistant mood disorders in particular major contributors to disability. In the long term, disability is pervasive and chronic but disappears when patients become asymptomatic. Depressive symptoms at levels of subthreshold depressive symptoms, minor depression/dysthymia, and major depressive disorder represent a continuum of depressive symptom severity in unipolar major depressive disorder, each level of which is associated with a significant stepwise increment in psychosocial disability (Judd et al., 2000). Adequate treatment with the objective of reaching remission in symptoms can reduce the degree of impairment to levels equal to community nondepressed samples (Miller et al., 1998). Unfortunately, the difficulty in attaining remission in many patients results in persistent functional impairment.

Work/Economic Consequences

Patients with severe mental illness have diminished earnings when compared to the general population. In 2001–2003, these patients had 12-month earnings averaging $16,306 less than other respondents with the same values for control variables (Kessler et al., 2008). Major depressive disorder, associated with significant economic burden, was estimated to cost $83.1 billion in the United States in 2000. Greenberg et al (2003) found that of the total burden, $26.1 billion was direct medical costs, $5.4 billion was suicide-related mortality costs, and $51.5 billion was workplace costs (wage-based value of days missed from work due to depression, as well as reduced productivity due to depression). A survey estimated that major depression was associated with 27.2 work-loss days per year, almost 70% due to reduced productivity (Kessler et al., 2006). Patients with treatment-resistant depression have twice the economic costs for employers compared to non-treatment-resistant depressed patients (Ivanova et al., 2010). Early-onset major depressive disorder causes substantial human capital loss, particularly in women, adversely affecting the final educational attainment and reducing future expected earnings by about 12%–18% (Berndt et al., 2000).

When considering schizophrenia in its relation to work-related/loss of productivity costs, it is key to bear in mind that close to 80% of patients with schizophrenia are unemployed (Thornicroft et al., 2004).

Health Care Costs

Crown et al (2002) reported that patients with treatment-resistant depression have 6 times the mean total medical cost than non-treatment-resistant patients, and 19 times the depression-related costs, including hospitalizations and medications.

Schizophrenia also has very onerous costs for health care systems. In 2002 an estimated $22.7 billion was spent in the United States in direct health care costs, including outpatient and inpatient care and medications. An additional $32.4 billion was calculated to be lost due to reduced productivity (Wu et al., 2005).

All of the anxiety disorders are associated with substantial economic and humanistic impact on patients and health care systems (Bereza, Machado, & Einarson, 2009). Generalized anxiety disorder, panic disorder, and posttraumatic stress disorder were associated with significant increases in medical costs (Marciniak et al., 2005; Olfson & Gameroff, 2007). Patients with general anxiety disorder are high utilizers of medical services (Wittchen, 2002). Even though the impact of social phobia is seen in the form of chronic educational, occupational, and social impairment (Lipsitz & Schneier, 2000), these patients also have significantly higher utilization and health care expenditure than normal controls (Acarturk et al., 2009).

There is also evidence that patients with personality disorders pose a high economic burden on society, a burden substantially higher than that found for depression or generalized anxiety disorder (Soeteman, Hakkaart-van Roijen, Verheul, & Busschbach, 2008).

Despite the clear demonstration that treatment-resistant mental disorders are major contributors to cost in health care, the money spent in their treatment continues to decrease. Mental health fell from 8% of all health expenditures in 1986 to 6% in 2003 (Mark, Levit, Buck, Coffey, & Vandivort-Warren, 2007). The costs of mental disorders are comparable to those of physical illnesses. The available evidence suggests that health care systems should rethink the allocation of budgets for research and development in psychiatric versus so-called medical illnesses (Smit et al., 2006).

Poor Understanding of Pathophysiology as a Contributor to Treatment Resistance

Although the major psychiatric disorders have long been recognized, the understanding of their individual pathophysiologies has been elusive. In the same way that the pathophysiology of other complex disorders such as cancer, diabetes, and coronary artery disease has remained elusive, the scientific community still struggles to understand the pathogenesis of the major mental disorders and the underlying processes that predispose, trigger, worsen, or render them resistant.

A better understanding of the neurobiological underpinnings of psychiatric disorders, guided by preclinical and clinical research, is clearly essential for the future development of specific targeted therapies that are more effective, achieve their effects more quickly, and are better tolerated than currently available treatments (Newberg, Catapano, Zarate, & Manji, 2008). In the past four decades the development of new treatments has, many times, been based on the proposed etiology for the disorders. For example, mood and anxiety disorders were approached within the framework of the monoamine hypothesis, schizophrenia was approached with a focus on the dopaminergic pathways, and targets for new drugs were largely developed with these systems in mind. These disease models had heuristic value but have evolved because the medications that were developed were only variations of previously known effective compounds, with safer profiles or more tolerability, but without increased efficacy and rate of response. The most efficacious single treatments for schizophrenia (clozapine), bipolar disorder (lithium), and depression (ECT) were discovered many years ago (Cade, 1949; Crilly, 2007; Lopez-Munoz, Alamo, Juckel, & Assion, 2007). The rapid advancements in molecular neurobiology and genomics together with newly discovered pathways and neurotransmitters, growth factors, and different signaling pathways will likely lead to the development of new treatments for these disorders (Martinowich, Manji, & Lu, 2007; Nemeroff, 2002).

If many neurological disorders from stroke to Parkinson disease are conceptualized as focal brain lesions, many psychiatric disorders can be understood as dysfunctions of brain circuits (Insel, 2009). Unlike Parkinson or Alzheimer disease, most psychiatric disorders lack any clear consensus on neuropathology, rare familial genetic causes, or highly penetrant vulnerability genes, providing no obvious starting points for molecular investigations (Krishnan & Nestler, 2010). The last years have witnessed a shift from a neurochemical pathology approach to a neurocircuitry approach, with structural and functional imaging (Drevets, Savitz, & Trimble, 2008; Graybiel & Rauch, 2000). With the development of new research and potentially therapeutic tools, this "circuit-based neurobiology" approach has been embraced. There are new promising ways of exploring these circuits in vivo, including deep brain stimulation and optogenetics (Deisseroth et al., 2006; Zhang, Aravanis, Adamantidis, de Lecea, & Deisseroth, 2007). By gaining more understanding of what lies behind the clinical symptoms of patients with severe treatment-resistant psychiatric disorders, we will be able to develop tomorrow's treatments that will not just be modifications of drugs that were discovered serendipitously six decades ago. It is important to note that the diagnostic categories of schizophrenia, bipolar disorder, and depression represent a heterogeneous collection of biologically distinct endophenotypes with their own unique pathophysiology. Personalized medicine in psychiatry is attempting to identify in individual patients the specific underlying cause(s) of their disorder and develop specific treatments for that person.

Final Considerations

Special consideration must be given to the problem of iatrogenesis. There are many treatment options that can cause significant adverse effects in patients, even when presented appropriately. When second-generation antipsychotics were introduced and a decreased risk for tardive dyskinesia was demonstrated compared to the older neuroleptics (Correll, Leucht, & Kane, 2004), the use of atypical antipsychotics became widespread. They were presented in many different conditions, sometimes off label and/or with little research support, even increasing the chance of a higher prevalence of tardive dyskinesia when used in combination with first-generation agents especially at older ages (Tarsy, Lungu, & Baldessarini, 2011). Adequate use of atypical antipsychotics is recommended for disorders other than primary psychotic disorders, but judicious use is encouraged (Nemeroff, 2005). A great deal of attention has focused in the past decade on the adverse cardiometabolic profile of certain atypical antipsychotics (Newcomer & Hennekens, 2007). As discussed earlier, patients with severe mental illness have 1.5 to 2 times the general population prevalence of diabetes, dyslipidemia, hypertension, and obesity (Fagiolini, Frank, Scott, Turkin, & Kupfer, 2005; McEvoy, et al., 2005). Clinicians need to be responsible prescribers of medications and treatments that have potential deleterious side effects. The misdiagnosis or rapid labeling of patients as treatment resistant might lead to treatment options that can bring irreversible consequences. In the recent years the advances in neurobiology and biotechnology made available certain treatment approaches that were unthinkable just a decade ago. Research in neuromodulation, including vagus nerve stimulation, repetitive transcranial magnetic stimulation, and deep brain stimulation, among other promising methods, has increased exponentially in the past decade, and there is genuine interest in the development of this field of psychiatry not only for the management of treatment-resistant patients but because it helps in the understanding of the complex pathophysiology of these disorders. However, there needs to be cautious optimism for the availability of these new therapeutic options. There are safety considerations involving both the short-term risk of neurosurgery itself (Terao et al., 2003) and in view of evidence of the long-term efficacy, long-term safety, and side-effect issues. In a follow-up trial 10 years after capsulotomy for severe refractory obsessive-compulsive disorder, a substantial number of patients (10 out of 25) had significant neuropsychiatric side effects, including problems with executive functioning, apathy, or disinhibition (Ruck et al., 2008). Although there is considerable evidence that deep brain stimulation is a highly effective treatment for refractory patients with obsessive-compulsive disorder (Dougherty et al., 2002), Tourette disorder (Maciunas et al., 2007), and depression (Kennedy et al., 2011), careful selection of patients is essential to ensure that there are no other confounding factors that will contribute to a poor response. There is justified concern in the scientific community that the widespread availability of these advanced technologies without adequate and careful research will place vulnerable patients at risk for not yet well-understood long-term consequences (Fins et al., 2011). A general consensus has been reached in which a cautious multidisciplinary approach promoting a careful selection of patients and a thorough follow-up is encouraged (Rabins et al., 2009). The scientific community and the psychiatric field in particular are still suffering from the consequences of psychosurgery in the 1950s (Hariz, Blomstedt, & Zrinzo, 2010).

Much remains to be done in the field of psychiatry to improve the care of patients with treatment-resistant disorders. We need to improve our diagnostic accuracy and identify comorbid conditions. More research is also needed to identify predictors of poor outcomes, including suicide and chronicity. Sadly, the majority of patients do not receive adequate treatment based on well-controlled clinical trials, and validated algorithms are rarely followed. Our understanding of the neurobiology of psychiatric disorders remains incomplete, and greater knowledge in this area will surely facilitate the development of novel effective pharmacotherapies, psychotherapies, and advanced somatic therapeutic options. Effective treatments are also needed for associated social dysfunction because we recognize that treatment will be incomplete if we do not consider the patient's full reinsertion in his or her environment as the goal of an effective treatment.

Disclosure Statement

P.R.P. has no conflicts of interest to disclose.

C.B.N. has received research grants from the National Institutes of Health and the Agency for Healthcare Research and Quality. He is a consultant at Xhale, Takeda, and SK PHarma and has financial interests in CeNeRx BioPharma, NovaDel Pharma Inc., PharmaNeuroBoost, ReVaax Pharma, and Xhale. He has sat on the scientific advisory boards of the following companies: American Foundation for Suicide Prevention (AFSP), CeNeRx BioPharma, National Alliance for Research on Schizophrenia and Depression, NovaDel Pharma Inc., Xhale, PharmaNeuroBoost, Anxiety Disorders Association of America, Skyland Trail, and AstraZeneca Pharamceuticals. He has sat on the board of directors of the following companies: AFSP, NoveDel Pharma Inc., Mt. Cook Pharma, and Skyland Trail.

References

Acarturk, C., Smit, F., de Graaf, R., van Straten, A., Ten Have, M., & Cuijpers, P. (2009). Economic costs of social phobia: A population-based study. *Journal of Affective Disorders, 115*(3), 421–429.

Albert, U., Bergesio, C., Pessina, E., Maina, G., & Bogetto, F. (2002). Management of treatment resistant obsessive-compulsive disorder. Algorithms for pharmacotherapy. *Panminerva Medicine, 44*(2), 83–91.

American Academy of Child and Adolescent Psychiatry. (1998). Practice parameters for the assessment and treatment of children and adolescents with obsessive-compulsive disorder. AACAP. *Journal of the American Academy of Child and Adolescent Psychiatry, 37*(Suppl 10), 27S–45S.

Andreasen, N. C., Carpenter, W. T., Jr., Kane, J. M., Lasser, R. A., Marder, S. R., & Weinberger, D. R. (2005). Remission in schizophrenia: Proposed criteria and rationale for consensus. *American Journal of Psychiatry, 162*(3), 441–449.

Ansseau, M., Dierick, M., Buntinkx, F., Cnockaert, P., De Smedt, J., Van Den Haute, M., & Vander Mijnsbrugge, D. (2004). High prevalence of mental disorders in primary care. *Journal of Affective Disorders, 78*(1), 49–55.

Barnes, T. R., & McEvedy, C. J. (1996). Pharmacological treatment strategies in the non-responsive schizophrenic patient. *International Clinical Psychopharmacology, 11*(Suppl 2), 67–71.

Bereza, B. G., Machado, M., & Einarson, T. R. (2009). Systematic review and quality assessment of economic evaluations and quality-of-life studies related to generalized anxiety disorder. *Clinical Therapeutics, 31*(6), 1279–1308.

Berndt, E. R., Koran, L. M., Finkelstein, S. N., Gelenberg, A. J., Kornstein, S. G., Miller, I. M., Keller, M. B. (2000). Lost human capital from early-onset chronic depression. *American Journal of Psychiatry, 157*(6), 940–947.

Bertolote, J. M., & Fleischmann, A. (2002). Suicide and psychiatric diagnosis: A worldwide perspective. *World Psychiatry, 1*(3), 181–185.

Bray, G. A., & Wilson, J. F. (2008). In the clinic. Obesity. *Annals of Internal Medicine, 149*(7), ITC4–1–15; quiz ITC14–16.

Brenner, H. D., Dencker, S. J., Goldstein, M. J., Hubbard, J. W., Keegan, D. L., Kruger, G., Midha, K. K. (1990). Defining treatment refractoriness in schizophrenia. *Schizophrenia Bulletin, 16*(4), 551–561.

Bunney, W. E., Jr., & Hamburg, D. A. (1963). Methods for reliable longitudinal observation of behavior. *Archives of General Psychiatry, 9*, 280–294.

Bushe, C. J., Taylor, M., & Haukka, J. (2010). Mortality in schizophrenia: A measurable clinical endpoint. *Journal of Psychopharmacology, 24*(Suppl 4), 17–25.

Bystritsky, A. (2006). Treatment-resistant anxiety disorders. *Molecular Psychiatry, 11*(9), 805–814.

Cade, J. F. (1949). Lithium salts in the treatment of psychotic excitement. *Medical Journal of Australia, 2*(10), 349–352.

Calabrese, J. R., Hirschfeld, R. M., Frye, M. A., & Reed, M. L. (2004). Impact of depressive symptoms compared with manic symptoms in bipolar disorder: Results of a U.S. community-based sample. *Journal of Clinical Psychiatry, 65*(11), 1499–1504.

Carney, R. M., & Freedland, K. E. (2009). Treatment-resistant depression and mortality after acute coronary syndrome. *American Journal of Psychiatry, 166*(4), 410–417.

Carney, R. M., Freedland, K. E., Rich, M. W., & Jaffe, A. S. (1995). Depression as a risk factor for cardiac events in established coronary heart disease: A review of possible mechanisms. *Annals of Behavioral Medicine, 17*(2), 142–149.

Churchill, R. (2010). No health without mental health: A role for the Cochrane Collaboration [editorial]. *The Cochrane Library*. Retrieved December 2011, from http://www.thecochranelibrary.com/details/editorial/859307/No-health-without-mental-health-a-role-for-the-Cochrane-Collaboration-by-Rachel-.html.

Compton, W. M., Conway, K. P., Stinson, F. S., & Grant, B. F. (2006). Changes in the prevalence of major depression and comorbid substance use disorders in the United States between 1991–1992 and 2001–2002. *American Journal of Psychiatry, 163*(12), 2141–2147.

Conley, R. R., & Kelly, D. L. (2001). Management of treatment resistance in schizophrenia. *Biological Psychiatry, 50*(11), 898–911.

Correll, C. U., Leucht, S., & Kane, J. M. (2004). Lower risk for tardive dyskinesia associated with second-generation antipsychotics: A systematic review of 1-year studies. *American Journal of Psychiatry, 161*(3), 414–425.

Crilly, J. (2007). The history of clozapine and its emergence in the US market: A review and analysis. *History of Psychiatry, 18*(1), 39–60.

Crown, W. H., Finkelstein, S., Berndt, E. R., Ling, D., Poret, A. W., Rush, A. J., & Russell, J. M. (2002). The impact of treatment-resistant depression on health care utilization and costs. *Journal of Clinical Psychiatry, 63*(11), 963–971.

Deisseroth, K., Feng, G., Majewska, A. K., Miesenbock, G., Ting, A., & Schnitzer, M. J. (2006). Next-generation optical technologies for illuminating genetically targeted brain circuits. *Journal of Neuroscience, 26*(41), 10380–10386.

Dickerson, F. B., Brown, C. H., Kreyenbuhl, J. A., Fang, L., Goldberg, R. W., Wohlheiter, K., & Dixon, L. B. (2006). Obesity among individuals with serious mental illness. *Acta Psychiatrica Scandinavia, 113*(4), 306–313.

Dixon, J. B., Dixon, M. E., & O'Brien, P. E. (2003). Depression in association with severe obesity: Changes with weight loss. *Archives of Internal Medicine, 163*(17), 2058–2065.

Dougherty, D. D., Baer, L., Cosgrove, G. R., Cassem, E. H., Price, B. H., Nierenberg, A. A., Rauch, S. L. (2002). Prospective long-term follow-up of 44 patients who received cingulotomy for treatment-refractory obsessive-compulsive disorder. *American Journal of Psychiatry, 159*(2), 269–275.

Drevets, W. C., Savitz, J., & Trimble, M. (2008). The subgenual anterior cingulate cortex in mood disorders. *CNS Spectrums, 13*(8), 663–681.

Elkis, H. (2007). Treatment-resistant schizophrenia. *Psychiatric Clinics of North America, 30*(3), 511–533.

Fagiolini, A., Frank, E., Scott, J. A., Turkin, S., & Kupfer, D. J. (2005). Metabolic syndrome in bipolar disorder: Findings from the Bipolar Disorder Center for Pennsylvanians. *Bipolar Disorders, 7*(5), 424–430.

Fagiolini, A., Kupfer, D. J., Houck, P. R., Novick, D. M., & Frank, E. (2003). Obesity as a correlate of outcome in patients with bipolar I disorder. *American Journal of Psychiatry, 160*(1), 112–117.

Faith, M. S., Matz, P. E., & Jorge, M. A. (2002). Obesity-depression associations in the population. *Journal of Psychosomatic Research, 53*(4), 935–942.

Fins, J. J., Mayberg, H. S., Nuttin, B., Kubu, C. S., Galert, T., Sturm, V., Schlaepfer, T. E. (2011). Misuse of the FDA's humanitarian device exemption in deep brain stimulation for obsessive-compulsive disorder. *Health Affairs (Millwood), 30*(2), 302–311.

Fleischhacker, W. W., Cetkovich-Bakmas, M., De Hert, M., Hennekens, C. H., Lambert, M., Leucht, S., Lieberman, J. A. (2008). Comorbid somatic illnesses in patients with severe mental disorders: Clinical, policy, and research challenges. *Journal of Clinical Psychiatry, 69*(4), 514–519.

Foa, E. B., & Kozak, M. J. (1996). Psychological treatment for obsessive-compulsive disorder. In M. R. Mavissakalian & R. F. Prien (Eds.), *Long-term treatments of anxiety disorders* (pp. 285–309). Washington, DC: American Psychiatric Press.

Fontaine, K. R., Redden, D. T., Wang, C., Westfall, A. O., & Allison, D. B. (2003). Years of life lost due to obesity. *Journal of the American Medical Association, 289*(2), 187–193.

Gijsman, H. J., Geddes, J. R., Rendell, J. M., Nolen, W. A., & Goodwin, G. M. (2004). Antidepressants for bipolar depression: A systematic review of randomized, controlled trials. *American Journal of Psychiatry, 161*(9), 1537–1547.

Goldstein, L. T., Goldsmith, S. J., Anger, K., & Leon, A. C. (1996). Psychiatric symptoms in clients presenting for commercial weight reduction treatment. *International Journal of Eating Disorders, 20*(2), 191–197.

Goodman, W. K., Ward, H. E., Kablinger, A. S., & Murphy, T. K. (2000). Biological approaches to treatment-resistant obsessive-compulsive disorder. In W. K. Goodman, M. V. Rudorfer, & J. D. Maser (Eds.), *Obsessive-compulsive disorder: Contemporary issues in management* (pp. 333–369). London: Erlbaum.

Graybiel, A. M., & Rauch, S. L. (2000). Toward a neurobiology of obsessive-compulsive disorder. *Neuron, 28*(2), 343–347.

Greenberg, P. E., Kessler, R. C., Birnbaum, H., Leong, S. A., Lowe, S. W., Berglund, P., & Corey-Lisle, P. K. (2003). The economic burden of depression in the United States: How did it change between 1990 and 2000? *Journal of Clinical Psychiatry, 64*(12), 1465–1476.

Gunderson, J. G., Weinberg, I., Daversa, M. T., Kueppenbender, K. D., Zanarini, M. C., Shea, M. T., Dyck, I. (2006). Descriptive and longitudinal observations on the relationship of borderline personality disorder and bipolar disorder. *American Journal of Psychiatry, 163*(7), 1173–1178.

Guy, W. (1970). Clinical Global Impression (CGI) Scale. In W. Guy & R. Bonato (Eds.), *Manual for the ECDEU Assessment Battery* (pp. 12.11–12.16). Chevy Chase, MD: National Institute of Mental Health.

Hariz, M. I., Blomstedt, P., & Zrinzo, L. (2010). Deep brain stimulation between 1947 and 1987: The untold story. *Neurosurgical Focus, 29*(2), E1.

Harvey, P. D., & Bellack, A. S. (2009). Toward a terminology for functional recovery in schizophrenia: Is functional remission a viable concept? *Schizophrenia Bulletin, 35*(2), 300–306.

Hennekens, C. H., Hennekens, A. R., Hollar, D., & Casey, D. E. (2005). Schizophrenia and increased risks of cardiovascular disease. *American Heart Journal, 150*(6), 1115–1121.

Holtzheimer, P. E., & Mayberg, H. S. (2011). Stuck in a rut: Rethinking depression and its treatment. *Trends in Neuroscience, 34*(1), 1–9.

Holtzheimer, P. E., III, & Mayberg, H. S. (2010). Deep brain stimulation for treatment-resistant depression. *American Journal of Psychiatry, 167*(12), 1437–1444.

Insel, T. R. (2009). Disruptive insights in psychiatry: Transforming a clinical discipline. *Journal of Clinical Investigation, 119*(4), 700–705.

Ivanova, J. I., Birnbaum, H. G., Kidolezi, Y., Subramanian, G., Khan, S. A., & Stensland, M. D. (2010). Direct and indirect costs of employees with treatment-resistant and non-treatment-resistant major depressive disorder. *Current Medical Research and Opinion, 26*(10), 2475–2484.

Juarez-Reyes, M. G., Shumway, M., Battle, C., Bacchetti, P., Hansen, M. S., & Hargreaves, W. A. (1995). Effects of stringent criteria on eligibility for clozapine among public mental health clients. *Psychiatric Services, 46*(8), 801–806.

Judd, L. L., Akiskal, H. S., Schettler, P. J., Endicott, J., Maser, J., Solomon, D. A., Keller, M. B. (2002). The long-term natural history of the weekly symptomatic status of bipolar I disorder. *Archives of General Psychiatry, 59*(6), 530–537.

Judd, L. L., Akiskal, H. S., Zeller, P. J., Paulus, M., Leon, A. C., Maser, J. D., Keller, M. B. (2000). Psychosocial disability during the long-term course of unipolar major depressive disorder. *Archives of General Psychiatry, 57*(4), 375–380.

Kane, J., Honigfeld, G., Singer, J., & Meltzer, H. (1988). Clozapine for the treatment-resistant schizophrenic. A double-blind comparison with chlorpromazine. *Archives of General Psychiatry, 45*(9), 789–796.

Karno, M., Golding, J. M., Sorenson, S. B., & Burnam, M. A. (1988). The epidemiology of obsessive-compulsive disorder in five US communities. *Archives of General Psychiatry, 45*(12), 1094–1099.

Kawachi, I. (1999). Physical and psychological consequences of weight gain. *Journal of Clinical Psychiatry, 60*(Suppl 21), 5–9.

Keck, P. E., & McElroy, S. L. (2003). Bipolar disorder, obesity, and pharmacotherapy-associated weight gain. *Journal of Clinical Psychiatry, 64*(12), 1426–1435.

Kellner, C. H., Knapp, R. G., Petrides, G., Rummans, T. A., Husain, M. M., Rasmussen, K., Fink, M. (2006). Continuation electroconvulsive therapy vs pharmacotherapy for relapse prevention in major depression: A multisite study from the Consortium for Research in Electroconvulsive Therapy (CORE). *Archives of General Psychiatry, 63*(12), 1337–1344.

Kennedy, S. H., Giacobbe, P., Rizvi, S. J., Placenza, F. M., Nishikawa, Y., Mayberg, H. S., & Lozano, A. M. (2011). Deep brain stimulation for treatment-resistant depression: Follow-up after 3 to 6 years. *American Journal of Psychiatry.*

Kessler, R. C., Akiskal, H. S., Ames, M., Birnbaum, H., Greenberg, P., Hirschfeld, R. M., Wang, P. S. (2006). Prevalence and effects of mood disorders on work performance in a nationally representative sample of U.S. workers. *American Journal of Psychiatry, 163*(9), 1561–1568.

Kessler, R. C., Berglund, P., Demler, O., Jin, R., Merikangas, K. R., & Walters, E. E. (2005). Lifetime prevalence and age-of-onset distributions of DSM-IV disorders in the National Comorbidity Survey Replication. *Archives of General Psychiatry, 62*(6), 593–602.

Kessler, R. C., Chiu, W. T., Demler, O., Merikangas, K. R., & Walters, E. E. (2005). Prevalence, severity, and comorbidity of 12-month DSM-IV disorders in the National Comorbidity Survey Replication. *Archives of General Psychiatry, 62*(6), 617–627.

Kessler, R. C., Heeringa, S., Lakoma, M. D., Petukhova, M., Rupp, A. E., Schoenbaum, M., Zaslavsky, A. M. (2008). Individual and societal effects of mental disorders on earnings in the United States: Results from the national comorbidity survey replication. *American Journal of Psychiatry, 165*(6), 703–711.

Kinon, B. J., Kane, J. M., Johns, C., Perovich, R., Ismi, M., Koreen, A., & Weiden, P. (1993). Treatment of neuroleptic-resistant schizophrenic relapse. *Psychopharmacology Bulletin, 29*(2), 309–314.

Kocsis, J. H., Gelenberg, A. J., Rothbaum, B., Klein, D. N., Trivedi, M. H., Manber, R., Thase, M. E. (2008). Chronic forms of major depression are still undertreated in the 21st century: Systematic assessment of 801 patients presenting for treatment. *Journal of Affective Disorders, 110*(1–2), 55–61.

Krishnan, V., & Nestler, E. J. (2010). Linking molecules to mood: New insight into the biology of depression. *American Journal of Psychiatry, 167*(11), 1305–1320.

Lasser, K., Boyd, J. W., Woolhandler, S., Himmelstein, D. U., McCormick, D., & Bor, D. H. (2000). Smoking and mental illness. *Journal of the American Medical Association, 284*(20), 2606–2610.

Liberman, R. P. (Ed.). (2008). *Recovery from disability: Manual of psychiatric rehabilitation*. Arlington, VA: American Psychiatric Publishing.

Lipsitz, J. D., & Schneier, F. R. (2000). Social phobia: Epidemiology and cost of illness. *Pharmacoeconomics*, *18*(1), 23–32.

Lopez-Munoz, F., Alamo, C., Juckel, G., & Assion, H. J. (2007). Half a century of antidepressant drugs: On the clinical introduction of monoamine oxidase inhibitors, tricyclics, and tetracyclics. Part I: Monoamine oxidase inhibitors. *Journal of Clinical Psychopharmacology*, *27*(6), 555–559.

Maciunas, R. J., Maddux, B. N., Riley, D. E., Whitney, C. M., Schoenberg, M. R., Ogrocki, P. J., Gould, D. J. (2007). Prospective randomized double-blind trial of bilateral thalamic deep brain stimulation in adults with Tourette syndrome. *Journal of Neurosurgery*, *107*(5), 1004–1014.

Mancebo, M. C., Eisen, J. L., Pinto, A., Greenberg, B. D., Dyck, I. R., & Rasmussen, S. A. (2006). The Brown Longitudinal Obsessive Compulsive Study: Treatments received and patient impressions of improvement. *Journal of Clinical Psychiatry*, *67*(11), 1713–1720.

Marciniak, M. D., Lage, M. J., Dunayevich, E., Russell, J. M., Bowman, L., Landbloom, R. P., & Levine, L. R. (2005). The cost of treating anxiety: The medical and demographic correlates that impact total medical costs. *Depression and Anxiety*, *21*(4), 178–184.

Marcus, S. C., & Olfson, M. (2010). National trends in the treatment for depression from 1998 to 2007. *Archives of General Psychiatry*, *67*(12), 1265–1273.

Mark, T. L., Levit, K. R., Buck, J. A., Coffey, R. M., & Vandivort-Warren, R. (2007). Mental health treatment expenditure trends, 1986–2003. *Psychiatric Services*, *58*(8), 1041–1048.

Martinowich, K., Manji, H., & Lu, B. (2007). New insights into BDNF function in depression and anxiety. *Nature Neuroscience*, *10*(9), 1089–1093.

Massion, A. O., Dyck, I. R., Shea, M. T., Phillips, K. A., Warshaw, M. G., & Keller, M. B. (2002). Personality disorders and time to remission in generalized anxiety disorder, social phobia, and panic disorder. *Archives of General Psychiatry*, *59*(5), 434–440.

McEvoy, J. P., Meyer, J. M., Goff, D. C., Nasrallah, H. A., Davis, S. M., Sullivan, L., Lieberman, J. A. (2005). Prevalence of the metabolic syndrome in patients with schizophrenia: Baseline results from the Clinical Antipsychotic Trials of Intervention Effectiveness (CATIE) schizophrenia trial and comparison with national estimates from NHANES III. *Schizophrenia Research*, *80*(1), 19–32.

Meltzer, H. Y. (1998). Suicide in schizophrenia: Risk factors and clozapine treatment. *Journal of Clinical Psychiatry*, *59*(Suppl 3), 15–20.

Michelson, D., Amsterdam, J. D., Quitkin, F. M., Reimherr, F. W., Rosenbaum, J. F., Zajecka, J., Beasley, C. M., Jr. (1999). Changes in weight during a 1-year trial of fluoxetine. *American Journal of Psychiatry*, *156*(8), 1170–1176.

Miller, I. W., Keitner, G. I., Schatzberg, A. F., Klein, D. N., Thase, M. E., Rush, A. J., Keller, M. B. (1998). The treatment of chronic depression, part 3: Psychosocial functioning before and after treatment with sertraline or imipramine. *Journal of Clinical Psychiatry*, *59*(11), 608–619.

Mokdad, A. H., Bowman, B. A., Ford, E. S., Vinicor, F., Marks, J. S., & Koplan, J. P. (2001). The continuing epidemics of obesity and diabetes in the United States. *Journal of the American Medical Association*, *286*(10), 1195–1200.

Murray, C. J., & Lopez, A. D. (1997). Alternative projections of mortality and disability by cause 1990–2020: Global Burden of Disease Study. *Lancet*, *349*(9064), 1498–1504.

Nemeroff, C. B. (2002). Recent advances in the neurobiology of depression. *Psychopharmacology Bulletin*, *36*(Suppl 2), 6–23.

Nemeroff, C. B. (2005). Use of atypical antipsychotics in refractory depression and anxiety. *Journal of Clinical Psychiatry*, *66*(Suppl 8), 13–21.

Newberg, A. R., Catapano, L. A., Zarate, C. A., & Manji, H. K. (2008). Neurobiology of bipolar disorder. *Expert Review of Neurotherapeutics*, *8*(1), 93–110.

Newcomer, J. W. (2007). Antipsychotic medications: Metabolic and cardiovascular risk. *Journal of Clinical Psychiatry*, *68*(Suppl 4), 8–13.

Newcomer, J. W., & Hennekens, C. H. (2007). Severe mental illness and risk of cardiovascular disease. *Journal of the American Medical Association*, *298*(15), 1794–1796.

Nierenberg, A. A., & Amsterdam, J. D. (1990). Treatment-resistant depression: Definition and treatment approaches. *Journal of Clinical Psychiatry*, *51*(Suppl), 39–47; discussion 48–50.

Nierenberg, A. A., Fava, M., Trivedi, M. H., Wisniewski, S. R., Thase, M. E., McGrath, P. J., Rush, A. J. (2006). A comparison of lithium and T(3) augmentation following two failed medication treatments for depression: A STAR*D report. *American Journal of Psychiatry*, *163*(9), 1519–1530; quiz 1665.

Nierenberg, A. A., & Wright, E. C. (1999). Evolution of remission as the new standard in the treatment of depression. *Journal of Clinical Psychiatry, 60*(Suppl 22), 7–11.

Ninan, P. T. (2001). Dissolving the burden of generalized anxiety disorder. *Journal of Clinical Psychiatry, 62* (Suppl 19), 5–10.

Nunes, E. V., & Levin, F. R. (2004). Treatment of depression in patients with alcohol or other drug dependence: A meta-analysis. *Journal of the American Medical Association, 291*(15), 1887–1896.

Olfson, M., & Gameroff, M. J. (2007). Generalized anxiety disorder, somatic pain and health care costs. *General Hospital Psychiatry, 29*(4), 310–316.

Palmer, B. A., Pankratz, V. S., & Bostwick, J. M. (2005). The lifetime risk of suicide in schizophrenia: A reexamination. *Archives of General Psychiatry, 62*(3), 247–253.

Pantelis, C., & Lambert, T. J. (2003). Managing patients with "treatment-resistant" schizophrenia. *Medical Journal of Australia, 178*(Suppl), S62–66.

Papakostas, G. I., Petersen, T., Pava, J., Masson, E., Worthington, J. J., 3rd, Alpert, J. E., Nierenberg, A. A. (2003). Hopelessness and suicidal ideation in outpatients with treatment-resistant depression: Prevalence and impact on treatment outcome. *Journal of Nervous and Mental Disease, 191*(7), 444–449.

Pickar, D., Owen, R. R., Litman, R. E., Konicki, E., Gutierrez, R., & Rapaport, M. H. (1992). Clinical and biologic response to clozapine in patients with schizophrenia. Crossover comparison with fluphenazine. *Archives of General Psychiatry, 49*(5), 345–353.

Pompili, M., Serafini, G., Innamorati, M., Lester, D., Shrivastava, A., Girardi, P., & Nordentoft, M. (2011). Suicide risk in first episode psychosis: A selective review of the current literature. *Schizophrenia Research, 129*(1), 1–11.

Rabins, P., Appleby, B. S., Brandt, J., DeLong, M. R., Dunn, L. B., Gabriels, L., Matthews, D. J. (2009). Scientific and ethical issues related to deep brain stimulation for disorders of mood, behavior, and thought. *Archives of General Psychiatry, 66*(9), 931–937.

Rasmussen, K. G., Mueller, M., Kellner, C. H., Knapp, R. G., Petrides, G., Rummans, T. A., CORE Group. (2006). Patterns of psychotropic medication use among patients with severe depression referred for electroconvulsive therapy: Data from the Consortium for Research on Electroconvulsive Therapy. *Journal of ECT, 22*(2), 116–123.

Ruck, C., Karlsson, A., Steele, J. D., Edman, G., Meyerson, B. A., Ericson, K., Svanborg, P. (2008). Capsulotomy for obsessive-compulsive disorder: Long-term follow-up of 25 patients. *Archives of General Psychiatry, 65*(8), 914–921.

Rudisch, B., & Nemeroff, C. B. (2003). Epidemiology of comorbid coronary artery disease and depression. *Biological Psychiatry, 54*(3), 227–240.

Rush, A. J., Trivedi, M. H., Wisniewski, S. R., Nierenberg, A. A., Stewart, J. W., Warden, D., Fava, M. (2006). Acute and longer-term outcomes in depressed outpatients requiring one or several treatment steps: A STAR*D report. *American Journal of Psychiatry, 163*(11), 1905–1917.

Saha, S., Chant, D., & McGrath, J. (2007). A systematic review of mortality in schizophrenia: Is the differential mortality gap worsening over time? *Archives of General Psychiatry, 64*(10), 1123–1131.

Simon, N. M., Otto, M. W., Wisniewski, S. R., Fossey, M., Sagduyu, K., Frank, E., Pollack, M. H. (2004). Anxiety disorder comorbidity in bipolar disorder patients: Data from the first 500 participants in the Systematic Treatment Enhancement Program for Bipolar Disorder (STEP-BD). *American Journal of Psychiatry, 161*(12), 2222–2229.

Smit, F., Cuijpers, P., Oostenbrink, J., Batelaan, N., de Graaf, R., & Beekman, A. (2006). Costs of nine common mental disorders: Implications for curative and preventive psychiatry. *Journal of Mental Health Policy and Economics, 9*(4), 193–200.

Soeteman, D. I., Hakkaart-van Roijen, L., Verheul, R., & Busschbach, J. J. (2008). The economic burden of personality disorders in mental health care. *Journal of Clinical Psychiatry, 69*(2), 259–265.

Solanki, R. K., Singh, P., & Munshi, D. (2009). Current perspectives in the treatment of resistant schizophrenia. *Indian Journal of Psychiatry, 51*(4), 254–260.

Sowden, G. L., Huffman, J. C. (2009). The impact of mental illness on cardiac outcomes: a review for the cardiologist. *International Journal of Cardiology, 132*(1), 30–37.

Stunkard, A. J., Fernstrom, M. H., Price, A., Frank, E., & Kupfer, D. J. (1990). Direction of weight change in recurrent depression. Consistency across episodes. *Archives of General Psychiatry, 47*(9), 857–860.

Tarsy, D., Lungu, C., & Baldessarini, R. J. (2011). Epidemiology of tardive dyskinesia before and during the era of modern antipsychotic drugs. *Handbook of Clinical Neurology, 100*, 601–616.

Terao, T., Takahashi, H., Yokochi, F., Taniguchi, M., Okiyama, R., & Hamada, I. (2003). Hemorrhagic complication of stereotactic surgery in patients with movement disorders. *Journal of Neurosurgery, 98*(6), 1241–1246.

Thase, M. E. (1996). The role of Axis II comorbidity in the management of patients with treatment-resistant depression. *Psychiatric Clinics of North America, 19*(2), 287–309.

Thornicroft, G., Tansella, M., Becker, T., Knapp, M., Leese, M., Schene, A., EPSILON Study Group. (2004). The personal impact of schizophrenia in Europe. *Schizophrenia Research, 69*(2–3), 125–132.

Tohen, M., Hennen, J., Zarate, C. M., Jr., Baldessarini, R. J., Strakowski, S. M., Stoll, A. L., Cohen, B. M. (2000). Two-year syndromal and functional recovery in 219 cases of first-episode major affective disorder with psychotic features. *American Journal of Psychiatry, 157*(2), 220–228.

Tondo, L., Baldessarini, R. J., Hennen, J., Minnai, G. P., Salis, P., Scamonatti, L., Mannu, P. (1999). Suicide attempts in major affective disorder patients with comorbid substance use disorders. *Journal of Clinical Psychiatry, 60* Suppl 2, 63–69; discussion 75–66, 113–116.

Trivedi, M. H., Rush, A. J., Wisniewski, S. R., Nierenberg, A. A., Warden, D., Ritz, L., STAR*D Study Team. (2006). Evaluation of outcomes with citalopram for depression using measurement-based care in STAR*D: Implications for clinical practice. *American Journal of Psychiatry, 163*(1), 28–40.

Walter, M., Gunderson, J. G., Zanarini, M. C., Sanislow, C. A., Grilo, C. M., McGlashan, T. H., Skodol, A. E. (2009). New onsets of substance use disorders in borderline personality disorder over 7 years of follow-ups: Findings from the Collaborative Longitudinal Personality Disorders Study. *Addiction, 104*(1), 97–103.

Warner, R. (2009). Recovery from schizophrenia and the recovery model. *Current Opinion in Psychiatry, 22*(4), 374–380.

Wieden, P. J., & Newcomer, J. W. (2007). Evidence of switching antipsychotic therapy to improve metabolic disturbances. *Journal of Clinical Psychiatry, 68*(5), e13.

Wingo, A. P., Baldessarini, R. J., Holtzheimer, P. E., & Harvey, P. D. (2010). Factors associated with functional recovery in bipolar disorder patients. *Bipolar Disorders, 12*(3), 319–326.

Wirshing, D. A. (2004). Schizophrenia and obesity: Impact of antipsychotic medications. *Journal of Clinical Psychiatry, 65*(Suppl 18), 13–26.

Wittchen, H. U. (2002). Generalized anxiety disorder: Prevalence, burden, and cost to society. *Depression and Anxiety, 16*(4), 162–171.

World Health Organization. (Ed.). (1999). *Figures and facts about suicide*. Geneva, Switzerland: Author.

World Health Organization. (2001). *The World Health report: 2001: Mental health: New understanding, new hope*. Geneva, Switzerland: Author.

World Health Organization. (2008). *The global burden of disease: 2004 update* (No. 978 92 4 156371 0). Geneva, Switzerland: Author.

Wu, E. Q., Birnbaum, H. G., Shi, L., Ball, D. E., Kessler, R. C., Moulis, M., & Aggarwal, J. (2005). The economic burden of schizophrenia in the United States in 2002. *Journal of Clinical Psychiatry, 66*(9), 1122–1129.

Yonkers, K. A., Bruce, S. E., Dyck, I. R., & Keller, M. B. (2003). Chronicity, relapse, and illness—course of panic disorder, social phobia, and generalized anxiety disorder: Findings in men and women from 8 years of follow-up. *Depression and Anxiety, 17*(3), 173–179.

Yonkers, K. A., Dyck, I. R., & Keller, M. B. (2001). An eight-year longitudinal comparison of clinical course and characteristics of social phobia among men and women. *Psychiatric Services, 52*(5), 637–643.

Yonkers, K. A., Dyck, I. R., Warshaw, M., & Keller, M. B. (2000). Factors predicting the clinical course of generalised anxiety disorder. *British Journal of Psychiatry, 176*, 544–549.

Yonkers, K. A., Warshaw, M. G., Massion, A. O., & Keller, M. B. (1996). Phenomenology and course of generalised anxiety disorder. *British Journal of Psychiatry, 168*(3), 308–313.

Zhang, F., Aravanis, A. M., Adamantidis, A., de Lecea, L., & Deisseroth, K. (2007). Circuit-breakers: Optical technologies for probing neural signals and systems. *Nature Reviews Neuroscience, 8*(8), 577–581.

Systematic Approach to Treatment-Resistant Depression
Psychopharmacology and Psychotherapy

K. Ryan Connolly and Michael E. Thase

Introduction

Depression is one of the world's greatest public health problems and, commensurate with its importance, over 50 years of dedicated research have yielded a dizzying number of pharmacologic, somatic, and psychosocial interventions. Such advances have resulted in the current state of practice, which sees about 50%–60% of patients responding to first-line therapies. Unfortunately, not all of these "responses" lead to a full remission of symptoms or a functional recovery, and only about one third of patients who begin treatment will enjoy a full remission of symptoms within the first 2 or 3 months (Fava & Davidson, 1996); incomplete remission likewise is associated with increased risks of subsequent relapse, chronicity, and poor psychosocial outcomes. Treatment-resistant depression (TRD) thus represents a pressing issue for all clinicians who work with people suffering from depression. Although there has never been a shortage of expert opinion about how to best approach the problem of TRD, a growing body of research is beginning to allow an evidence-based approach to be formulated, including some hierarchical algorithms based on level of evidence of efficacy and risk-benefit appraisals. This chapter will provide an overview of our view of the state of the art circa 2011.

Diagnostic Approach

Treatment-resistant depression is not a diagnosis per se, but rather a description of one aspect of an individual's clinical course. Assessment of a depressed person who has not responded to one or more standard strategies should start with confirmation that he or she is indeed suffering from major depressive disorder (MDD) and that the patient's depression is indeed resistant to the treatment(s) that has thus far been recommended. Though admittedly clichéd advice, one should begin this exercise with the understanding that MDD is a very heterogeneous condition and that a large number of patients who received treatment with antidepressants actually do not suffer from MDD. Similarly, many patients who are said to have not "responded" to a particular treatment either could not tolerate or did not adhere to an adequate trial of that medication, falsely inflating their perceived level of treatment resistance.

The broader family of depressive disorders also are a highly comorbid set of conditions, including some conditions in which the affective syndrome is a consequence of an antecedent medical disorder or a medication. The depressive syndrome that precedes detection of carcinoma of the head of the pancreas is one such prototypic condition, and thyroid disease, cerebrovascular disease, dementia, syphilis, encephalitis, central nervous system tumors, and many other metabolic/endocrine illnesses have been associated with secondary depressive syndromes that are not particularly responsive to antidepressants and should be considered in a differential diagnosis and, if possible, excluded (Privitera & Lyness, 2007). In addition to the exclusion of medical conditions that may cause secondary depressive disorders, clinicians also should consider whether medical comorbidities are optimally treated: Even when not causing depressive symptoms per se, the overall burden of a patient's medical illnesses has been associated with increasing levels of depression severity and a lower likelihood of response to standard therapies (Iosifescu, 2007).

In addition to general medical comorbidities, psychiatric comorbidities that are not particularly responsive to antidepressant therapies also should be systematically assessed and, if necessary, addressed in the treatment plan. Substance use disorders, for example, can both lead to depressive syndromes and, even when clearly secondary to the depressive disorder, reduce responsiveness to standard therapies. This is particularly important because people with substance abuse problems are often hesitant to volunteer details of their alcohol or drug use and will not volunteer this information unless asked. Other psychiatric diagnoses should also be evaluated for and treated, because (much like the case with general medical illnesses) an increased burden of Axis I comorbidities is also associated with a more severe and chronic course of depression (Kessler et al., 2005).

With respect to the heterogeneity of major depressive episodes, special attention should also be paid to historical details and signs and symptoms that are suggestive of bipolar disorder (BPD). While a conventional diagnostic interview is likely to be sufficient to diagnose a patient with a history of an unequivocal episode of mania, at least one half of those who will ultimately be found to have BPD will present with depression as the initial episode and others with less clear-cut histories will not be able to differentiate periods of mood elevation from times of "normal" (or an idealized normal) functioning. It is estimated that about 30% of patients with BPD have at some time been diagnosed as suffering from MDD (Correa et al., 2010; Hirschfeld et al., 2003). Yet another subset of depressed patients with no history of manic episodes or distinct periods of hypomania present with selected characteristics that are suggestive of BPD, such as family history, frequent depressive recurrence, early age of onset, and reverse neurovegetative features. As a poor or adverse response to antidepressants is sometimes included among these so-called soft signs of a bipolar spectrum of illness, this issue is particularly germane to the assessment of people with TRD (Correa et al., 2010; Hirschfeld et al., 2003).

Finally, careful screening for psychotic symptoms may reveal a reason for nonresponse to standard antidepressants in a significant minority of depressed patients, particularly among those with high symptom severity. This is not only because the psychotic subtype of MDD is

TABLE 2.1 Thase and Rush Staging Method

Stage 0	Any medication trials, to date, judged to be inadequate
Stage I	Failure of at least one adequate trial of one major class of antidepressants
Stage II	Failure of at least two adequate trials of at least two distinctly different classes of antidepressants
Stage III	Stage II resistance plus failure of an adequate trial of a TCA
Stage IV	Stage III resistance plus failure of an adequate trial of an MAOI
Stage V	Stage IV resistance plus a course of bilateral electroconvulsive therapy

MAOIs, monoamine oxidase inhibitors; TCA, tricyclic antidepressants.
Source: Adapted from Thase and Rush (1997).

relatively nonresponsive to antidepressant monotherapy (as compared to nonpsychotic forms of MDD), but psychotic or psychotic-like symptoms also may be indicators of other conditions that are typically more treatment resistant (i.e., schizoaffective disorder, dissociative disorders, borderline personality disorder, posttraumatic stress disorder). With respect to psychotic episodes of MDD, it is fair to say that one should not be considered to be truly treatment resistant until there have been adequate trials of at least one combined antidepressant-antipsychotic regimen and electroconvulsive therapy (ECT).

Staging

Since the original scheme proposed by Thase and Rush, first proposed in 1995 and revised in 1997, several additional TRD staging systems have been published (see Tables 2.1–2.4). Though there is no agreed-upon definition of TRD, what these staging methods all share is the idea that treatment resistance can be conceptualized along a continuum, which—to some

TABLE 2.2 The European Staging Method

Nonresponder to (specify) TCA, SSRI, MAOI, SNRI, ECT, other
No response to one adequate antidepressant trial
Duration of trial: 6–8 weeks
Treatment-resistant depression
Resistance to two or more adequate antidepressant trials
Duration of trial:
  TRD1: 12–16 weeks
  TRD2: 18–24 weeks
  TRD3: 24–32 weeks
  TRD4: 30–40 weeks
  TRD5: 36 weeks–1 year
Chronic resistant depression
Resistance to several antidepressant trials, including augmentation strategy
Duration of trial(s): at least 12 months

ECT, electroconvulsive therapy; MAOIs, monoamine oxidase inhibitors; SNRIs, serotonin–norepinephrine reuptake inhibitors; SSRIs, selective serotonin reuptake inhibitors; TCA, tricyclic antidepressants; TRD, treatment-resistant depression.
Source: Adapted from Sourey et al (1999).

TABLE 2.3 Massachusetts General Hospital Staging Method

—No response to each adequate (at least 6 weeks of an adequate dosage of an antidepressant) trial of a marketed antidepressant generates an overall score of resistance (1 point per trial).

—Optimization of dose, optimization of duration, and augmentation or combination for each trial (based on the Massachusetts General Hospital or Antidepressant Treatment Response Questionnaire) increase the overall score (0.5 point per trial per optimization strategy).

—Electroconvulsive therapy increases the overall score by three points.

Source: Adapted from Fava (2003).

extent—can be described with respect to a hierarchy of medications. Also common is the idea that a treatment trial can be called a failure only after an adequate dose of medication is given for an adequate length of time. At this point the role for staging the extent of treatment resistance is mainly clinical, because their reliability has not been fully assessed, though standardized definitions would be helpful in the construction of clinical trials tailored specifically for TRD (Ruhe et al., 2011). Nevertheless, it should be noted that the minimum working classification for TRD used in studies intended for review by regulatory authorities such as the US Food and Drug Administration (FDA) is a history of nonresponse to at least two adequate trials of antidepressants during the current depressive episode.

TABLE 2.4 Maudsley Staging Parameters and Suggested Scoring Conventions

Parameter/Dimension	Parameter Specification	Score
Duration	Acute (≤12 months)	1
	Subacute (13–24 months)	2
	Chronic (>24 months)	3
Symptoms severity	Subsyndromal	
	Syndromal	
	Mild	2
	Moderate	3
	Severe without psychosis	4
	Severe with psychosis	5
Treatment failures		
Antidepressants	Level 1: 1–2 medications	1
	Level 2: 3–4 medications	2
	Level 3: 5–6 medications	3
	Level 4: 7–10 medications	4
	Level 5: >10 medications	5
Augmentation	Not used	0
	Used	1
Electroconvulsive therapy	Not used	0
	Used	1
Total		(15)

Source: Adapted from Fekadu et al (2009).

Goals and Expectations for Treatment

The primary goal of the acute phase of treatment of MDD is a complete remission of symptoms. Patients who experience only a partial response are increasingly understood to have prognoses and functional outcomes little better than patients who did not respond at all (Judd et al., 2000; Miller et al., 1998). The goal of complete remission is lofty, and it certainly makes the prospects of successful goal attainment in TRD less likely. Furthermore, estimates for the prognosis for remission in this population are sobering: Once a patient has failed an antidepressant trial, each subsequent trial becomes less likely to succeed. In the series of trials conducted under the auspices of STAR*D, for example, remission rates after one failure were around 30% irrespective of the treatment chosen, and again 30% after two failures; subsequent trials became much less successful with 15%–20% remission rates (Rush et al., 2006a). While these numbers may not—at first blush—appear promising, it is important to remember that the vast majority of people with MDD eventually recover: About 80% of patients will recover from an index major depressive episode within 2 years, with over 90% recovering within 10 years. The approach to TRD, then, is essentially one of persistence and ongoing engagement; if the clinician and patient can patiently tolerate successive attempts at treatment, they should eventually be rewarded with a successful outcome. The following sections will review the evidence that will allows for a systematic approach that places the options with the greatest chance of success in the forefront of treatment.

Pharmacologic Treatment Approach

A number of empirically supported strategies to relieve TRD exist and are detailed in current treatment guidelines (American Psychiatric Association [APA], 2010; Institute for Clinical Systems Improvement [ICSI], 2011; Lam et al., 2009; Mahli et al., 2009). Those with the strongest evidence of efficacy are as follows:

- Lithium augmentation
- Augmentation with second-generation antipsychotics
- Augmentation with thyroid hormone
- Switching to another antidepressant

In addition, augmentation with psychostimulants is not infrequently practiced, as is combination therapy with two or more antidepressants; these strategies will be reviewed, though it should be noted that they are supported by less evidence than the options listed previously.

Switching to a Second Antidepressant

Evidence

After the failure of a first-line antidepressant (currently the selective serotonin reuptake inhibitors [SSRIs], serotonin–norepinephrine reuptake inhibitors [SNRIs], and bupropion), the intuitive reaction would be to try another. But is there a way to determine which one has the best chance of success?

One time-honored approach is to switch to a different class of medication, with the hope that a depression that is resistant to one mechanism may respond to another. However, surprisingly few studies with newer antidepressants support this strategy. Switching to an SNRI, rather than a second SSRI, after the failure of an SSRI has been compared in two double-blind clinical trials with mixed results. In one trial of 122 hospitalized or partial hospital patients, a switch to venlafaxine resulted in a 20% greater remission rate than a switch to paroxetine (Poirier and Boyer 1999). In a larger trial of 422 depressed outpatients, however, venlafaxine was not superior to citalopram (Lenox-Smith and Jiang, 2008). This question was also approached in the less highly controlled ARGOS and STAR*D trials, which enrolled large numbers of patients in "real-world" clinical settings to evaluate sequential open-label, albeit randomized strategies for SSRI nonresponders. The ARGOS trial compared switching to venlafaxine, mirtazapine, or a second SSRI among over 3,000 SSRI nonresponders and found an 8% advantage in remission rates for those receiving venlafaxine as compared to the other options (Baldomero et al., 2005). The STAR*D level II trial compared switching to venlafaxine with switches to sertraline or bupropion among 488 subjects with depression resistant to citalopram; here venlafaxine showed a similar numerical advantage over the SSRI sertraline (7% difference in remission rates) and a somewhat smaller advantage compared to switching to bupropion (4% difference in remission rates). However, neither of these differences was statistically significant, nor were they consistently evident on secondary outcome measures (Rush et al., 2006a).

Much the same has been found in trials that examined switches to bupropion or mirtazapine after SSRI nonresponse; at present there is no evidence to suggest that either of these is a better choice than a second SSRI (Ruhe et al., 2006; Rush et al., 2006b). At this point, there is little evidence to guide treatment among the current, widely prescribed antidepressants after one failure, and almost none to guide selection in more treatment-resistant cases. It seems prudent, then, to base treatment selection on adverse effects (e.g., bupropion for a patient who developed marked sexual dysfunction on an SSRI) or particular depression symptoms (e.g., mirtazapine for a depression with reduced sleep and appetite) and to try several first-line antidepressants before moving on to less frequently used medications.

Once the first-line antidepressants have been exhausted, clinicians often move on to "classical" options such as the tricyclic antidepressants (TCAs) and monoamine oxidase inhibitors (MAOIs). Perhaps because of their formidable adverse effect profiles, these medications are often viewed as "the big guns" to be brought out when other medications have failed. However, it is not clear at this point that these agents are any more effective than the current first-line medications. TCAs are at least as effective as newer medications for treatment-resistant depression, but they have been only seldom compared in well-conducted trials and none has so far found them to be superior (Neirenberg et al., 2003; Fava et al., 2006). Even fewer data exist for the MAOIs among patients who have not responded to at least several trials of newer antidepressants. While data suggest that MAOIs may be particularly effective for treatment of TCA-resistant depression and for patients with prominent reversed vegetative symptoms, no trials convincingly demonstrate a benefit of MAOIs in TRD over first-line treatments and, in STAR*D, the performance of tranylcypromine was particularly disappointing (McGrath et al., 2006; Thase et al., 1992).

Recommendations for Switching to a New Antidepressant

In a sense, the data thus far to guide the selection of a second-choice antidepressant are both frustratingly sparse and liberating: At first glance any choice seems as good as any other. On the other hand, it seems intuitively unreasonable to try all of the SSRIs before trying a different class of antidepressants. To provide useful clinical guidance, we therefore offer the following recommendations once the decision to switch to a new antidepressant is made (also see Table 2.5):

- After the failure of two agents in the same class, a trial of an agent in a different class should be tried. While it remains unclear why some patients have differential responses to SSRIs, a switch to "something different" may help to preserve both patient and clinical morale in the face of serial failures, and it may well succeed where previous trials failed.
- Comorbidities, when present, should be taken into account during medication selection. Many of the currently available antidepressants differ in their additional indications; thus, bupropion may be a fine second-line agent for a patient with uncomplicated depression, whereas the TCA clomipramine may be better for a patient with obsessive-compulsive disorder who has not responded to vigorous trials with SSRIs or SNRIs.
- Adverse effect profiles must also be weighed, just as with initial treatment selection; though venlafaxine after a failure of sertraline is in general a fine option, for an older patient with significant cardiovascular disease, this may not be the case.
- For clear cases of "atypical features" depression, a course of MAOI may be considered earlier in the course than otherwise, based on clinical experience and earlier clinical trial data (APA, 2010).
- "Softer" indicators should not be ignored either: Patient preference and family history of response to a given agent are far from established predictors of response but may at least increase patient adherence and optimism.

Augmentation

While it is increasingly clear that the goal of treatment should be a full remission of symptoms, rather than a partial response, clinicians are understandably loath to abandon a medication that has shown some benefit, particularly after one or more complete failures. At such a point an agent that might augment the partially effective antidepressant can be an attractive option to increase the odds of response while maintaining the gains already made. Historically, lithium salts and thyroid hormones have been used as augmentation agents, while more recently the second-generation antipsychotics have garnered much attention in this role. Psychostimulants and modafinil have also been investigated as augmentation agents. Though augmentation of a partial antidepressant response seems the most natural indication for these agents, it is notable that the clinical trials that have examined them have focused almost exclusively on the case of *complete* nonresponse, making the decision of when to switch and when to augment somewhat less certain.

Lithium

Lithium has been used to augment TCAs and MAOIs since the 1960s (Zall et al., 1968); early experiences suggested that this could occur in as little as 48 hours (de Montigny et al., 1981).

TABLE 2.5 First-Line Antidepressants

Drug	Year Introduced in the United States	US FDA Indications	P450 Interactions	Recommended Dose Range for Major Depressive Disorder	Notes
Selective Serotonin Reuptake Inhibitors					
Fluoxetine	1987	MDD, OCD, bulimia nervosa, PMDD, panic disorder	Inhibits: 2D6, 2C19	20–80 mg daily	Nonlinear pharmacokinetics; very long half-life allows weekly dosing
Sertraline	1992	MDD, OCD, panic disorder, PTSD, PMDD	Inhibits: 2C9, 2D6 (to a lesser extent than fluoxetine or paroxetine)	50–200 mg daily	
Paroxetine	1993	MDD, OCD, panic disorder, social phobia, GAD, PTSD	Inhibits: 2d6	20–50 mg daily 20–62.5 mg daily (controlled-release)	Nonlinear pharmacokinetics; has appreciable anticholinergic side effects[a]
Fluvoxamine	1994	OCD	Inhibits: 1A2, 2C9, 2C19	Not indicated	Twice-daily dosing
Citalopram	1998	MDD	Inhibits: 2D6 (very weakly)	20–60 mg daily	Racemic mixture: *R*-citalopram may inhibit efficacy of *S*-citalopram[b]
Escitalopram	2003	MDD, GAD	Inhibits: 2D6 (very weakly)	10–20 mg daily	*S* enantiomer of citalopram
Serotonin-Norepinephrine Reuptake Inhibitors					
Venlafaxine	1994	MDD, GAD, panic disorder, SAD	Nonsignificant	75–375 mg in 2–3 divided doses (immediate-release); 75–225 mg (extended-release)	May cause hypertension

Duloxetine	2004	MDD, GAD, diabetic neuropathy, fibromyalgia	Moderate inhibitor of 2D6	60–120 mg daily	Nonlinear kinetics
Desvenlafaxine	2008	MDD	Nonsignificant	50 mg daily	Primary active metabolite of venlafaxine
Novel Antidepressants					
Bupropion	1985	MDD, SAD, smoking cessation	Substrate of cytochrome P450 2B6 and 2D6; modestly inhibits 2D6	100–150 mg three times daily (immediate release); 150–200 mg twice daily (sustained release; 300–450 mg daily (extended-release hydrochloride)	Likely works by inhibition of norepinephrine reuptake, dopamine reuptake (to a lesser extent), and likely other mechanisms. No sexual adverse effects
Mirtazapine	1997	MDD	Substrate of 2D6, 1A2, 3A4, 2C9; weak competitive inhibition of 2D6	15–45 mg daily at bedtime	Acts by blockade of α_2 adrenergic and $5HT_2$ and $5HT_3$ serotonergic receptors. Low incidence of sexual adverse effects, low incidence of nausea. Risks of weight gain and somnolence

Note. First-line antidepressants remain the best option for a switch after an initial treatment failure.

[a]Stahl, 1998.

[b]Kasper et al., 2009, GAD, generalized anxiety disorder; MDD, major depressive disorder; OCD, obsessive-compulsive disorder; PMDD, premenstrual dysphoric disorder; PTSD, posttraumatic stress disorder; SAD, social anxiety disorder.

Source: Information from Preskorn SH. Clinical pharmacology of selective serotonin reuptake inhibitors. Professional Communications Ltd., Pfizer, USA; http://medicine.iupui.edu/clinpharm/ddis/table.asp (retrieved 9/6/2010); and package inserts.

Though this dramatic effect was not replicated in more subsequent studies, it has since become clear that lithium can significantly augment the action of TCAs, as borne out by eight of ten randomized trials that, when pooled, show an NNT of 4 for lithium augmentation (dosed to a plasma level of 0.6–1.0 mEql/L) over placebo (Crossley and Bauer, 2007).

When lithium augmentation was a preferred option for TRD, it was debated as to whether lithium actually potentiated the effect of tricyclic antidepressants or whether lithium itself had antidepressant effects for a subset of patients with so-called pseudounipolar depression (Kupfer et al., 1975). There was also speculation that the effects of lithium might be better viewed as an accelerator of response to antidepressant medications. In either case, the exact mechanism by which lithium would exert these properties was obscure, a limitation that—despite 30 years of additional research—is still true. Moreover, although it is increasingly clear that the effects of lithium administration on the brain are diverse, the initially proposed mechanism of TCA augmentation, that of increased serotonin neurotransmission, remains a viable hypothesis (Bschor et al., 2003; de Montigny et al., 1983).

This hypothesis is interesting as it suggests that lithium may not be as useful to augment SSRIs with their already extremely potent effects of serotonergic neurotransmission; indeed, there have been very few trials that specifically examined this combination. The majority of reports have been open or uncontrolled, and they have tended to show a relatively modest beneficial effect for this combination (Delgado et al., 1988; Fava et al., 1994; Ontiveros et al., 1991). The lone randomized, placebo-controlled trial by Baumann and colleagues found a large benefit of this combination in 24 patients for whom citalopram monotherapy had proved ineffective—60% versus 14% response with lithium and placebo augmentation, respectively, though the small number of subjects must be noted (Baumann et al., 1996).

Overall, we can be confident that lithium effectively augments the antidepressant efficacy of TCAs, though more evidence is needed before such definitive claims can be made about its activity in combination with SSRIs or other first-line antidepressants.

Triiodothyronine

Like lithium, thyroid augmentation is best studied in patients who have not benefited from a course of therapy with a tricyclic antidepressant. Rather than the T_4 that is typically used to treat hypothyroidism, however, T_3 (triiodothyronine) was the form of thyroid hormone first studied for this purpose because, as it is the active form of thyroid hormone in the brain, it was presumed to have a more rapid onset of action (Altshuler et al., 2001). The first such study was undertaken by Prange and colleagues in 1969. This placebo-controlled study found T_3 effective at improving and accelerating antidepressant response to imipramine (Prang et al., 1969). Since this classic trial, numerous others have investigated the potential role of T_3 in improving antidepressant response.

A 1996 meta-analysis by Aronson and colleagues (1996) focused on the efficacy of T_3 augmentation in patients who had not responded to TCAs. They concluded that, as compared to placebo-treated patients, those who received augmentation with thyroid hormone were twice as likely to respond, with a pooled NNT of 4.3, comparable to the effect observed in the meta-analysis of lithium augmentation reviewed earlier (Aronson et al., 1996).

As with lithium augmentation, the question remains as to whether the success of adding T_3 to TCAs can be replicated in treatment with newer antidepressants; this topic was reviewed in a 2008 meta-analysis (Cooper-Kazaz et al., 2008). To date, the single trial that demonstrated a statistically significant benefit over placebo actually did not test thyroid augmentation but rather evaluated coadministration of T_3 from the outset of therapy with sertraline (maximum dose: 100 mg/day; Cooper-Kazaz & Lerer, 2008). Interestingly, remitters showed lower baseline T_3 and a greater suppression of TSH than did nonremitters, suggesting that this agent may have been useful only in patients with suboptimal thyroid functioning.

Like lithium, T_3 is an effective augmenter of TCAs; the evidence for augmentation of newer antidepressants is even sparser, however, and the trials that do exist have not thus far shown much support for T_3 in this indication. We do, however, continue to favor this strategy for patients with low normal baseline thyroid function studies or borderline high TSH levels.

Lithium Versus T_3

Lithium and T_3 augmentation were directly compared as part of the STAR*D study. In this trial, 142 patients who failed to respond to two sequential trials of modern antidepressants (i.e., citalopram, followed by sertraline, bupropion, or venlafaxine XR) were randomized to receive either T_3 (25–50 μg) or lithium (450–900 mg) augmentation (Nierenberg et al., 2006). In this trial, 15.9% of the patients treated with lithium augmentation remitted, as compared to 24.7% of the patients treated with thyroid augmentation. Although this difference is on the border of clinical significance, it was not statistically significant. Moreover, secondary analyses suggested that the trend favoring thyroid augmentation was likely attributable to the fact that it was better tolerated and easier for the STAR*D physicians to implement than lithium augmentation. It should be noted, however, that the primary outcome in this study was remission (specified as ≤7 on the 17-item Hamilton Depression Rating Scale, HDRS); a far more stringent criteria than response (50% reduction in symptoms), which had been the typical outcome measure in the prior studies discussed earlier. Another factor to consider is the level of treatment resistance shown in the study population; the subjects in the STAR*D trial had continued depressive symptoms without remission after two antidepressant treatments, while the level of treatment resistance was generally not specified in the earlier studies.

Second-Generation Antipsychotics

The second-generation antipsychotics (SGAs) have been the focus of much study as to their potential role in the treatment of depressive disorders. Given their currency, these studies have the advantage of studying augmentation of current, first-line antidepressants. Furthermore, as there is significant commercial interest in bringing new strategies for the treatment of depression to market, many of the studies of the SGAs have followed the conventions required for regulatory review of novel antidepressant medications. As a result, the studies utilize more standardized definitions of treatment-resistant depression, are well controlled, are large enough to ensure adequate statistical power to reliably detect even modest antidepressant benefits, and they tend to be conducted in sufficient number to permit replication. On one hand, these methodological features make an evaluation of the evidence much easier; on the other, the apparent "weight of the evidence" favoring adjunctive SGA therapy over older standards has been explicitly skewed by the commercial potential of these compounds: More evidence of efficacy is not synonymous with more effective.

The neuropharmacologic rationale for the use of SGAs to augment SSRIs or SNRIs is based on the broad receptor binding profiles of this class of medications (Meltzer & Massey, 2011; Papakostas & Shelton, 2008). Like some antidepressants (trazodone, nefazodone, mirtazapine), olanzapine, aripiprazole and risperidone inhibit to $5\text{-}HT_{2A}$ receptors (Meltzer & Massey, 2011). Ziprasidone and aripiprazole are also $5\text{-}HT_{1A}$ partial agonists, a pharmacologic effect that also may confer antidepressant efficacy (Papakostas & Shelton, 2008). In addition, quetiapine has been shown to inhibit norepinephrine reuptake, although not with the potency of secondary amine TCAs such as nortriptyline (Jensen et al., 2008). In 2011, aripiprazole and quetiapine have been FDA approved for use as adjuncts to antidepressant medications and fixed doses of the combination of olanzapine and fluoxetine (OFC, Symbyax) have been approved for treatment of patients who have not responded to adequate courses of antidepressant therapy.

Aripiprazole

Aripiprazole was the first SGA to be specifically approved by the FDA for use as an adjunct to first-line antidepressants. This approval was based on the results of two positive randomized clinical trials (Berman et al., 2007; Marcus et al., 2008). These trials enrolled patients who had a history of nonresponse to at least one but no more than three trials of SSRIs or venlafaxine. In both trials, patients were next treated for 8 additional weeks with their doctor's choice of fluoxetine, sertraline, paroxetine, citalopram, or venlafaxine XR in combination with a single-blind placebo. Nonresponders were then randomized to either aripiprazole (2–20 mg/day; modal dose: 10 mg/day) or placebo for an additional 6 weeks. Both trials documented statistically significant efficacy on the primary dependent measure (the Montgomery-Åsberg Depression Rating Scale [MADRS]), and a pooled analysis of these trials (total $n = 749$) showed a significant advantage for aripiprazole for remission rates, with an NNT of 10 for remission (Thase et al., 2006). A third trial of 349 patients using almost exactly the same methods fully replicated the aforementioned results (Berman et al., 2009). Aripiprazole was again superior to placebo in producing remission, this time with an NNT of 6. Across the three studies, it was noteworthy that the groups receiving active adjunctive therapy separated from those receiving placebo after 1–2 weeks of therapy, with little evidence of additional efficacy at doses above 10 mg/day.

Although adjunctive aripiprazole was generally well tolerated and all three studies reported high completion rates, about one third of the patients taking active aripiprazole experienced akathisia and restlessness. Average weight gain on active adjunctive aripiprazole ranged between about 1 to 2 kg across 6 weeks of double-blind therapy.

Given three positive, and no negative or failed trials, aripiprazole has a very strong evidence base as an antidepressant augmentation agent. The optimal duration of therapy and the actual longer term risks of problematic weight gain, dyslipidemia and other metabolic complications, and ultimately tardive dyskinesia have not been systematically evaluated.

Quetiapine

Quetiapine has been studied as an adjunct to antidepressants in two large placebo-controlled random controlled trials and several smaller studies. While its putative mechanism as a treatment for depression was unknown before these studies began, it has since been discovered that n-desalkylquetiapine (now known as norquetiapine) is a moderately potent inhibitor of the norepinephrine transporter (Jensen et al., 2008).

Three small trials of quetiapine were included in an early meta-analysis of antipsychotic augmentation of antidepressant treatment; these trials all demonstrated benefit over placebo, but were also quite small, with 15, 36 and 58 subjects (see Papakostas et al., 2007). Two much larger trials have subsequently been published; these focused on the newer extended-release formulation of quetiapine (QXR; Bauer et al., 2009; El-Khalili et al., 2010).

The first trial evaluated the efficacy of either 150 or 300 mg doses of QXR, compared to placebo augmentation, in 493 subjects over 8 weeks; all patients had a history of an inadequate response to an adequate trial of a standard antidepressant (predominantly SSRIs and SNRIs), which they were taking at a stable dose at the time of study entry (Bauer et al., 2009). The 300 mg dose of QXR showed a statistically significant improvement in MADRS compared to placebo with an NNT for remission of 8. Both QXR groups experienced significant elevations in body weight, triglycerides, LDL, and Hemoglobin A1C. The second multisite trial studied 446 outpatients using a similar design (El-Khalili et al., 2010). The 300 mg dose of quetiapine was again found to be statistically superior to placebo in reducing MADRS total scores, with an NNT of 12 for remission. As with the first trial, metabolic outcomes were significantly different between the medication and placebo groups. Increases in glucose and body weight were again seen, as well as a dose-dependent increase in LDL and triglycerides; an overall shift from fewer than three to at least three metabolic risk factors for cardiovascular disease was seen in the groups receiving quetiapine.

Quetiapine appears to be an effective adjunctive strategy for patients who are refractory to first-line antidepressants, and, although a dose–response relationship has not been definitively established, to our eyes the 300 mg/day dose may have a subtle advantage as compared to the 150 mg/day dose. The efficacy must be balanced, however, with the risks of sedation, weight gain, and other metabolic adverse effects, which may well be greater than those associated with adjunctive aripiprazole. The optimal duration of adjunctive therapy and the actual longer terms risks of problematic weight gain, dyslipidemia and other metabolic complications, and ultimately tardive dyskinesia have not been systematically evaluated for this indication.

Olanzapine

Although not the first SGA to be approved for adjunctive therapy, olanzapine was the first to be systematically studied as an adjunct to SSRI treatment, with a specific focus on use in combination with fluoxetine (referred to as OFC). The first such trial, by Shelton et al (2001) was a small but well-controlled trial of 28 patients that showed promising results of olanzapine added to fluoxetine. This led to a series of four larger scale studies trials, which—in aggregate—provided sufficient evidence of the efficacy of OFC to lead to FDA approval of this strategy.

In the first of the larger trials to be published, an 8-week, double-blind study, patients with a history of nonresponse to one SSRI were treated with nortriptyline, with dose escalation up to 175 mg/day. Five hundred nonresponders to nortriptyline monotherapy were then randomized to switch to olanzapine, fluoxetine, or OFC or to continue on nortriptyline. This trial failed to find an advantage for OFC, or any significant difference among the therapies, with numeric trends actually favoring the group receiving ongoing nortriptyline therapy on some analyses (Shelton et al., 2005).

A second large trial recruited 483 depressed patients who reported resistance to one SSRI (Corya et al., 2006). Participants first received a 7-week course of therapy with venlafaxine immediate release (mean 226 mg/day), with nonresponders randomly assigned to 12 weeks of additional therapy with OFC, olanzapine, fluoxetine, a low dose of OFC (1 mg olanzapine/5 mg fluoxetine), or continued therapy with venlafaxine. The low-dose group was intended to serve as an active placebo-control condition. The only significant difference in efficacy seen was between OFC and olanzapine alone. As was the case with nortriptyline in the previous trial, the patients who continued to receive venlafaxine had relatively good outcomes. Moreover, the patients who received low-dose OFC also did unexpectedly well. As a result of these several difficult-to-interpret results, this might be considered a failed trial.

Most recently, another pair of large trials addressed this issue; these trials were identical in design and were pooled and analyzed together for greater statistical power (Thase et al., 2007). Depressed patients with a history of one prior unsuccessful course of SSRI therapy were recruited and treated prospectively for 8 weeks with fluoxetine (mean dose 47.4 mg/ day). The first trial, which randomized 638 patients, showed no benefit of OFC compared to fluoxetine alone. The second trial, which randomized 675 patients, found a significant effect favoring OFC over both monotherapies. The greater efficacy of OFC was confirmed in the pooled analysis of the two studies, with an NNT of 10 (Thase et al., 2007). Efficacy of OFC as compared to both ongoing therapy with fluoxetine and olanzapine monotherapy was confirmed in a comprehensive metaanalysis of the total Lilly clinical trial database (Trivedi et al., 2009). In this analysis, the benefit of treatment with these combinations was reliably demonstrated after 1–2 weeks of therapy.

It should also be noted that olanzapine was associated with significantly greater weight gain and increase in total cholesterol compared to fluoxetine alone. With the increasing understanding of how commonly these effects, as well as impairment of blood glucose control, are seen with SGAs in general and olanzapine in particular, a careful risk/benefit appraisal will weigh these risks with the potential for clinical benefit. It should also be noted that rather than strictly an augmentation therapy, it is the proprietary combination of olanzapine and fluoxetine that has been studied as a treatment for TRD; it has not been shown that olanzapine augments other antidepressants.

The optimal duration of OFC therapy has not been determined. Likewise, the actual longer term risks of problematic weight gain, dyslipidemia and other metabolic complications, and ultimately tardive dyskinesia have not be systematically evaluated for this indication (Goodwin et al., 2009).

Risperidone

Two placebo-controlled studies have evaluated the utility of adjunctive risperidone for acute phase therapy and a third trial has evaluated continuation-phase therapy after an open-label course of adjunctive treatment (Keitner et al., 2009; Mahmoud et al., 2007). The first trial of risperidone as an augmentation agent demonstrated a significant increase in response and remission rates among 268 patients who had not benefited from a course of antidepressant monotherapy after 4 weeks (Mahmoud et al., 2007). Subjects were randomized to risperidone or placebo augmentation for another 4 weeks; risperidone-treated patients showed a significantly higher remission rate, with an NNT of 7.

The second trial, a placebo-controlled study of 97 nonresponders to SSRIs and other first-line antidepressants, also demonstrated a significant advantage of risperidone, with an NNT of 3.6 for remission (Keitner et al., 2009). Interestingly, the risperidone group showed significantly more rapid improvement in the first 2 weeks of the trial; by the fourth week this more rapid rate of improvement had slowed and both groups were seen to be improving at the same rate. As was the case with the first trial, the brevity of the study is a limitation and, given the apparent difference in speed of response, it is possible that risperidone may accelerate response without ultimately increasing the likelihood of response or remission.

The third trial sought to evaluate the long-term efficacy of risperidone augmentation in a placebo-controlled discontinuation design (Rapaport et al., 2006). In this trial, 241 responders to open-label risperidone augmentation of citalopram were next randomized to either continued risperidone or placebo augmentation, in blinded fashion, with time to relapse as the primary outcome. At the end of 24 weeks, there were no significant differences seen between the two groups.

Risperidone has been found to improve antidepressant responses in two, relatively short randomized, controlled trials. Its lack of efficacy in a longer-term trial and the short-term nature of the other studies leaves risperidone with significantly weaker support as an antidepressant augmentation agent, and at this time no further study of this indication is planned.

Other Second-Generation Psychotics

There are currently too few data to evaluate whether ziprasidone, paliperidone, lurasidone, asenapine, or iloperidone offer clinical utility as augmentation agents.

Modafinil and Stimulants

Modafinil is a wakefulness-promoting agent that likely works through the modulation of serotonin, histamine, dopamine and orexin neurotransmission (Minzenberg & Carter, 2008). Modafinil has been evaluated for the treatment of patients with partial response to antidepressants and who evinced "persistent symptoms of fatigue and sleepiness" in two large, 6-week randomized, controlled trials ($n = 447$) that were pooled and analyzed together (Fava et al., 2007). Though not seen in the individual trials, the pooled analysis demonstrated significant improvements in fatigue and sleepiness, as well as overall depression (NNT for response was 9, remission rates not reported). This suggests that the benefit of this modafinil in TRD may be small in this persistently fatigued, sleepy population; its benefit in patients without these residual symptoms is unknown and the drug did not have demonstrable benefits on the so-called core symptoms of depression (Fava et al., 2007).

Classical psychostimulants (methylphenidate and amphetamine compounds) have long been used clinically as augmentation agents due to their ability to increase alertness and elevate mood. However, the results of a meta-analysis by the Cochrane collaboration found that there are little data in the form of clinical trials to support this use (Candy et al., 2008). Furthermore, two more recent trials of an extended-release form of methylphenidate failed to show significant efficacy for this use (Patkar et al., 2006; Ravindran et al., 2008).

So, despite their long history of use, there is not adequate empirical support to recommend stimulants for adjunctive therapy for antidepressant nonresponders.

Other Augmentation Strategies

In addition to the agents described earlier, two agents with $5HT_{1A}$ agonist activity, pindolol and buspirone, have been studied as augmentation agents. Though pindolol has shown efficacy at accelerating antidepressant response, and buspirone is often used clinically as an augmentation agent, both have failed to show efficacy in well-controlled trials and cannot be recommended on the basis of the empirical literature (Appleberg et al., 2001; Ballesteros & Callado, 2004; Landen et al., 1998).

Recommendations

Overall, we recommend augmentation in cases of partial response and, when urgency of symptomatic benefit is of paramount importance, we recommend adjunctive therapy with SGAs when the initial antidepressant therapy has been sufficiently well tolerated to justify continued administration. Choice of augmentation agent should be personalized for the likely risks and benefits to an individual patient (see Table 2.6).

- Of all currently available augmentation options, the SGAs currently have the most support for use with newer generation antidepressants, and they are the only FDA-approved options for this indication. However, the NNTs observed in controlled studies hover around 10, which is on the border of clinical significance, an observation that essentially cries out for comparisons of these more costly strategies against older standards. The SGAs are also associated with variable rates of serious metabolic adverse effects, EPS and somnolence, and, when effective, the optimal duration of therapy has not been established. We therefore guardedly recommend aripiprazole and quetiapine for adjunctive therapy; it is our clinical impression that patients with decreased appetite and insomnia may more easily tolerate quetiapine augmentation, while those more sensitive to sedation and weight gain may benefit more from aripiprazole. Given the lack of evidence of olanzapine as an adjunct to medications other than fluoxetine, we do not recommend this as a "first-line" augmentation agent, though recognize that OFC is an effective option for patients who have not responded to fluoxetine monotherapy.
- Lithium remains a useful and inexpensive option. With demonstrated efficacy as an augmenter of TCA action, we consider it to be the first line to augment a partial response to TCAs. Given the long-term risks of thyroid, cardiovascular, and renal adverse effects, and the sparser evidence for augmentation of newer agents, lithium should be reserved for when SGAs are contraindicated or have been unsuccessful or intolerable or for when there is a high index of suspicion that the depressive episode falls within the bipolar spectrum.
- T_3 remains another useful and inexpensive option for TCA augmentation, and it is arguably safer and better tolerated. Its use with newer antidepressants is, however, even less supported by evidence and should be reserved for when other options have been exhausted or, potentially, in cases of subclinical or clinical hypothyroidism comorbid with depression.

TABLE 2.6 Augmentation Agents

Medication	Augmentation Dose	Notable Adverse Effects	Notes
Aripiprazole[a]	5–20 mg/day	Akathisia	First line for augmentation; expensive
Quetiapine[a]	150–300 mg/day	Sedation, weight gain, increase in lipids and blood glucose	First line for augmentation; expensive
Olanzapine[a]	3–12 mg/day (in combination with 25–50 mg fluoxetine)	weight gain, increase in lipids and blood glucose	Only approved/studied with fluoxetine. Not preferred first line for augmentation
Lithium	Sufficient for blood level of 0.4–0.8 mEq/L	Decline in renal and thyroid function, arrhythmia, weight gain, sedation	Weaker evidence for augmentation of non-TCA antidepressants
Triidothyronine (T$_3$)	25–50 µg/day	Tachycardia, nervousness, arrhythmia	Weaker evidence for augmentation of non-TCA antidepressants
Modafinil	100–400 mg/day	Headache, insomnia, anxiety	Only studied in patients with persistent sleepiness/fatigue

Note. Information taken from respective manufacturer's package inserts.
[a]All SGAs are considered to pose some risk for weight gain and metabolic adverse effects: olanzapine>quetiapine>aripiprazole. All SGAs carry a warning for increased risk of death when used in elders with dementia, and all also have a theoretical risk or tardive dyskinesia.
TCA, tricyclic antidepressant.

- Stimulants are surprisingly understudied, and modafinil seems to have only a modest augmenting effect. These options should likely be reserved when other options are exhausted or when comorbidities (sleep apnea, narcolepsy, attention-deficit/hyperactivity disorder) indicate their use.

Combination Therapy

A third strategy for addressing TRD, similar to augmentation, is the addition of a second first-line antidepressant agent to an existing antidepressant regimen. This strategy is more likely to be used when there is a partial response to a first agent that a clinician is unwilling to risk losing by changing course entirely. While some combinations make no logical sense (e.g., two SSRIs), others offer presumably complementary mechanisms that could potentially improve treatment (e.g., mirtazapine and venlafaxine, as they both increase serotonergic and adrenergic neutrotransmission, but by different mechanisms, with the added possibility of mirtazapine lessening venlafaxine side effects through blockade of 5HT3 receptors). Theoretical downsides of this include multiplying side effects, increasing medication burden and the possibility of unnecessary polypharmacy (i.e., when the patient responds to the addition of the second agent, it is unclear if the first needs to be continued). In any case, these combinations, despite their frequent clinical use, are surprisingly understudied in clinical trials (Thase, 2011), although some data do exist to help guide clinical practice.

Mirtazapine Combinations

Mirtazapine is an antagonist at serotonin 5HT$_{2A}$ and 5HT3 receptors and adrenergic α2 receptors (de Boer, 1996) and is currently the best-studied antidepressant in combinations, with four clinical trials reporting on its use (Blier et al., 2009, 2010; Carpenter et al., 2002;

McGrath et al., 2006). The first study, by Carpenter and colleagues, randomized 26 subjects who had not responded to an optimized antidepressant trial to receive either mirtazapine augmentation at 30 mg or placebo augmentation (Carpenter et al., 2002). After 4 weeks, subjects who received adjunctive mirtazapine showed significantly better remission rates on the HDRS, with an NNT of 3. Two others by Blier et al have examined the use of such a combination from the initiation of therapy and have found that the combination of mirtazapine with another antidepressant (SSRI, bupropion, venlafaxine) is often more effective than either agent alone, with an NNT of 3 to 5 (Blier et al., 2009, 2010). The combination of mirtazapine and venlafaxine was also studied in the STAR*D level 4 trial of 109 patients that had previously had three unsuccessful medication trials, where it was compared to monotherapy with the MAOI tranylcypromine (McGrath et al., 2006). A numerical but not statistical advantage in remission rates was seen with the combination, though it must be noted that tranylcypromine may have suffered a dosing disadvantage.

Bupropion Combinations

Although bupropion is one of the most commonly used antidepressants for combination therapy, there are no placebo-controlled randomized, controlled trials of this strategy. The combination of bupropion and citalopram was studied in the STAR*D level 2 trial, where it was compared to augmentation with buspirone (Trivedi et al., 2006)). After 12 weeks of treatment, both groups showed an HDRS remission rate of 30%, although bupropion therapy showed some modest advantages on secondary outcome measures.

Mianserin Combinations

Similar to mirtazapine (although not available in the United States), mianserin blocks 5HT2 and α-adrenergic receptors, and it has been studied as an adjunct to other antidepressants in two random controlled trials (Ferreri et al., 2001; Maes et al., 1999). Maes and colleagues found that coinitiation of the combination of mianserin and fluoxetine was markedly superior to fluoxetine alone or fluoxetine plus pindolol in a group of 31 subjects (Maes et al., 1999). Rather than coinitiation, Ferreri and colleagues (2001) evaluated the addition of mianserin in the case of nonresponse to an ongoing antidepressant trial. This trial randomized 104 patients who had not responded to 6 weeks of fluoxetine treatment to further treatment with fluoxetine, a switch to mianserin, or a switch to a combination of the two. After 6 weeks, the combination group showed a significant improvement in remission rates compared to the other groups, with an NNT of 4 for remission over fluoxetine alone.

Desipramine Combinations

The combination of desipramine and fluoxetine has also been studied, by Nelson et al (2004), but like those of the Blier group, this study investigated the coinitiation of the combination from treatment outset. In this study, the combination of desipramine and fluoxetine was significantly more effective than either fluoxetine or desipramine alone and the advantage of the combined treatment strategy was large and clinically meaningful. However, it is noteworthy that, although the patients were not selected specifically for a history of treatment resistance, the two monotherapies were essentially ineffective and the study was quite small, with 12–14 subjects per arm.

Recommendations

At this point, the role of combination therapy with antidepressants is somewhat unclear, as there is little evidence to speak of for their efficacy in TRD. As it stands, mirtazapine seems to be relatively well supported as an adjunct to commonly used medications and may be as useful as any of the augmentation strategies mentioned earlier in the case of partial response, particularly in patients that can tolerate weight gain and somnolence, or who are particularly adverse to the idea of sexual adverse effects. For those for whom these side effects are unacceptable, we do favor the use of bupropion, despite the lack of evidence from properly controlled randomized controlled trials.

Psychotherapy

Psychotherapy is increasingly accepted as one of the first-line therapies for MDD, both singly and in combination with antidepressants (APA, 2010). Most of the work in TRD has used the newer time-limited models of therapy, such as cognitive-behavioral therapy (CBT) and its several variants (behavioral activation [BA] or cognitive-behavioral analysis system of psychotherapy [CBASP]). Beyond ensuring the opportunity to provide ongoing social support patients with more chronic, unremitting depressive disorders, which can be life saving in and of itself, these focused psychotherapies are tailored to target deficits in productive or reinforcing behaviors (i.e., behavioral activation strategies), problem solving, or amelioration of specific symptoms (i.e., negative cognitions, insomnia, or anxiety). Other time-limited therapies, such as interpersonal psychotherapy (IPT), focus on identifying and working through problems in relationships (i.e., role transitions, role disputes, or unresolved grief), whereas CBASP guides patients to be more specific in identifying their goals within relationships and to practice more productive ways of interacting with significant others. Despite such promise, however, only a handful of good-quality studies have specifically addressed the utility of psychotherapy using sequential treatment models and operationally defined levels of TRD.

As part of the STAR*D level 2 trials for patients who had not responded to an adequate trial of citalopram, Thase and colleagues (2007) compared a switch to CBT versus a switch to another antidepressant medication and CBT augmentation to medication augmentation in patients who had an unsatisfactory response to citalopram. In this trial, patients were randomized to receive either CBT or a change in pharmacotherapy. The CBT protocol consisted of up to 16 individual sessions over 12 weeks. Those allocated to the CBT arms could receive it either alone or in combination with ongoing citalopram therapy; outcomes thus were contrasted between the two CBT arms and either the three-medication switch strategies (i.e., bupropion-SR, sertraline, or venlafaxine XR) or the two-medication augmentation options (i.e., bupropion-SR or buspirone). At the end of the study, all treatment groups experienced a remission rate of approximately 30%, with no significant differences between the groups; the only notable difference seen in the study was the significantly faster remission with medication augmentation compared to CBT augmentation (55.3 vs. 40.1 days, $p = .022$). Interestingly, although CBT monotherapy was significantly better tolerated than the medication switching options, the side effect experiences of the patients receiving it in combination with citalopram therapy were not significantly different from the group receiving adjunctive medication strategies.

One large-scale randomized controlled trial of CBT evaluated patients who had responded to standard antidepressant therapy but who had too many residual symptoms to be considered in remission (Paykel et al., 1999). In this trial, 158 incompletely remitted patients with MDD receiving continuation phase pharmacotherapy were randomly assigned to receive either clinical management or 18 sessions of CBT over 20 weeks; longer term data up to 68 weeks were also collected. After 20 weeks, both groups showed a reduction in HDRS of approximately 9 points, with no significant difference between groups; however, subjects receiving CBT did show significantly reduced risk of relapse, as well as better social functioning and self-esteem and reduced guilt and hopelessness (Paykel et al., 1999; Scott et al., 2000).

In a smaller randomized controlled trial of incompletely remitted patients, Kennedy and colleagues randomized 44 antidepressant-treated patients to receive 8 further weeks of either Cognitive Therapy (12 sessions) or lithium augmentation (0.4–1.0 mEq/L; Kennedy et al., 2003). No significant differences were seen between the groups during this short trial, with final remission rates of 38% for lithium augmentation and 26% for Cognitive Therapy.

In another small preliminary study, Harley and colleagues (2008) randomized 24 patients with unsatisfactory response to ongoing antidepressant medication to either 16 weekly sessions of a dialectical behavior therapy (DBT) skills group or a waitlist condition; DBT primarily has been evaluated as a treatment of borderline personality disorder. The group receiving DBT showed significant improvements in HDRS and Beck Depression Inventory (BDI) total scores, with effect sizes (Cohen's d) of 1.45 and 1.31, respectively, suggesting that further study of this treatment is warranted.

Several studies of CBASP, the only form of psychotherapy specifically developed for treatment of chronic depressions, are also germane to this discussion. In the first large-scale study of CBASP, 681 patients with chronic depression (defined as an episode lasting at least 2 years or "double depression") to 12 weeks of treatment with nefazodone (up to 600 mg/d), 16–20 sessions of the Cognitive Behavioral Analysis System of Psychotherapy (CBASP), or the combination of the two treatments (Keller et al., 2000). Though this patient group had been, on average, depressed for an average of 8 years, relatively few patients in this study actually had treatment-resistant depression. The two monotherapies produced remission rates of about 30%, whereas the combination resulted in a remission rate of 48%, or an NNT of about 5. Patients in the monotherapy conditions who did not respond were subsequently offered a switch to the alternate treatment (Schatzberg et al., 2005). In this partial crossover trial, both treatment groups experienced significant improvements in depressive symptoms; the group switched from nefazodone to CBASP had a significantly higher treatment completion rate and, as a result, a significantly higher response rate in the intent-to-treat analysis (57% versus 42%). However, a subsequent larger scale trial of chronic depression that included pharmacotherapy nonresponders and incompletely remitted patients (Kocsis et al., 2009) failed to confirm that CBASP was a particularly effective sequential treatment option as compared to either a supportive psychotherapy or an alternate course of antidepressant medication.

Recommendations

As is often the case in treatment-resistant populations, the literature for psychotherapy in TRD is sparser that one might hope. However, it thus far seems that systematic and evidence-based psychotherapy may offer equivalent efficacy as many medication options for this difficult population. More intriguingly, the hypothesis that psychotherapy, presumably by virtue of its different mechanism of action, may offer additive benefits has some limited empirical support in this population. As such, we recommend that—in addition to the pharmacotherapy recommendations earlier—any patient suffering from TRD be offered a course of evidence-based psychotherapy, as it currently seems to offer no risk other than cost, and it likely represents a safe adjunct or alternative therapy for patients too often failed by medication alone.

Clinical Practice Recommendations

1. When faced with the failure of a treatment for depression, clinicians should pause to reconfirm their diagnosis in order to rule out misdiagnosis and to identify complicating diagnoses that may hinder ultimate remission.
2. The level of treatment resistance should be staged to help guide treatment and prognosis. It is important to differentiate treatment trials that ended due to nonadherence or intolerance from truly failed trials of adequate dose and duration.
3. After a complete failure of a first-line antidepressant (i.e., less than 20%–25% improvement in symptom burden), usually the next step should be to select another first-line medication; at this point in treatment, combinations and augmentation add unnecessarily to adverse effect burden. Potential exceptions to this general rule might include patients for whom urgency may warrant use of an adjunctive SGA or for whom there is a strong index of suspicion of bipolar disorder.
4. After two failures of first-line antidepressants, other classes of medications should be tried. Switching should continue until at least a partial response is achieved or until a patient has failed to respond to both TCAs and/or MAOIs. Medication choice should be personalized as discussed earlier.
5. If a partial response is achieved, one should consider adjunctive or combination strategies.
6. Augmentation/combination should begin with aripiprazole, quetiapine, or mirtazapine if the primary antidepressant is a current, first-line medication. If the primary medication is a TCA, then lithium or thyroid augmentation is preferable.
7. Given the relatively low likelihood of response with any of these medication options after three or more trials, a discussion of a switch to ECT or another neuromodulation therapy (see next chapter) should not be delayed until all other options have been exhausted.
8. Though it represents a viable switching or augmentation strategy in its own right, we recommend all patients with TRD be offered an evidence-based psychotherapy when possible, as its effects may be additive and certainly seem not to hinder the use of other treatments.

Finally, it must be noted that the evidence to guide clinicians who treat TRD patients is limited and frequently exhausted in clinical practice. It is therefore important to remain optimistic and creative when necessary, and to remember to maintain and provide hope to balance the sobering prognoses often faced with this patient population. As further research continues to add to the present body of knowledge, and new treatments continue to be introduced, clinicians must remain hopeful, diligent, and secure in the knowledge than sooner or later, nearly every patient with TRD can be helped.

Disclosure Statement

K.R.C. has no conflicts of interest to disclose.

During the past three years, M.E.T. has consulted with Aldolor, Alkermes, AstraZeneca, Bristol-Myers Squibb, Dey Pharmaceuticals, Eli Lilly & Co., Forest Laboratories, Gerson Lehman Group, GlaxoSmithKline, Guidepoint Global, H. Lundbeck A/S, MedAvante, Inc., Merck (Organon; Schering-Plough), Neuronetics Inc., Novartis, Otsuka, Ortho-McNeil (Johnson & Johnson), PamLab, Pfizer (Wyeth), PharmaNeuroboost, Rexahn, Roche Inc, Shire US Inc., Supernus, Takeda, and Transcept. During the same time period, Dr. Thase has received honoraria for talks funded by AstraZeneca, Bristol-Myers Squibb, Dey Pharmaceuticals, Eli Lilly & Company, Merck, and Pfizer. During the past three years, Dr. Thase has received grants from the Agency for Healthcare Research and Quality, Eli Lilly & Co., Forest Pharmaceuticals, GlaxoSmithKline, the National Institute of Mental Health, Otsuka Pharmaceuticals, and Pfizer Pharmaceuticals.

References

Altshuler LL, Bauer M, Frye MA, Gitlin MJ, Mintz J, Szuba MP, Leight KL, Whybrow PC. Does thyroid supplementation accelerate tricyclic antidepressant response? A review and meta-analysis of the literature. *Am J Psychiatry* 2001;158:1617–1622.

American Psychiatric Association. *Practice Guideline for Treatment of Patients with Major Depressive Disorder.* 3rd ed. Retrieved February 2011, from http://www.psychiatryonline.com/pracGuide/pracGuideTopic_7.aspx

Aronson R, Offman HJ, Joffe RT, Naylor CD. Triiodothyronine augmentation in the treatment of refractory depression. A meta-analysis. *Arch Gen Psychiatry* 1996;53:842–848.

Baldomero EB, Ubago JG, Cercos CL, Ruiloba JV, Calvo CG, Lopez RP. Venlafaxine extended release versus conventional antidepressants in the remission of depressive disorders after previous antidepressant failure: ARGOS study. *Depress Anxiety* 2005;22(2):68–76.

Ballesteros J, Callado LF. Effectiveness of pindolol plus serotonin uptake inhibitors in depression: A meta-analysis of early and late outcomes from randomised controlled trials. *J Affect Disord* 2004;79(1–3):137–147.

Bauer M, Pretorius HW, Constant EL, Earley WR, Szamosi J, Brecher M. Extended-release quetiapine as adjunct to an antidepressant in patients with major depressive disorder: Results of a randomized, placebo-controlled, double-blind study. *J Clin Psychiatry* 2009;70:540–549.

Baumann P, Nil R, Souche A, Montaldi S, Baettig D, Lambert S, Uehlinger C, Kasas A, Amey M, Jonzier-Perey M. A double-blind, placebo-controlled study of citalopram with and without lithium in the treatment of therapy-resistant depressive patients: A clinical, pharmacokinetic, and pharmacogenetic investigation. *J Clin Psychopharmacol* 1996;16:307–314.

Berman RM, Fava M, Thase ME, Trivedi MH, Swanink R, McQuade RD, Carson WH, Adson D, Taylor L, Hazel J, Marcus RN. Aripiprazole augmentation in major depressive disorder: A double-blind, placebo-controlled study in patients with inadequate response to antidepressants. *CNS Spectr* 2009;14:197–206.

Berman RM, Marcus RN, Swanink R, McQuade RD, Carson WH, Corey-Lisle PK, Khan A. The efficacy and safety of aripiprazole as adjunctive therapy in major depressive disorder: A multicenter, randomized, double-blind, placebo-controlled study. *J Clin Psychiatry* 2007;68:843–853.

Blier P, Gobbi G, Turcotte JE, de Montigny C, Boucher N, Hébert C, Debonnel G. Mirtazapine and paroxetine in major depression: A comparison of monotherapy versus their combination from treatment initiation. *Eur Neuropsychopharmacol* 2009;19:457–465.

Blier P, Ward HE, Tremblay P, Laberge L, Hébert C, Bergeron R. Combination of antidepressant medications from treatment initiation for major depressive disorder: A double-blind randomized study. *Am J Psychiatry* 2010;167:281–288.

Bschor T, Lewitzka U, Sasse J, Adli M, Koberle U, Bauer M. Lithium augmentation in treatment-resistant depression: Clinical evidence, serotonergic and endocrine mechanisms. *Pharmacopsychiatry* 2003;36(Suppl 3): S230–234.

Candy M, Jones L, Williams R, Tookman A, King M. Psychostimulants for depression. *Cochrane Database Syst Rev* 2008;(2):CD006722.

Carpenter LL, Yasmin S, Price LH. A double-blind, placebo-controlled study of antidepressant augmentation with mirtazapine. *Biol Psychiatry* 2002;51:183–188.

Cooper-Kazaz R, Lerer B. Efficacy and safety of triiodothyronine supplementation in patients with major depressive disorder treated with specific serotonin reuptake inhibitors. *Int J Neuropsychopharmacol* 2008;11: 685–699.

Cooper-Kazaz R, Apter JT, Cohen R, Karagichev L, Muhammed-Moussa S, Grupper D, Drori T, Newman ME, Sackeim HA, Glaser B, Lerer B. Combined treatment with sertraline and liothyronine in major depression: A randomized, double-blind, placebo-controlled trial. *Arch Gen Psychiatry* 2007;64:679–688.

Correa R, Akiskal H, Gilmer W, Nierenberg AA, Trivedi M, Zisook S. Is unrecognized bipolar disorder a frequent contributor to apparent treatment resistant depression? *J Affect Disord* 2010;127:10–18.

Corya SA, Williamson D, Sanger TM, Briggs SD, Case M, Tollefson G. A randomized, double-blind comparison of olanzapine/fluoxetine combination, olanzapine, fluoxetine, and venlafaxine in treatment-resistant depression. *Depress Anxiety* 2006;23:364–372.

Crossley NA, Bauer M. Acceleration and augmentation of antidepressants with lithium for depressive disorders: Two meta-analyses of randomized, placebo-controlled trials. *J Clin Psychiatry* 2007;68(6):935–940.

de Boer T. The pharmacologic profile of mirtazapine. *J Clin Psychiatry* 1996;57(Suppl 4): 19–25.

De Montigny C, Cournoyer G, Morissette R, Langlois R, Caille G. Lithium carbonate addition in tricyclic antidepressant-resistant unipolar depression. correlations with the neurobiologic actions of tricyclic antidepressant drugs and lithium ion on the serotonin system. *Arch Gen Psychiatry* 1983;40:1327–1334.

De Montigny C, Grunberg F, Mayer A, Deschenes JP. Lithium induces rapid relief of depression in tricyclic antidepressant drug non-responders. *Br J Psychiatry* 1981;138:252–256.

Delgado PL, Price LH, Charney DS, Heninger GR. Efficacy of fluvoxamine in treatment-refractory depression. *J Affect Disord* 1988;15:55–60.

El-Khalili N, Joyce M, Atkinson S, Buynak RJ, Datto C, Lindgren P, Eriksson H. Extended-release quetiapine fumarate (quetiapine XR) as adjunctive therapy in major depressive disorder (MDD) in patients with an inadequate response to ongoing antidepressant treatment: A multicentre, randomized, double-blind, placebo-controlled study. *Int J Neuropsychopharmacol* 2010;13(7):917–932.

Fava M, Davidson KG. Definition and epidemiology of treatment-resistant depression. *Psychiatr Clin North Am* 1996;19(2):179–200.

Fava M, Rosenbaum JF, McGrath PJ, Stewart JW, Amsterdam JD, Quitkin FM. Lithium and tricyclic augmentation of fluoxetine treatment for resistant major depression: A double-blind, controlled study. *Am J Psychiatry* 1994;151:1372–1374.

Fava M, Rush AJ, Wisniewski SR, Nierenberg AA, Alpert JE, McGrath PJ, Thase ME, Warden D, Biggs M, Luther JF, Niederehe G, Ritz L, Trivedi MH. A comparison of mirtazapine and nortriptyline following two consecutive failed medication treatments for depressed outpatients: A STAR*D report. *Am J Psychiatry* 2006;163(7):1161–1172.

Fava M, Thase ME, DeBattista C, Doghramji K, Arora S, Hughes RJ. Modafinil augmentation of selective serotonin reuptake inhibitor therapy in MDD partial responders with persistent fatigue and sleepiness. *Ann Clin Psychiatry* 2007;19(3):153–159.

Ferreri M, Lavergne F, Berlin I, Payan C, Puech AJ. Benefits from mianserin augmentation of fluoxetine in patients with major depression non-responders to fluoxetine alone. *Acta Psychiatr Scand* 2001;103(1):66–72.

Goodwin G, Fleischhacker W, Arango C, Baumann P, Davidson M, de Hert M, Falkai P, Kapur S, Leucht S, Licht R, Naber D, O'Keane V, Papakostas G, Vieta E, Zohar J. Advantages and disadvantages of combination treatment with antipsychotics ECNP consensus meeting, March 2008, Nice. *Eur Neuropsychopharmacol* 2009;19(7):520–532.

Harley R, Sprich S, Safren S, Jacobo M, Fava M. Adaptation of dialectical behavior therapy skills training group for treatment-resistant depression. *J Nerv Ment Dis* 2008;196:136–143.

Hirschfeld RM, Calabrese JR, Weissman MM, Reed M, Davies MA, Frye MA, Keck PE Jr, Lewis L, McElroy SL, McNulty JP, Wagner KD. Screening for bipolar disorder in the community. *J Clin Psychiatry* 2003;64:53–59.

Institute for Clinical Systems Improvement. *Guideline for Major Depression in Adults in Primary Care*. Retrieved March 2011 from, http://www.icsi.org/guidelines_and_more/gl_os_prot/behavioral_health/depression_5/ depression__major__in_adults_in_primary_care_4.html

Iosifescu DV. Treating depression in the medically ill. *Psychiatr Clin North Am* 2007;30:77–90.

Jensen NH, Rodriguiz RM, Caron MG, Wetsel WC, Rothman RB, Roth BL. N-desalkylquetiapine, a potent norepinephrine reuptake inhibitor and partial 5-HT1A agonist, as a putative mediator of quetiapine's antidepressant activity. *Neuropsychopharmacology* 2008;33:2303–2312.

Judd LL, Paulus MJ, Schettler PJ, Akiskal HS, Endicott J, Leon AC, Maser JD, Mueller T, Solomon DA, Keller MB. Does incomplete recovery from first lifetime major depressive episode herald a chronic course of illness? *Am J Psychiatry* 2000;157:1501–1504.

Keitner GI, Garlow SJ, Ryan CE, Ninan PT, Solomon DA, Nemeroff CB, Keller MB. A randomized, placebo-controlled trial of risperidone augmentation for patients with difficult-to-treat unipolar, non-psychotic major depression. *J Psychiatr Res* 2009;43:205–214.

Keller MB, McCullough JP, Klein DN, Arnow B, Dunner DL, Gelenberg AJ, Markowitz JC, Nemeroff CB, Russell JM, Thase ME, Trivedi MH, Zajecka J. A comparison of nefazodone, the cognitive behavioral-analysis system of psychotherapy, and their combination for the treatment of chronic depression. *N Engl J Med* 2000;342:1462–1470.

Kennedy SH, Segal ZV, Cohen NL, Levitan RD, Gemar M, Bagby RM. Lithium carbonate versus cognitive therapy as sequential combination treatment strategies in partial responders to antidepressant medication: An exploratory trial. *J Clin Psychiatry* 2003;64:439–444.

Kessler RC, Berglund P, Demler O, Jin R, Merikangas KR, Walters EE. Lifetime prevalence and age-of-onset distributions of DSM-IV disorders in the national comorbidity survey replication. *Arch Gen Psychiatry* 2005;62:593–602.

Kocsis JH, Gelenberg AJ, Rothbaum BO, Klein DN, Trivedi MH, Manber R, Keller MB, Leon AC, Wisniewski SR, Arnow BA, Markowitz JC, Thase ME, for the REVAMP Investigators. Cognitive Behavioral Analysis System of Psychotherapy and brief supportive psychotherapy for augmentation of antidepressant nonresponse in chronic depression. The REVAMP trial. *Arch Gen Psychiatry* 2009;66(11):1178–1188.

Kupfer DJ, Pickar D, Himmelhoch JM, Detre TP. Are there two types of unipolar depression? *Arch Gen Psychiatry* 1975;32:866–871.

Lam RW, Kennedy SH, Grigoriadis S, McIntyre RS, Milev R, Ramasubbu R, Parikh SV, Patten SB, Ravindran AV, Canadian Network for Mood and Anxiety Treatments (CANMAT). Canadian Network for Mood and Anxiety Treatments (CANMAT) clinical guidelines for the management of major depressive disorder in adults. III. Pharmacotherapy. *J Affect Disord* 2009;117(Suppl 1):S26–S43.

Landen M, Bjorling G, Agren H, Fahlen T. A randomized, double-blind, placebo-controlled trial of buspirone in combination with an SSRI in patients with treatment-refractory depression. *J Clin Psychiatry* 1998;59(12):664–668.

Lenox-Smith AJ, Jiang Q. Venlafaxine extended release versus citalopram in patients with depression unresponsive to a selective serotonin reuptake inhibitor. *Int Clin Psychopharmacol* 2008;23(3):113–119.

Maes M, Libbrecht I, van Hunsel F, Campens D, Meltzer HY. Pindolol and mianserin augment the antidepressant activity of fluoxetine in hospitalized major depressed patients, including those with treatment resistance. *J Clin Psychopharmacol* 1999;19:177–182.

Mahmoud RA, Pandina GJ, Turkoz I, Kosik-Gonzalez C, Canuso CM, Kujawa MJ, Gharabawi-Garibaldi GM. Risperidone for treatment-refractory major depressive disorder: A randomized trial. *Ann Intern Med* 2007;147:593–602.

Malhi GS, Adams D, Porter R, Wignall A, Lampe L, O'Connor N, Paton M, Newton LA, Walter G, Taylor A, Berk M, Mulder RT; Northern Sydney Central Coast Mental Health Drug & Alcohol; NSW Health Clinical Redesign Program; CADE Clinic, University of Sydney. Clinical practice recommendations for depression. *Acta Psychiatr Scand Suppl* 2009;439:8–26.

Marcus RN, McQuade RD, Carson WH, Hennicken D, Fava M, Simon JS, Trivedi MH, Thase ME, Berman RM. The efficacy and safety of aripiprazole as adjunctive therapy in major depressive disorder: A second multicenter, randomized, double-blind, placebo-controlled study. *J Clin Psychopharmacol* 2008;28:156–165.

McGrath PJ, Stewart JW, Fava M, Trivedi MH, Wisniewski SR, Nierenberg AA, Thase ME, Davis L, Biggs MM, Shores-Wilson K, Luther JF, Niederehe G, Warden D, Rush AJ. Tranylcypromine versus venlafaxine plus mirtazapine following three failed antidepressant medication trials for depression: A STAR*D report. *Am J Psychiatry* 2006;163:1531–1541.

McGrath PJ, Stewart JW, Harrison W, Quitkin FM. Treatment of tricyclic refractory depression with a monoamine oxidase inhibitor antidepressant. *Psychopharmacol Bull* 1987;23(1):169–172.

McGrath PJ, Stewart JW, Harrison W, Quitkin FM. Treatment of tricyclic refractory depression with a monoamine oxidase inhibitor antidepressant. *Psychopharmacol Bull* 1987;23:169–172.

Meltzer HY, Massey BW. The role of serotonin receptors in the action of atypical antipsychotic drugs. *Curr Opin Pharmacol* 2011;11:59–67.

Miller IW, Keitner GI, Schatzberg AF, Klein DN, Thase ME, Rush AJ, Markowitz JC, Schlager DS, Kornstein SG, Davis SM, Harrison WM, Keller MB. The treatment of chronic depression, part 3: Psychosocial functioning before and after treatment with sertraline or imipramine. *J Clin Psychiatry* 1998;59:608–619.

Minzenberg MJ, Carter CS. Modafinil: A review of neurochemical actions and effects on cognition. *Neuropsychopharmacology* 2008;33(7):1477–1502.

Nelson JC, Mazure CM, Jatlow PI, Bowers MB Jr, Price LH. Combining norepinephrine and serotonin reuptake inhibition mechanisms for treatment of depression: A double-blind, randomized study. *Biol Psychiatry* 2004;55:296–300.

Nierenberg AA, Fava M, Trivedi MH, Wisniewski SR, Thase ME, McGrath PJ, Alpert JE, Warden D, Luther JF, Niederehe G, Lebowitz B, Shores-Wilson K, Rush AJ. A comparison of lithium and T(3) augmentation following two failed medication treatments for depression: A STAR*D report. *Am J Psychiatry* 2006;163: 1519–1530.

Nierenberg AA, Papakostas GI, Petersen T, Kelly KE, Iacoviello BM, Worthington JJ, Tedlow J, Alpert JE, Fava M. Nortriptyline for treatment-resistant depression. *J Clin Psychiatry* 2003;64(1):35–39.

Ontiveros A, Fontaine R, Elie R. Refractory depression: The addition of lithium to fluoxetine or desipramine. *Acta Psychiatr Scand* 1991;83:188–192.

Papakostas GI, Shelton RC. Use of atypical antipsychotics for treatment-resistant major depressive disorder. *Curr Psychiatry Rep* 2008;10:481–486.

Papakostas GI, Shelton RC, Smith J, Fava M. Augmentation of antidepressants with atypical antipsychotic medications for treatment-resistant major depressive disorder: A meta-analysis. *J Clin Psychiatry* 2007;68:826–831.

Patkar AA, Masand PS, Pae CU, Peindl K, Hooper-Wood C, Mannelli P, Ciccone P. A randomized, double-blind, placebo-controlled trial of augmentation with an extended release formulation of methylphenidate in outpatients with treatment-resistant depression. *J Clin Psychopharmacol* 2006;26(6):653–656.

Paykel ES, Scott J, Teasdale JD, Johnson AL, Garland A, Moore R, Jenaway A, Cornwall PL, Hayhurst H, Abbott R, Pope M. Prevention of relapse in residual depression by cognitive therapy: a controlled trial. *Arch Gen Psychiatry* 1999;56(9):829–835.

Poirier MF, Boyer P. Venlafaxine and paroxetine in treatment-resistant depression. Double-blind, randomised comparison. *Br J Psychiatry* 1999;175:12–16.

Prange AJ Jr, Wilson IC, Rabon AM, Lipton MA. Enhancement of imipramine antidepressant activity by thyroid hormone. *Am J Psychiatry* 1969;126:457–469.

Privitera, MR, Lyness, JM. Depression. In: Duthie E Jr, Katz PR, Malone ML, eds. *The Practice of Geriatrics*. 4th ed. New York: W.B. Saunders; 2007:Chapter 27; 345–358.

Rapaport MH, Gharabawi GM, Canuso CM, Mahmoud RA, Keller MB, Bossie CA, Turkoz I, Lasser RA, Loescher A, Bouhours P, Dunbar F, Nemeroff CB. Effects of risperidone augmentation in patients with treatment-resistant depression: Results of open-label treatment followed by double-blind continuation. *Neuropsychopharmacology* 2006;31:2505–2513.

Ravindran AV, Kennedy SH, O'Donovan MC, Fallu A, Camacho F, Binder CE. Osmotic-release oral system methylphenidate augmentation of antidepressant monotherapy in major depressive disorder: Results of a double-blind, randomized, placebo-controlled trial. *J Clin Psychiatry* 2008;69(1):87–94.

Ruhe HG, van Rooijen G, Spijker J, Peeters FP, Schene AH. Staging methods for treatment resistant depression. A systematic review. *J Affect Disord* 2011; [Epub ahead of print].

Rush AJ, Trivedi MH, Wisniewski SR, Nierenberg AA, Stewart JW, Warden D, Niederehe G, Thase ME, Lavori PW, Lebowitz BD, McGrath PJ, Rosenbaum JF, Sackeim HA, Kupfer DJ, Luther J, Fava M. Acute and longer-term outcomes in depressed outpatients requiring one or several treatment steps: A STAR*D report. *Am J Psychiatry* 2006;163(11):1905–1917.

Rush AJ, Trivedi MH, Wisniewski SR, Stewart JW, Nierenberg AA, Thase ME, Ritz L, Biggs MM, Warden D, Luther JF, Shores-Wilson K, Niederehe G, Fava M, STAR*D Study Team. Bupropion-SR, sertraline, or venlafaxine-XR after failure of SSRIs for depression. *N Engl J Med* 2006;354(12):1231–1242.

Ruhe HG, Huyser J, Swinkels JA, Schene AH. Switching antidepressants after a first selective serotonin reuptake inhibitor in major depressive disorder: A systematic review. *J Clin Psychiatry* 2006;67:1836–1855.

Schatzberg AF, Rush AJ, Arnow BA, Banks PL, Blalock JA, Borian FE, Howland R, Klein DN, Kocsis JH, Kornstein SG, Manber R, Markowitz JC, Miller I, Ninan PT, Rothbaum BO, Thase ME, Trivedi MH, Keller MB. Chronic depression: Medication (nefazodone) or psychotherapy (CBASP) is effective when the other is not. *Arch Gen Psychiatry* 2005;62(5):513–520.

Scott J, Teasdale JD, Paykel ES, Johnson AL, Abbott R, Hayhurst H, Moore R, Garland A. Effects of cognitive therapy on psychological symptoms and social functioning in residual depression. *Br J Psychiatry* 2000;177: 440–446.

Shelton RC, Tollefson GD, Tohen M, Stahl S, Gannon KS, Jacobs TG, Buras WR, Bymaster FP, Zhang W, Spencer KA, Feldman PD, Meltzer HY. A novel augmentation strategy for treating resistant major depression. *Am J Psychiatry* 2001;158:131–134.

Shelton RC, Williamson DJ, Corya SA, Sanger TM, Van Campen LE, Case M, Briggs SD, Tollefson GD. Olanzapine/fluoxetine combination for treatment-resistant depression: A controlled study of SSRI and nortriptyline resistance. *J Clin Psychiatry* 2005;66:1289–1297.

Thase ME. Antidepressant combinations: widely used, but far from empirically validated. *Can J Psychiatry* 2011;56(6):317–323.

Thase ME, Corya SA, Osuntokun O, Case M, Henley DB, Sanger TM, Watson SB, Dube S. A randomized, double-blind comparison of olanzapine/fluoxetine combination, olanzapine, and fluoxetine in treatment-resistant major depressive disorder. *J Clin Psychiatry* 2007;68:224–236.

Thase ME, Frank E, Mallinger AG, Hamer T, Kupfer DJ. Treatment of imipramine-resistant recurrent depression, III: Efficacy of monoamine oxidase inhibitors. *J Clin Psychiatry* 1992;53(1):5–11.

Thase ME, Friedman ES, Biggs MM, Wisniewski SR, Trivedi MH, Luther JF, Fava M, Nierenberg AA, McGrath PJ, Warden D, Niederehe G, Hollon SD, Rush AJ. Cognitive therapy versus medication in augmentation and switch strategies as second-step treatments: A STAR*D report. *Am J Psychiatry* 2007;164:739–752.

Thase ME, Trivedi MH, Nelson JC, Fava M, Swanink R, Tran QV, Pikalov A, Yang H, Carlson BX, Marcus RN, Berman RM. Examining the efficacy of adjunctive aripiprazole in major depressive disorder: A pooled analysis of 2 studies. *Prim Care Companion J Clin Psychiatry* 2008;10:440–447.

Trivedi MH, Fava M, Wisniewski SR, Thase ME, Quitkin F, Warden D, Ritz L, Nierenberg AA, Lebowitz BD, Biggs MM, Luther JF, Shores-Wilson K, Rush AJ, STAR*D Study Team. Medication augmentation after the failure of SSRIs for depression. *N Engl J Med* 2006;354:1243–1252.

Trivedi MH, Thase ME, Osuntokun O, Henley DB, Case M, Watson SB, Campbell GM, Corya SA. An integrated analysis of olanzapine/fluoxetine combination in clinical trials of treatment-resistant depression. *J Clin Psychiatry* 2009;70(3):387–396.

Zall H, Therman PG, Myers JM. Lithium carbonate: A clinical study. *Am J Psychiatry* 1968;125(4):549–555.

Management of Treatment-Resistant Depression

Somatic Nonpharmacological Therapies

Paul E. Holtzheimer

Introduction

Somatic, nonpharmacological therapies are among the oldest available treatments for severe psychiatric illness. Modern attempts at ablative surgery for disabling mental disorders occurred as early as 1891 (Burckhardt, 1891), and electroconvulsive therapy was introduced in the late 1930s (Bini, 1938). Development of these therapies was jointly driven by the severity of the disorders being treated and the lack of pharmacological or psychotherapeutic interventions.

As psychotropic medications and evidence-based psychotherapies emerged in the 1950s and 1960s, the use of somatic, nonpharmacological therapies diminished. However, over the past few decades, interest in these treatments has increased. This has been guided by a growing recognition of the limits of medications and psychotherapy for treating severe psychiatric illness, including treatment-resistant depression (TRD), as well as improved models of the neural systems involved in regulating mood, thought, and behavior (spurred by a rapidly developing neuroimaging database).

This chapter will first review the somatic, nonpharmacological therapies currently available for the treatment of depression and TRD, including electroconvulsive therapy (ECT), ablative neurosurgery, vagus nerve stimulation (VNS), and transcranial magnetic stimulation (TMS). Subsequently, emerging therapies will be discussed, including transcranial direct current stimulation (tDCS), magnetic seizure therapy (MST), direct cortical stimulation (DCS), and deep brain stimulation (DBS). In a summary section, these various treatments will be assessed with regard to where each might fit into the broader TRD treatment repertoire.

Current Strategies

Electroconvulsive Therapy

Description

Ugo Cerletti and Lucio Bini first reported on the use of ECT to treat "schizophrenia" in 1938 (Bini, 1938). Since then, ECT has become established as one of the most effective treatments for depression, including TRD. ECT involves delivering electricity through the brain, between scalp electrodes, to induce a generalized seizure. Over several weeks, a series of seizures are given two to three times per week. ECT is performed under general anesthesia with complete sedation and muscle paralysis to limit the physical effects of the seizure. Each seizure typically lasts 25–60 seconds. Standard electrode placements for ECT include bitemporal (with one electrode placed over each temporal lobe), bifrontal (with electrodes placed over the left and right prefrontal cortex), and right unilateral (with one electrode placed over the right temporal lobe and the other over the vertex). Typical stimulation parameters include 500–800 milliamperes (mA) given at 20–130 Hz with a 0.3 millisecond (ultrabrief) to 2.0 millisecond pulse width for 0.5–8.0 seconds.

Efficacy

ECT is broadly viewed as the most effective acute treatment for a major depressive episode (Fink, 2001; The UK ECT Review Group, 2003), with remission rates well over 40%–50%, even in TRD patients (Prudic et al., 1996; Kellner et al., 2006; Sackeim et al., 2009); in less resistant patients, remission rates approach 80%–90%. Multiple open and blinded controlled trials have helped confirm the efficacy of ECT (Grunhaus et al., 2000; Grunhaus et al., 2003; Kho et al., 2003; The UK ECT Review Group, 2003). Largely due to stigma, ECT is often not considered until a patient has failed multiple other antidepressant treatments. Given its efficacy and overall tolerability (Rose et al., 2003), it may be that ECT should be offered earlier for TRD patients. In patients at higher risk for suicide, for example, ECT should be considered sooner than at its more conventional "last resort" position (Kellner et al., 2005).

A number of treatment factors appear to influence the efficacy of ECT. In one meta-analysis, bilateral ECT was found to be more effective than unilateral ECT (The UK ECT Review Group, 2003), though the true difference in efficacy is likely small since individual studies have not consistently shown this (Sackeim et al., 2000, 2008; Kellner et al., 2010). For optimal efficacy, bilateral ECT needs to be delivered at 2–3 times the seizure threshold (Sackeim et al., 2008), but unilateral ECT may need to be delivered at 6–12 times seizure threshold (McCall et al., 2000; Sackeim et al., 2008). A seizure duration of at least 25 seconds is generally considered necessary for an efficacious treatment (Price et al., 1978; ECT Task Force of the American Psychiatric Association, 2001).

ECT is clearly established as an acute treatment for depression. However, relapse of depression following a successful ECT course remains problematic, with 40%–84% of patients relapsing within 6 months even following full remission (Bourgon and Kellner, 2000; Sackeim, Haskett et al., 2001; Kellner et al., 2006). Certain medication regimens may help decrease the likelihood of relapse after ECT. For example, Sackeim, Haskett, and colleagues (2001) found that a combination of nortriptyline and lithium following successful ECT was superior in preventing depressive relapse compared to nortriptyline alone and placebo. Continuation and/or maintenance ECT (continued delivery of ECT treatments at increasing intervals over time) may be implemented to help minimize depressive relapse following successful ECT. Despite some evidence supporting continuation ECT (Trevino et al., 2010), its long-term efficacy has not been sufficiently established (Kellner et al., 2006).

Safety

Relative contraindications to ECT include severe cardiovascular conditions and conditions affecting the central nervous system such as increased intracranial pressure, recent cerebral infarction or bleeding, cerebral angioma, or aneurysm. Serious adverse events are rare with ECT but include cardiovascular, cerebrovascular, or pulmonary complications (usually related to anesthesia). One study found the mortality rate associated with ECT to be about 2 per 100,000 treatments (Shiwach et al., 2001), and patients treated with ECT have a lower 3-year mortality rate compared to depressed patients with inadequate antidepressant treatment (Avery and Winokur, 1976). Minor side effects of ECT include headaches, nausea, muscle aches, and fatigue. ECT is deemed to have a favorable risk/benefit ratio in the elderly (ECT Task Force of the American Psychiatric Association, 2001) and has been used safely in children and pregnant women (Black et al., 1985; Bertagnoli and Borchardt, 1990; Ghaziuddin et al., 1996; Rey and Walter, 1997; ECT Task Force of the American Psychiatric Association, 2001; Pinette and Wax, 2010).

Cognitive impairments are common with ECT and represent the side effects of greatest concern to patients and providers. Cognitive side effects of ECT include transient postictal confusion, short-term anterograde amnesia, and retrograde amnesia that can occasionally be quite pronounced and long lasting, especially for autobiographical memory (Lisanby et al., 2000; Sackeim et al., 2007; Moreines et al., 2011). Certain treatment modifications may help minimize or at least reduce the cognitive side effects of ECT, including using ultrabrief pulse (0.3 ms) instead of standard brief pulse (1–2 ms) stimulation (Sackeim et al., 2008), using unilateral instead of bilateral electrode placement (Sackeim et al., 2008) (though not all studies have shown this (Kellner et al., 2010), giving treatment two instead of three times per week and using the lowest necessary dose of ECT (typically achieved by determining the seizure threshold and treating relative to that).

Mechanism

ECT influences many neural systems, though its mechanisms of action are largely unknown. Human and animal studies have found ECT to be associated with the expression of neurotrophic factors, increased neurogenesis, enhanced synaptic connectivity, neurotransmitter changes, alterations in intracellular signaling, and the secretion of hormones, neuropeptides, and endogenous opioids (Madsen et al., 2000; Coyle and Duman, 2003; Wahlund and von Rosen, 2003; Altar et al., 2004; Madsen et al., 2005). ECT affects brain activity in regions implicated in the pathophysiology of depression (Krystal et al., 2000; Henry et al., 2001; Nobler et al., 2001; Wahlund and von Rosen, 2003; Takano et al., 2007; Mayberg, 2009).

Ablative Surgery

Description

Ablative neurosurgery is one of the oldest and most invasive of the currently available treatments for TRD, and prior to the emergence of the first antidepressant medications in the 1950s (Kuhn, 1958; Bailey et al., 1959; Kiloh et al., 1960), ablative procedures (such as the prefrontal leucotomy (Jasper, 1995) were the only treatment option for patients with severe, life-threatening depression unresponsive to ECT. With the rise of psychopharmacology, rates of ablative procedures for severe psychiatric illness decreased significantly. However, facilitated by the development of stereotactic neurosurgical techniques that allowed more focal ablation with fewer side effects (Sachdev and Sachdev, 1997; Hariz et al., 2010), neurosurgery remained an option for a small group of severely ill patients, including those with severe TRD.

Ablative procedures in use today include capsulotomy (a lesion in the anterior limb of the internal capsule), cingulotomy (a lesion in the dorsal anterior cingulate), subcaudate tractotomy (a lesion in thalamocortical white matter tracts inferior to the anterior striatum), and limbic leucotomy (which combines a subcaudate tractotomy with a cingulotomy) (Marino Junior and Cosgrove, 1997). These are generally accomplished by making a radiofrequency lesion at the neural target under local or general anesthesia using stereotactic neurosurgical techniques. The Gamma Knife approach may also be used.

Efficacy

No controlled data exist for ablative procedures in TRD patients. The efficacy for these procedures in open-label, naturalistic studies of TRD patients has been judged to be between 22% and 75% (Sachdev and Sacher, 2005; Shields et al., 2008; Steele et al., 2008; Christmas et al., 2010). However, no standard definition of efficacy has been used across studies, such that it is difficult to assess the differential efficacy of each approach.

Safety

Adverse events associated with ablative neurosurgery include risks associated with the surgical procedure itself (intracranial hemorrhage, infection, and complications from anesthesia) as well as side effects associated with the lesion. Known side effects of these procedures include epilepsy, cognitive abnormalities, and personality changes (Sachdev and Sacher, 2005; Shields et al., 2008; Moreines et al., 2011). Again, it is difficult to compare the relative safety of these procedures.

Mechanism

Ablation for severe psychiatric illness was largely based on early neuroanatomical models of mood regulation, such as the Papez circuit (Papez, 1937), that hypothesized these disorders were caused by abnormally increased and unregulated information outflow from the thalamus to the prefrontal cortices. Thus, the rationale for ablation was to sever the white matter connections between the thalamus and the prefrontal cortex in an attempt to decrease this abnormal communication. Modulation of activity within a mood regulation neural network continues to be the driving theory behind modern ablative procedures for TRD, though the neuroanatomical models used have been much refined due to advances in structural and functional neuroimaging over the past several decades.

Vagus Nerve Stimulation

Description

VNS first emerged as a potential treatment for medication-refractory epilepsy and was initially approved by the US Food and Drug Administration (FDA) in 1997 for this indication (Ben-Menachem, 2002). VNS was later approved by the US FDA for the adjunctive long-term treatment of chronic or treatment-resistant major depression not responding to at least four antidepressant medications. With VNS, an electrode is attached to the left vagus nerve and connected to an implanted programmable pulse generator/battery pack (IPG) implanted in the chest wall. Programming is performed using an external wand. Typical stimulation parameters include 0.25 milliamperes current, 20–30 Hz, 250–500 ms pulse width, and an on/off cycle of 30 seconds on every 3–5 minutes.

Efficacy

The initial rationale for VNS in the treatment of depression was primarily based on modest mood improvements seen in nondepressed epileptic patients treated with VNS (Elger et al., 2000; Harden et al., 2000). Further justification included the mood stabilizing effects of certain anticonvulsant medications and the possible anticonvulsant effects of other antidepressant treatments, such as ECT (Sackeim, 1999; George et al., 2003).

An initial open study in 60 nonepileptic TRD patients found a 31% response rate (defined as a >50% decreased in Hamilton Depression Rating Scale [HDRS] score) and a 15% remission rate (HDRS <8) after 10 weeks of VNS treatment (Sackeim, Rush et al., 2001). These response and remission rates were similar at 1 year (Marangell et al., 2002) and were somewhat greater 2 years postsurgery (Nahas et al., 2005). Confirming these results, a European multicenter open-label study of VNS in TRD patients demonstrated a 37% response and 17% remission rate after 3 months of chronic stimulation and a 53% response and 33% remission rate after 1 year (Schlaepfer et al., 2008).

A pivotal, multicenter, double-blind, sham-controlled study of VNS in patients that had failed 2–6 antidepressant medications in the current episode did not find statistically significant antidepressant effects for 10 weeks of active VNS versus sham (no stimulation following surgery) (Rush, Marangell et al., 2005). At the end of the 10-week double-blind period, response rate was only 15% with active VNS versus 10% with sham. Following this double-blind study, all patients received open, active VNS combined with treatment as usual (TAU). After 1 year of stimulation (VNS + TAU), response rate was 27% and remission rate was 16% (Rush, Sackeim et al., 2005), and these rates were statistically significantly greater than the 13% response and 7% remission rates seen in a second TRD cohort treated with TAU but never receiving VNS (George et al. 2005). The 1-year relapse rate following successful VNS + TAU was roughly 25%–35% (Sackeim et al., 2007) versus about 60% following successful TAU alone (Dunner et al., 2006). (In the open-label European study, relapse was >50% in the year following response, though the long-term [2 year] benefits appeared to be more substantial; Bajbouj et al., 2010.)

Safety

VNS surgery is generally well tolerated, and side effects of chronic stimulation are modest (Ben-Menachem, 2001). Common side effects of chronic VNS include voice changes, hoarseness, and coughing that usually occur only during the 30-second "on" period of stimulation and can diminish in severity over time. In general, VNS appears to have no significant cognitive side effects, though higher stimulation intensity may be associated with some modest cognitive impairments (Helmstaedter et al., 2001; Moreines et al., 2011). The published data suggest that over 80% of VNS patients choose to continue stimulation over time.

Mechanism

The potential mechanisms of action of VNS in epilepsy and depression are currently unknown. The vagus nerve has extensive connections throughout the brain, so it is not unreasonable that VNS could affect higher level brain systems involved in the regulation of mood, thought, and behavior. These effects are partially corroborated by neuroimaging data (Chae et al., 2003; Conway et al., 2006; Kosel et al., 2011). Other potential mechanisms of action for VNS include alteration of the activity of γ-aminobutyric acid (GABA) (Ben-Menachem et al., 1995; Marrosu et al., 2003), dopamine (Carpenter et al., 2004), and norepinephrine (Lechner et al., 1997; Krahl et al., 1998; Hassert et al., 2004; Groves et al., 2005) systems, though these data are not unequivocal (Carpenter et al., 2004). Also, these effects have not consistently been associated with therapeutic response (Ben-Menachem et al., 1995). The mechanisms of action of VNS remain an active area of investigation (Nemeroff et al., 2006).

Transcranial Magnetic Stimulation

Description

TMS is a noninvasive brain stimulation technique approved by the US FDA for the treatment of depression in patients that have failed one antidepressant medication during the current episode. TMS uses an electromagnetic coil placed against the scalp to generate a rapidly changing magnetic field that induces a depolarizing electrical current in the underlying cortex. Single-pulse TMS is used in the study of a number of neural functions (Anand and Hotson, 2002).

Repetitive TMS (rTMS) delivers a train of stimuli at a set frequency. High-frequency rTMS refers to stimulation delivered at ≥5 Hz stimulation, while low-frequency rTMS denotes rTMS delivered at ≤1 Hz stimulation. These two types of rTMS appear to have unique physiological effects with high-frequency rTMS leading to an increase in motor cortical excitability (Pascual-Leone et al., 1994) and low-frequency resulting in a decrease in motor cortical excitability (Chen et al., 1997). Stimulation intensity is typically defined relative to the resting motor threshold (MT) for the small muscles in the hand; motor threshold is defined as the stimulation intensity needed to evoke a motor response in about half of a series of trials. The most commonly studied intensities for rTMS have been 80%–120% of motor threshold.

During an rTMS treatment session, multiple stimulation trains are given. A standard treatment course involves daily sessions (each lasting about an hour) for 3–6 weeks. Patients are awake during treatment, and no anesthesia is required. The types of rTMS most commonly studied for the treatment of depression include high-frequency rTMS (generally 5 Hz–20 Hz) applied to the left dorsolateral prefrontal cortex (DLPFC) and low-frequency rTMS (generally 1 Hz) applied to the right DLPFC. Only high-frequency left DLPFC rTMS has been approved by the US FDA for the treatment of depression.

Efficacy

The use of rTMS to treat depression was primarily based on early neuroimaging data suggesting a role for the DLPFC (especially the left side) in the pathophysiology of depression (Baxter et al., 1989) and the demonstration of mood changes following rTMS in healthy controls (George et al., 1996; Pascual-Leone et al., 1996). Testing of rTMS for the treatment of depression began in 1993 (Hoflich et al., 1993). Since then, there have been multiple open-label and controlled trials of rTMS as a treatment for TRD (often defined as failure of at least one or two antidepressant medications in the current episode). Taken together, these studies have consistently demonstrated statistically significant antidepressant effects for both high-frequency rTMS applied to the left DLPFC and low-frequency rTMS applied to the right DLPFC (Holtzheimer et al., 2001; Burt et al., 2002; Kozel and George, 2002; Fitzgerald et al., 2003; Martin et al., 2003; Schutter, 2010). Although the antidepressant effect size for rTMS has been moderately strong (Cohen's d = 0.4–0.8), response and remission rates (20%–40% and 10%–20%, respectively) have generally been low. rTMS has been approved by the US FDA for the treatment of depression not responding to a single antidepressant medication in the current episode.

The effectiveness of rTMS for depression has been validated by two multicenter, triple-blind, randomized, sham-controlled studies (one industry-sponsored, one federally funded). The industry-sponsored study tested 4–6 weeks of high-frequency left DLPFC rTMS as monotherapy in 301 medication-free depressed patients not responding to at least one antidepressant medication (O'Reardon et al., 2007). Stimulation parameters included 10 Hz stimulation at 120% MT. This study found antidepressant effects that approached statistical significance (p = .057) on the primary outcome measure (a decrease in Montgomery-Asberg Depression Rating Scale [MADRS; Montgomery et al., 1985] score after 4 weeks of treatment). Statistically significant antidepressant benefit was demonstrated for active rTMS on most secondary measures. Compared to sham, 6 weeks of active rTMS was associated with a statistically significantly higher response rate (24% vs. 12%) and remission rate (14% vs. 6%) (O'Reardon et al., 2007). Level of treatment resistance predicted antidepressant effects such that active rTMS was associated with statistically significant antidepressant effects only in patients that had failed no more than one adequate antidepressant medication in the current episode; for more resistant patients, there was no statistically significant benefit of active rTMS (Lisanby et al., 2009); these findings led to the FDA decision to approve rTMS for patients who had failed only a single antidepressant medication in the current episode. In an open-label extension phase of this study, 6 weeks of active rTMS was associated with a 43% response and 20% remission rate in patients previously receiving sham; in patients that had received active rTMS during the blinded phase of the study, continued open-label rTMS was associated with a 26% response and 11% remission rate (Avery et al., 2008).

A four-site National Institute of Mental Health (NIMH)–funded randomized, sham-controlled study of 199 patients used eligibility criteria and stimulation parameters similar to the industry-sponsored study mentioned earlier. This study demonstrated statistically significant antidepressant effects for active rTMS (George et al., 2010). Response rates were 15% with active rTMS compared to 5% with sham rTMS; remission rates were 14% with active rTMS versus 5% with sham rTMS (similar to the industry-sponsored study). These data also suggested that rTMS was more effective in patients with a lower degree of medication resistance.

High-frequency left DLPFC rTMS has also been compared to ECT in a small number of studies with mixed results (Grunhaus et al., 2000; Pridmore et al., 2000; Janicak et al., 2002; Grunhaus et al., 2003; Schulze-Rauschenbach et al., 2005; Rosa et al., 2006; Eranti et al., 2007; Knapp et al., 2008). Low-frequency right DLPFC ECT was found to be inferior to ECT as an antidepressant treatment (Hansen et al., 2011). In general, the current data suggest rTMS is not as effective as ECT for the treatment of depression (Fitzgerald, 2007).

The maintenance of benefit following an acute course of rTMS is largely unknown. Smaller studies have suggested that relapse rates following successful rTMS are similar to those following ECT (Dannon et al., 2002; Avery et al., 2006), but they suggest a repeat course of rTMS may have benefit in patients that relapse (Demirtas-Tatlidede et al., 2008). In the industry-sponsored study described earlier (O'Reardon et al., 2007), 10% of patients relapsed in the 24 weeks following successful rTMS, and a total of 38% of patients met criteria for symptomatic worsening (Janicak et al., 2010); all patients had been placed on maintenance pharmacotherapy following the acute rTMS course. Of note, a repeat acute course of adjunctive rTMS led to symptomatic improvement in 84% of these patients (Janicak et al., 2010).

Limited data have been reported on the use of rTMS in special populations (the elderly, children/adolescents, and pregnant/postpartum women). Open studies of rTMS in elderly depressed patients have found mixed results (Figiel et al., 1998; Abraham et al., 2007; Milev et al., 2009). A double-blind, sham-controlled study in older TRD patients failed to show statistically significant antidepressant effects for rTMS, though stimulation parameters were not optimal based on current standards (Manes et al., 2001). However, rTMS has shown benefit for poststroke depression (Jorge et al., 2004) and vascular depression (Fabre et al., 2004; Jorge et al., 2008)—studies that largely sampled from an older population. Greater prefrontal atrophy in older adults may explain these mixed results since the ability of rTMS to affect cortical function and have antidepressant effects likely decreases with increasing distance from the TMS coil (Kozel et al., 2000; Nahas et al., 2001; Mosimann et al., 2002). By correcting intensity for difference in scalp-cortical distance between the DLPFC and the motor cortex (where motor threshold is determined), it may be possible for rTMS to be as effective in older adults as it is in younger adults. rTMS has been used in children and adolescents without serious adverse events and with some indication of antidepressant efficacy (Walter et al., 2001; Quintana, 2005; Loo et al., 2006; Bloch et al., 2008; Croarkin et al., 2010; D'Agati et al., 2010). rTMS has also been used safely in depressed pregnant and postpartum women with a suggestion of efficacy (Nahas et al., 1999; Klirova et al., 2008; Garcia et al., 2010; Zhang et al., 2010; Kim et al., 2011). However, the safety of TMS and rTMS in these special populations has not been established.

A number of demographic, clinical, and treatment parameters may affect the antidepressant efficacy of rTMS. As in the aforementioned study, older age may be a negative predictive factor for efficacy. Psychotic depression has been shown to respond better to ECT than rTMS (Grunhaus et al., 2000). Patients with depressive episodes longer than 2–4 years duration may be less likely to respond to rTMS (Holtzheimer et al., 2004; Lisanby et al., 2009). Higher treatment intensity (>100%), a greater number of total TMS pulses over the course of treatment, and longer treatment courses (at least 3–6 weeks, though possibly longer) may be associated with greater antidepressant efficacy (Boutros et al., 2002; Padberg et al., 2002; Gershon et al., 2003; Avery et al., 2008).

Several groups have investigated ways of optimizing rTMS as a treatment for depression. Although less studied than high-frequency left DLPFC rTMS, low-frequency right DLPFC rTMS has also consistently demonstrated antidepressant effects that appear to be equal to those left-sided rTMS (Burt et al., 2002; Fitzgerald et al., 2003; Fitzgerald, Hoy et al., 2009; Pallanti et al., 2010; Rossini et al., 2010). However, it is less clear whether patients who do not respond to high-frequency left DLPFC rTMS are more likely to respond to low-frequency right DLPFC rTMS, or vice versa (Fitzgerald et al., 2003; Fitzgerald, McQueen et al., 2009). Combination rTMS (providing both left high-frequency and right low-frequency rTMS during the same session) has been tested with mixed results (Conca et al., 2002; Dragasevic et al., 2002; Loo, Mitchell et al., 2003; Hausmann et al., 2004; Fitzgerald et al., 2006; McDonald et al., 2006); these data generally do not suggest that combination rTMS is more effective that unilateral rTMS. The adjunctive use of rTMS with concurrently started medications has been explored, again with mixed results, suggesting that adjunctive rTMS might increase the speed of antidepressant response but that the overall antidepressant efficacy may be no greater (Herwig et al., 2003; Hansen et al., 2004; Poulet et al., 2004; Rossini et al., 2005; Rumi et al., 2005; Bretlau et al., 2008; Pallanti et al., 2010). Theta-burst rTMS, which typically involves delivering a 50-Hz burst of rTMS pulses 5 times per second (i.e., at 5 Hz), has been evaluated with encouraging but very preliminary results (Chistyakov et al., 2010; Holzer and Padberg, 2010; Wu et al., 2010). In an attempt to hasten the efficacy of rTMS and increase its availability for patients, an open-label study of accelerated rTMS was conducted (15 standard rTMS treatment sessions were delivered over 2 days in an inpatient setting) (Holtzheimer et al., 2010); this study found antidepressant efficacy similar to other open-label rTMS studies: Response and remission rates were 43% and 29%, respectively, immediately following treatment, and were maintained over the next 6 weeks; side effects were similar to those seen with daily rTMS. Finally, with the goal of targeting deeper brain structures beyond the superficial prefrontal cortex, TMS systems are being designed to provide "deep TMS" (Zangen et al., 2005; Levkovitz et al., 2007; Fadini et al., 2009; Levkovitz et al., 2009; Harel et al., 2011).

Safety

Common side effects of rTMS include pain at the site of stimulation and headaches, though most patients tolerate treatments very well (O'Reardon et al., 2007; George et al., 2010). There are no cognitive side effects associated with rTMS for depression (Loo et al., 2001; Martis et al., 2003; Hausmann et al., 2004; O'Reardon et al., 2007; George et al., 2010). While transient auditory threshold increases have been reported with rTMS (Loo et al., 2001), this can be eliminated with the use of foam earplugs. The use of rTMS has been associated with the emergence of hypomania and mania (Garcia-Toro, 1999; Nedjat and Folkerts, 1999; Dolberg et al., 2001; Sakkas et al., 2003; Huang et al., 2004; Gijsman, 2005; Rachid et al., 2006; Xia et al., 2008; Chang et al., 2010). However, neither hypomania nor mania was observed in either of the large, multicenter clinical trials (including about 400 patients); thus, the rate of treatment-emergent mania with rTMS in TRD patients is likely very low.

Although high-frequency rTMS can induce a generalized seizure in epileptic and non-epileptic individuals (Wassermann, 1998), seizure risk is extremely low when stimulation parameters are maintained within suggested safety guidelines (Wassermann, 1998); no confirmed seizure has occurred in any study of rTMS for depression that has followed these guidelines. Low-frequency rTMS does not appear to increase the risk of seizure (Wassermann, 1998). However, as rTMS use expands into the community, there may be instances where patients with a higher baseline seizure risk are being treated. Therefore, rTMS providers should be cognizant of factors that might decrease the seizure threshold, such as a past history of seizures, certain proconvulsant concomitant medications (e.g., Mufti et al., 2010), or recent taper of benzodiazepines or anticonvulsants. All rTMS providers should be trained in the basic initial management of a patient with a generalized seizure.

Mechanism

The mechanism of action of rTMS is largely unknown. Preclinical studies suggest rTMS may induce physiological and behavioral effects in animals similar to those elicited with established antidepressant treatments (Muller et al., 2000; Post and Keck, 2001). An initial hypothesis proposed that high-frequency stimulation would increase the activity of the underlying hypoactive prefrontal cortex leading to antidepressant efficacy. This was supported by imaging studies showing left prefrontal hypoactivity to be the most consistent finding in depressed patients versus controls, and studies showing that high-frequency rTMS led to increased cortical excitability when given over the motor cortex. However, attempts to "target" rTMS by focusing on prefrontal areas with relative hypoactivity have not been successful (Herwig et al., 2003; Paillere Martinot et al., 2010). Rather than acting on a single brain region, it is more likely that rTMS acts via modulation of activity within a network of brain regions involved in mood regulation, with the DLPFC as an inroad into this network. This broad hypothesis concerning mechanism of action is supported by numerous imaging studies demonstrating that rTMS effects brain activity changes in multiple regions involved in the regulation of mood, thought, and behavior (Conca et al., 2000; Speer et al., 2000; Strafella et al., 2001; Nadeau et al., 2002; Loo, Sachdev et al., 2003; Mayberg, 2003; Michael et al., 2003; Fregni, Ono et al., 2006; Fitzgerald et al., 2007; Luborzewski et al., 2007; Kito et al., 2008; Baeken et al., 2009; Li et al., 2010).

Emerging Strategies

Transcranial Direct Current Stimulation

Description

tDCS is a noninvasive technique that delivers direct current electricity to the cortex via two scalp electrodes. Similar to rTMS, a series of treatment sessions are provided over consecutive days for 1 or more weeks. It is thought that tDCS modulates cortical excitatory tone rather than causing neuronal depolarization directly. Either cathodal or anodal stimulation can be delivered, and these are thought to have differential neurophysiological effect.

Efficacy

Current data on tDCS include a small number of relatively small open- and sham-controlled studies (Nitsche et al., 2009). Five sessions of tDCS applied to the left DLPFC have shown mixed antidepressant efficacy in sham-controlled studies with one study finding a statistically significant antidepressant benefit (Fregni, Boggio et al., 2006), but another failing to replicate this (Loo et al., 2010). A third sham-controlled study using 10 sessions demonstrated antidepressant efficacy for active tDCS (Boggio et al., 2008). A large, multicenter study of tDCS compared to sertraline using a sham- and placebo-controlled design is currently underway (Brunoni et al., 2011).

Safety

Adverse events associated with tDCS appear to be relatively minor (Poreisz et al., 2007). A common side effect is an uncomfortable scalp sensation during stimulation. Nausea, headaches, dizziness, concentration difficulties, and visual phenomena have also been reported. At least one case of hypomania has been associated with the use of tDCS for depression (Arul-Anandam et al., 2010).

Mechanism

As with other focal neuromodulation techniques, tDCS is thought to exert its antidepressant effects via functional changes within a neural network of brain regions involved in mood regulation. The basic mechanism of action of tDCS is believed to arise from a change in spontaneous neural firing. Anodal stimulation appears to increase cortical excitability and lead to an increase in spontaneous neural firing in the underlying cortex, while cathodal stimulation leads to decreased cortical excitability and a lower spontaneous firing rate for cortical neurons (Murphy et al., 2009; Zaghi et al., 2010). Thus, it is thought that tDCS can affect the plasticity of the neural networks involved and lead to either enhanced or weakened connectivity between brain regions. Given this, it has also been hypothesized that tDCS might be most effective when combined with another antidepressant therapy, such as psychotherapy (Murphy et al., 2009).

Magnetic Seizure Therapy

Description

With ECT, fewer cognitive side effects but equivalent efficacy may be achieved with more focal stimulation approaches (e.g., right unilateral versus bitemporal) (Lisanby, 2007; Sackeim et al., 2008). Magnetic seizure therapy (MST) aims to provide an ECT-like treatment by inducing a series of seizures using highly focal stimulation with a TMS machine. As with ECT, patients are treated under general anesthesia. A TMS machine is generally set to its maximum intensity output to optimize the likelihood of generating a seizure. Unfortunately, machines typically used for providing rTMS are not able, even at the maximum output, to generate a seizure in all patients nor reliably stimulate above seizure threshold. Therefore, newer machines have been developed that allow higher intensity stimulation.

Efficacy

Clinical data on MST in TRD patients are limited at this time. Early testing has supported feasibility and suggested antidepressant effects (Kosel et al., 2003; Lisanby et al., 2003; Kayser et al., 2008). One small controlled trial found that ECT was more effective than MST (White et al., 2006), and another small trial found similar antidepressant effects for both MST and ECT (Kayser et al., 2010).

Safety

The general risks of MST are similar to those associated with ECT and mostly relate to complications from anesthesia. As hypothesized, MST as currently delivered appears to have a superior cognitive safety profile compared to ECT (Kosel et al., 2003; Lisanby et al., 2003; White et al., 2006; Kayser et al., 2008; Kayser et al., 2010).

Mechanism

The mechanism of action of MST is unknown but is proposed to be similar to that of ECT, although there may be subtle differences in the neurophysiologic effects of MST compared to ECT (Cycowicz et al., 2008; Cycowicz et al., 2009; Rowny et al., 2009).

Direct Cortical Stimulation

Description

DCS uses epidural or subdural electrodes to directly stimulate the cortex. Stimulation is driven by a subcutaneously implanted pulse generator/battery (IPG). One or more cortical electrodes can be implanted and used for stimulation. Stimulation can either be monopolar (with the IPG serving as the cathode) or bipolar (with different electrodes serving as anode and cathode).

Efficacy

Data on DCS for TRD are currently to one small, open-label pilot study (Nahas et al., 2010). In this study, DCS electrodes were implanted over the medial and lateral prefrontal cortices bilaterally. Five severely ill TRD patients were enrolled, and each had failed at least four adequate treatments in the current episode. Three out of five patients were in remission following 7 months of chronic, intermittent stimulation.

Safety

The risks of DCS include the risks of surgery (hemorrhage, infection, and complications from anesthesia) and potential risks from acute and chronic cortical stimulation. In the pilot study mentioned earlier (Nahas et al., 2010), one patient required explantation due to a scalp infection. Otherwise, the DCS procedure and chronic stimulation were well tolerated.

Mechanism

If DCS is found to have antidepressant effects, its mechanism will likely be similar to that of TMS, though chronic stimulation may induce different changes in the neural networks involved in TRD. This has not yet been explored in either humans or animal models.

Deep Brain Stimulation

Description

With DBS, an electrode is inserted into a specific brain region (either unilaterally or bilaterally) through a burr hole in the skull using stereotactic neurosurgical techniques. Each electrode array can contain several distinct contacts that can be used to provide monopolar or bipolar stimulation. As with VNS and DCS, the electrodes are connected via subcutaneous wires to an IPG that controls stimulation and provides the power supply for the system.

DBS is an established treatment for patients with severe, treatment-resistant Parkinson disease (PD), essential tremor, and dystonia. DBS has largely replaced ablative surgery in these conditions as it can be adjusted to achieve maximal benefit with a minimum of side effects and can be turned off or completely removed in the case of severe, unwanted side effects. DBS of the anterior internal capsule (as a potential replacement for capsulotomy; this target is also referred to as the ventral capsule/ventral striatum [VC/VS]) has shown potential safety and efficacy for patients with severe treatment-refractory obsessive-compulsive disorder (OCD) based on a multicenter open-label case series of 26 patients (Greenberg et al., 2010). VC/VS DBS for OCD is FDA-approved via a Humanitarian Device Exemption in the United States.

Efficacy

The data on DBS for TRD are currently limited to relatively small, open-label, uncontrolled studies. The first report of DBS for TRD described the results of 6 months of chronic bilateral subcallosal cingulate (SCC) DBS in six patients with severe TRD (all patients had failed at least four adequate antidepressant treatments in the current epidosde) (Mayberg et al., 2005). Four of six patients were responders, and three were remitters. This cohort was expanded to 20 patients and demonstrated a 60% response rate after 6 months of chronic SCC DBS and a 55% response rate after 1 year (Lozano et al., 2008). Antidepressant effects were largely maintained between 6 and 12 months, with 72% of 6-month responders still meeting response criteria at 12 months (three additional patients achieved response by 12 months). With a range of long-term follow-up of 3–6 years for these patients, 64.3% are responders (Kennedy et al., 2011). Of note, two patients committed suicide in the long-term follow-up period; neither suicide was deemed to be related to DBS.

Three other reports have described antidepressant efficacy for SCC DBS. A case study reported antidepressant benefit for right unilateral (but not bilateral) SCC DBS (Guinjoan et al., 2010). An open-label study of eight TRD patients found an 87.5% response and a 37.5% remission rate at 6 months and then a 62.5% response and 50% remission rate at 1 year (Puigdemont et al., 2011). Finally, an open-label study of chronic SCC DBS in 17 TRD patients (seven with bipolar II disorder) demonstrated a 41% response and 18% remission rate at 6 months, a 36% response and 36% remission rate at 1 year, and a 92% response and 58% remission rate at 2 years (Holtzheimer et al., 2012). This study included a 4-week blinded sham lead-in period. Compared to baseline, patients were mildly improved following the sham period, but this may have been due to benefits associated with the DBS surgery itself. Bipolar depressed patients showed similar improvements as the unipolar depressed patients, and there were no episodes of hypomania or mania identified. Importantly, no patient achieving remission with SCC DBS had a spontaneous relapse over the period of follow-up. However, with blinded discontinuation in three patients, all three had a return/worsening of depressive symptoms over 2–3 weeks (with a return of antidepressant efficacy with reinitiation of stimulation); a similar worsening of depression was seen with battery depletions with a return of antidepressant effects with battery replacement. As with the earlier studies, SCC DBS was not associated with acute or chronic adverse effects.

Based on antidepressant effects seen in OCD patients with VC/VS DBS, a three-center, open-label pilot study of VC/VS DBS for TRD patients without OCD was performed. Following 6 months of chronic stimulation in 15 TRD patients, 40% of patients achieved response and 27% achieved remission (Malone et al., 2009). At last follow-up (24 ± 15 months after onset of stimulation, with a range of 6–51 months), there was a 53% response rate and a 33% remission rate.

The nucleus accumbens (Nacc) is a subcortical structure that comprises the majority of the VS aspect of the VC/VS DBS target. Based on its role in reward processing (and possibly anhedonia), this region was targeted in 10 TRD patients in an open-label, uncontrolled pilot study of chronic DBS (Bewernick et al., 2010). Following 12 months of stimulation, 50% of patients were responders. No neuropsychological deficits were associated with chronic stimulation, and improvements across a number of domains were identified (Grubert et al., 2011). Long-term follow-up in these patients (with the addition of one more subject) found that 5 of 11 patients (45%) remained responders at last follow-up (up to 4 years of chronic stimulation; Thomas Schlaepfer, personal communication).

Case reports have described potential antidepressant efficacy of DBS of the inferior thalamic peduncle (which contains thalamo-cortical projection fibers) (Jimenez et al., 2005) and the habenula (which is involved in modulation of monoaminergic neurotransmission) (Sartorius et al., 2010).

Safety

As with other invasive neurosurgical approaches, the serious adverse events of DBS are primarily related to the surgical procedure: intracranial hemorrhage, infection, and complications from anesthesia. Side effects of acute and chronic stimulation appear to relate primarily to the target for DBS. In the SCC DBS studies, there were no adverse events associated with acute or chronic stimulation, and there were no negative cognitive effects (Mayberg et al., 2005; Lozano et al., 2008; McNeely et al., 2008; Kennedy et al., 2011; Holtzheimer et al., in press). For the VC/VS and Nacc targets, adverse effects of acute stimulation included hypomania, anxiety, perseverative speech, autonomic symptoms, and involuntary facial movements; these were mostly reversible with a stimulation parameter change. No cognitive side effects were described for either target with chronic stimulation.

Mechanism

The general putative mechanism for DBS for TRD is modulation of activity within a neural network involved in mood regulation and persistent depression. The choice of the SCC target was based on a converging neuroanatomical database that supported a critical role for Brodmann Area 25 (BA25; located within the SCC) in a neural network involved in depression and antidepressant response (Mayberg, 2009). The rationale for the VC/VS target emerged from data in OCD patients showing that many patients experienced significant improvement in comorbid depression (Greenberg et al., 2010). The Nacc target was supported by its being a part of the VC/VS target and the role of the Nacc in reward processing and possibly anhedonia (Schlaepfer and Lieb, 2005; Schlaepfer et al., 2008). The support for the ITP target comes from the more traditional model of abnormal thalamic outflow to the prefrontal cortices as the primary pathophysiology of TRD (Jimenez et al., 2007). Support for the habenula target comes from the role of this structure in the modulation of monoaminergic neurotransimission (Sartorius and Henn, 2007; Sartorius et al., 2010).

Conceptualizing a Role for Somatic, Nonpharmacological Therapies for Treatment-Resistant Depression

It is expected that most of the therapies discussed in this chapter, especially those that are more invasive, would serve as adjuncts to established medication and psychotherapeutic approaches to TRD. To this end, it is important to emphasize that medications and psychotherapy are currently and should remain first-line therapies for depression. It is also recognized that a mediation switch, various medication combinations, and/or the combination of medication(s) with psychotherapy can be efficacious in TRD, especially in earlier stages of resistance (Thase and Rush, 1997; Thase et al., 1997; Rush et al., 2006; Thase et al., 2007). Therefore, the role of somatic, nonpharmacological therapies for TRD must be carefully considered within the context of already established medication and psychotherapeutic approaches.

In approaching the treatment decision-making process for a depressed patient, it is important to consider the distinct phases of treatment: acute versus maintenance (Kupfer, 1991). The acute phase of treatment is focused on getting the patient out of the depressed episode. The maintenance phase is then focused on preventing future episodes. It is possible that different treatments may be uniquely designed for each of these phases of treatment. A second consideration is the level of TRD being treated; some treatments may be more or less effective than others at different stages of treatment resistance.

Considering the acute phase of treatment, ECT, TMS, tDCS, and MST have all shown at least preliminary acute efficacy in TRD patients. However, the long-term efficacy of these treatments is not clear, and the efficacy of maintenance treatment is suggested but not confirmed (Bourgon and Kellner, 2000; Sackeim, Haskett et al., 2001; Kellner et al., 2006; Janicak et al., 2010; Trevino et al., 2010). Following the failure of an adequate trial of a single antidepressant medication, or possibly the intolerance of several medications (though this is not an FDA-approved indication), TMS would be a reasonable treatment option. If tDCS demonstrates safety and efficacy in depressed patients, it is likely that it would also be an appropriate treatment at this stage. For patients that have failed two or more medications, ECT and MST (presuming efficacy and safety are established) would be more appropriate for acute treatment.

By design, the more invasive therapies (ablation, VNS, DCS, DBS) should be considered as maintenance treatments, though they may also have some acute efficacy. Among these, VNS may be appropriate for patients that have failed 4–6 antidepressant medications in the current episode (with six treatments being the upper limit for inclusion into the pivotal trial). DCS and DBS may be appropriate for patients that have failed 4 or more adequate treatments in the current episode. Ablative neurosurgery may still be an option for some patients, though it is expected that DBS would largely supplant ablation as a treatment for TRD (as has been the case in movement disorders). Furthermore, it should be noted that DBS is not simply virtual ablation (McIntyre and Thakor, 2002; McIntyre et al., 2004), such that the efficacy of DBS at certain targets (e.g., the SCC, ITP, and habenula) may not predict efficacy of ablation of these targets.

Summary

Somatic, nonpharmacological therapies for TRD are among the oldest modern treatments available in psychiatry but also represent a cutting edge of treatment development. As the neuroanatomical models of psychiatric disease have improved, and the techniques for modulating neural systems have become more refined, the ability to directly and focally alter neural network activity has advanced tremendously. The growing database on the various strategies discussed in this chapter is highly encouraging. Yet enthusiasm must be tempered with caution based on the very preliminary nature of the data to date. So focal neuromodulation will likely continue to be an active and exciting research area, and it is hoped that emerging strategies will represent novel and more effective antidepressant treatments. Still, clinicians should introduce these treatments into practice carefully, being aware of the relative strengths and weaknesses supporting each intervention.

Disclosure Statement

P.E.H. has received grant funding from the Dana Foundation, Greenwall Foundation, NARSAD, NIMH (K23 MH077869), National Institutes of Health Loan Repayment Program, Northstar, Inc., Stanley Medical Research Institute, and Woodruff Foundation; he has received consulting fees from St. Jude Medical Neuromodulation.

References

Abraham, G., R. Milev, L. Lazowski, et al. (2007). Repetitive transcranial magnetic stimulation for treatment of elderly patients with depression—an open label trial. *Neuropsychiatr Dis Treat* 3(6): 919–924.

Altar, C. A., P. Laeng, L. W. Jurata, et al. (2004). Electroconvulsive seizures regulate gene expression of distinct neurotrophic signaling pathways. *J Neurosci* 24(11): 2667–2677.

Anand, S., & J. Hotson. (2002). Transcranial magnetic stimulation: Neurophysiological applications and safety. *Brain Cogn* 50(3): 366–386.

Arul-Anandam, A. P., C. Loo & P. Mitchell. (2010). Induction of hypomanic episode with transcranial direct current stimulation. *J ECT* 26(1): 68–69.

Avery, D. H., P. E. Holtzheimer, 3rd, W. Fawaz et al. (2006). A controlled study of repetitive transcranial magnetic stimulation in medication-resistant major depression. *Biol Psychiatry* 59(2): 187–194.

Avery, D. H., K. E. Isenberg, S. M. Sampson, et al. (2008). Transcranial magnetic stimulation in the acute treatment of major depressive disorder: Clinical response in an open-label extension trial. *J Clin Psychiatry* 69(3): 441–451.

Avery, D., & G. Winokur (1976). Mortality in depressed patients treated with electroconvulsive therapy and antidepressants. *Arch Gen Psychiatry* 33(9): 1029–1037.

Baeken, C., R. De Raedt, C. Van Hove et al. (2009). HF-rTMS treatment in medication-resistant melancholic depression: Results from 18FDG-PET brain imaging. *CNS Spectr* 14(8): 439–448.

Bailey, S. D., L. Bucci, E. Gosline et al. (1959). Comparison of iproniazid with other amine oxidase inhibitors, including W-1544, JB-516, RO 4-1018, and RO 5-0700. *Ann N Y Acad Sci* 80: 652–668.

Bajbouj, M., A. Merkl, T. E. Schlaepfer et al. (2010). Two-year outcome of vagus nerve stimulation in treatment-resistant depression. *J Clin Psychopharmacol* 30(3): 273–281.

Baxter, L. R., Jr., J. M. Schwartz, M. E. Phelps et al. (1989). Reduction of prefrontal cortex glucose metabolism common to three types of depression. *Arch Gen Psychiatry* 46(3): 243–250.

Ben-Menachem, E. (2001). Vagus nerve stimulation, side effects, and long-term safety. *J Clin Neurophysiol* 18(5): 415–418.

Ben-Menachem, E. (2002). Vagus-nerve stimulation for the treatment of epilepsy. *Lancet Neurol* 1(8): 477–482.

Ben-Menachem, E., A. Hamberger, T. Hedner et al. (1995). Effects of vagus nerve stimulation on amino acids and other metabolites in the CSF of patients with partial seizures. *Epilepsy Res* 20(3): 221–227.

Bertagnoli, M. W., & C. M. Borchardt (1990). A review of ECT for children and adolescents. *J Am Acad Child Adolesc Psychiatry* 29(2): 302–307.

Bewernick, B. H., R. Hurlemann, A. Matusch et al. (2010). Nucleus accumbens deep brain stimulation decreases ratings of depression and anxiety in treatment-resistant depression. *Biol Psychiatry* 67(2): 110–116.

Bini, L. (1938). Experimental researches on epileptic attacks induced by the electric current. *Am J Psychiatry* 94: 172–174.

Black, D. W., J. A. Wilcox & M. Stewart (1985). The use of ECT in children: Case report. *J Clin Psychiatry* 46(3): 98–99.

Bloch, Y., N. Grisaru, E. V. Harel et al. (2008). Repetitive transcranial magnetic stimulation in the treatment of depression in adolescents: An open-label study. *J ECT* 24(2): 156–159.

Boggio, P. S., S. P. Rigonatti, R. B. Ribeiro et al. (2008). A randomized, double-blind clinical trial on the efficacy of cortical direct current stimulation for the treatment of major depression. *Int J Neuropsychopharmacol* 11(2): 249–254.

Bourgon, L. N., & C. H. Kellner (2000). Relapse of depression after ECT: A review. *J ECT* 16(1): 19–31.

Boutros, N. N., R. Gueorguieva, R. E. Hoffman et al. (2002). Lack of a therapeutic effect of a 2-week sub-threshold transcranial magnetic stimulation course for treatment-resistant depression. *Psychiatry Res* 113(3): 245–254.

Bretlau, L. G., M. Lunde, L. Lindberg et al. (2008). Repetitive transcranial magnetic stimulation (rTMS) in combination with escitalopram in patients with treatment-resistant major depression: a double-blind, randomised, sham-controlled trial. *Pharmacopsychiatry* 41(2): 41–47.

Brunoni, A. R., L. Valiengo, A. Baccaro et al. (2011). Sertraline vs. ELectrical Current Therapy for Treating Depression Clinical Trial—SELECT TDCS: Design, rationale and objectives. *Contemporary Clinical Trials* 32(1): 90–98.

Burckhardt, G. (1891). On cortical resection as a contribution to the operative treatment of psychosis. *Psychiatrie psychischgerichtliche Medizin* 47: 463–548.

Burt, T., S. H. Lisanby & H. A. Sackeim (2002). Neuropsychiatric applications of transcranial magnetic stimulation: A meta-analysis. *Intl J Neuropsychopharmacol* 5(1): 73–103.

Carpenter, L. L., F. A. Moreno, M. A. Kling et al. (2004). Effect of vagus nerve stimulation on cerebrospinal fluid monoamine metabolites, norepinephrine, and gamma-aminobutyric acid concentrations in depressed patients. *Biol Psychiatry* 56(6): 418–426.

Chae, J. H., Z. Nahas, M. Lomarev et al. (2003). A review of functional neuroimaging studies of vagus nerve stimulation (VNS). *J Psychiatr Res* 37(6): 443–455.

Chang, C. H., S. J. Chen & H. C. Tsai (2010). Manic episode following a combined treatment of repetitive transcranial magnetic stimulation and venlafaxine. *J Neuropsychiatry Clin Neurosci* 22(2): E18–E19.

Chen, R., J. Classen, C. Gerloff et al. (1997). Depression of motor cortex excitability by low-frequency transcranial magnetic stimulation. *Neurology* 48(5): 1398–1403.

Chistyakov, A. V., O. Rubicsek, B. Kaplan et al. (2010). Safety, tolerability and preliminary evidence for antidepressant efficacy of theta-burst transcranial magnetic stimulation in patients with major depression. *Int J Neuropsychopharmacol* 13(3): 387–393.

Christmas, D., M. S. Eljamel, S. Butler et al. (2010). Long term outcome of thermal anterior capsulotomy for chronic, treatment refractory depression. *J Neurol Neurosurg Psychiatry* 82(6): 594–600.

Conca, A., J. Di Pauli, W. Beraus et al. (2002). Combining high and low frequencies in rTMS antidepressive treatment: Preliminary results. *Hum Psychopharmacol* 17(7): 353–356.

Conca, A., H. Fritzsche, W. Peschina et al. (2000). Preliminary findings of simultaneous 18F-FDG and 99mTc-HMPAO SPECT in patients with depressive disorders at rest: Differential correlates with ratings of anxiety. *Psychiatry Res* 98(1): 43–54.

Conway, C. R., Y. I. Sheline, J. T. Chibnall et al. (2006). Cerebral blood flow changes during vagus nerve stimulation for depression. *Psychiatry Res* 146(2): 179–184.

Coyle, J. T., & R. S. Duman. (2003). Finding the intracellular signaling pathways affected by mood disorder treatments. *Neuron* 38(2): 157–160.

Croarkin, P. E., C. A. Wall, S. M. McClintock et al. (2010). The emerging role for repetitive transcranial magnetic stimulation in optimizing the treatment of adolescent depression. *J ECT* 26(4): 323–329.

Cycowicz, Y. M., B. Luber, T. Spellman et al. (2008). Differential neurophysiological effects of magnetic seizure therapy (MST) and electroconvulsive shock (ECS) in non-human primates. *Clin EEG Neurosci* 39(3): 144–149.

Cycowicz, Y. M., B. Luber, T. Spellman et al. (2009). Neurophysiological characterization of high-dose magnetic seizure therapy: Comparisons with electroconvulsive shock and cognitive outcomes. *J ECT* 25(3): 157–164.

D'Agati, D., Y. Bloch, Y. Levkovitz et al. (2010). rTMS for adolescents: Safety and efficacy considerations. *Psychiatry Res* 177(3): 280–285.

Dannon, P. N., O. T. Dolberg, S. Schreiber et al. (2002). Three and six-month outcome following courses of either ECT or rTMS in a population of severely depressed individuals—preliminary report. *Biol Psychiatry* 51(8): 687–690.

Demirtas-Tatlidede, A., D. Mechanic-Hamilton, D. Z. Press et al. (2008). An open-label, prospective study of repetitive transcranial magnetic stimulation (rTMS) in the long-term treatment of refractory depression: Reproducibility and duration of the antidepressant effect in medication-free patients. *J Clin Psychiatry* 69(6): 930–934.

Dolberg, O. T., S. Schreiber & L. Grunhaus. (2001). Transcranial magnetic stimulation-induced switch into mania: A report of two cases. *Biol Psychiatry* 49(5): 468–470.

Dragasevic, N., A. Potrebic, A. Damjanovic et al. (2002). Therapeutic efficacy of bilateral prefrontal slow repetitive transcranial magnetic stimulation in depressed patients with Parkinson's disease: An open study. *Mov Disord* 17(3): 528–532.

Dunner, D. L., A. J. Rush, J. M. Russell et al. (2006). Prospective, long-term, multicenter study of the naturalistic outcomes of patients with treatment-resistant depression. *J Clin Psychiatry* 67(5): 688–695.

ECT Task Force of the American Psychiatric Association. (2001). *The practice of electroconvulsive therapy*. Washington, DC: American Psychiatric Press.

Elger, G., C. Hoppe, P. Falkai et al. (2000). Vagus nerve stimulation is associated with mood improvements in epilepsy patients. *Epilepsy Res* 42(2–3): 203–210.

Eranti, S., A. Mogg, G. Pluck et al. (2007). A randomized, controlled trial with 6-month follow-up of repetitive transcranial magnetic stimulation and electroconvulsive therapy for severe depression. *Am J Psychiatry* 164(1): 73–81.

Fabre, I., A. Galinowski, C. Oppenheim et al. (2004). Antidepressant efficacy and cognitive effects of repetitive transcranial magnetic stimulation in vascular depression: An open trial. *Int J Geriatr Psychiatry* 19(9): 833–842.

Fadini, T., L. Matthaus, H. Rothkegel et al. (2009). H-coil: Induced electric field properties and input/output curves on healthy volunteers, comparison with a standard figure-of-eight coil. *Clin Neurophysiol* 120(6): 1174–1182.

Figiel, G. S., C. Epstein, W. M. McDonald et al. (1998). The use of rapid-rate transcranial magnetic stimulation (rTMS) in refractory depressed patients. *J Neuropsychiatry Clin Neurosci* 10(1): 20–25.

Fink, M. (2001). Convulsive therapy: A review of the first 55 years. *J Affect Disord* 63(1–3): 1–15.

Fitzgerald, P. B. (2007). Repetitive transcranial magnetic stimulation is not as effective as electroconvulsive therapy for major depression. *Evid Based Ment Health* 10(3): 78.

Fitzgerald, P. B., J. Benitez, A. de Castella et al. (2006). A randomized, controlled trial of sequential bilateral repetitive transcranial magnetic stimulation for treatment-resistant depression. *Am J Psychiatry* 163(1): 88–94.

Fitzgerald, P. B., T. L. Brown, N. A. Marston et al. (2003). Transcranial magnetic stimulation in the treatment of depression: A double-blind, placebo-controlled trial. *Arch Gen Psychiatry* 60(10): 1002–1008.

Fitzgerald, P. B., K. Hoy, Z. J. Daskalakis et al. (2009). A randomized trial of the anti-depressant effects of low- and high-frequency transcranial magnetic stimulation in treatment-resistant depression. *Depress Anxiety* 26(3): 229–234.

Fitzgerald, P. B., S. McQueen, S. Herring et al. (2009). A study of the effectiveness of high-frequency left prefrontal cortex transcranial magnetic stimulation in major depression in patients who have not responded to right-sided stimulation. *Psychiatry Res* 169(1): 12–15.

Fitzgerald, P. B., A. Sritharan, Z. J. Daskalakis et al. (2007). A functional magnetic resonance imaging study of the effects of low frequency right prefrontal transcranial magnetic stimulation in depression. *J Clin Psychopharmacol* 27(5): 488–492.

Fregni, F., C. R. Ono, C. M. Santos et al. (2006). Effects of antidepressant treatment with rTMS and fluoxetine on brain perfusion in PD. *Neurology* 66(11): 1629–1637.

Fregni, F., P. S. Boggio, M. A. Nitsche et al. (2006). Treatment of major depression with transcranial direct current stimulation. *Bipolar Disord* 8(2): 203–204.

Garcia, K. S., P. Flynn, K. J. Pierce et al. (2010). Repetitive transcranial magnetic stimulation treats postpartum depression. *Brain Stimul* 3(1): 36–41.

Garcia-Toro, M. (1999). Acute manic symptomatology during repetitive transcranial magnetic stimulation in a patient with bipolar depression. *Br J Psychiatry* 175: 491.

George, M. S., S. H. Lisanby, D. Avery et al. (2010). Daily left prefrontal transcranial magnetic stimulation therapy for major depressive disorder: A sham-controlled randomized trial. *Arch Gen Psychiatry* 67(5): 507–516.

George, M. S., A. J. Rush, L. B. Marangell et al. (2005). A one-year comparison of vagus nerve stimulation with treatment as usual for treatment-resistant depression. *Biol Psychiatry* 58(5): 364–373.

George, M. S., A. J. Rush, H. A. Sackeim et al. (2003). Vagus nerve stimulation (VNS): Utility in neuropsychiatric disorders. *Int J Neuropsychopharmacol* 6(1): 73–83.

George, M. S., E. M. Wassermann, W. A. Williams et al. (1996). Changes in mood and hormone levels after rapid-rate transcranial magnetic stimulation (rTMS) of the prefrontal cortex. *J Neuropsychiatry Clin Neurosci* 8(2): 172–180.

Gershon, A. A., P. N. Dannon & L. Grunhaus (2003). Transcranial magnetic stimulation in the treatment of depression. *Am J Psychiatry* 160(5): 835–845.

Ghaziuddin, N., C. A. King, M. W. Naylor et al. (1996). Electroconvulsive treatment in adolescents with pharmacotherapy-refractory depression. *J Child Adolesc Psychopharmacol* 6(4): 259–271.

Gijsman, H. J. (2005). Mania after transcranial magnetic stimulation in PTSD. *Am J Psychiatry* 162(2): 398; author reply 398–400.

Greenberg, B. D., L. A. Gabriels, D. A. Malone, Jr. et al. (2010). Deep brain stimulation of the ventral internal capsule/ventral striatum for obsessive-compulsive disorder: Worldwide experience. *Mol Psychiatry* 15: 64–79.

Groves, D. A., E. M. Bowman & V. J. Brown (2005). Recordings from the rat locus coeruleus during acute vagal nerve stimulation in the anaesthetised rat. *Neurosci Lett* 379(3): 174–179.

Grubert, C., R. Hurlemann, B. H. Bewernick et al. (2011). Neuropsychological safety of nucleus accumbens deep brain stimulation for major depression: Effects of 12-month stimulation. *World J Biol Psychiatry* 12(7): 516–527.

Grunhaus, L., P. N. Dannon, S. Schreiber et al. (2000). Repetitive transcranial magnetic stimulation is as effective as electroconvulsive therapy in the treatment of nondelusional major depressive disorder: an open study. *Biol Psychiatry* 47(4): 314–324.

Grunhaus, L., S. Schreiber, O. T. Dolberg et al. (2003). A randomized controlled comparison of electroconvulsive therapy and repetitive transcranial magnetic stimulation in severe and resistant nonpsychotic major depression. *Biol Psychiatry* 53(4): 324–331.

Guinjoan, S. M., H. S. Mayberg, E. Y. Costanzo et al. (2010). Asymmetrical contribution of brain structures to treatment-resistant depression as illustrated by effects of right subgenual cingulum stimulation. *J Neuropsychiatry Clin Neurosci* 22(3): 265–277.

Hansen, P. E., B. Ravnkilde, P. Videbech et al. (2011). Low-frequency repetitive transcranial magnetic stimulation inferior to electroconvulsive therapy in treating depression. *J ECT* 27(1): 26–32.

Hansen, P. E., P. Videbech, K. Clemmensen et al. (2004). Repetitive transcranial magnetic stimulation as add-on antidepressant treatment. The applicability of the method in a clinical setting. *Nord J Psychiatry* 58(6): 455–457.

Harden, C. L., M. C. Pulver, L. D. Ravdin et al. (2000). A pilot study of mood in epilepsy patients treated with vagus nerve stimulation. *Epilepsy Behav* 1(2): 93–99.

Harel, E. V., A. Zangen, Y. Roth et al. (2011). H-coil repetitive transcranial magnetic stimulation for the treatment of bipolar depression: an add-on, safety and feasibility study. *World J Biol Psychiatry* 12(2): 119–126.

Hariz, M. I., P. Blomstedt & L. Zrinzo (2010). Deep brain stimulation between 1947 and 1987: The untold story. *Neurosurg Focus* 29(2): E1.

Hassert, D. L., T. Miyashita & C. L. Williams (2004). The effects of peripheral vagal nerve stimulation at a memory-modulating intensity on norepinephrine output in the basolateral amygdala. *Behav Neurosci* 118(1): 79–88.

Hausmann, A., G. Kemmler, M. Walpoth et al. (2004). No benefit derived from repetitive transcranial magnetic stimulation in depression: A prospective, single centre, randomised, double blind, sham controlled add on trial. *J Neurol Neurosurg Psychiatry* 75(2): 320–322.

Hausmann, A., A. Pascual-Leone, G. Kemmler et al. (2004). No deterioration of cognitive performance in an aggressive unilateral and bilateral antidepressant rTMS add-on trial. *J Clin Psychiatry* 65(6): 772–782.

Helmstaedter, C., C. Hoppe & C. E. Elger (2001). Memory alterations during acute high-intensity vagus nerve stimulation. *Epilepsy Res* 47(1–2): 37–42.

Henry, M. E., M. E. Schmidt, J. A. Matochik et al. (2001). The effects of ECT on brain glucose: A pilot FDG PET study. *J ECT* 17(1): 33–40.

Herwig, U., Y. Lampe, F. D. Juengling et al. (2003). Add-on rTMS for treatment of depression: A pilot study using stereotaxic coil-navigation according to PET data. *J Psychiatr Res* 37(4): 267–275.

Hoflich, G., S. Kasper, A. Hufnagel et al. (1993). Application of transcranial magnetic stimulation in treatment of drug-resistant major depression—A report of two cases. *Human Psychopharmacology* 8: 361–365.

Holtzheimer, P. E., 3rd, J. Russo & D. H. Avery (2001). A meta-analysis of repetitive transcranial magnetic stimulation in the treatment of depression. *Psychopharmacol Bull* 35(4): 149–169.

Holtzheimer, P. E., M. E. Kelley, R. E. Gross et al. (2012). Subcallosal cingulate deep brain stimulation for treatment-resistant unipolar and bipolar depression. *Arch Gen Psychiatry* 69(2): 150–158.

Holtzheimer, P. E., 3rd, W. M. McDonald, M. Mufti et al. (2010). Accelerated repetitive transcranial magnetic stimulation for treatment-resistant depression. *Depress Anxiety* 27(10): 960–963.

Holtzheimer, P. E., 3rd, J. Russo, K. H. Claypoole et al. (2004). Shorter duration of depressive episode may predict response to repetitive transcranial magnetic stimulation. *Depress Anxiety* 19(1): 24–30.

Holzer, M., & F. Padberg (2010). Intermittent theta burst stimulation (iTBS) ameliorates therapy-resistant depression: A case series. *Brain Stimul* 3(3): 181–183.

Huang, C. C., T. P. Su & I. K. Shan (2004). A case report of repetitive transcranial magnetic stimulation-induced mania. *Bipolar Disord* 6(5): 444–445.

Janicak, P. G., S. M. Dowd, B. Martis et al. (2002). Repetitive transcranial magnetic stimulation versus electroconvulsive therapy for major depression: Preliminary results of a randomized trial. *Biol Psychiatry* 51(8): 659–667.

Janicak, P. G., Z. Nahas, S. H. Lisanby et al. (2010). Durability of clinical benefit with transcranial magnetic stimulation (TMS) in the treatment of pharmacoresistant major depression: Assessment of relapse during a 6-month, multisite, open-label study. *Brain Stimul* 3(4): 187–199.

Jasper, H. H. (1995). A historical perspective. The rise and fall of prefrontal lobotomy. *Adv Neurol* 66: 97–114.

Jimenez, F., F. Velasco, R. Salin-Pascual et al. (2005). A patient with a resistant major depression disorder treated with deep brain stimulation in the inferior thalamic peduncle. *Neurosurgery* 57(3): 585–593; discussion 585–593.

Jimenez, F., F. Velasco, R. Salin-Pascual et al. (2007). Neuromodulation of the inferior thalamic peduncle for major depression and obsessive compulsive disorder. *Acta Neurochir Suppl* 97(Pt 2): 393–398.

Jorge, R. E., D. J. Moser, L. Acion et al. (2008). Treatment of vascular depression using repetitive transcranial magnetic stimulation. *Arch Gen Psychiatry* 65(3): 268–276.

Jorge, R. E., R. G. Robinson, A. Tateno et al. (2004). Repetitive transcranial magnetic stimulation as treatment of poststroke depression: A preliminary study. *Biol Psychiatry* 55(4): 398–405.

Kayser, S., B. Bewernick, N. Axmacher et al. (2008). Magnetic seizure therapy of treatment-resistant depression in a patient with bipolar disorder. *J ECT* 25(2): 137–140.

Kayser, S., B. H. Bewernick, C. Grubert et al. (2010). Antidepressant effects, of magnetic seizure therapy and electroconvulsive therapy, in treatment-resistant depression. *J Psychiatr Res* 45(5): 569–576.

Kellner, C. H., M. Fink, R. Knapp et al. (2005). Relief of expressed suicidal intent by ECT: A consortium for research in ECT study. *Am J Psychiatry* 162(5): 977–982.

Kellner, C. H., R. Knapp, M. M. Husain et al. (2010). Bifrontal, bitemporal and right unilateral electrode placement in ECT: Randomised trial. *Br J Psychiatry* 196: 226–234.

Kellner, C. H., R. G. Knapp, G. Petrides et al. (2006). Continuation electroconvulsive therapy vs pharmacotherapy for relapse prevention in major depression: A multisite study from the Consortium for Research in Electroconvulsive Therapy (CORE). *Arch Gen Psychiatry* 63(12): 1337–1344.

Kennedy, S. H., P. Giacobbe, S. J. Rizvi et al. (2011). Deep brain stimulation for treatment-resistant depression: Follow-up after 3 to 6 years. *Am J Psychiatry* 168(5): 502–510.

Kho, K. H., M. F. van Vreeswijk, S. Simpson et al. (2003). A meta-analysis of electroconvulsive therapy efficacy in depression. *J ECT* 19(3): 139–147.

Kiloh, L. G., J. P. Child & G. Latner. (1960). A controlled trial of iproniazid in the treatment of endogenous depression. *Journal of Mental Science* 106(444): 1139–1144.

Kim, D. R., N. Epperson, E. Pare et al. (2011). An open label pilot study of transcranial magnetic stimulation for pregnant women with major depressive disorder. *J Womens Health (Larchmt)* 20(2): 255–261.

Kito, S., K. Fujita & Y. Koga. (2008). Regional cerebral blood flow changes after low-frequency transcranial magnetic stimulation of the right dorsolateral prefrontal cortex in treatment-resistant depression. *Neuropsychobiology* 58(1): 29–36.

Klirova, M., T. Novak, M. Kopecek et al. (2008). Repetitive transcranial magnetic stimulation (rTMS) in major depressive episode during pregnancy. *Neuro Endocrinol Lett* 29(1): 69–70.

Knapp, M., R. Romeo, A. Mogg et al. (2008). Cost-effectiveness of transcranial magnetic stimulation vs. electroconvulsive therapy for severe depression: A multi-centre randomised controlled trial. *J Affect Disord* 109(3): 273–285.

Kosel, M., H. Brockmann, C. Frick et al. (2011). Chronic vagus nerve stimulation for treatment-resistant depression increases regional cerebral blood flow in the dorsolateral prefrontal cortex. *Psychiatry Res* 191(3): 153–159.

Kosel, M., C. Frick, S. H. Lisanby et al. (2003). Magnetic seizure therapy improves mood in refractory major depression. *Neuropsychopharmacology* 28(11): 2045–2048.

Kozel, F. A., & M. S. George (2002). Meta-analysis of left prefrontal repetitive transcranial magnetic stimulation (rTMS) to treat depression. *Journal of Psychiatric Practice* 8(5): 270–275.

Kozel, F. A., Z. Nahas, C. deBrux et al. (2000). How coil-cortex distance relates to age, motor threshold, and antidepressant response to repetitive transcranial magnetic stimulation. *J Neuropsychiatry Clin Neurosci* 12(3): 376–384.

Krahl, S. E., K. B. Clark, D. C. Smith et al. (1998). Locus coeruleus lesions suppress the seizure-attenuating effects of vagus nerve stimulation. *Epilepsia* 39(7): 709–714.

Krystal, A. D., M. West, R. Prado et al. (2000). EEG effects of ECT: Implications for rTMS. *Depress Anxiety* 12(3): 157–165.

Kuhn, R. (1958). The treatment of depressive states with G 22355 (imipramine hydrochloride). *Am J Psychiatry* 115(5): 459–464.

Kupfer, D. J. (1991). Long-term treatment of depression. *J Clin Psychiatry* 52(Suppl): 28–34.

Lechner, S. M., A. L. Curtis, R. Brons et al. (1997). Locus coeruleus activation by colon distention: Role of corticotropin-releasing factor and excitatory amino acids. *Brain Res* 756(1–2): 114–124.

Levkovitz, Y., E. V. Harel, Y. Roth et al. (2009). Deep transcranial magnetic stimulation over the prefrontal cortex: Evaluation of antidepressant and cognitive effects in depressive patients. *Brain Stimul* 2(4): 188–200.

Levkovitz, Y., Y. Roth, E. V. Harel et al. (2007). A randomized controlled feasibility and safety study of deep transcranial magnetic stimulation. *Clin Neurophysiol* 118(12): 2730–2744.

Li, C. T., S. J. Wang, J. Hirvonen et al. (2010). Antidepressant mechanism of add-on repetitive transcranial magnetic stimulation in medication-resistant depression using cerebral glucose metabolism. *J Affect Disord* 127 (1–3): 219–229.

Lisanby, S. H. (2007). Electroconvulsive therapy for depression. *N Engl J Med* 357(19): 1939–1945.

Lisanby, S. H., M. M. Husain, P. B. Rosenquist et al. (2009). Daily left prefrontal repetitive transcranial magnetic stimulation in the acute treatment of major depression: Clinical predictors of outcome in a multisite, randomized controlled clinical trial. *Neuropsychopharmacology* 34(2): 522–534.

Lisanby, S. H., B. Luber, T. E. Schlaepfer et al. (2003). Safety and feasibility of magnetic seizure therapy (MST) in major depression: randomized within-subject comparison with electroconvulsive therapy. *Neuropsychopharmacology* 28(10): 1852–1865.

Lisanby, S. H., J. H. Maddox, J. Prudic et al. (2000). The effects of electroconvulsive therapy on memory of autobiographical and public events. *Arch Gen Psychiatry* 57(6): 581–590.

Loo, C. K., P. B. Mitchell, V. M. Croker et al. (2003). Double-blind controlled investigation of bilateral prefrontal transcranial magnetic stimulation for the treatment of resistant major depression. *Psychol Med* 33(1): 33–40.

Loo, C., T. McFarquhar & G. Walter. (2006). Transcranial magnetic stimulation in adolescent depression. *Australas Psychiatry* 14(1): 81–85.

Loo, C., P. Sachdev, H. Elsayed et al. (2001). Effects of a 2- to 4-week course of repetitive transcranial magnetic stimulation (rTMS) on neuropsychologic functioning, electroencephalogram, and auditory threshold in depressed patients. *Biol Psychiatry* 49(7): 615–623.

Loo, C. K., P. S. Sachdev, W. Haindl et al. (2003). High (15 Hz) and low (1 Hz) frequency transcranial magnetic stimulation have different acute effects on regional cerebral blood flow in depressed patients. *Psychol Med* 33(6): 997–1006.

Loo, C. K., P. Sachdev, D. Martin et al. (2010). A double-blind, sham-controlled trial of transcranial direct current stimulation for the treatment of depression. *Int J Neuropsychopharmacol* 13(1): 61–69.

Lozano, A. M., H. S. Mayberg, P. Giacobbe et al. (2008). Subcallosal cingulate gyrus deep brain stimulation for treatment-resistant depression. *Biol Psychiatry* 64(6): 461–467.

Luborzewski, A., F. Schubert, F. Seifert et al. (2007). Metabolic alterations in the dorsolateral prefrontal cortex after treatment with high-frequency repetitive transcranial magnetic stimulation in patients with unipolar major depression. *J Psychiatr Res* 41(7): 606–615.

Madsen, T. M., A. Treschow, J. Bengzon et al. (2000). Increased neurogenesis in a model of electroconvulsive therapy. *Biol Psychiatry* 47(12): 1043–1049.

Madsen, T. M., D. D. Yeh, G. W. Valentine et al. (2005). Electroconvulsive seizure treatment increases cell proliferation in rat frontal cortex. *Neuropsychopharmacology* 30(1): 27–34.

Malone, D. A., Jr., D. D. Dougherty, A. R. Rezai et al. (2009). Deep brain stimulation of the ventral capsule/ventral striatum for treatment-resistant depression. *Biol Psychiatry* 65(4): 267–275.

Manes, F., R. Jorge, M. Morcuende et al. (2001). A controlled study of repetitive transcranial magnetic stimulation as a treatment of depression in the elderly. *Int Psychogeriatr* 13(2): 225–231.

Marangell, L. B., A. J. Rush, M. S. George et al. (2002). Vagus nerve stimulation (VNS) for major depressive episodes: one year outcomes. *Biol Psychiatry* 51(4): 280–287.

Marino Junior, R., & G. R. Cosgrove. (1997). Neurosurgical treatment of neuropsychiatric illness. *Psychiatr Clin North Am* 20(4): 933–943.

Marrosu, F., A. Serra, A. Maleci et al. (2003). Correlation between GABA(A) receptor density and vagus nerve stimulation in individuals with drug-resistant partial epilepsy. *Epilepsy Res* 55(1–2): 59–70.

Martin, J. L., M. J. Barbanoj, T. E. Schlaepfer et al. (2003). Repetitive transcranial magnetic stimulation for the treatment of depression: Systematic review and meta-analysis. *Br J Psychiatry* 182: 480–491.

Martis, B., D. Alam, S. M. Dowd et al. (2003). Neurocognitive effects of repetitive transcranial magnetic stimulation in severe major depression. *Clin Neurophysiol* 114(6): 1125–1132.

Mayberg, H. S. (2003). Modulating dysfunctional limbic-cortical circuits in depression: Towards development of brain-based algorithms for diagnosis and optimised treatment. *Br Med Bull* 65: 193–207.

Mayberg, H. S. (2009). Targeted electrode-based modulation of neural circuits for depression. *J Clin Invest* 119(4): 717–725.

Mayberg, H. S., A. M. Lozano, V. Voon et al. (2005). Deep brain stimulation for treatment-resistant depression. *Neuron* 45(5): 651–660.

McCall, W. V., D. M. Reboussin, R. D. Weiner et al. (2000). Titrated moderately suprathreshold vs fixed high-dose right unilateral electroconvulsive therapy: acute antidepressant and cognitive effects. *Arch Gen Psychiatry* 57(5): 438–444.

McDonald, W. M., K. Easley, E. H. Byrd et al. (2006). Combination rapid transcranial magnetic stimulation in treatment refractory depression. *Neuropsychiatr Dis Treat* 2(1): 85–94.

McIntyre, C. C., M. Savasta, L. Kerkerian-Le Goff et al. (2004). Uncovering the mechanism(s) of action of deep brain stimulation: Activation, inhibition, or both. *Clin Neurophysiol* 115(6): 1239–1248.

McIntyre, C. C., & N. V. Thakor. (2002). Uncovering the mechanisms of deep brain stimulation for Parkinson's disease through functional imaging, neural recording, and neural modeling. *Crit Rev Biomed Eng* 30(4–6): 249–281.

McNeely, H. E., H. S. Mayberg, A. M. Lozano et al. (2008). Neuropsychological impact of Cg25 deep brain stimulation for treatment-resistant depression: Preliminary results over 12 months. *J Nerv Ment Dis* 196(5): 405–410.

Michael, N., M. Gosling, M. Reutemann et al. (2003). Metabolic changes after repetitive transcranial magnetic stimulation (rTMS) of the left prefrontal cortex: A sham-controlled proton magnetic resonance spectroscopy (1H MRS) study of healthy brain. *Eur J Neurosci* 17(11): 2462–2468.

Milev, R., G. Abraham, G. Hasey et al. (2009). Repetitive transcranial magnetic stimulation for treatment of medication-resistant depression in older adults: A case series. *J ECT* 25(1): 44–49.

Montgomery, S. A., N. Smeyatsky, M. de Ruiter et al. (1985). Profiles of antidepressant activity with the Montgomery-Asberg Depression Rating Scale. *Acta Psychiatr Scand Suppl* 320: 38–42.

Moreines, J. L., S. M. McClintock & P. E. Holtzheimer. (2011). Neuropsychologic effects of neuromodulation techniques for treatment-resistant depression: A review. *Brain Stimul* 4(1): 17–27.

Mosimann, U. P., S. C. Marre, S. Werlen et al. (2002). Antidepressant effects of repetitive transcranial magnetic stimulation in the elderly: Correlation between effect size and coil-cortex distance. *Arch Gen Psychiatry* 59(6): 560–561.

Mufti, M. A., P. E. Holtzheimer, 3rd, C. M. Epstein et al. (2010). Bupropion decreases resting motor threshold: A case report. *Brain Stimul* 3(3): 177–180.

Muller, M. B., N. Toschi, A. E. Kresse et al. (2000). Long-term repetitive transcranial magnetic stimulation increases the expression of brain-derived neurotrophic factor and cholecystokinin mRNA, but not neuropeptide tyrosine mRNA in specific areas of rat brain. *Neuropsychopharmacology* 23(2): 205–215.

Murphy, D. N., P. Boggio & F. Fregni. (2009). Transcranial direct current stimulation as a therapeutic tool for the treatment of major depression: Insights from past and recent clinical studies. *Curr Opin Psychiatry* 22(3): 306–311.

Nadeau, S. E., K. J. McCoy, G. P. Crucian et al. (2002). Cerebral blood flow changes in depressed patients after treatment with repetitive transcranial magnetic stimulation: Evidence of individual variability. *Neuropsychiatry Neuropsychol Behav Neurol* 15(3): 159–175.

Nahas, Z., B. S. Anderson, J. Borckardt et al. (2010). Bilateral epidural prefrontal cortical stimulation for treatment-resistant depression. *Biol Psychiatry* 67(2): 101–109.

Nahas, Z., L. B. Marangell, M. M. Husain et al. (2005). Two-year outcome of vagus nerve stimulation (VNS) for treatment of major depressive episodes. *J Clin Psychiatry* 66(9): 1097–1104.

Nahas, Z., M. A. Molloy, P. L. Hughes et al. (1999). Repetitive transcranial magnetic stimulation: Perspectives for application in the treatment of bipolar and unipolar disorders. *Bipolar Disord* 1(2): 73–80.

Nahas, Z., C. C. Teneback, A. Kozel et al. (2001). Brain effects of TMS delivered over prefrontal cortex in depressed adults: Role of stimulation frequency and coil-cortex distance. *J Neuropsychiatry Clin Neurosci* 13(4): 459–470.

Nedjat, S., & H. W. Folkerts. (1999). Induction of a reversible state of hypomania by rapid-rate transcranial magnetic stimulation over the left prefrontal lobe. *J ECT* 15(2): 166–168.

Nemeroff, C. B., H. S. Mayberg, S. E. Krahl et al. (2006). VNS therapy in treatment-resistant depression: Clinical evidence and putative neurobiological mechanisms. *Neuropsychopharmacology* 31(7): 1345–1355.

Nitsche, M. A., P. S. Boggio, F. Fregni et al. (2009). Treatment of depression with transcranial direct current stimulation (tDCS): A review. *Exp Neurol* 219(1): 14–19.

Nobler, M. S., M. A. Oquendo, L. S. Kegeles et al. (2001). Decreased regional brain metabolism after ECT. *Am J Psychiatry* 158(2): 305–308.

O'Reardon, J. P., H. B. Solvason, P. G. Janicak et al. (2007). Efficacy and safety of transcranial magnetic stimulation in the acute treatment of major depression: A multisite randomized controlled trial. *Biol Psychiatry* 62(11): 1208–1216.

Padberg, F., P. Zwanzger, M. E. Keck et al. (2002). Repetitive transcranial magnetic stimulation (rTMS) in major depression: Relation between efficacy and stimulation intensity. *Neuropsychopharmacology* 27(4): 638–645.

Paillere Martinot, M. L., A. Galinowski, D. Ringuenet et al. (2010). Influence of prefrontal target region on the efficacy of repetitive transcranial magnetic stimulation in patients with medication-resistant depression: A [(18) F]-fluorodeoxyglucose PET and MRI study. *Int J Neuropsychopharmacol* 13(1): 45–59.

Pallanti, S., S. Bernardi, A. Di Rollo et al. (2010). Unilateral low frequency versus sequential bilateral repetitive transcranial magnetic stimulation: Is simpler better for treatment of resistant depression? *Neuroscience* 167(2): 323–328.

Papez, J. W. (1937). A proposed mechanism of emotion. *Arch Neurol Psychiatry* 38: 725–743.

Pascual-Leone, A., M. D. Catala & A. Pascual-Leone Pascual. (1996). Lateralized effect of rapid-rate transcranial magnetic stimulation of the prefrontal cortex on mood. *Neurology* 46(2): 499–502.

Pascual-Leone, A., J. Valls-Sole, E. M. Wassermann et al. (1994). Responses to rapid-rate transcranial magnetic stimulation of the human motor cortex. *Brain* 117(Pt 4): 847–858.

Pinette, M. G., & J. R. Wax. (2010). The management of depression during pregnancy: A report from the American Psychiatric Association and the American College of Obstetricians and Gynecologists. *Obstet Gynecol* 115(1): 188–189; author reply 189.

Poreisz, C., K. Boros, A. Antal et al. (2007). Safety aspects of transcranial direct current stimulation concerning healthy subjects and patients. *Brain Res Bull* 72(4–6): 208–214.

Post, A., & M. E. Keck. (2001). Transcranial magnetic stimulation as a therapeutic tool in psychiatry: What do we know about the neurobiological mechanisms? *J Psychiatr Res* 35(4): 193–215.

Poulet, E., J. Brunelin, C. Boeuve et al. (2004). Repetitive transcranial magnetic stimulation does not potentiate antidepressant treatment. *Eur Psychiatry* 19(6): 382–383.

Price, T. R., T. B. Mackenzie, G. J. Tucker et al. (1978). The dose-response ratio in electroconvulsive therapy a preliminary study. *Arch Gen Psychiatry* 35(9): 1131–1136.

Pridmore, S., R. Bruno, Y. Turnier-Shea et al. (2000). Comparison of unlimited numbers of rapid transcranial magnetic stimulation (rTMS) and ECT treatment sessions in major depressive episode. *Int J Neuropsychopharmacol* 3(2): 129–134.

Prudic, J., R. F. Haskett, B. Mulsant et al. (1996). Resistance to antidepressant medications and short-term clinical response to ECT. *Am J Psychiatry* 153(8): 985–992.

Puigdemont, D., R. Perez-Egea, M. J. Portella et al. (2011). Deep brain stimulation of the subcallosal cingulate gyrus: Further evidence in treatment-resistant major depression. *Int J Neuropsychopharmacol*: 1–13. [Epub ahead of print].

Quintana, H. (2005). Transcranial magnetic stimulation in persons younger than the age of 18. *J ECT* 21(2): 88–95.

Rachid, F., J. Golaz, G. Bondolfi et al. (2006). Induction of a mixed depressive episode during rTMS treatment in a patient with refractory major depression. *World J Biol Psychiatry* 7(4): 261–264.

Rey, J. M., & G. Walter. (1997). Half a century of ECT use in young people. *Am J Psychiatry* 154(5): 595–602.

Rosa, M. A., W. F. Gattaz, A. Pascual-Leone et al. (2006). Comparison of repetitive transcranial magnetic stimulation and electroconvulsive therapy in unipolar non-psychotic refractory depression: A randomized, single-blind study. *Int J Neuropsychopharmacol* 9(6): 667–676.

Rose, D., P. Fleischmann, T. Wykes et al. (2003). Patients' perspectives on electroconvulsive therapy: Systematic review. *BMJ* 326(7403): 1363.

Rossini, D., A. Lucca, L. Magri et al. (2010). A symptom-specific analysis of the effect of high-frequency left or low-frequency right transcranial magnetic stimulation over the dorsolateral prefrontal cortex in major depression. *Neuropsychobiology* 62(2): 91–97.

Rossini, D., L. Magri, A. Lucca et al. (2005). Does rTMS hasten the response to escitalopram, sertraline, or venlafaxine in patients with major depressive disorder? A double-blind, randomized, sham-controlled trial. *J Clin Psychiatry* 66(12): 1569–1575.

Rowny, S. B., Y. M. Cycowicz, S. M. McClintock et al. (2009). Differential heart rate response to magnetic seizure therapy (MST) relative to electroconvulsive therapy: A nonhuman primate model. *Neuroimage* 47(3): 1086–1091.

Rumi, D. O., W. F. Gattaz, S. P. Rigonatti et al. (2005). Transcranial magnetic stimulation accelerates the antidepressant effect of amitriptyline in severe depression: A double-blind placebo-controlled study. *Biol Psychiatry* 57(2): 162–166.

Rush, A. J., L. B. Marangell, H. A. Sackeim et al. (2005). Vagus nerve stimulation for treatment-resistant depression: a randomized, controlled acute phase trial. *Biol Psychiatry* 58(5): 347–354.

Rush, A. J., H. A. Sackeim, L. B. Marangell et al. (2005). Effects of 12 months of vagus nerve stimulation in treatment-resistant depression: A naturalistic study. *Biol Psychiatry* 58(5): 355–363.

Rush, A. J., M. H. Trivedi, S. R. Wisniewski et al. (2006). Acute and longer-term outcomes in depressed outpatients requiring one or several treatment steps: A STAR*D report. *Am J Psychiatry* 163(11): 1905–1917.

Sachdev, P., & J. Sachdev. (1997). Sixty years of psychosurgery: Its present status and its future. *Aust N Z J Psychiatry* 31(4): 457–464.

Sachdev, P., & J. Sacher. (2005). Long-term outcome of neurosurgery for treatment of resistant depression. *J Neuropsychiatry Clin Neurosci* 17(4): 478–485.

Sackeim, H. A. (1999). The anticonvulsant hypothesis of the mechanisms of action of ECT: Current status. *J ECT* 15(1): 5–26.

Sackeim, H. A., S. K. Brannan, A. John Rush et al. (2007). Durability of antidepressant response to vagus nerve stimulation (VNSTM). *Int J Neuropsychopharmacol* 10(6): 817–826.

Sackeim, H. A., E. M. Dillingham, J. Prudic et al. (2009). Effect of concomitant pharmacotherapy on electroconvulsive therapy outcomes: Short-term efficacy and adverse effects. *Arch Gen Psychiatry* 66(7): 729–737.

Sackeim, H. A., R. F. Haskett, B. H. Mulsant et al. (2001). Continuation pharmacotherapy in the prevention of relapse following electroconvulsive therapy: A randomized controlled trial. *JAMA* 285(10): 1299–1307.

Sackeim, H. A., J. Prudic, D. P. Devanand et al. (2000). A prospective, randomized, double-blind comparison of bilateral and right unilateral electroconvulsive therapy at different stimulus intensities. *Arch Gen Psychiatry* 57(5): 425–434.

Sackeim, H. A., J. Prudic, R. Fuller et al. (2007). The cognitive effects of electroconvulsive therapy in community settings. *Neuropsychopharmacology* 32(1): 244–254.

Sackeim, H. A., J. Prudic, M. S. Nobler et al. (2008). Effects of pulse width and electrode placement on the efficacy and cognitive effects of electroconvulsive therapy. *Brain Stimul* 1(2): 71–83.

Sackeim, H. A., A. J. Rush, M. S. George et al. (2001). Vagus nerve stimulation (VNS) for treatment-resistant depression: Efficacy, side effects, and predictors of outcome. *Neuropsychopharmacology* 25(5): 713–728.

Sakkas, P., P. Mihalopoulou, P. Mourtzouhou et al. (2003). Induction of mania by rTMS: Report of two cases. *Eur Psychiatry* 18(4): 196–198.

Sartorius, A., & F. A. Henn. (2007). Deep brain stimulation of the lateral habenula in treatment resistant major depression. *Med Hypotheses* 69(6): 1305–1308.

Sartorius, A., K. L. Kiening, P. Kirsch et al. (2010). Remission of major depression under deep brain stimulation of the lateral habenula in a therapy-refractory patient. *Biol Psychiatry* 67(2): e9–e11.

Schlaepfer, T. E., M. X. Cohen, C. Frick et al. (2008). Deep brain stimulation to reward circuitry alleviates anhedonia in refractory major depression. *Neuropsychopharmacology* 33(2): 368–377.

Schlaepfer, T. E., C. Frick, A. Zobel et al. (2008). Vagus nerve stimulation for depression: Efficacy and safety in a European study. *Psychol Med* 38(5): 651–661.

Schlaepfer, T. E., & K. Lieb. (2005). Deep brain stimulation for treatment of refractory depression. *Lancet* 366(9495): 1420–1422.

Schulze-Rauschenbach, S. C., U. Harms, T. E. Schlaepfer et al. (2005). Distinctive neurocognitive effects of repetitive transcranial magnetic stimulation and electroconvulsive therapy in major depression. *Br J Psychiatry* 186: 410–416.

Schutter, D. J. (2010). Quantitative review of the efficacy of slow-frequency magnetic brain stimulation in major depressive disorder. *Psychol Med* 40(11): 1789–1795.

Shields, D. C., W. Asaad, E. N. Eskandar et al. (2008). Prospective assessment of stereotactic ablative surgery for intractable major depression. *Biol Psychiatry* 64(6): 449–454.

Shiwach, R. S., W. H. Reid & T. J. Carmody. (2001). An analysis of reported deaths following electroconvulsive therapy in Texas, 1993–1998. *Psychiatr Serv* 52(8): 1095–1097.

Speer, A. M., T. A. Kimbrell, E. M. Wassermann et al. (2000). Opposite effects of high and low frequency rTMS on regional brain activity in depressed patients. *Biol Psychiatry* 48(12): 1133–1141.

Steele, J. D., D. Christmas, M. S. Eljamel et al. (2008). Anterior cingulotomy for major depression: Clinical outcome and relationship to lesion characteristics. *Biol Psychiatry* 63(7): 670–677.

Strafella, A. P., T. Paus, J. Barrett et al. (2001). Repetitive transcranial magnetic stimulation of the human prefrontal cortex induces dopamine release in the caudate nucleus. *J Neurosci* 21(15): RC157.

Takano, H., N. Motohashi, T. Uema et al. (2007). Changes in regional cerebral blood flow during acute electroconvulsive therapy in patients with depression: positron emission tomographic study. *Br J Psychiatry* 190: 63–68.

Thase, M. E., E. S. Friedman, M. M. Biggs et al. (2007). Cognitive therapy versus medication in augmentation and switch strategies as second-step treatments: A STAR*D report. *Am J Psychiatry* 164(5): 739–752.

Thase, M. E., J. B. Greenhouse, E. Frank et al. (1997). Treatment of major depression with psychotherapy or psychotherapy-pharmacotherapy combinations. *Arch Gen Psychiatry* 54(11): 1009–1015.

Thase, M., & A. Rush. (1997). When at first you don't succeed: Sequential strategies for antidepressant nonresponders. *J Clin Psychiatry* 58(Suppl 13): 23–29.

The UK ECT Review Group. (2003). Efficacy and safety of electroconvulsive therapy in depressive disorders: A systematic review and meta-analysis. *The Lancet* 361: 799–808.

Trevino, K., S. M. McClintock & M. M. Husain. (2010). A review of continuation electroconvulsive therapy: Application, safety, and efficacy. *J ECT* 26(3): 186–195.

Wahlund, B., & D. von Rosen. (2003). ECT of major depressed patients in relation to biological and clinical variables: A brief overview. *Neuropsychopharmacology* 28(Suppl 1): S21–26.

Walter, G., J. M. Tormos, J. A. Israel et al. (2001). Transcranial magnetic stimulation in young persons: A review of known cases. *J Child Adolesc Psychopharmacol* 11(1): 69–75.

Wassermann, E. M. (1998). Risk and safety of repetitive transcranial magnetic stimulation: Report and suggested guidelines from the International Workshop on the Safety of Repetitive Transcranial Magnetic Stimulation, June 5-7, 1996. *Electroencephalogr Clin Neurophysiol* 108(1): 1–16.

White, P. F., Q. Amos, Y. Zhang et al. (2006). Anesthetic considerations for magnetic seizure therapy: A novel therapy for severe depression. *Anesth Analg* 103(1): 76–80, table of contents.

Wu, C. C., C. H. Tsai, M. K. Lu et al. (2010). Theta-burst repetitive transcranial magnetic stimulation for treatment-resistant obsessive-compulsive disorder with concomitant depression. *J Clin Psychiatry* 71(4): 504–506.

Xia, G., P. Gajwani, D. J. Muzina et al. (2008). Treatment-emergent mania in unipolar and bipolar depression: focus on repetitive transcranial magnetic stimulation. *Int J Neuropsychopharmacol* 11(1): 119–130.

Zaghi, S., M. Acar, B. Hultgren et al. (2010). Noninvasive brain stimulation with low-intensity electrical currents: Putative mechanisms of action for direct and alternating current stimulation. *Neuroscientist* 16(3): 285–307.

Zangen, A., Y. Roth, B. Voller et al. (2005). Transcranial magnetic stimulation of deep brain regions: Evidence for efficacy of the H-coil. *Clin Neurophysiol* 116(4): 775–779.

Zhang, X., K. Liu, J. Sun et al. (2010). Safety and feasibility of repetitive transcranial magnetic stimulation (rTMS) as a treatment for major depression during pregnancy. *Arch Womens Ment Health* 13(4): 369–370.

Treatment-Resistant Bipolar Disorder

Mark A. Frye

Introduction

Bipolar disorder is a mood disorder characterized by recurrent episodes of mania, hypomania, and depression. The symptom range associated with the illness is broad, and treatment response or mood stabilization can be complex given multiple points of therapeutic intervention (i.e., acute mania, acute bipolar depression, maintenance, or recurrence prevention) and optimal management of clinical variables (i.e., rapid cycling, comorbidity, treatment emergent switch) that make functional recovery elusive.

From a treatment perspective, the pharmacopoeia has evolved substantially since the approval of lithium carbonate in 1970. At present, there are ten approved drugs, used as monotherapy, for acute mania, including lithium, a first-generation antipsychotic (chlorpromazine), two anticonvulsants (divalproex sodium, divalproex sodium extended release, carbamazepine extended release), and six atypical antipsychotics (olanzapine, risperidone, quetiapine, quetiapine extended release, aripiprazole, ziprasidone, and asenapine). Combination therapy, by definition resistant to lithium or divalproex monotherapy, has been approved for olanzapine, quetiapine, risperidone, and aripiprazole. Bipolar depression approvals only include quetiapine extended release (bipolar I and II depression) and the combination of olanzapine/fluoxetine (bipolar I). Seven maintenance treatments are approved and include lithium, lamotrigine, olanzapine, risperidone injectable, and aripiprazole monotherapy as well as quetiapine extended release, risperidone injectable, and ziprasidone adjunct to lithium or divalproex sodium. Despite these therapeutic advances, treatment resistance broadly defined as inefficacy and/or poor tolerability contributing to nonadherence continues to be a substantial clinical problem.

Classification of Treatment Resistance

Despite interest in development and initial validation of treatment-resistant depression scales in major depressive disorder (i.e., Maudsley Staging model or Thase-Rush criteria;

Ruhe et al., 2011), there has been no consensus or widespread development of a treatment resistance scale in bipolar disorder. The Maudsley or Thase-Rush criteria are useful and the concept is clinically valuable as it focuses the clinician's assessment on the duration and severity of the index episode of major depression versus the lifelong course of illness; the scale also reinforces the assessment of whether treatment interventions for the index episode were of adequate dose and duration avoiding inflation of treatment resistance by review of all lifetime past pharmacotherapies.

While there is lack of standardization as to quantifying treatment resistance or failure to achieve remission related to specific pharmacotherapies, there is an increasing recognition of the importance of staging the illness (Kapczinski et al., 2009). Prior to treatment intervention, the illness severity needs to be assessed; this is essentially the first part of the resistance assessment. Staging the illness as latent or with subthreshold symptoms, Stage I (bipolar disorder with interepisode recovery with no Axis I, II, or III comorbidity), Stage II (rapid cycling and or comorbidities), and Stage III (cognitive and function decline) allow for studying underlying disease mechanisms and provides the baseline assessment to better understand the subsequent treatment intervention outcome.

In bipolar disorder treatment resistance, it is generally assumed that there has been lack of optimal mood stabilization in acute episode of mania or bipolar depression or lack of recurrent mood episode prevention. Whether side effect burden and subsequent non-adherence is a component of a treatment resistance scale remains to be determined. While all antimanic combination regulatory trials focused on nonresponse, one placebo-controlled evaluation of adjunctive donepezil, a reversible acetyl-cholinesterase inhibitor approved for use in Alzheimer disease (Eden Evins et al., 2006) and an open-label adjunctive trial of the antiarrhythmia drug mexiletine (Schaffer et al., 2000) included treatment intolerance in the study design.

Recent work by Pacchiarotti and colleagues (2009) has proposed criteria for treatment bipolar I depression resistance, refractoriness, and intractability. Treatment resistance was defined as nonremission despite adequate dose and duration of lithium treatment, lamotrigine augmentation of ongoing mood stabilization, or full dose (600 mg or greater) quetiapine monotherapy. Refractoriness was defined as further failure to reach remission with olanzapine/fluoxetine or lamotrigine quetiapine combination treatments. Intractability was defined as further failure to achieve remission with adjunctive antidepressant, modafinil, or pramipexole combinations therapies. Finally, involutional bipolar I depression was failure to achieve remission with a course of electroconvulsive therapy. Bipolar II depression had similar gradation of treatment failure, but it included monoamine oxidase inhibitor antidepressants in the definition of intractability. This scale, yet to be fully developed or validated and based on evidence base data for treatment response, is an important step in assessing treatment resistance in bipolar disorder.

Correlates of Treatment Resistance

Nonmood correlates to treatment resistance are not infrequent or inconsequential in the overall management in this patient population. Bipolar treatment-resistant patients tend to be on complicated polypharmacy regimens with significant access I, II, and III comorbidity.

In reviewing treating resistance, it is advisable, at least once, to carefully review the past psychiatric history to confirm a bipolar diagnosis. Confirmation of a bipolar diathesis would rule out other Axis I and II disorders whose symptoms were misattributed to bipolar disorder and as such, pseudo bipolar treatment resistance. For example, the false-positive rate of the Mood Disorder Questionnaire (MDQ), a screening instrument for bipolar disorder, has been reported up to 30% based on symptom overlap with attention-deficit/hyperactivity disorder, substance use disorders, and borderline personality disorder (Zimmerman et al., 2010a, 2010b). Once the diagnosis is confirmed, current symptoms should be reviewed to confirm the primary reason for current treatment are symptoms of bipolar disorder versus additional Axis I, II, or III clinical concerns (i.e., emphasis on the comorbidity).

A careful review of treatment adherence of the current medication combination is needed prior to assessing level of resistance. Severity of both mania and depression and complicated polypharmacotherapy (i.e., combination mood stabilizers) have both been associated with nonadherence (Keck et al., 1996; Sajatovic et al., 2011) and would thus suggest more educational based tools for remediation versus additional pharmacotherapy. Recent work has provided more detailed psychosocial and illness severity risk factors that extend far beyond the focus of the clinic (Sajatovic et al., 2011). In this small, mixed-model quantitative and qualitative interview of 20 poorly adherent community based bipolar patients, nonadherence was most common in minorities, unmarried individuals, and those with comorbid substance use disorders. Furthermore, the most common reasons for nonadherence were forgetting, side effects, long-term treatment recommendation, and disorganized home environment or specifically a person in the patient's social network advising against medications.

Clinical correlates of treatment resistance primarily related to bipolar disorder have focused on long-term course of illness measures such as age of onset and comorbidity. Initial work from the Stanley Bipolar Network reported that both lifetime and current Axis I comorbidity were associated with earlier age at onset of affective symptoms and syndromal bipolar disorder (McElroy et al., 2001); current comorbidity, relevant to the discussion of resistance, was associated with cycle acceleration and more severe episodes over time. Further work from this group prospectively followed 529 adult bipolar outpatients to assess 1-year outcome based on illness onset in childhood/adolescence versus adulthood (Post et al., 2010). The younger onset group, in comparison to the adulthood onset group, exhibited significantly greater severity of mania and depression, greater number of episodes, more days depressed, and more days with ultradian cycling. Even after 4 years follow-up, the differences in severity and duration of depression remained significantly different. Delays to first treatment were associated with more time depressed, greater severity of depression, more ultradian cycling, and greater number of episodes. Thus, it is not surprising to see greater treatment resistance in the depressive phase of illness.

Treatment-Resistant Mania

Treatment-resistant mania unresponsive to Food and Drug Administration (FDA)-approved treatments (lithium, carbamazepine, divalproex sodium, olanzapine, quetiapine, risperidone, risperidone long-term injection, ziprasidone, aripiprazole, asenapene, and lurasidone) will require combination treatment. A recent meta-analysis reviewing more than 16,000 patients from 68 controlled acute mania trials suggests overall efficacy was superior for antipsychotic drugs, specifically risperidone, olanzapine, and haloperidol, in comparison to mood stabilizers; gabapentin, lamotrigine, and topiramate were no better than placebo (Cipriani et al., 2011). Thus, if acute mania has not responded to lithium, divalproex, or carbamazepine, antipsychotic monotherapy should be considered. Haloperidol must be considered in treatment-resistant mania given this efficacy profile. However, it is important to remember that typical antipsychotics, in comparison to atypical antipsychotics, have a greater risk of tardive dyskinesia. There may be additional risk for tardive dyskinesia in bipolar patients. In comparison to studies evaluating patients with schizophrenia, a number of studies in bipolar disorder have reported higher rates of extrapyramidal symptoms, including tardive dyskinesia; furthermore, typical antipsychotic treatment, in comparison to lithium, has been associated with greater postmanic episode depressive symptom severity and depressive episode recurrence (Frye et al., 1998).

Several of the FDA-approved monotherapies (olanzapine, risperidone, quetiapine, aripirazole) do have additional indications in combination as adjunct to lithium or divalproex sodium (reviewed in Ketter, 2009). It is increasingly recognized that complex combination pharmacotherapy is often needed to achieve optimal outcomes (Frye et al., 2000). However, outside of regulatory studies of adjunctive atypical antipsychotic to lithium or divalproex sodium, combination studies of lithium maintenance with lamotrigine (van der Loos et al., 2009), carbamazepine (Denicoff et al., 1997), and divalproex (Geddes et al., 2010), as well as divalproex sodium with haloperidol (Muller-Oerlinghausen et al., 2000), there is little additional evidence base, in this case for mania, as to specific combinations available to guide clinicians. Several novel treatments have been evaluated in small, controlled pilot studies that warrant further investigation.

Tamoxifen is an anti-estrogen receptor protein kinase C inhibitor approved for use in the prophylaxis of breast cancer. Given its PKC inhibition, this compound was evaluated as a novel treatment for treatment-resistant mania (Yildez et al., 2008). The first 3-week placebo-controlled investigation of manic inpatients ($n = 66$) reported significant improvement in manic symptoms with tamoxifen (80 mg daily) versus placebo. The second study, a 6-week placebo-controlled study of lithium maintained manic inpatients ($n = 40$) again found significant antimanic effect with adjunctive tamoxifen 80 mg daily (Amrollahi et al., 2011).

There is increasing interest in reexamining the purinergic system and its dysregulation in bipolar disorder. In the first 8-week, placebo-controlled study, 82 *DSM-IV* confirmed manic inpatients (91% psychotic) with a Young Mania Rating Scale score (YMRS) of 20 were randomized to upper therapeutic level lithium (1.0–1.2 mmol/L) + haloperidol 10 mg daily + the hypouricemic agent allopurinol 300 mg daily or lithium + haloperidol + placebo (Akhondzadeh et al., 2006). There was a significant reduction in manic symptoms with allopurinol versus placebo. In a larger 4-week confirmatory study, 180 manic inpatients were randomized to lithium plus allopurinol 600 mg daily ($n = 60$), dipyridamole 200 mg daily ($n = 60$), or placebo ($n = 60$; Machado-Vieira, 2008). Again, adjunctive allopurinol was associated with greater reduction in manic symptom severity and greater remission rate than placebo. In this case, there was a significant correlation between reduction in plasma uric acid level and manic symptom severity.

Despite the negative trials of gabapentin (Pande et al., 2000) and topiramate (Delbello, 2005; Kushner et al., 2006) in acute mania, there have been positive trials with anticonvulsants other than divalproex sodium and carbamazepine. Phenytoin has been evaluated in two placebo-controlled studies; phenytoin 300–400 mg daily adjunct to haloperidol was associated with significant improvement in acute mania ($n = 30$) and similar dosing to ongoing mood stabilization ($n = 23$) was associated with reduced mood episode recurrence (Mishory et al., 2000, 2003). Oxcarbazepine, a keto-congener of carbamazepine, has been evaluated in four studies (one placebo controlled, three comparison, total $n = 51$) of acute mania or maintenance. In general the data suggest similar effectiveness to haloperidol and lithium (Yatham, 2004). Oxcarbazepine is generally thought to have greater tolerability and fewer drug interactions, though not zero, compared to the FDA-approved carbamazepine. It is unclear how many carbamazepine nonresponders for acute mania would, in fact, subsequently respond to oxcarbazepine. Other less studied compounds with limited impression or controlled negative studies include verapamil; Janicak et al., 1998), zonisamide (McElroy et al., 2005), and levetiracetam (Grunze et al., 2003). Finally, electroconvulsive therapy (ECT), where during the course of treatment seizure threshold increases, two controlled studies, comparing ECT to lithium and ECT to lithium + haloperidol, reported significant benefits for acute mania (Mukherjee et al., 1988; Small et al. 1998).

While there is no current FDA approval for clozapine in bipolar disorder, there is a general clinical sense of significant therapeutic benefit, particularly in treatment-resistant cases. In a 3-week open, randomized evaluation of mania resistant to lithium, subjects who were randomized to adjunctive clozapine ($n = 15$, mean dose 166 mg daily) in comparison to the FDA-approved chlorpromazine ($n = 12$, mean dose 310 mg daily) exhibited a greater reduction in manic symptoms as measured by the Young Mania Rating Scale score (YMRS) at week 2. While there was no significant difference at study endpoint, the accelerating or rapid stabilizing antimanic response can be clinically meaningful (Barbini et al., 1997). Finally, in a group of treatment-resistant bipolar patients ($n = 38$), adding on clozapine, in comparison to treatment as usual, was associated with significant reduction in total medication use (i.e., polypharmacy) and significant improvement in symptoms of mania, positive and negative symptoms (Suppes et al., 1999).

Bipolar Depression and Rapid Cycling

Given the predominance of depression in bipolar disorder, it is particularly noteworthy that only 2 FDA-approved treatments are currently available for depression versus 10 for acute mania and 6 for maintenance. Presently, olanzapine/fluoxetine combination and quetiapine monotherapy are the only FDA-approved treatments for bipolar depression. The recent meta-analysis of lamotrigine for bipolar depression clearly, despite absence of FDA approval for acute episodes, suggests effectiveness (Geddes et al., 2010). The antidepressant benefit reported for quetiapine and olanzapine/fluoxetine is not generalizable to other atypical antipsychotics, with negative studies for ziprasidone and aripiprazole (Frye, 2011).

Most compelling is recognizing that all of the unimodal FDA-approved antidepressants for major depressive disorder are used off label in bipolar depression with relatively little evidence base to warrant their widespread use (Baldessarini et al., 2007). A recent meta-analysis of 15 studies in bipolar depression comparing antidepressants of all classes (serotonin reuptake inhibitors, dual action serotonin norepinephrine reuptake inhibitors, tricyclic antidepressants, monoamine oxidase inhibitors, bupropion) versus placebo or active comparator (n = 2,373) reported nonsignificant benefits of antidepressant versus placebo (response: RR = 1.18 [95% CI, 0.99–1.4; p = .06]; remission: RR = 1.20 [95% CI, 0.98–1.47, p = .09]; Sidor and MacQueen, 2010). However, antidepressants with different mechanism may have meaningful clinical differences, particularly in treatment-resistant cases. For example, paroxetine is arguably the most rigorously studied selective serotonin reuptake inhibitor in bipolar depression (Nemeroff, 2001; Sachs, 2007; McElroy, 2010). While study design (monotherapy vs. adjunctive placebo-controlled, tricyclic or bupropion comparator), duration (8-week, 26-week), outcome measure (response or durable recovery), and presence of treatment resistance (Nemeroff et al., 2001) were all different, all studies failed to show significant difference from placebo. Conversely, in now classic controlled studies of monoamine oxidase inhibitors, including a double-blind crossover of imipramine resistant anergic bipolar depression, tranylcypromine proved to be highly efficacious and rapid in treating depressive symptoms (Himmelhoch et al., 1982; Thase et al., 1992).

Treatment resistance was not reported in all of these studies and there may be merit in considering these agents for bipolar depression not responsive to mood stabilization. For example, in a group of treatment-resistant (i.e., an inadequate response to mood stabilization therapy) bipolar depressed patients (n = 174), a 10-week double-blind trial compared treatment with sertraline (mean dose 192 mg), venlafaxine (195 mg), or bupropion (285 mg; Post et al., 2006). While not placebo controlled, response rates (defined as a 50% reduction in the Inventory for Depressive Symptoms) were approximately 50% for each antidepressant. Longer term data on antidepressant use in bipolar depression are limited. In a randomized 1-year continuation of the 10-week trial described earlier, over two thirds of patients who had an initial response to an antidepressant maintained their response (Altshuler et al., 2009). The potential benefits of adjunctive antidepressant treatment needs to be weighed against the potential of antidepressant-induced mania, which appears to have a number of illness (i.e., mixed depression, substance abuse comorbidity) and treatment intervention (venlafaxine, tricyclic antidepressants) risk factors (Vieta et al., 2002; Post et al., 2006; Frye et al., 2009).

In contrast to novel drug development in mania, which has focused primarily on atypical and anticonvulsant compounds, novel drug development in bipolar depression has had broader candidate compounds (modafinil/armodafinil, pramipexole, ketamine, riluzole, omega 3 fatty acid) that may prove to be useful for treatment-resistant bipolar depression. Modafinil, approved to improve wakefulness in patients with excessive sleepiness associated with narcolepsy, sleep apnea, and shift work sleep disorder, has been evaluated in bipolar treatment-resistant depression (Frye et al., 2007). In a 6-week, randomized, double-blind, placebo-controlled study of bipolar I/II (n = 85) depressed patients inadequately responsive to a mood stabilizer with or without concurrent antidepressant therapy, adjunctive modafinil (n = 41, mean dose 170 mg) in comparison to placebo (n = 44) was associated with a greater decrease in depressive symptoms and higher response (44% vs. 23%) and remission (39% vs. 18%) rates, respectively. There was no difference between these two groups in treatment-emergent hypomania or hospitalization for mania. This positive pilot study prompted a larger placebo-controlled study of the enantiomer armodafinil (Calabrese et al., 2010). In this 8-week, multicenter, randomized, double-blind, placebo-controlled study, subjects who were randomized to adjunctive armodafinil 150 mg ($n = 128$), versus placebo ($n = 129$), showed greater improvement in depressive symptoms as measured by the Inventory for Depression Symptoms (IDS). However, none of the secondary outcome measures had significant treatment group differences with further investigation underway.

Pramipexole is a partial D2/D3 agonist approved for Parkinson disease and has been evaluated in two 6-week, randomized, double-blind, placebo-controlled studies ($n = 22$ BPI/II, $n = 21$ BPII) as adjunct treatment to mood stabilizers (Goldberg et al., 2004; Zarate et al., 2004). Dosed well below the average dosing for Parkinson disease (1.7 mg vs. 4.5 mg), response rates were significantly higher in both studies for pramipexole versus placebo (67% vs. 20% and 60% vs. 9%). While one bipolar I subject developed psychotic mania, there was no difference in switch rate to hypomania in the bipolar II study. A lack of commercial interest in the development of pramipexole has led to its relegation to generic formulation only, despite its scientific appeal as a putative psychotropic for treatment-resistant bipolar depression.

Glutamatergic modulation (i.e., lamotrigine, ketamine, riluzole) is increasingly being studied in treatment-resistant bipolar depression. Ketamine is an N-methyl D aspartate glutamate receptor antagonist that has had renewed interest in being evaluated as a rapid-acting antidepressant. Eighteen lithium or divalproex treatment-resistant bipolar depressed subjects were randomized to intravenous infusion of ketamine hydrochloride (0.5 mg/kg) or placebo on 2 separate testing days 2 weeks apart (Diazgranados et al., 2010). Depressive symptomatology was significantly improved in subjects receiving ketamine compared to placebo. Seventy-one percent of subjects responded to ketamine versus 6% responding to placebo. Generally, the medication was well tolerated, though there were transient adverse effects with associated symptoms that fully cleared prior to study observation. Riluzole, an FDA-approved medication for amyotrophic lateral sclerosis, was administered in a 6-week open-label trial in 14 patients with treatment-resistant bipolar depression with 60% having failed two or more prior treatments (Brennan et al., 2010). Riluzole (mean dose 181.8 mg daily) was associated with significant reduction in depression rating scale scores as measured by the Hamilton Depression Rating Scale with evidence, as well, of an increased glutamine to glutamate ratio associated with treatment.

A number of lines of evidence from epidemiological surveys, biochemical, and clinical studies suggest a possible link between omega-3 fatty acid consumption and mood disorders (Frangou et al., 2006). In this first 12-week double-blind, placebo-controlled study, 75 outpatients with bipolar depression were randomized to adjunctive EPA 1 gram, EPA 2 grams, or placebo. Patients in both EPA treatment groups displayed significantly greater reductions in HDRS total scores compared with patients receiving placebo. However, the interpretation of these findings is limited by changes in patients' medication regimens allowed during the trial for symptom worsening. A secondary biomarker study showed statistically significant increases in N-acetyl aspartate (NAA) in those subjects randomized to EPA, suggesting a possible neurotrophic role of omega 3 fatty acids in bipolar disorder (Frangou et al, 2007). The second placebo-controlled study was longer in trial duration (4 months), utilized a higher dose of EPA (6 g/d), and stratified randomization in outpatients with bipolar depression based on the presence ($n = 59$) or absence of rapid cycling ($n = 57$). There were no significant differences in baseline to endpoint change in symptoms of depression, mania, or switch (Keck et al., 2006). In a post-hoc analysis of this study, younger patients did better on medication, while older patients actually did better on placebo. These two controlled studies suggest further investigation.

There are additional controlled studies suggesting efficacy for treatment-resistant bipolar depression with focused psychotherapies (collaborative care as the control intervention; Miklovitz, 2006), antioxidant N-acetyl cysteine (Berk et al., 2008), and sleep deprivation in combination with the beta blocker/5HT 1A antagonist pindolol (Smeraldi et al., 1999). It is increasingly likely that treatment-resistant bipolar disorder may have important gender differences in illness burden and or treatment response. In a multicenter, 6-week, double-blind, randomized, placebo-controlled fixed-dose trial assessing efficacy of levothyroxine (300 µg/d) adjunctive to continuing mood stabilizer and/or antidepressant medication in adult bipolar treatment-resistant patients ($n = 62$), there was no significant difference in treatment outcome in depression as measured by the Hamilton Rating Scale for Depression score (Bauer, 2010). However, a secondary analysis revealed statistically significant improvement for the bipolar women, but not men, suggesting thyroid abnormalities, already known to be more prevalent in women, and thyroid therapeutic interventions may be gender specific.

Early open trials of transcranial magnetic stimulation in treatment-resistant bipolar depression look promising The first 3-week open-label trial of repetitive transcranial stimulation ($n = 11$, 1 Hz, 110% motor threshold, 300 stimuli/day) was associated with 55% rate of response and 36% rate of remission (Dell'Osso et al., 2009). The second study, a 4-week open-label study ($n = 19$, 20 Hz, 1,680 stimuli/day) was associated with a 63% rate of response and a 53% rate of remission (Harel et al., 2011). Further study with parameters optimal for remission without mood switch need to be further evaluated. Also, deep brain stimulation may prove to be an important future therapeutic intervention for bipolar disorder and is currently being investigated (Tye et al., 2009). Preliminary investigation of subcallosal cingulate DBS for treatment resistant depression (n = 17) which included a single blind sham stimulation phase, 24 week open label active stimulation, and 2-year follow up phase reported response/remission rates of 41% / 18% at 24 weeks and 92% / 58% at 2 year follow up respectively; bipolar depressed patients had similar response / remission rates to the unipolar depressed patients with no induction of mania or hypomania (Holtzheimer et al., 2012).

Conclusion

Treatment resistance is contributing to substantial morbidity and mortality in bipolar disorder. It will be imperative to develop consensus nomenclature not only on the course and outcome (response, remission, recurrence, mood switch) in bipolar disorder (Tohen et al., 2010) but also to develop validated and standardized measures of treatment resistance. Staging the illness with careful assessment of Axis I, II, and III comorbidity, quantification of allostatic burden (Kapczinski et al., 2009), and the proposals for depressive resistance, refractoriness, and intractability (Pacchiarotti et al., 2009) are important first steps in future treatment resistance research. It is increasingly recognized that complex combination pharmacotherapy is often needed to achieve optimal outcomes in treatment-resistant bipolar disorder (Frye et al., 2000). This is an artful combination of evidence-based decision making, primarily focused on mood stabilizers, anticonvulsants, atypical antipsychotic, judicious use of antidepressants, and novel compounds and individualized treatment considerations for patients.

Disclosure Statement

M. A. F. receives grant support from Pfizer, National Alliance for Schizophrenia and Depression (NARSAD), National Institute of Mental Health (NIMH), National Institute of Alcohol Abuse and Alcoholism (NIAAA), and the Mayo Foundation.

References

Akhondzadeh S, Milajerdi MR, Amini H, Tehrani-Doost M. Allopurinol as an adjunct to lithium and haloperidol for treatment of patients with acute mania: a double-blind randomized, placebo controlled trial. *Bipolar Disorder* 2006; 8: 485–489.

Altshuler LL, Post RM, Hellemann G, Leverich GS, Nolen WA, Frye MA, Keck PE Jr, Kupka RW, Grunze H, McElroy SL, Sugar CA, Suppes T. Impact of antidepressant continuation after acute positive or partial treatment response for bipolar depression: a blinded, randomized study. *J Clin Psychiatry* 2009; 70: 450–457.

Amrollahi Z, Rezaei F, Salehi B, Modabbernia AH, Maroufi A, Esfandiari GE, Naderi M, Ghebleh F, Ahmadi-Abhari SA, Sadeghi M, Tabrizi M, Akhondzadeh S. Double-blind, randomized, placebo-controlled 6-week study on the efficacy of tamoxifen adjunctive to lithium in acute bipolar mania. *J Affective Disord* 2011; 129: 327–331.

Baldessarini RJ, Leahy L, Arcona S, Gause D, Zhang W, Hennen J. Patterns of psychotropic drug prescription for U.S. patients with diagnoses of bipolar disorders. *Psychiatric Services* 2007; 58(1): 85–91.

Barbini B, Scherillo P, Benedetti F, Crespi G, Colombo C, Smeraldi E. Response to clozapein in acute mania is more rapid than that of chlorpromazine. *Int Clin Psychopharmaoclogy* 1997; 12: 109–112.

Bauer M. Gender differences in response to thyroid hormone: a randomized, placebo-controlled study of levothyroxine as add-on treatment in bipolar depression. Presented at the Biannual Meeting of the International Society for Bipolar Disorder, Sao Paulo, Brazil, March 2010.

Berk M, Copolov DL, Dean O, Lu K, Jeavons S, Schapkaitz I, Anderson-Hunt M, Bush AI. N-acetyl cysteine for depressive symptoms in bipolar disorder—a double-blind randomized placebo-controlled trial. *Biol Psychiatry* 2008; 64: 468–475.

Brennan BP, Hudson JI, Jensen JE, McCarthy J, Roberts JL, Prescot AP, Cohen BM, Pope HG, Jr, Renshaw PF, Ongur D. Rapid enhancement of glutamatergic neurotransmission in bipolar depression following treatment with riluzole. *Neuropsychopharmacology* 2010; 35: 834–846.

Calabrese JR, Ketter TA, Youakim JM, Tiller JM, Yang R, Frye MA. Adjunctive armodafinil for major depressive episodes associated with bipolar I disorder: a randomized, multicenter, double-blind, placebo-controlled, proof-of-concept study. *J Clin Psychiatry* 2010; 71: 1363–1370.

Cipriani A, Barbui C, Salanti G, Rendell J, Brown R, Stockton S, Purgato M, Spineli LM, Goodwin GM, Geddes JR. Comparative efficacy and acceptability of antimanic drugs in acute mania: a multiple-treatments meta-analysis. *Lancet* 2011; 378: 1306–1315.

Delbello MP, Findling RL, Kushner S, Wang D, Olson WH, Capece JA, Fazzio L, Rosenthal NR. A pilot controlled trial of topiramate for mania in children and adolescents with bipolar disorder. *JAACAP* 2005; 44: 539–547.

Dell'Osso B, Mundo E, D'Urso N, Pozzoli S, Buoli M, Ciabatti M, Rosanova M, Massimini M, Bellina V, Mariotti M, Altamura AC. Augmentative repetitive navigated transcranial magentic stimulation (rTMS) in drug-resistant bipolar depression. *Bipolar Disord* 2009; 11: 76–81.

Denicoff KD, Smith-Jackson EE, Disney ER, Ali SO, Leverich GS, Post RM. Comparative prophylactic efficacy of lithium, carbamazepine, and the combination in bipolar disorder. *J Clin Psychiatry* 1997; 58(11): 470–478.

Diazgranados N, Ibrahim L, Brutsche NE, Newberg A, Kronstein P, Khalife S, Kammerer WA, Quezado Z, Luckenbaugh DA, Salvadore G, Machado-Vieira R, Manji HK, Zarate CA, Jr A randomized add-on trial of an N-methyl-D-aspartate antagonist in treatment-resistant bipolar depression. *Arch Gen Psychiatry* 2010; 67: 793–802.

Eden Evins A, Demopulos C, Nierenberg A, Culhane MA, Eisner L, Sachs G. A double-blind, placebo-controlled trial of adjunctive donepezil in treatment-resistant mania. *Bipolar Disord* 2006; 8: 75–80.

Frangou S, Lewis M, McCrone P. Efficacy of ethyl-eicosapentaenoic acid in bipolar depression: randomized double-blind placebo-controlled study. *Br J Psychiatry* 2006; 188: 46–50.

Frangou S, Lewis M, Wollard J, Simmons A. Preliminary in vivo evidence of increase N-acetyl aspartate following eicosapentaenoic acid treatment in patients with bipolar disorder. *J Clin Psychopharmacology* 2007; 21: 435–439.

Frye MA. Clinical practice. Bipolar disorder: a focus on depression. *N Engl J Med* 2011; 364(1): 51–59

Frye MA, Grunze H, Suppes T, McElroy SL, Keck PE, Walden J, Leverich GS, Altshuler LL, Nakelsky S, Hwang S, Mintz J, Post RM. A placebo-controlled evaluation of adjunctive modafinil in the treatment of bipolar depression. *Am J Psychiatry* 2007; 164(8): 1242–1249.

Frye MA, Helleman G, McElroy SL, Altshuler LL, Black DO, Keck PE Jr, Nolen WA, Kupka R, Leverich GS, Grunze H, Mintz J, Post RM, Suppes T. Correlates of treatment-emergent mania associated with antidepressant treatment in bipolar depression. *Am J Psychiatry* 2009, 166: 164–172.

Frye MA, Ketter TA, Altshuler LL, Denicoff K, Dunn RT, Kimbrell TA, Cora-Locatelli G, Post RM. Clozapine in bipolar disorder: treatment implications for other atypical antipsychotics. *J Affect Disord* 1998; 48: 91–104.

Frye MA, Ketter TA, Leverich GS, Huggins T, Lantz C, Denicoff KD, Post RM. The increasing use of polypharmacotherapy for refractory mood disorders: 22 years of study. *J Clin Psychiatry* 2000; 61: 9–15.

Geddes JR, Calabrese JR, Goodwin GM. Lamotrigine for treatment of bipolar depression: independent meta-analysis and meta-regression of individual patient data from five randomized trials. *Br J Psychiatry* 2009; 194(1): 4–9.

Geddes JR, Goodwin GM, Rendell J, Azorin JM, Cipriani A, Ostacher MJ, Morris R, Alder N, Jusczak E, The BALANCE Investigators. Lithium plus valproate combination therapy versus monotherapy for relapse prevention in bipolar I disorder (BALANCE): a randomized open label trial. *Lancet* 2010; 375: 385–395.

Goldberg JF, Burdick KE, Endick CJ. Preliminary randomized, double-blind, placebo-controlled trial of pramipexole added to mood stabilizers for treatment-resistant bipolar depression. *Am J Psychiatry* 2004; 161(3): 564–566.

Grunze H, Langosch J, Born C, Schaub G, Walden J. Levetiracetam in the treatment of acute mania: an open add on study with an on-off-on design. *J Clin Psychiatry* 2003; 64: 781–784.

Harel EV, Zangen A, Roth Y, Reti I, Braw Y, Levkovits Y. H-coil repetitive transcranial magnetic stimulation for the treatment of bipolar depression: an add-on safety and feasibility study. *World J Biol Psychiatry* 2011; 12: 119–126.

Himmelhoch JM, Fuchs CZ, Symons BJ. A double blind study of tranylcypromine treatment of major anergic depression. *J Nerv Mental Disease* 1982; 170: 628–634.

Holtzheimer PE, Kelley ME, Gross RE, Filkowski MM, Garlow SJ, Barrocas A, Wint D, Craighead MC, Kozarsky J, Chismar R, Moreines JL, Mewes K, Posse PR, Gutman DA, Mayberg HS. Subcallosal cingulate deep brain stimulation for treatment resistant unipolar and bipolar depression. *Arch Gen Psychiatry* 2012, [Epbu ahead of print]

Janicak PG, Sharma PP, Pandey G, and Davis JM. Verapamil for the treatment of acute mania: a double-blind, placebo-controlled study. *Am J Psychiatry* 1998; 155: 972–973.

Kapczinski F, Dias W, Kauer-Sant'Anna M, Frey BN, Grassi-Oliveira R, Colom F, Berk M. Clinical implications of a staging model for bipolar disorder. *Expert Rev Neurother* 2009; 9: 957–966.

Keck PE Jr, McElroy SL, Strakowski SM, Stanton SP, Kizer DL, Balistereri TM, Bennett JA, Tugrul KC, West SA. Factors associated with pharmacologic noncompliance in patients with mania. *J Clin Psychiatry* 1996; 57: 292–297.

Keck PE, Mintz J, McElroy SL, Freeman MP, Suppes T, Frye MA, Altshuler LL, Kupka R, Nolen WA, Leverich GS, Denicoff KD, Grunze H, Duan N, Post RM. Double-blind randomized, placebo-controlled trials of Ethyl-eicosapentanoate in the treatment of bipolar depression and rapid cycling bipolar disorder. *Biol Psychiatry* 2006; 60: 1020–1022.

Ketter TA, ed. Handbook of diagnosis and treatment of bipolar disorder. American Psychiatry Association, DC, Amazon.com 2009.

Kushner SF, Khan A, Olson WH. Topiramate monotherapy in the management of acute mania: results of four double-blind placebo controlled trials. *Bipolar Disord* 2006; 8: 15–27.

Machado-Vieira R, Soares JC, Lara DR, Luckenbaugh DA, Busnello JV, Marca G, Cunha A, Souza DO, Zarate CA, Kapczinski F. A double blind randomized placebo controlled 4-week study on the efficacy and safety of the purinergic agents allopurinol and didyridamole adjunctive to lithium in acute bipolar mania. *J Clin Psychiatry* 2008; 69(8): 1237–1245.

McElroy SL, Altshuler LL, Suppes T, Keck PE, Jr, Frye MA, Denicoff KD, Nolen WA, Kupka RW, Leverich GS, Rochussen JR, Rush AJ, Post RM. Axis I psychiatric comorbidity and its relationship to historical illness variables in 288 patients with bipolar disorder. *Am J Psychiatry* 2001; 158: 420–426.

McElroy SL, Suppes T, Keck PE, Black D, Frye M, Altshuler LL, Nolen WA, Kupka RW, Leverich GS, Walden J, Grunze H, Post RM. Open label adjunctive zonisamide in the treatment of bipolar disorder: a prospective trial. *J Clin Psychiatry* 2005; 66: 617–624.

McElroy SL, Weisler RH, Chang W, Olausson B, Paulsson B, Bretcher M, Agambaram V, Merideth C, Nordenhem A, Young AH. A double-blind, placebo-controlled study of quetiapine and lithium monotherapy in adults in the acute phase of bipolar depresssion (Embolden I). *J Clin Psychiatry* 2010; 71: 163–174.

Miklowitz DJ, Otto MW, Frank E, Reilly-Harrington NA, Wisniewski SR, Kogan JN, Nierenberg AA, Calabrese JR, Marangell LB, Gyulai L, Araga M, Gonzalez JM, Shirley ER, Thase ME, Sachs GS. Psychosocial treatments for bipolar depression: a 1-year randomized trial from the Systematic Treatment Enhancement Program. *Arch Gen Psychiatry* 2007; 64: 419–426.

Mishory A, Winokur M, Bersudsky Y. Prophylactic effect of phenytoin in bipolar disorder: a controlled study. *Bipolar Disord* 2003; 5: 464–467.

Mishory A, Yaroslavsky Y, Bersudsky Y, Belmaker RH. Phenytoin as an antimanic anticonvulsant: a controlled study. *Am J Psychiatry* 2000; 157: 463–465.

Mukherjee S, Sackeim HA, Lee C. Unilateral ECT in teh treatment of manic episodes. *Convulsive Therapy* 1988; 4: 74–80.

Muller-Oerlinghausen B, Retzow A, Henn FA, Giedke H, Walden J. Valproate as an adjunct to neuroleptic medications for the treatment of acute episodes of mania: a prospective, randomized, double-blind, placebo-controlled, multicenter study. European Valproate Mania Study Group. *J Clin Psychopharmacology* 2000; 20: 195–203.

Nemeroff CB, Evans DL, Gyulai L, Sachs GS, Bowden CL, Gergel IP, Oakes R, Pitts CD: Double-blind, placebo-controlled comparison of imipramine and paroxetine in the treatment of bipolar depression. *Am J Psychiatry* 2001; 6: 906–912.

Pacchiarotti I, Mazzarini L, Colom F, Sanchez-Moreno J, Girardi P, Kotzalidis GD, Vieta E. Treatment-resistant bipolar depression: towards a new definition. *Acta Psychiatr Scand* 2009; 120: 429–440.

Pande AC, Crockatt JG, Janney CA, Werth JL, Tsaroucha G. Gabapentin in bipolar disorder: a placebo controlled trial of adjunctive therapy. Gabapentin Bipolar Disorder Study Group. *Bipolar Disord* 2000; 2: 249–255.

Post RM, Altshuler LL, Leverich GS, Frye MA, Nolen WA, Kupka RW, Suppes T, McElroy S, Keck PE, Denicoff KD, Grunze H, Walden J, Kitchen CM, Mintz J. Mood switch in bipolar depression: comparison of adjunctive venlafaxine, bupropion and sertraline. *Brit J Psychiatry* 2006; 189: 124–131.

Post RM, Leverich GS, Kupka RW, Keck PE, Jr, McElroy SL, Altshuler LL, Frye MA, Luckenbaugh DA, Rowe M, Grunze H, Suppes T, Nolen WA. Early-onset bipolar disorder and treatment delay are risk factors for poor outcome in adulthood. *J Clin Psychiatry* 2010; 71: 864–872.

Ruhe HG, van Rooijen G, Spiiker J, Peeters FP, Schene AH. Staging methods for treatment resistant depression: a systematic review. *J Affect Disord* 2011. [Epub ahead of print].

Sachs GS, Nierenberg AA, Calabrese JR, Marangell LB, Wisniewski SR, Gyulai L, Friedman ES, Bowden CL, Fossey MD, Ostacher MJ, Ketter TA, Patel J, Hauser P, Rapport D, Martinez JM, Allen MH, Miklowitz DJ, Otto MW, Dennehy EB, Thase ME: Effectiveness of adjunctive antidepressant treatment for bipolar depression. *N Engl J Med* 2007; 356(17): 1711–1722.

Sajatovic M, Levin J, FeuntesCAsiano E, Cassidy KA, Tatsuoka C, Jenkiins JH. Illness experience and reasons for nonadherence among individuals with bipolar disorder who are poorly adherent with medication. *Compr Psychiatry* 2011; 52: 280–287.

Schaffer A, Levitt AJ, Joffe RT. Mexiletine in treatment-resistant bipolar disorder. *J Affect Disord* 2000; 57: 249–253.

Sidor MM, Macqueen GM. Antidepressants for the acute treatment of bipolar depression: a systematic review and meta-analysis. *J Clin Psychiatry* 2011; 72: 156–167.

Small JG, Klapper MH, Kellams JJ, Miller MJ, Milstein V, Sharpley PH, Small IF. Electroconvulsive treatment compared with lithium in the management of manic states. *Arch Gen Psychiatry* 1998; 45: 727–732.

Smeraldi E, Benedetti F, Barbini B, Campori E, Colombo C. Sustained antidepressant effect of sleep deprivation combined with pindolol in bipolar depression. A placebo-controlled trial. *Neuropsychopharmacology* 1999; 20(4): 380–385.

Suppes T, Webb A, Paul B, Carody T, Kraemer H, Rush AJ. Clinical outcome in a randomized 1-year trial of clozapine versus treatment as usual for patients with treatment resistance and a history of mania. *Am J Psychiatry* 1999; 156: 1164–1169.

Thase ME, Mallinger AG, McKnight D, Himmelhoch J. Treatment of imipramine-resistant recurrent depression, IV: a double-blind crossover study of tranylcypromine for anergic bipolar depression. *Am J Psychiatry* 1992; 149: 195–198.

Tohen M, Frank E, Bowden CL, Colom F, Ghaemi SN, Yatham LN, Malhi GS, Calabrese JR, Nolen WA, Vieta E, Kapczinski F, Goodwin GM, Suppes T, Sachs GS, Chengappa KR, Grunze H, Mitchell PB, Kanba S, Berk M. The International Society for Bipolar Disorders (ISBD) Task Force report on the nomenclature of course and outcome in bipolar disorders. *Bipolar Disord* 2009; 11: 453–473.

Tye SJ, Frye MA, Lee KH. Disrupting disordered neurocircuitry: treating refractory psychiatric illness with neuromodulation. *Mayo Clin Proc* 2009; 84: 522–532.

van der Loos MD, Mulder PG, Hartong EG, Blom MB, Vergouwen AC, de Keyzer HJ, Notten PJ, Luteijn ML, Timmermans MA, Vieta E, Nolen WA, LamLit Study Group. Efficacy and safety of lamotrigine as add-on treatment to lithium in bipolar depression: a multicenter, double-blind, placebo-controlled trials. *J Clin Psychiatry* 2009; 70: 223–231.

Vieta E, Martinex-Aran A, Goikolea JN, Torrent C, Colom F, Benabarre A, Reinares M. A randomized trial comparing paroxetine and venlafaxine in the treatment of bipolar depressed patients taking mood stabilizers. *J Clin Psychiatry* 2002; 63: 508–512.

Yatham LN. New anticonvulsants in the treatment of bipolar disorder. *J Clin Psychiatry* 2004: 65S: 28–35.

Yildiz A, Gulervuz S, Ankerst DP, Ongur D, Renshaw PF. Protein kinase C inhibition in the treatment of mania: a double-blind, placebo-controlled trial of Tamofen. *Arch Gen Psychiatry* 2008; 65: 255–263.

Zarate CA, Payne JL, Singh J, Quiroz JA, Luckenbaugh DA, Denicoff KD, Charney DS, Manji HK. Pramipexole for bipolar II depression: a placebo-controlled proof of concept study. *Biol Psychiatry* 2004; 56(1): 54–60.

Zimmerman M, Galione JN, Ruggero CJ, Chelminski I, Young D, Dairymple K, McGlinchey JB. Screening for bipolar disorder and finding borderline personality disorder. *J Clin Psychiatry* 2010b; 71: 1212–1214.

Zimmerman M, Gallone JN, Chelminski I, Young D, Dairymple K. Psychiatric diagnoses in patients who screen positive on the Mood Disorder Questionnaire: implications for using the scale as a case-finding instrument for bipolar disorder. *Psychiatry Res* 2010a. [Epub ahead of print].

Assessment and Management of Treatment Resistance in Panic Disorder

R. Bruce Lydiard

Introduction

Panic disorder (PD) is a severe and potentially disabling anxiety disorder that affects 3.5%–5% of individuals in the United States during their lives (American Psychiatric Association [APA], 2000; Kessler et al., 2006). Panic attacks are characterized by a sudden surge of physical symptoms accompanied by cognitive symptoms, including fear of dying or losing control/going crazy, with at least four symptoms (Table 5.1).

For the diagnosis of PD, the individual experiences a change in behavior and/or cognition that persists for at least 1 month. It is characterized by recurrent unexpected panic attacks (see Table 5.2), at least one of which is followed by ≥ 1 month of one or more of the following: (a) concern over having more attacks; (b) worrying about the implications of the attacks (e.g., having a heart attack, losing control, or "going crazy"); and (c) significant change in behavior related to the attacks (help seeking, fearful avoidance) (APA, 2000). PD most frequently appears in the late teens or early twenties and affects women twice as often as men. A significant percentage of affected individuals exhibit fear and avoidance of situations in which they may be unable to escape or which may be embarrassing should another attack occur (agoraphobia; APA, 2000). The avoidance behavior can interfere with work, social, and family functioning (or all of these); and it can range from mild to completely disabling. PD rarely occurs alone but typically co-occurs with other anxiety disorders, depression, or for some, alcohol/substance abuse disorders (Bolton et al., 2006; Kessler et al., 2006; Mueller & Swift, 1992; Zimmerman et al., 2003). Comorbid agoraphobia and other psychiatric disorders represent a significant treatment challenge and appear to contribute to increasingly poor outcome as they accrue (Bruce et al., 2005; Keller & Hanks, 1993). In the published treatment research literature, patients with comorbid disorders were typically excluded, thus limiting extrapolation of many research findings to clinical practice. Findings from the

TABLE 5.1 *DSM-IV-TR* Diagnostic Criteria for Panic Attack

A discrete period of intense fear or discomfort, in which four (or more) of the following symptoms developed abruptly and reached a peak within 10 minutes:
1. Palpitations, pounding heart, or accelerated heart rate
2. Sweating
3. Trembling or shaking
4. Sensations of shortness of breath or smothering
5. Feeling of choking
6. Chest pain or discomfort
7. Nausea or abdominal distress
8. Feeling dizzy, unsteady, light-headed, or faint
9. Derealization (feelings of unreality) or depersonalization (being detached from oneself)
10. Fear of losing control or going crazy
11. Fear of dying
12. Paresthesias (numbness or tingling sensations)
13. Chills or hot flushes

National Comorbidity Study indicated that while 96.1% of individuals with PD with agoraphobia sought treatment within the past year, nearly half received suboptimal treatment (Kessler et al., 2006).

This chapter will focus on the assessment and management of inadequate treatment outcome in PD. The term "treatment resistance" for PD has not been formalized. Much of the extant literature consists of reports including small groups of patients and case reports on treatment of PD patients with "unsatisfactory" response to one or several treatments, often without defining the degree of improvement or the treatments received. Likewise, there has been no consensus on what constitutes "adequate treatment" with medications or psychosocial treatment such as cognitive-behavioral therapy (CBT), although some suggestions have been offered (APA, 2009).

Following a brief discussion of relevant neurobiology, some general principles for optimizing treatment for PD will be discussed. Finally, a differential diagnostic approach to systematic evaluation of unsatisfactory treatment outcome in PD will be outlined.

Panic Disorder: Relevant Neurobiology

Gorman and colleagues proposed a neuroanatomic fear network model that integrates the empirical evidence that both pharmacotherapy and CBT were effective in the treatment of PD (Gorman et al., 2000). This model proposes that in PD and other anxiety disorders, there

TABLE 5.2 *DSM-IV TR* Diagnostic Criteria for Panic Disorder

1. Recurrent unexpected panic attacks
2. At least one of the attacks has been followed by 1 month (or more) of one or more of the following:
   —persistent concern about having additional attacks
   —worry about the implication of the attack or its consequences
   —a significant change in behavior related to the attacks
3. The panic attacks are not due to the direct physiological effects of a substance or a general medical condition.
4. The panic attacks are not better accounted for by another mental disorder, such as social phobia, obsessive-compulsive disorder, posttraumatic stress disorder, or separation anxiety disorder.

is an abnormally sensitized "fear network" in which the central nucleus of the amygdala functions as the "alarm button." When activated, it initiates panic attacks via projections to key nuclei in the brainstem, thalamus, and hypothalamus. Under normal conditions, inhibitory effects from the hippocampus and medial prefrontal cortex (mPFC) modulate the excitability of amygdala and other lower brain nuclei. Failure of effective inhibition results in panic attacks, fearful avoidance, other panic-related symptoms, and functional impairment. This model predicts that pharmacotherapy exerts therapeutic effects by normalizing the reactivity of the amygdala and brainstem areas within the fear network to suppress panic attacks, followed in turn by decreased anticipatory anxiety and reduction in conditioned fear behaviors. CBT is predicted to work "upstream" by normalizing distorted cognitions, enhancing the ability of the higher cortical structures to exert inhibitory effects on lower brain structures, and reducing panic attacks and related learned fear responses.

Corticotropin-releasing factor (CRF) is an anxiogenic neuropeptide that plays an important role in mediating the stress response, fear, arousal, depression, and anxiety (Binder & Nemeroff, 2010; Coplan & Lydiard, 1998; Stout, Owens, & Nemeroff, 2003; Weiss et al., 1994). Preclinical research has shown that effective antipanic drug treatments exert direct or indirect effects to diminish CRF activity, synthesis, or postsynaptic reactivity to CRF release (Stout et al., 2003).

Other neurobiological findings in persons with PD include abnormally low occipital lobe concentrations of the inhibitory neurotransmitter gamma-amino-butyric acid (GABA) (Goddard et al., 2001b), reduced response of individuals with PD to acute benzodiazepine (BZD) administration (Goddard et al., 2004; Roy-Byrne et al., 1990), reduced density of brain BZD receptors (Bremner et al., 2000), and hypothalamic-pituitary-adrenal axis hyperreactivity in response to experimental contextual external cues suggesting novelty or future challenge (Abelson et al., 2007).

Imaging studies have suggested mPFC abnormalities in PD, including reduced mPFC anatomic volume (Sobanski et al., 2010) and abnormally low mPFC metabolic activity (Sakai et al., 2005). Patients with PD who had achieved remission with treatment showed persistent unstable mPFC responses to experimental emotional conflict stimuli along with activation of lower limbic and brainstem structures (Chechko et al., 2009), suggesting that this is a trait rather than state condition. A recent summary of imaging studies examining PD treatment effects on brain function in PD provided evidence consistent with the theorized CBT facilitation of enhanced cortical function and inhibitory effects on lower structures (de Carvalho, Rosenthal, & Nardi, 2010). The imaging studies examining changes after antidepressant treatment of PD were more complex but overlapped with areas affected by CBT treatment (Prasko et al, 2004; Sim, Kang, & Yu, 2010).

General Principles for Optimizing Treatment of Panic Disorder

The Initial Evaluation

The initial assessment should include a thorough psychiatric history to confirm the diagnosis of PD and screening for comorbid psychiatric disorders, including other anxiety disorders and depression. A history of any prior treatment and outcomes should be obtained. Assessment of patient safety, including current and past suicidal ideation, self-injury, family history of suicide, current psychosocial stressors, and current protective factors (family and friends, spirituality and religious belief, and problem-solving skill), is essential (APA, 2009). Psychosocial and developmental history, including childhood adversity, family psychiatric history, and general review of symptoms, should be included.

A medical history and current medications, including asthma treatments (steroids, bronchodilators), sedative-hypnotic-alcohol use (withdrawal), substance abuse history (cannabis, stimulants), usual caffeine intake (including soft drinks, energy drinks, tea, and coffee), over-the-counter medications including decongestants (pseudoephedrine, phenylpropanolamine), and any alternative or herbal treatments that can cause anxiety, should be completed (Simon & Fischmann 2005; Zaubler & Katin, 1996). The medical workup should include a complete physical examination, complete blood count, thyroid function tests, urinalysis, urine screen for abused drugs, electrolytes and liver function tests, and electrocardiogram. Certain presentations should encourage more thorough assessment. These include PD onset over age 40, true vertigo, timing of anxiety clearly related to meals, loss of consciousness, amnestic episodes, and panic attacks without fear (Zaubler & Katon, 1996).

The Therapeutic Alliance

Establishing and maintaining credibility with the patient is a key strategy for successful treatment outcome. Educating the patient about PD at each opportunity can promote compliance with treatment.

Evidence that the risk for PD can be inherited may help to reduce the patient's sense of failure to manage panic symptoms on his or her own. Particularly at the beginning of treatment, being available and encouraging questions will help foster a sense of trust. Review the available empirically proven treatment options, including pros and cons of each. It is advisable to inform the patient that there are several options beyond the initial treatment and that it is not uncommon to try more than one treatment or treatment modality in order to find the best "fit" for that individual. Assuring the patient that there is always flexibility in the treatment process can enhance compliance. If possible, include significant others in this discussion.

Assessment and Documentation of Baseline Severity and Change with Treatment

To determine whether a patient has improved, assessing the initial severity of the illness with standardized instruments will allow for effective assessment of severity and change during treatment (APA, 2009). Measurement of panic attack frequency was used as the primary outcome measure of many earlier treatment studies. It has been shown that panic attack frequency correlates poorly with global improvement and other measures of panic-related symptoms (Michelson et al., 1999) and is not adequate as a main outcome measure. The Panic Disorder Severity Scale (PDSS) (Shear et al., 2001) is a clinically useful, validated rating for PD assessment (Furukawa et al., 2009). The PDSS assesses frequency of panic attacks, degree of distress related to the attacks, anticipatory anxiety, phobic avoidance, and illness interference with work and social functioning. For depression, validated self-rating scales for depression such as Hospital Anxiety and Depression Scale (HADS) (Zigmond & Snaith, 1983) or Quick Inventory of Depressive Symptomatology (QUIDS) (Bernstein et al., 2007) can supplement the initial clinical interview and help track progress at subsequent meetings.

Choice of Treatment

Patient Factors

The choice of the initial treatment involves a collaborative interchange between patient and clinician, the wishes and beliefs of the patient, the orientation and expertise of the clinician, and the severity of the PD. The two first-line treatment choices recommended in the American Psychiatric Association Treatment Guidelines for PD (APA, 2009) include pharmacotherapy and psychosocial therapy such as CBT, usually with exposure. Attention to whether the most distressing panic symptoms for that patient are physiological (e.g., cardiorespiratory, gastrointestinal, neurological) or more psychological concerns (fear of going crazy, catastrophic interpretation, distorted cognition) may inform the choice of initial treatment (APA, 2009) (see Figure 5.1).

Pharmacotherapy

The selective serotonin reuptake inhibitors (SSRIs), serotonin-norepinephrine reuptake inhibitors (SNRIs), tricyclic antidepressants (TCAs), traditional monoamine oxidase inhibitors (MAOIs), and the benzodiazepines (BZDs) are approximately equally efficacious in the treatment of panic disorder (APA, 2009; Otto et al., 2001; Stein et al., 2010). Treatment choice is guided by the individual's prior treatment history, concurrent medical and psychiatric conditions, the pharmacokinetic and pharmacodynamic properties of the individual agent (half-life, drug-drug interactions, side effects), and cost and availability.

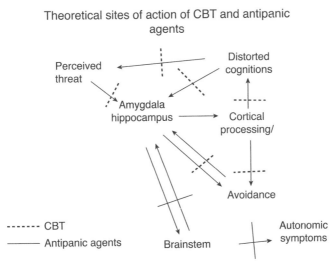

FIGURE 5.1 Cognitive-behavioral therapy (CBT) and pharmacotherapy target different brain areas.

Antidepressants

Based on their breadth of efficacy, tolerability, ease of administration, and safety in overdose compared to older agents, the SSRIs and SNRIs are recommended as the first-line treatment for patients with PD with or without comorbidity (APA, 2009; Stein et al., 2010). Most are available as inexpensive generic agents. SSRIs available in the United States include sertraline, paroxetine, fluoxetine, fluvoxamine, citalopram, and escitalopram. All have been shown in multicenter studies to be effective for treating PD (Stein et al., 2010). Fluoxetine, sertraline, and paroxetine have received Food and Drug Administration (FDA) approval. The SNRI venlafaxine also has FDA approval for PD, and it is generally considered as equivalent in efficacy to SSRIs for the treatment of PD.

Tricyclic Antidepressants

Imipramine (IMI) is the most well studied (Cross-National Collaborative Panic Study Group, 1992). Clomipramine, a TCA with potent inhibitor of serotonin reuptake, is effective in the treatment of PD and has a greater breadth of efficacy than the other TCAs (Hoffart et al., 1993; Lecrubier, 1998). While TCAs are as effective as SSRIS for PD, the predictable side effect burden and danger in overdose limit enthusiasm for their use unless first-line treatments fail.

Monoamine Oxidase Inhibitors

The traditional nonselective agents such as phenelzine and tranylcypromine have not been studied in *DSM*-defined PD but are effective in individuals with phobic avoidance with panic attacks (Lydiard & Ballenger, 1987). These older nonselective MAOIs are rarely used due to their side effect burden, toxicity in overdose, and potential for hypertensive crisis after tyramine ingestion. For treatment-resistant PD they should be kept in mind as an alternative for the rare patient who is unresponsive to other pharmacotherapy (Buch & Wagner, 2007). The selective MAO-A inhibitor selegiline has not been studied in PD. The reversible MAOI (moclobemide), which is unavailable in the United States, was not reliably superior to placebo in clinical trials (Stein et al., 2010).

Other Antidepressants

There are insufficient data on the efficacy of mirtazapine and nefazodone (Stein et al., 2010). Data for bupropion show mixed results in open-label studies, and it is not recommended (Sheehan et al., 1983; Simon et al., 2003) as first-line treatment. Bupropion may be coprescribed to address depression or sexual side effects of antidepressant treatment (Labbate et al., 1997).

Benzodiazepines

The most well studied BZDs are alprazolam and clonazepam. Other less well studied BZDs, including lorazepam and diazepam, are also effective for PD (APA, 2009; Lydiard et al., 2001). Controlled studies in very large PD patient samples confirmed the efficacy of alprazolam to be comparable to imipramine (Cross-National Collaborative Panic Study Group, 1992). Alprazolam is effective and well tolerated, reducing panic attack frequency and severity within the first several days of treatment. Due to the short half-life of alprazolam, multiple daily doses are necessary. For some patients "interdose rebound" can be bothersome (Herman, Brotman, & Rosenbaum, 1987). Clonazepam is twice as potent as alprazolam, and it has efficacy equal to alprazolam (Tesar et al., 1991); both are FDA approved for PD. The long-elimination half-life of clonazepam has the advantage of simplifying treatment to once- or twice-daily administration (Herman et al., 1987). This reduces the severity of withdrawal following abrupt discontinuation, presumably by avoiding wide fluctuations in plasma levels.

Daily administration of BZDs invariably results in the development of physiologic dependence and the appearance of withdrawal upon discontinuation. When treatment is interrupted abruptly, withdrawal symptoms appear. These discontinuation symptoms are less pronounced with clonazepam due to a more gradual decline in plasma concentrations than is observed with more rapidly excreted agents such as alprazolam or lorazepam. For many clinicians and patients, use of the BZDs can be limited by concerns over physiological dependence and also largely unfounded concern over the potential for abuse of BZDs (DuPont, Greene, & Lydiard, 2010). Clinicians should specifically distinguish between "addiction" (nonmedical use) and "physiological dependence" (iatrogenic), as the two terms are unfortunately used interchangeably (Dupont, 1997). Moreover, the empirical evidence indicates that risk for misuse in anxious patients without a history of substance abuse is very low (DuPont, 1997). With long-term use, there is no evidence suggesting dose escalation (Lepola, Rimon, & Riekkinen, 1993; Nagy et al., 1993; Pollack et al., 1993; Rickels & Schweizer, 1998; Rickels et al., 1993). An early pharmaco-epidemiologic study that assessed BZD use or abuse patterns in the United States concluded that *underutilization* of BZDs was a greater problem than the rare cases of abuse of BZDs by anxious individuals (Uhlenhuth et al., 1988).

Unwanted effects of BZDs include sedation, ataxia, fatigue, and subjective memory difficulty. The latter concern—memory disruption—remains controversial (Otto, Bruce, & Deckersbach, 2005) despite evidence to the contrary (DuPont et al., 2010; Gladsjo et al., 2001).

Anticonvulsants

One multicenter, placebo-controlled study of gabapentin supported its efficacy in the treatment of panic disorder (Pande et al., 2000). Sodium valproate (VPA) has been shown to benefit, although the support for its use is limited to open studies (Woodman & Noyes, 1994) and has been reported to be useful for patients with comorbid bipolar disorder and for PD complicated by alcohol abuse (Brady, Sonne, & Lydiard, 1994; Perugi et al., 2010). Evidence for other anticonvulsants such as tiagabine, vigabatrin, and levetiracetam is limited to open-label reports for PD (Lydiard, 2003).

Other Agents

Buspirone, a nonbenzodiazepine anxiolytic, is ineffective as monotherapy for PD (Sheehan, Raj, & Sheehan, 1990).

There is limited, uncontrolled information suggesting beneficial effects from olanzapine (Hollifield et al., 2005; Sepede et al., 2006) and augmentation with risperidone (Simon et al., 2006) in treatment-resistant PD. There is no evidence to support long-term treatment

(Depping et al., 2010). The decision to use second-generation antipsychotics should be limited to severely ill patients for whom no other treatment has been effective.

Cognitive-Behavioral Therapy

CBT treatment has been shown to be as effective for PD as pharmacotherapy in acute treatment, with more durable benefits (Barlow, 2001). It provides an alternative for patients who do not wish to receive medication treatment (APA, 2009). The standard components of CBT for PD include cognitive-restructuring interventions, exposure, and arousal reduction. For patients for whom discontinuation of BZDs is planned, CBT has been shown to significantly increase the likelihood of successful discontinuation (Otto et al., 2010).

CBT treatment requires professional training for optimal results. It is generally provided in 12–16 weekly sessions (Barlow, 2001). Some studies have shown that PD patients with comorbid depression and other anxiety respond well to CBT directed at PD, with eventual significant improvement in both PD and comorbid disorders (Allen et al., 2010; Craske et al., 2007). Others reported less benefit in comorbid patients (Woody et al., 1999).

Adequate Intensity of Treatment

Antidepressants

Adequate dosing is essential for effective treatment of PD. About three-fourths of apparent PD treatment failures are due to inadequate dosage and/or duration of treatment with antipanic medication (Cowley et al. 1997; Roy-Byrne et al., 1999; Simon et al., 2002). The recommended dosage for antipanic medications is mainly derived from fixed-dose (or "dose-finding") studies completed during the process of obtaining FDA approval. If one or more of several fixed doses of medication is found to be statistically significantly superior to placebo, the *Physicians Desk Reference* (PDR) will refer to that dose or range of doses as the "usually effective" or "target" dose. For example, the "target dose" listed in the PDR for paroxetine is noted to be 40 mg daily even though many patients receiving lower doses benefitted. For sertraline the range recommended therapeutic doses of 50–200 mg daily was based on the *lack* of statistical differences between drug groups (50, 100, or 200 mg daily) in pivotal clinical trials. There is no information about efficacy of dosages higher than those studied during drug development in PD studies. Thus, the true optimal dose for a given patient may be higher than the "recommended" dose or range. This must be determined by gradually advancing the dose until full therapeutic effect or limiting side effects occur.

SSRI/SNRI and TCA-induced activation is common during initiation of treatment. This should be explained prior to initiating treatment. Advising the patient that this reaction is not dangerous, and may even suggest that the diagnosis of panic disorder is correct, may help shift the perception of this side effect to a more positive experience. For patients who experience activation from even small initial doses, reducing the dose by dissolving capsules in fruit juice in order to administer a tolerable dose of a few milligrams can be accomplished, with very gradual dose adjustments as tolerated.

TCAs should be reserved for patients with a poor response to at least two first-line agents. Empirical data for the TCAs are limited to imipramine. Mavissakalian and Perel (1989) reported that patients whose daily oral IMI dose was at or above a threshold of about 150 mg oral showed better rates of response versus lower doses. These investigators also reported that patients that achieved steady-state plasma concentrations of (IMI + desipramine combined) in the 125–150 ng/ml range experienced an optimal balance between benefits and side effects reported at higher doses (Mavissakalian & Perel, 1995). For more severely ill patients with comorbid depression, higher doses or levels may be necessary. In addition to targeting plasma levels, TCA levels can also be useful in confirming compliance.

Benzodiazepines

For most patients, doses of alprazolam in the range of 1.5 to 5 mg daily are sufficient (Lesser et al., 1992; Lydiard et al., 1992). A dose-finding study comparing several dosages of clonazepam versus placebo suggested that the "optimal" dose for clonazepam is approximately 2–4 mg daily. For clinical use, clonazepam appears to be about twice as potent as alprazolam (Tesar et al., 1991).

When there is an inadequate response, adherence with treatment is unclear, or if an individual patient appears to require higher levels than expected, plasma levels of BZDs are clinically useful. Fixed-dose studies of alprazolam show that each oral dose of 1 mg is associated with 10 ng/ml at steady-state plasma levels. Maximal clinical improvement with a tolerable side effects burden appeared to be in the 20–60 ng/ml range (correlating with 2–6 mg daily dose) (Lesser et al., 1992). For the occasional patients who appear to require an unusually high oral dose of alprazolam to achieve the desired therapeutic effect, plasma levels are helpful in determining whether patients are rapid metabolizers or are among those who need unusually high doses to achieve therapeutic plasma levels.

Adequate treatment also requires an appropriate duration of treatment at an effective dose. The available information from the published literature indicates that for uncomplicated PD, improvement in panic attack frequency is usually observable within 4–6 weeks for antidepressants and for BZDs often within the first week. For more highly comorbid patients, the response may be slower and the observation for response should be accordingly longer: 8–12 weeks. When it appears that further benefit at a given dose is unlikely, a systematic dose increase with observation at appropriate (8–12 week) intervals can avoid adverse effects and optimize benefit. Table 5.3 shows recommendations based on the published literature (APA, 2009; Stein et al., 2010). If the upper limit of the dosage range shown is reached, and there is clinically significant partial response with tolerable side effects, gradually increasing the dose and close monitoring for improvement and tolerability of side effects is a reasonable strategy. The psychiatrist can address medicolegal concerns by documenting the rationale for prescribing higher dosages, that risks and benefits have been discussed, and that the patient understands and agrees. If the psychiatrist or patient has significant concerns about higher dosages, referral for consultation to a psychiatrist with an expertise in anxiety disorders can help reassure the patient and the clinician.

Cognitive-Behavioral Therapy

The adequacy of CBT treatment "dose" is a function of the number of sessions, the protocol being used, and the skill of the therapist. Manualized treatments have substantially standardized CBT. The number of CBT sessions suggested by experts as adequate should be

TABLE 5.3 Dosage Ranges for Antipanic Medications

Agents	(T1/2,hr)	Suggested Dosage Range (mg/d)	Initial Dose (mg/d)
SSRIs/SNRIs			
Fluoxetine	24–72	20–40	5–10
Citalopram	35	20–40	5
Sertraline	24	100–200	12.5–25
Paroxetine	21	20–40	5–10
Escitalopram	27–32	10–20	5
Fluvoxamine	15	100–200	25
Venlafaxine	5–11	150–225	12.5
Benzodiazepines			
Alprazolam[a]	6–12	2–6	0.5–1
Lorazepam[a]	8–12	2–8	1.5–2
Clonazepam	18–50	1–4	0.25–0.5
Tricyclics			
Imipramine[b]	12–24	150–300	10
Clomipramine	11–20	50–150	10
Desipramine	28–36	100–200	10
MAOIs			
Phenelzine	—	45–60	15
Tranylcypromine	—	30–40	10

Note. Some patients will require higher doses than recommended range.
[a]Multiple divided doses necessary.
[b]Plasma levels can guide treatment.
MAOIs, monoamine oxidase inhibitors; SNRIs, serotonin–norepinephrine reuptake inhibitors; SSRIs, selective serotonin reuptake inhibitors.

12–16 weekly sessions (Barlow, 2001). Effective CBT in some published studies can be accomplished in as few as 5 sessions (Pollack et al., 2008).

Differential Diagnosis for Inadequate Response to Initial Treatment

Persistent Panic Attacks

The first item on the differential diagnosis for persistent unexpected panic attacks is inadequate intensity of treatment. If unexpected panic attacks persist, and pharmacotherapy has been sufficient in dose and duration, adding CBT is a good strategy. For attacks that appear to be primarily stimulus bound, consider other anxiety disorders such as social anxiety disorder (SAD), generalized anxiety disorder (GAD), posttraumatic stress disorder (PTSD), or obsessive-compulsive disorder (OCD), each of which can be associated with panic attacks (Craske et al., 2010; Jack, Heimberg, & Mennin, 1999). Disorder-specific CBT (with exposure if indicated) should be added to treatment. Increasing the dose of the antidepressant and/or adding a BZD may be useful. Switching to a different SSRI or SNRI with efficacy for the comorbid anxiety disorder may be required (see Table 5.4).

TABLE 5.4 Differential Diagnosis for Inadequate Treatment Response in Panic Disorder

Persistent Symptom(s)	Differential Diagnosis	Suggested Approach
Persistent panic attacks	Unexpected	Inadequate treatment intensity: Adjust accordingly Partial response: —Increase dose and observe —Augment with second agent —CBT/exposure —Imipramine with plasma levels No response: —Reconsider diagnosis —Switch to different agent or CBT
	Situationally bound	Agoraphobia: —add CBT/exposure
	Situationally bound	Related to PTSD, social anxiety, OCD: —Disorder-specific CBT —Increase AD dose —Add BZD
	Medical condition or treatment Caffeine excess	Address as indicated
Persistent nonpanic anxiety	Residual anticipatory anxiety	Add/increase dose BZD Add CBT
	Antidepressant-related activation	Adjust dosage Add BZD, beta blocker
	Interdose BZD rebound	Long-acting BZD
	Psychosocial stress	Patient education Environmental hygiene Adjust treatment plan as needed
	Alcohol/substance abuse	Assess, treat, or refer
	Generalized anxiety disorder	Increase antidepressant dose Add or increase BZD Disorder-specific CBT
Residual avoidance	Agoraphobia	CBT/exposure
	Social anxiety, PTSD, OCD	Disorder-specific CBT/exposure
Other psychiatric disorders	Depression	Increase antidepressant treatment Add CBT
	Bipolar disorder	Mood stabilizer ± BZD Discontinue antidepressant if possible
Nonadherence	Inadequate patient or family understanding	Education information resources
	Sexual dysfunction or weight gain	Bupropion, sildenafil, switch agents

CBT, cognitive-behavioral therapy; OCD, obsessive compulsive disorder; PTSD, posttraumatic stress disorder.

Persistent Nonpanic Anxiety

Comorbid anxiety disorders such as SAD, GAD, or PTSD contribute to overall anxiety symptoms. If the patient is receiving an intermediate half-life BZD such as alprazolam or lorazepam, interdose rebound may cause recurrent periodic anxiety or even panic attacks. Review current medications and any new medications, including alternative or herbal remedies that the patient may not have shared with the provider. Previously undetected alcohol and/or substance abuse can worsen PD and interfere with treatment (Otto et al., 1992; Robinson et al., 2009). Although there is evidence that SSRIs and CBT alone may benefit anxiety in alcohol-dependent patients, they may not meaningfully enhance long-term relapse risk (Schade et al., 2007). Review of initially reported medical problems, possible new medical problems, or changes in treatment that may have any potential contribution to anxiety should be completed, and treatment should be adjusted accordingly. Intolerance to antidepressants, as noted earlier, can promote anxiety.

Comorbid Mood Disorder

In community studies, PD is often associated with comorbid major depression. When depression and PD coexist, both disorders are more severe, more persistent, and less likely to respond to standard treatments (Keller & Hanks, 1993; Kessler et al., 1998; Roy-Byrne et al., 2000). There are no established guidelines for this important subgroup of patients, but it is clear that treatment intensity should be maximized for patients with PD and comorbid depression who have only partially responded to initial treatment. For such patients, increasing the dose of antidepressant incrementally and observing for improvement is often helpful.

For patients with depression who do not respond to aggressive pharmacotherapy with first-line antidepressants or CBT, using imipramine with targeted plasma levels is a reasonable consideration. For some patients, improvement can be maintained with gradually switching to an SSRI or SNRI and tapering imipramine.

There is significant co-occurrence of PD and bipolar disorder (Doughty et al., 2004 Goodwin & Hoven, 2002; Kilbane et al., 2009; Simon & Fischmann 2005). Coexisting PD and bipolar disorder predicts poor prognosis for both conditions (El-Mallakh & Hollifield, 2008; Lee & Dunner, 2008). Comorbid bipolar II disorder may be overlooked during the initial evaluation, as these patients often fail to identify periods of hypomania as problematic. In addition, a positive family history for cyclic mood changes can help increase the index of suspicion. Because antidepressant treatment causes mood instability, the treatment prescribed should include reduction or discontinuation of antidepressant treatment if possible, and adding a mood stabilizer. Limited data suggest VPA treatment (Woodman & Noyes, 1994) may be a good choice. VPA has been reported to be beneficial in patients with comorbid PD and bipolar disorder, including a subgroup further complicated by alcohol abuse (Brady et al., 1994; Perugi et al., 2002, 2010). Short-term atypical antipsychotics have been reported to be beneficial for some patients (Menaster, 2005; Oruc & Cavaljuga, 2003). The risk of antipsychotic treatment must be considered in the context of the severity and functional impairment of the individual patient.

Residual Phobic Avoidance

The differential diagnosis for residual avoidance includes evaluation of whether there was insufficient exposure for agoraphobia or if there may be concurrent anxiety disorder with related avoidance (SAD, PTSD, OCD). If avoidance is being driven by a comorbid anxiety disorder, disorder-specific CBT should be added. If social avoidance due to demoralization or social withdrawal secondary to depressed mood appears to be promoting avoidance, the appropriate course of action should be pursued.

Other Factors

New onset or worsening of preexisting psychosocial stress can exacerbate PD and interfere with PD treatment. Reassessment should include asking about new problems, interpersonal difficulties, and occupational or family stressors. Noncompliance with treatment can result from lack of sufficient patient understanding of the principles of treatment, including compliance with medication administration or behavioral changes prescribed. Some patients or significant others require refresher information sessions about the nature of the illness and/or the requirements for adequate treatment.

The Next Step: After the First Treatment Fails

If the issues of diagnosis, treatment intensity, and other factors noted earlier have been addressed, and unsatisfactory response is apparent, it makes sense to change the treatment. The options are to augment the initial treatment agent or modality or switch to a different treatment agent or modality. The empirical literature in this area is very limited. The majority of published studies reporting beneficial effects from treatment changes included patient samples that were not carefully characterized. The only published study to date that prospectively studied SSRI treatment resistance and that used state-of-the-art methods was inconclusive due to its small sample (Simon et al., 2009). However, it did support the concept that supplementing pharmacotherapy with CBT, increased dose of the initial agent, or adding a BZD were all equally effective, though there were very limited increases in remission. While not as illuminating as would be hoped, the study is a model for future research with sufficiently large sample sizes and adequate statistical power.

Augmentation of Pharmacotherapy

Several augmentation strategies that have been reported to improve inadequate response in PD have been reported, but none has been intensively studied. Lacking empirical proof, there is substantial clinical experience suggesting that adding a BZD can be beneficial. Pindolol, a β-adrenergic antagonist with 5HT1a agonist properties that has been shown to be useful as an augmenting agent in resistant depression in some studies, has been shown in one small controlled study to benefit patients who had not responded to 20 mg fluoxetine for 8 weeks (Hirschman et al, 2000; Herman, Brotman, & Rosenbaum, 1987). The dose (Michelson et al., 1998) and duration of SSRI treatment in that study may have been inadequate. One case series reported that combining an SSRI and TCA was helpful for patients unreponsive to either alone (Tiffon et al., 1994). There are limited uncontrolled data supporting the utility of mirtazapine for PD as an augmenting strategy (APA, 2009; Carli et al., 2002). Uncontrolled reports have suggested the utility of addition of atypical neuroleptics in treatment-resistant PD (Hollifield et al., 2005; Simon et al., 2006). However, this practice should be considered only for very severely ill and treatment-resistant PD patients. Repetitive transcranial magnetic stimulation as an augmentation treatment was shown to be beneficial in a small group of PD patients who were unresponsive to SSRIs (Prasko et al., 2007), though this approach is probably not practical or widely available, and it is expensive in cost.

Finally, there is evidence that the addition of CBT to augment inadequately effective drug treatment for PD has been shown to be an effective strategy (Heldt et al., 2006; Otto et al., 1999; Pollack et al., 1994).

Augmentation of Cognitive-Behavioral Therapy

There are only limited data regarding the addition of pharmacotherapy to partial responders to CBT. Clomipramine augmentation of unsuccessful behavioral treatment for hospitalized patients has been reported to be effective (Hoffart et al., 1993). For outpatients who were inadequately responsive to CBT, adding the SSRI paroxetine has been shown to be an effective strategy (Kampman et al., 2002).

The literature on combined treatments has generally suggested a slight advantage for combined medication and psychotherapy over either monotherapy alone. Following treatment discontinuation, combined treatments were comparable to psychotherapy alone, and slightly better than medication alone (Barlow et al., 2000; Furukawa, Watanabe, & Churchill, 2007). There are a few studies that have examined combining clonazepam initially with SSRI treatment and tapering the clonazepam after a few weeks, and they showed faster onset with the combination (Goddard et al., 2001a; Pollack et al., 2003).

Switching Treatment

If there is no response with the initial monotherapy, switching treatments is indicated. For pharmacotherapy, switching to a different first-line treatment (a different SSRI or to an SNRI) is recommended. After two SSRIs or an SSRI and an SNRI, second-line pharmacotherapy such as TCAs or benzodiazepines is warranted (APA, 2009). When switching from one SSRI or SNRI antidepressant to another, it is common practice to add the second agent and gradually increase the dose with gradual up-titration to a moderate dose treatment (for example, 150 mg sertraline or venlafaxine) and then gradually down-titrating the initially prescribed agent. Careful additional upward titration during or after the process of cross-titration can avoid SSRI discontinuation symptoms. The process takes several weeks and requires careful observation.

For patients who are considered appropriate and willing to follow a low-tyramine diet, the older MAOIs may be beneficial. There is no empirical basis beyond the older published literature, but one recent report suggested benefits from phenelzine after other treatments were unhelpful (Buch & Wagner, 2007). Use of these older MAOIs should be undertaken by psychiatrists familiar with their use and the management of their side effects. Introducing these agents requires tapering and discontinuation of other antidepressants for at least 2 weeks prior to initiating treatment, longer with fluoxetine.

With the exception of one controlled study of psychodynamic psychotherapy for PD (Milrod et al., 2007), there is no alternative to individual or group CBT that has been empirically shown to be effective for PD. Other approaches that enhance treatment adherence, provide more information, or otherwise support the individual should be made based on the psychiatrist's knowledge of the patient.

Conclusions

Treatment of PD has evolved and improved substantially as our understanding of the neurobiology and neurobiological substrates of anxiety have expanded. The optimal treatment must still be individualized for each patient. A systematic, differential diagnostic approach to the evaluation and optimal treatment of PD has been presented. As research provides more information on optimizing treatment, additional advances in providing relief for the many individuals who suffer from PD will be made. Undertreatment of PD remains a major problem. The most important of the identified factors for promoting adequate treatment of PD is insufficient intensity of treatment.

Disclosure Statement

R.B.L. has no financial conflicts.

References

Abelson JL, Khan S, Liberzon I, Young EA. HPA axis activity in patients with panic disorder: Review and synthesis of four studies. *Depress Anxiety* 2007;24(1):66–76.

Allen LB, White KS, Barlow DH, Shear MK, Gorman JM, Woods SW. Cognitive-Behavior Therapy (CBT) for panic disorder: Relationship of anxiety and depression comorbidity with treatment outcome. *J Psychopathol Behav Assess* 2010;32(2):185–192.

American Psychiatric Association. Diagnostic and Statistical Manual for Mental Disorders, 4th ed, rev. Washington, DC: American Psychiatric Association; 2000.

American Psychiatric Association. Practice Guidelines for the Treatment of Persons with Disorder, 2nd ed. Washington, DC: American Psychiatric Association; 2009.

Barlow DH. Clinical Handbook of Psychological Disorders: A Step-by-Step Treatment Manual. New York: Guilford Press; 2001.

Barlow DH, Gorman JM, Shear MK, Woods SW. Cognitive-behavioral therapy, imipramine, or their combination for panic disorder: A randomized controlled trial. *JAMA* 2000;283(19):2529–2536.

Bernstein IH, Rush AJ, Carmody TJ, Woo A, Trivedi MH. Clinical vs. self-report versions of the quick inventory of depressive symptomatology in a public sector sample. *J Psychiatr Res* 2007;3–4:239–246.

Binder EB, Nemeroff CB. The CRF system, stress, depression and anxiety-insights from human genetic studies. *Mol Psychiatry* 2010;15:574–588.

Bolton J, Cox B, Clara I, Sareen J. Use of alcohol and drugs to self-medicate anxiety disorders in a nationally representative sample. *J Nerv Ment Dis* 2006;194(11):818–825.

Brady KT, Sonne S, Lydiard RB. Valproate treatment of comorbid panic disorder and affective disorders in two alcoholic patients. *J Clin Psychopharmacol* 1994;14(1):81–82.

Bremner JD, Innis RB, White T, Fujita M, Silbersweig D, Goddard AW, Staib L, Stern E, Cappiello A, Woods S, Baldwin R, Charney DS. SPECT [I-123]iomazenil measurement of the benzodiazepine receptor in panic disorder. *Biol Psychiatry* 2000;47(2):96–106.

Bruce SE, Yonkers KA, Otto MW, Eisen JL, Weisberg RB, Pagano M, Shea MT, Keller MB. Influence of psychiatric comorbidity on recovery and recurrence in generalized anxiety disorder, social phobia, and panic disorder: A 12-year prospective study. *Am J Psychiatry* 2005;162(6):1179–1187.

Buch S, Wagner M. Successful use of phenelzine in treatment-resistant panic disorder. *J Clinical Psychiatry* 2007;68(2):335–336.

Carli V, Sarchiapone M, Camardese G, Romano L, DeRisio S. Mirtazapine in the treatment of panic disorder. *Arch Gen Psychiatry* 2002;59(7):661–662.

Chechko N, Wehrle R, Erhardt A, Holsboer F, Czisch M, Samann PG. Unstable prefrontal response to emotional conflict and activation of lower limbic structures and brainstem in remitted panic disorder. *PLoS One* 2009;4(5):e5537.

Coplan JD, Lydiard RB. Brain circuits in panic disorder. *Biol Psychiatry* 1998;44:1264–1276.

Cowley DS, Ha EH, Roy-Byrne PP. Determinants of pharmacologic treatment failure in panic disorder. *J Clin Psychiatry* 1997;58(12):555–561; quiz 62-3.

Craske MG, Farchione TJ, Allen LB, Barrios V, Stoyanova M, Rose R. Cognitive behavioral therapy for panic disorder and comorbidity: More of the same or less of more? *Behav Res Ther* 2007;45(6):1095–1109.

Craske MG, Kircanski K, Epstein A, Wittchen H, Pine DS, Lewis-Fernández R, Hinton D. Panic disorder: A review of DSM-IV panic disorder and proposals for DSM-V. *Depress Anxiety* 2010;27:93–112.

Cross-National Collaborative Panic Study Group. Drug treatment of panic disorder. Comparative efficacy of alprazolam, imipramine, and placebo. *Br J Psychiatry* 1992;161:191–202.

de Carvalho MR, Rozenthal M, Nardi AE. The fear circuitry in panic disorder and its modulation by cognitive-behaviour therapy interventions. *World J Biol Psychiatry* 2010;11:188–198.

Depping AM, Komossa K, Kissling W, Leucht S. Second-generation antipsychotics for anxiety disorders. *Cochrane Database Syst Rev* 2010(12):CD008120.

Doughty CJ, Wells JE, Joyce PR, Olds RJ, Walsh AE. Bipolar-panic disorder comorbidity within bipolar disorder families: A study of siblings. *Bipolar Disord* 2004;6(3):245–252.

DuPont RL. Panic disorder and addiction: The clinical issues of comorbidity. *Bull Menninger Clin* 1997;61 (2 Suppl A):A54–A65.

Dupont RL, Greene. W, Lydiard RB. Sedatives and hypnotics: Clinical use and abuse. 2010. [accessed May 1, 2011]. Available at: http://www.uptodate.com/contents/sedatives-and-hypnotics-clinical-use-and-abuse.

El-Mallakh RS, Hollifield M. Comorbid anxiety in bipolar disorder alters treatment and prognosis. *Psychiatr Q* 2008;79(2):139–150.

Furukawa TA, Katherine Shear M, Barlow DH, Gorman JM, Woods SW, Money R, Etschel E, Engel RR, Leucht S. Evidence-based guidelines for interpretation of the Panic Disorder Severity Scale. *Depress Anxiety* 2009;26(10):922–929.

Furukawa TA, Watanabe N, Churchill R. Combined psychotherapy plus antidepressants for panic disorder with or without agoraphobia. *Cochrane Database Syst Rev* 2007(1):CD004364.

Gladsjo JA, Rapaport MH, McKinney R, Auerbach M, Hahn T, Rabin A, Oliver T, Haze A, Judd LL. Absence of neuropsychologic deficits in patients receiving long-term treatment with alprazolam-XR for panic disorder. *J Clin Psychopharmacol* 2001;21(2):131–138.

Goddard AW, Brouette T, Almai A, Jetty P, Woods SW, Charney D. Early coadministration of clonazepam with sertraline for panic disorder. *Arch Gen Psychiatry* 2001a;58(7):681–686.

Goddard AW, Mason GF, Almai A, Rothman DL, Behar KL, Petroff OA, Charney DS, Krystal JH. Reductions in occipital cortex GABA levels in panic disorder detected with 1h-magnetic resonance spectroscopy. *Arch Gen Psychiatry* 2001b;58(6):556–561.

Goddard AW, Mason GF, Appel M, Rothman DL, Gueorguieva R, Behar KL, Krystal JH. Impaired GABA neuronal response to acute benzodiazepine administration in panic disorder. *A J Psychiatry* 2004;161(12):2186–2193.

Goodwin RD, Hoven CW. Bipolar-panic comorbidity in the general population: Prevalence and associated morbidity. *J Affect Disord* 2002;70(1):27–33.

Gorman JM, Kent JM, Sullivan GM, Coplan JD. Neuroanatomical hypothesis of panic disorder, revised. *A J Psychiatry* 2000;157(4):493–505.

Heldt E, Gus Manfro G, Kipper L, Blaya C, Isolan L, Otto MW. One-year follow-up of pharmacotherapy-resistant patients with panic disorder treated with cognitive-behavior therapy: Outcome and predictors of remission. *Behav Res Ther* 2006;44(5):657–665.

Herman JB, Brotman AW, Rosenbaum JF. Rebound anxiety in panic disorder patients treated with shorter-acting benzodiazepines. *J Clin Psychiatry* 1987;48 (Suppl):22–28.

Hirschmann S, Dannon PN, Iancu I, Dolberg OT, Zohar J, Grunhaus L. Pindolol augmentation in patients with treatment-resistant panic disorder: A double-blind, placebo-controlled trial. *J Clin Psychopharmacol* 2000;20(5):556–559.

Hoffart A, Due-Madsen J, Lande B, Gude T, Bille H, Torgersen S. Clomipramine in the treatment of agoraphobic inpatients resistant to behavioral therapy. *J Clin Psychiatry* 1993;54(12):481–487.

Hollifield M, Thompson PM, Ruiz JE, Uhlenhuth EH. Potential effectiveness and safety of olanzapine in refractory panic disorder. *Depress Anxiety* 2005;21(1):33–40.

Jack MS, Heimberg RG, Mennin DS. Situational panic attacks: impact on distress and impairment among patients with social phobia. *Depress Anxiety* 1999;10:110–118.

Kampman M, Keijsers GP, Hoogduin CA, Hendriks GJ, A randomized, double-blind, placebo-controlled study of the effects of adjunctive paroxetine in panic disorder patients unsuccessfully treated with cognitive-behavioral therapy alone. *J Clin Psychiatry.* 2002;63:772–777.

Keller MB, Hanks DL. Course and outcome in panic disorder. *Prog Neuropsychopharmacol Biol Psychiatry* 1993;17(4):551–570.

Kessler RC, Chiu WT, Jin R, Ruscio AM, Shear K, Walters EE. The epidemiology of panic attacks, panic disorder, and agoraphobia in the National Comorbidity Survey Replication. *Arch Gen Psychiatry* 2006;63(4): 415–424.

Kessler RC, Stang PE, Wittchen HU, Ustun TB, Roy-Burne PP, Walters EE. Lifetime panic-depression comorbidity in the National Comorbidity Survey. *Arch Gen Psychiatry* 1998;55(9):801–808.

Kilbane EJ, Gokbayrak NS, Galynker I, Cohen L, Tross S. A review of panic and suicide in bipolar disorder: Does comorbidity increase risk? *J Affect Disord* 2009;115(1-2):1–10.

Labbate LA, Grimes JB, Hines A, Pollack MH. Bupropion treatment of serotonin reuptake antidepressant-associated sexual dysfunction. *Ann Clin Psychiatry* 1997;9(4):241–245.

Lecrubier Y. The impact of comorbidity on the treatment of panic disorder. *J Clin Psychiatry* 1998;59(Suppl 8): 11–14; discussion 15–16.

Lee JH, Dunner DL. The effect of anxiety disorder comorbidity on treatment resistant bipolar disorders. *Depress Anxiety* 2008;25(2):91–97.

Lepola UM, Rimon RH, Riekkinen PJ. Three-year follow-up of patients with panic disorder after short-term treatment with alprazolam and imipramine. *Int Clin Psychopharmacol* 1993;8(2):115–118.

Lesser IM, Lydiard RB, Antal E, Rubin RT, Ballenger JC, DuPont R. Alprazolam plasma concentrations and treatment response in panic disorder and agoraphobia. *A J Psychiatry* 1992;149(11):1556–1562.

Lydiard RB. The role of GABA in anxiety disorders. *J Clin Psychiatry* 2003;(64 Suppl 3):21–27.

Lydiard RB, Ballenger JC. Antidepressants in panic disorder and agoraphobia. *J Affect Disord* 1987(13): 153–168.

Lydiard RB, Lesser IM, Ballenger JC, Rubin RT, Laraia M, DuPont R. A fixed-dose study of alprazolam 2 mg, alprazolam 6 mg, and placebo in panic disorder. *J Clin Psychopharmacol* 1992;12(2):96–103.

Lydiard RB, Otto MW, Milrod B. Panic Disorder. In: Gabbard GO, editor. Treatments of Psychiatric Disorders. Washington, DC: American Psychiatric Association; 2001, p. 247–282.

Mavissakalian MR, Perel JM. Imipramine dose-response relationship in panic disorder with agoraphobia. Preliminary findings. *Arch Gen Psychiatry.* 1989;46(2):127–131.

Mavissakalian MR, Perel JM. Imipramine treatment of panic disorder with agoraphobia: Dose ranging and plasma level-response relationships. *A J Psychiatry* 1995;152(5):673–682.

Menaster M. Efficacy of quetiapine in panic disorder with agoraphobia and obsessive-compulsive disorder in a patient with bipolar disorder. *Psychiatry (Edgmont)* 2005;2(9):17–18.

Michelson D, Lydiard RB, Pollack MH, Tamura RN, Hoog SL, Tepner R, Demitrack MA, Tollefson GD. Outcome assessment and clinical improvement in panic disorder: Evidence from a randomized controlled trial of fluoxetine and placebo. The Fluoxetine Panic Disorder Study Group. *A J Psychiatry* 1998;155(11):1570–1577.

Michelson D, Pollack M, Lydiard RB, Tamura R, Tepner R, Tollefson G. Continuing treatment of panic disorder after acute response: Randomised, placebo-controlled trial with fluoxetine. The Fluoxetine Panic Disorder Study Group. *Br J Psychiatry* 1999;174:213–218.

Milrod B, Leon AC, Busch F, Rudden M, Schwalberg M, Clarkin J, Aronson A, Singer M, Turchin W, Klass ET, Graf E, Teres JJ, Shear MK. A randomized controlled clinical trial of psychoanalyticpsychotherapy for panic disorder. *Am J Psychiatry* 2007;164:265–272.

Mueller TI, Swift RM. Comorbidity of panic disorder and substance use disorders. *R I Med* 1992;75(5): 277–280.

Nagy LM, Krystal JH, Charney DS, Merikangas KR, Woods SW. Long-term outcome of panic disorder after short-term imipramine and behavioral group treatment: 2.9-year naturalistic follow-up study. *J Clin Psychopharmacol* 1993;13(1):16–24.

Oruc L, Cavaljuga S. Olanzapine in treatment of patients with bipolar 1 disorder and panic comorbidity: a case study. *Bosn J Basic Med Sci* 2003;3(4):67–69.

Otto MW, Bruce SE, Deckersbach T. Benzodiazepine use, cognitive impairment, and cognitive-behavioral therapy for anxiety disorders: Issues in the treatment of a patient in need. *J Clin Psychiatry* 2005;66(Suppl 2):34–38.

Otto MW, McHugh RK, Simon NM, Farach FJ, Worthington JJ, Pollack MH. Efficacy of CBT for benzodiazepine discontinuation in patients with panic disorder: Further evaluation. *Behav Res Ther* 2010;48(8):720–727.

Otto MW, Pollack MH, Penava SJ, Zucker BG. Group cognitive behavior therapy for patients failing to respond to pharmacotherapy for panic disorder: A clinical case series. *Behav Res Ther* 1999;37:763–770.

Otto MW, Pollack MH, Sachs GS, O'Neil CA, Rosenbaum JF. Alcohol dependence in panic disorder patients. *J Psychiatr Res* 1992;26(1):29–38.

Otto MW, Tuby KS, Gould RA, McLean RY, Pollack MH. An effect-size analysis of the relative efficacy and tolerability of serotonin selective reuptake inhibitors for panic disorder. *A J Psychiatry* 2001;158(12):1989–1992.

Pande AC, Pollack MH, Crockatt J, Greiner M, Chouinard G, Lydiard RB, Taylor CB, Dager SR, Shiovitz T. Placebo-controlled study of gabapentin treatment of panic disorder. *J Clin Psychopharmacol* 2000;20(4): 467–471.

Perugi G, Frare F, Toni C, Tusini G, Vannucchi G, Akiskal HS. Adjunctive valproate in panic disorder patients with comorbid bipolar disorder or otherwise resistant to standard antidepressants: A 3-year "open" follow-up study. *Eur Arch Psychiatry Clin Neurosci* 2010;260(7):553–560.

Perugi G, Toni C, Frare F, Ruffolo G, Moretti L, Torti C, Akiskal HS. Effectiveness of adjunctive gabapentin in resistant bipolar disorder: Is it due to anxious-alcohol abuse comorbidity? *J Clin Psychopharmacol* 2002; 22(6):584–591.

Pollack MH, Otto MW, Kaspi SP, Hammerness PG, Rosenbaum JF. Cognitive behavior therapy for treatment-refractory panic disorder. *J Clin Psychiatry* 1994;55(5):200–205.

Pollack MH, Otto MW, Roy-Byrne PP, Coplan JD, Rothbaum BO, Simon NM, Gorman JM. Novel treatment approaches for refractory anxiety disorders. *Depress Anxiety* 2008;25(6):467–476.

Pollack MH, Otto MW, Tesar GE, Cohen LS, Meltzer-Brody S, Rosenbaum JF. Long-term outcome after acute treatment with alprazolam or clonazepam for panic disorder. *J Clin Psychopharmacol* 1993;13(4):257–263.

Pollack MH, Simon NM, Worthington JJ, Doyle AL, Peters P, Toshkov F, Otto MW. Combined paroxetine and clonazepam treatment strategies compared to paroxetine monotherapy for panic disorder. *J Psychopharmacol* 2003;17(3):276–282.

Praško J, Horácek J, Zálesky R, Kopecek M, Novák T, Pašková B, L. S, Belohlávek O, Höschl C. The change of regional brain metabolism (18FDG PET) in panic disorder during the treatment with cognitive behavioral therapy or antidepressants. *Neuro Endocrinol Lett* 2004;5:340–348.

Prasko J, Zalesky R, Bares M, Horacek J, Kopecek M, Novak T, Paskova B. The effect of repetitive transcranial magnetic stimulation (rTMS) add on serotonin reuptake inhibitors in patients with panic disorder: A randomized, double blind sham controlled study. *Neuro Endocrinol Lett* 2007;28(1):33–38.

Rickels K, Schweizer E. Panic disorder: Long-term pharmacotherapy and discontinuation. *J Clin Psychopharmacol* 1998;18(6 Suppl 2):12S–8S.

Rickels K, Schweizer E, Weiss S, Zavodnick S. Maintenance drug treatment for panic disorder. II. Short- and long-term outcome after drug taper. *Arch Gen Psychiatry* 1993;50(1):61–68.

Robinson J, Sareen J, Cox BJ, Bolton J. Self-medication of anxiety disorders with alcohol and drugs: Results from a nationally representative sample. *J Anxiety Disord* 2009;23(1):38–45.

Roy-Byrne PP, Cowley DS, Greenblatt DJ, Shader RI, Hommer D. Reduced benzodiazepine sensitivity in panic disorder. *Arch Gen Psychiatry* 1990;47(6):534–538.

Roy-Byrne PP, Stang P, Wittchen HU, Ustun B, Walters EE, Kessler RC. Lifetime panic-depression comorbidity in the National Comorbidity Survey. Association with symptoms, impairment, course and help-seeking. *Br J Psychiatry* 2000;176:229–235.

Roy-Byrne PP, Stein MB, Russo J, Mercier E, Thomas R, McQuaid J, Katon WJ, Craske MG, Bystritsky A, Sherbourne CD. Panic disorder in the primary care setting: Comorbidity, disability, service utilization, and treatment. *J Clin Psychiatry* 1999;60(7):492–499; quiz 500.

Sakai Y, Kumano H, Nishikawa M, Sakano Y, Kaiya H, Imabayashi E. Cerebral glucose metabolism associated with a fear network in panic disorder. *Neuroreport* 2005;21:927–931.

Schade A, Marquenie LA, van Balkom AJ, Koeter MW, de Beurs E, van Dyck R, van den BW. Anxiety disorders: Treatable regardless of the severity of comorbid alcohol dependence. *Eur Addict Res* 2007;13:109–115.

Sepede G, De Berardis D, Gambi F, Campanella D, La Rovere R, D'Amico M, Cicconetti A, Penna L, Peca S, Carano A, Mancini E, Salerno RM, Ferro FM. Olanzapine augmentation in treatment-resistant panic disorder: A 12-week, fixed-dose, open-label trial. *J Clin Psychopharmacol* 2006;26(1):45–49.

Shear MK, Rucci P, Williams J, Frank E, Grochocinski V, Vander Bilt J, Houck P, Wang T. Reliability and validity of the Panic Disorder Severity Scale: Replication and extension. *J Psychiatr Res* 2001;35(5):293–296.

Sheehan DV, Ballenger J, Jacobsen G. Treatment of endogenous anxiety with phobic, hysterical, and hypochondriacal symptoms. *Arch Gen Psychiatry* 1980;37(1):51–59.

Sheehan DV, Davidson J, Manschreck T, Van Wyck Fleet J. Lack of efficacy of a new antidepressant (bupropion) in the treatment of panic disorder with phobias. *J Clin Psychopharmacol* 1983;3(1):28–31.

Sheehan DV, Raj AB, Sheehan KH, Soto S. Is buspirone effective for panic disorder? *J Clin Psychopharmacol* 1990;10(1):3–11.

Sim H-B, Kang E-H, Yu B-H. Changes in cerebral cortex and limbic brain functions after short-term paroxetine treatment in panic disorder: An [18F]FDG-PET pilot study. *Psychiatry Investig* 2010;3:215–219.

Simon NM, Emmanuel N, Ballenger J, Worthington JJ, Kinrys G, Korbly NB, Farach FJ, Pollack MH. Bupropion sustained release for panic disorder. *Psychopharmacol Bull* 2003;37(4):66–72.

Simon NM, Fischmann D. The implications of medical and psychiatric comorbidity with panic disorder. *J Clin Psychiatry* 2005;66(Suppl 4):8–15.

Simon NM, Hoge EA, Fischmann D, Worthington JJ, Christian KM, Kinrys G, Pollack MH. An open-label trial of risperidone augmentation for refractory anxiety disorders. *J Clin Psychiatry* 2006;67(3):381–385.

Simon NM, Otto MW, Worthington JJ, Hoge EA, Thompson EH, Lebeau RT, Moshier SJ, Zalta AK, Pollack MH. Next-step strategies for panic disorder refractory to initial pharmacotherapy: A 3-phase randomized clinical trial. *J Clin Psychiatry* 2009;70(11):1563–1570.

Simon NM, Safren SA, Otto MW, Sharma SG, Lanka GD, Pollack MH. Longitudinal outcome with pharmacotherapy in a naturalistic study of panic disorder. *J Affect Disord* 2002;69(1–3):201–208.

Sobanski T, Wagner G, Peikert G, Gruhn U, Schluttig K, Sauer H, Schlosser R. Temporal and right frontal lobe alterations in panic disorder: A quantitative volumetric and voxel-based morphometric MRI study. *Psychol Med* 2010;40(11):1879–1886.

Stein MB, Steckler T, Lightfoot JD, Hay E, Goddard GW. Pharmacologic treatment of panic disorder. In: Stein MB, Steckler T, editors. Current Topics in Behavioral Neurosciences. Heidelberg, Germany: Springer-Verlag; 2010, p. 470–481.

Stout SC, Owens MJ, Nemeroff CB. Regulation of corticotropin-releasing factor neuronal systems and hypothalamic-pituitary-adrenal axis activity by stress and chronic antidepressant treatment. *J Pharmacol Exp Ther* 2003;300:1085–1092.

Tesar GE, Rosenbaum JF, Pollack MH, Otto MW, Sachs GS, Herman JB, Cohen LS, Spier SA. Double-blind, placebo-controlled comparison of clonazepam and alprazolam for panic disorder. *J Clin Psychiatry* 1991;52(2):69–76.

Tiffon L, Coplan JD, Papp LA, Gorman JM. Augmentation strategies with tricyclic or fluoxetine treatment in seven partially responsive panic disorder patients. *J Clin Psychiatry* 1994;55(2):66–69.

Uhlenhuth EH, DeWit H, Balter MB, Johanson CE, Mellinger GD. Risks and benefits of long-term benzodiazepine use. *J Clin Psychopharmacol* 1988;8(3):161–167.

Weiss JM, Stout JC, Aaron MF, Quan N, Owens MJ, Butler PD, Nemeroff CB. Depression and anxiety: Role of the locus coeruleus and corticotropin-releasing factor. *Brain Res Bull* 1994;35(5–6):561–572.

Woodman CL, Noyes R, Jr. Panic disorder: Treatment with valproate. *J Clin Psychiatry* 1994;55(4):134–136.

Woody S, McLean PD, Taylor S, Koch WJ. Treatment of major depression in the context of panic disorder. *J Affect Disord* 1999;53(2):163–174.

Zaubler TS, Katon W. Panic disorder and medical comorbidity: A review of the medical and psychiatric literature. *Bull Menninger Clin* 1996;60(2 Suppl A):A12–A38.

Zigmond A, Snaith RP. The Hospital Anxiety and Depression Scale. *Acta Psychiatr Scand* 1983;67:361–370.

Zimmermann P, Wittchen HU, Hofler M, Pfister H, Kessler RC, Lieb R. Primary anxiety disorders and the development of subsequent alcohol use disorders: A 4-year community study of adolescents and young adults. *Psychol Med* 2003;33(7):1211–1222.

Treatment-Resistant Posttraumatic Stress Disorder

Kerry-Ann Louw and Dan J. Stein

Introduction

Posttraumatic stress disorder (PTSD) is a prevalent and disabling condition (Kessler, Sonnega, Bromet, Hughes, & Nelson, 1995). The lifetime prevalence ranges from 6.8% to 12.3% in the general adult population in the United States (Kessler, Chiu, Demler, Merikangas, & Waters, 2005; Kessler et al., 1995; Resnick, Kilpatrick, Dansky, Sanders, & Best, 1993). PTSD has considerable comorbidity with other anxiety disorders, depression, and substance use disorders and an association with increased use of health services (Baldwin et al., 2005). The degree of impairment and disability of PTSD is comparable to other seriously impairing mental disorders (Kessler, 2000).

Given that PTSD represents an important public health problem, it is crucial that effective management and preventive strategies are developed. Fortunately, there have been significant advances in our understanding of PTSD symptoms and their underlying psychobiology (Heim & Nemeroff, 2009). In addition, there is growing evidence supporting the safety and efficacy of pharmacotherapeutic and psychotherapeutic interventions in the treatment of PTSD (Cloitre, 2009; Stein, Ipser, & McAnda, 2009). Unfortunately, a significant proportion of individuals with PTSD do not respond to first-line treatments.

While some of the burden of PTSD may be due to underdiagnosis and undertreatment, such resistance to treatment is also a significant contributor to its negative health impact. This chapter will begin with an overview of the assessment and diagnosis of PTSD and of recent work on its neurobiological underpinnings. Current treatment options, possible factors underlying treatment resistance, and proposed strategies for managing treatment resistance will then be discussed.

Assessment and Diagnosis

The diagnosis of PTSD begins with establishing a history of trauma that is followed by onset of symptoms that fall into three clusters: reexperiencing, avoidance of reminders of the event, and hyperarousal (American Psychiatric Association, 2000). The definition of what constitutes a traumatic event has evolved; in *DSM-IV* a traumatic event is defined as actual or threatened death, serious injury, or threat to the physical integrity of self or others (American Psychiatric Association, 2000). It is important to emphasize that relatively rare but highly traumatizing events (e.g., rape, assault) are very strongly associated with subsequent PTSD, but that the vast majority of traumatic events and PTSD are due to less common events that are more weakly associated with PTSD (e.g., motor vehicle accidents).

It is noteworthy that the vast majority of individuals have experienced traumatic events. Typically, PTSD symptoms experienced after such an event decline over time. Some individuals may meet criteria for acute stress disorder. In a minority of individuals, symptoms persist for longer (greater than a month) and PTSD criteria are met. In the past, PTSD was conceptualized as a normal reaction to an abnormal event, but given data on what kinds of trauma lead to PTSD, and given data on the psychobiology of PTSD (see later discussion), the current view is that PTSD is a pathological response to trauma (Yehuda & McFarlane, 1995).

The risk factors associated with the likelihood of developing PTSD can occur before, during, and after the traumatic event (Brewin, Andrews, & Valentine, 2000; Kroll, 2003). Factors present before the trauma that predict poorer outcome include lower socioeconomic status, female gender, substance misuse, the presence of family or personal history of a psychiatric illness, and a history of parental neglect (Bisson, 2007; Brewin et al., 2000). In addition to the fact that certain kinds of trauma have a higher conditional probability of PTSD (see earlier), other risk factors during exposure to the trauma include duration, severity, and proximity of the trauma, as well as peritraumatic responses such as dissociation (Brewin et al., 2000). Risk factors present after the trauma include lack of social support and additional life stress (Brewin et al., 2000).

Once it has developed, the course of PTSD is often chronic and persisting (Wittchen, Gloster, Beesdo, Schonfeld, & Perkonigg, 2009). In longitudinal studies it has been shown that PTSD symptoms develop shortly after the trauma, subside in many survivors, and persist in others beyond 3 months in the form of chronic PTSD (Peleg & Shalev, 2006). In the United States National Co-morbidity Survey (NCS) over one third of individuals reported having PTSD 6 years after they developed it (Kessler et al., 1995). This chronic form of PTSD is associated with greater morbidity, psychiatric comorbidity, and treatment resistance (Shalev, 2009).

In patients presenting with PTSD, it is important to assess symptom severity, comorbidity, and the various risk factors mentioned earlier. A range of symptom severity measures exist; the Clinician Administered PTSD Scale (CAPS) is the current gold standard in pharmacotherapy trials. The most common comorbid disorders in PTSD are depression, substance use disorders, and other anxiety disorders (Kessler et al., 1995). A range of other symptoms should also be assessed; these include aggression and suicidality (Davidson, Hughes, Blazer, & George, 1991).

Psychobiology of Posttraumatic Stress Disorder

As emphasized earlier, PTSD is increasingly regarded as a pathological condition mediated by dysfunctional psychobiological systems (Yehuda & McFarlane, 1995). Neural networks that regulate fear and stress responses involve the hippocampus, amygdala, and prefrontal cortex (Heim & Nemeroff, 2009). Several neurotransmitters and neuropeptides have been implicated in these circuits. Neurobiological changes in these systems may be responsible for specific features of PTSD such as altered mechanisms of learning and extinction, and sensitization to stress and arousal (Heim & Nemeroff, 2009). A better understanding of these systems is relevant to explaining why certain treatments work and in guiding future targets for pharmacotherapy; these are briefly reviewed in this section.

A key anatomic structure involved in PTSD is the hippocampus. Animal studies show that the hippocampus is implicated in the control of stress responses, declarative and episodic memory, and contextual aspects of fear conditioning (Heim & Nemeroff, 2009). Reduced hippocampal volume and abnormal hippocampal function is a consistent imaging finding in PTSD sufferers (Bremner et al., 1995; Karl et al., 2006). Reduced volume has been thought to be the result of atrophy secondary to chronic stress and glucocorticoid exposure (Heim & Nemeroff, 2009). An alternative view, however, is that reduced hippocampal volume is a risk factor for, rather than a result of, PTSD (Gilbertson et al., 2002). Hippocampal dysfunction may promote activation of stress responses and contribute to impaired extinction of conditioned fear (Heim & Nemeroff, 2009).

Animal studies indicate that the amygdala is involved in emotional processing and the coordination of the automatic threat response (Matthew, Price, & Charney, 2008). Connections between the amygdala and hippocampus are implicated in context conditioning while connections between the amygdala and prefrontal cortex modulate stress responsiveness and mediate extinction of fear memory (Heim & Nemeroff, 2009). The amygdala-cortical pathways also encode the emotional salience and aversiveness of the memories (Ressler & Mayberg, 2007). Brain imaging studies confirm that the amygdala also plays an important role in modulating emotions and fear conditioning in humans (Phelps & LeDoux, 2005). Furthermore, amygdala hyperresponsiveness is seen in imaging studies of PTSD sufferers (Liberzon & Sripada, 2008; Shin, Rauch, & Pitman, 2006), consistent with enhanced fear conditioning.

Basic findings suggest that the prefrontal cortex exerts inhibitory control over the amygdala, therefore diminishing the stress response (Shin et al., 2006). Patients with PTSD may have decreased volumes of the frontal cortex (Rauch et al., 2003) and reduced activation of the prefrontal cortex (Shin et al., 2006). Decreased activity in the medial prefrontal regions of patients with PTSD suggests a failure of higher cortical structures to suppress amygdala processing. During treatment, it might be hypothesized that enhancing cortical control over fear circuits could improve symptoms of PTSD (Shalev, 2009).

The neurotransmitters and neuropeptides involved in these stress and fear response circuits include noradrenaline, serotonin, and glutamate. Noradrenaline (NA) (norepinephrine), a centrally acting catecholamine that mediates the central nervous and autonomic nervous system responses to stress, is thought to play a role in modulating and increasing amygdala activation and enhancing fear conditioning (Geracioti et al., 2001; Ravindra & Stein, 2009). Increased levels of NA may be linked to decreased activity in the prefrontal cortex, with reduced extinction of the fear response (Ravindra & Stein, 2009). Consistent with such a view, the NA system has been found to be hyperactive in individuals with PTSD (Geracioti et al., 2001; Ravindra & Stein, 2009).

The response of PTSD symptoms to selective serotonin inhibitors (SSRIs) indirectly implicates the serotonin system in PTSD (Ravindra & Stein, 2009). Serotonin is thought to play a role in amygdala and hypothalamic-pituitary-adrenal (HPA) axis modulation (Ravindra & Stein, 2009). There are also important interactions between serotonergic and the NA systems. Animal studies suggest that long-term treatment with SSRIs promotes hippocampal neurogenesis (Duman, Nakagawa, & Malberg, 2001) and decreases HPA axis responsiveness (Jensen et al., 1999). Consistent with this, brain imaging studies in humans suggest that SSRIs promote hippocampal neurogenesis (Vermetten, Vythilingam, Southwick, Charney, & Bremner, 2003).

Glutamate, the primary excitatory neurotransmitter in the central nervous system (CNS), is thought to play a role in the initiation and maintenance of the HPA stress response and in the formation of memory through long-term potentiation (Ravindra & Stein, 2009). Memory formation is considered a key process in PTSD, and long-term potentiation possibly contributes to consolidation of trauma memories in PTSD (Heim & Nemeroff, 2009). In animal studies, pretreatment with glutamatergic NMDA-receptor antagonists has been shown to decrease stress responsiveness (Jezova, Tokarev, & Rusnak, 1995; Tokarev & Jezova, 1997), and the partial NMDA receptor antagonist D-cycloserine has been shown to improve the extinction of fear (Heim & Nemeroff, 2009). D-cycloserine has also been shown to improve anxiety symptoms in patients with phobias undergoing exposure therapy (Heim & Nemeroff, 2009), this may be linked to improved fear extinction.

A range of other neurotransmitter and neuroendocrine systems have been shown to be involved in PTSD. PTSD studies consistently reveal reduced cortisol levels, raised corticotrophin-releasing factor (CRF) and hypersuppression of cortisol in low-dose dexamethasone suppression tests (Heim & Nemeroff, 2009; Martin, Ressler, Binder, & Nemeroff, 2009), reflecting hypersensitivity of the negative feedback system of the HPA axis (Yehuda, 2002). Prospective studies have shown that low cortisol at the time of exposure to psychological trauma predicts the development of PTSD (Resnick, Yehuda, Ptiman, & Foy, 1995; Yehuda, McFarlanlane, & Shaylev, 1998). This may reflect a preexisting risk factor for biological failure to contain the stress response at the time of trauma (Yehuda, 2002).

Dopamine, a catecholamine involved in modulating mesolimbic reward pathways, has also been implicated in fear conditioning (Heim & Nemeroff, 2009). There is evidence in humans that stress exposure induces mesolimbic dopamine release, which may impact on HPA axis responses (Heim & Nemeroff, 2009). Genetic variations in the dopaminergic system have also been implicated in moderating risk for PTSD (Heim & Nemeroff, 2009).

Gamma-aminobutyric acid (GABA), the principal inhibitory neurotransmitter in the CNS, exerts anxiolytic effects and dampens behavioral and physiological responses to stress, in part by inhibiting the NA and CRF circuits involved in fear and stress responses (Heim & Nemeroff, 2009). GABA acts on GABAA receptors, part of the GABAA/Benzodiazepine (BZ) receptor complex. Brain imaging studies show decreased BZ receptor binding in the cortex, thalamus, and hippocampus of patients with PTSD, suggesting that decreased density or affinity of the BZ receptor may play a role in PTSD (Heim & Nemeroff, 2009).

Gene variants in many of these molecular systems may contribute to the risk of developing PTSD after trauma exposure (Heim & Nemeroff, 2009). PTSD has a heritability range of 30% to 40% (Martin et al., 2009). The key role of the traumatic event in PTSD and the importance of environmental factors have made linkage and candidate gene studies difficult, and research has focused on gene–environment interactions (Broekman, Olff, & Boer, 2007). A potential gene–childhood interaction between the stress-related gene FKBP5 and childhood trauma has been studied as a predictor of severity of adult PTSD symptoms (Binder et al., 2008). The data showed that four single-nucleotide polymorphisms of the FKBP5 gene interacted with severity of child abuse as a predictor of adult PTSD symptoms (Binder et al., 2008). Emerging research on genetic variations in psychobiological systems that determine responses to trauma and risk for developing PTSD have potential implications for predicting the need for and the response to treatment.

Current Treatments

In this section we describe current pharmacological and psychotherapeutic treatments. We briefly summarize the findings of meta-analyses, clinical guidelines, and some data from individual clinical trials.

Pharmacotherapy

Several meta-analyses of PTSD pharmacotherapy have been published (Stein, Ipser, & McAnda, 2009). The most recent and comprehensive analysis summarized 37 short-term randomized control trials (RCTs) of pharmacotherapy for PTSD and concluded that medications are effective in treating the three symptom clusters of PTSD (Ipser & Stein, 2011). The largest body of evidence for treatment over the short term existed for the SSRIs and venlafaxine. The longer term use of SSRIs was shown to improve efficacy and prevent relapse, which supports the consensus that treatment of chronic PTSD should be continued for at least a year.

On the other hand, some reviews of the literature have expressed skepticism about the data on PTSD treatment. A review of the literature undertaken by the Institute of Medicine emphasized that there is currently insufficient evidence to determine the value of pharmacotherapy (Committee on Treatment of Posttraumatic Stress Disorder, 2008). This review emphasized that the database of trials on PTSD was relatively small, and that effect sizes of different medications were not large. However, the report cautions that even though studies meeting their research design criteria were unavailable, this does not mean that current interventions are ineffectual or harmful.

On the basis of different approaches to synthesizing the literature, clinical guidelines have reached somewhat different viewpoints regarding pharmacotherapy of PTSD. Most treatment guidelines, including the American Psychiatric Association guidelines (American Psychiatric Association, 2004), emphasize the SSRIs and selective noradrenergic reuptake inhibitors (SNRIs) as first-line treatment of PTSD (Stein, Ipser, & McAnda, 2009). The National Institute for Health and Clinical Excellence (NICE) guidelines, on the other hand, recommend psychotherapy as a first-line intervention above any medical treatment, and they note that if medication is provided, paroxetine and mirtazepine are recommended for the treatment of PTSD in primary care and phenelzine and amitriptyline in specialist care (National Institute for Health and Clinical Excellence, 2005). NICE used a 0.5 cutoff to decide whether an effect size was clinically significant; however, in the case of a disabling condition and relatively treatment-resistant disorder like PTSD, this may be an overly conservative threshold.

Individual trials have studied a broad range of agents. The most studied are the SSRIs (see Table 6.1) and of these paroxetine and sertraline have FDA approval. While most SSRI studies have focused on short-term treatment, there are also positive data from longer term relapse prevention studies (Davidson et al., 2001). Other classes of medications that have been studied include the SNRIs, tricyclic antidepressants (TCAs), monoamine oxidase inhibitors (MAOIs), antipsychotics, and adrenergic suppressors. We briefly review these trials in the section on "Alternative Agents."

Psychotherapy

A number of different psychotherapies have been shown to be efficacious for PTSD (Cloitre, 2009). A Cochrane review of RCTs of psychological treatments supported the use of individual trauma-focused cognitive-behavioral therapy (TFCBT), eye movement desensitisation and reprocessing (EMDR), stress management, and group TFCBT as efficacious treatments of PTSD (Bisson & Andrew, 2007). Other non-trauma-focused psychological treatments did not reduce PTSD symptoms as significantly.

NICE guidelines recommend TFCBT and EMDR as first-line treatments (National Institute for Health and Clinical Excellence, 2005). Non-trauma-focused therapies are considered second-line treatments along with pharmacotherapy. IOM guidelines recommend exposure therapies as first-line and EMDR, cognitive restructuring, coping skills, and group therapy as second-line choices (Committee on Treatment of Posttraumatic Stress Disorder, 2008).

TFCBT has the largest individual trial research base (Shalev, 2009). Sessions occur over 4–12 weeks with components including education, relaxation, exposure, and cognitive restructuring (Bisson, 2007). Cognitive therapy and prolonged exposure are the components associated with the largest effects (Shalev, 2009). Cognitive therapy aims at addressing and correcting cognitive distortions. Prolonged exposure is done through imagined or in vivo exposure, and it aims at promoting processing of the memory and reduction of avoidance and distress associated with the memory. A meta-analysis of 14 RCTs of TFCBT showed a greater reduction in PTSD symptoms in patients receiving TFCBT versus those receiving treatment as usual (Bisson & Andrew, 2007). TFCBT is efficacious when delivered individually or in groups (Bisson & Andrew, 2007).

EMDR involves the recalling and visualizing of traumatic experiences while making repeated eye movements. It has been shown to be efficacious in five individual trials (Bisson & Andrew, 2007; Davidson & Parker, 2001).

Stress management combines CBT components, but the focus is not on the trauma. Three trials have shown efficacy above treatment as usual (Bisson & Andrew, 2007). However, due to the low numbers in these studies (N = 86), further trials are warranted.

TABLE 6.1 SSRI Placebo-Controlled Drug Studies in Posttraumatic Stress Disorder

Medication	Study	Population	Comparison Group	N	Duration of Trial (Weeks)	Results
Sertraline	(Brady et al., 2000)	Civilians	Placebo	187	12	Sertraline superior to placebo
Sertraline	(Davidson, Pearlstein, et al., 2001)	Civilians	Placebo	208	28	Sertraline superior to placebo
Sertraline	(Davidson, Rothbaum, et al., 2001)	Civilians	Placebo	96	12	Sertraline superior to placebo
Sertraline	(Zohar et al., 2002)	Veterans	Placebo	42	10	Numeric but no statistical superiority of sertraline over placebo
Sertraline	(Tucker et al., 2003)	Civilians	Placebo Citalopram	58	10	No superiority of citalopram or sertraline over placebo
Sertraline	(Brady et al., 2005)	Civilians	Placebo	94	12	No superiority of sertraline over placebo
Sertraline	(Davidson, et al., 2006)	Civilians	Placebo Venlafaxine	538	12	Sertraline superior to placebo on secondary measures
Sertraline	(Friedman, Marmar, Baker, Sikes, & Farfel, 2007)	Veterans	Placebo	129	12	No superiority of sertraline over placebo
Paroxetine	(Marshall, Beebe, Oldham, & Zaninelli, 2001)	Mostly civilians	Placebo	551	12	Paroxetine superior to placebo
Paroxetine	(Tucker et al., 2001)	Mostly civilians	Placebo	307	12	Paroxetine superior to placebo
Paroxetine	(Stein, Davidson, Seedat, & Beebe, 2003)	Mostly civilians	Placebo	322	12	Paroxetine superior to placebo
Paroxetine	(Marshall et al., 2007)	Civilians	Placebo	70	10	Paroxetine superior to placebo
Fluoxetine	(van der Kolk et al., 1994)	Civilians	Placebo	64	5	Fluoxetine superior to placebo
Fluoxetine	(Connor, Sutherland, Tupler, Malik, & Davidson, 1999)	Civilians	Placebo	53	12	Fluoxetine superior to placebo
Fluoxetine	(Martenyi, Brown, Zhang, Prakash, & Koke, 2002)	Mostly veterans	Placebo	301	12	Fluoxetine superior to placebo
Fluoxetine	(Martenyi, Brown, Zhang, Koke, & Prakash, 2002)	Veterans	Placebo	131	24	Fluoxetine superior to placebo in relapse prevention
Fluoxetine	(Davidson et al., 2005)	Civilians	Placebo	62	24	Fluoxetine superior to placebo in relapse prevention
Fluoxetine	(Hertzberg, Feldman, Beckhan, Kudler, & Davidson, 2000)	Veterans	Placebo	12	12	No superiority of fluoxetine over placebo
Fluoxetine	(Martenyi, Brown, & Caldwell, 2007)	Civilians	Placebo	411	12	No superiority of fluoxetine over placebo
Fuoxetine	(van der Kolk et al., 2007)	Civilians	Placebo	88	8	No superiority of fluoxetine over placebo
Citalopram	(Tucker et al., 2003)	Civilians	Placebo Sertraline	58	10	No superiority of citalopram or sertraline over placebo

Assessment of Treatment Resistance

Treatment resistance in PTSD can be defined as failure to respond optimally to first-line treatments. Only 30% of PTSD patients receiving an SSRI achieve complete remission after 12 weeks of treatment (Brady et al., 2000; Davidson, Rothbaum, van der Kolk, Sikes, & Farfel, 2001; Marshall, Beebe, Oldham, & Zaninelli, 2001; Tucker et al., 2001). A further 55% of the partial responders may achieve full remission after a further 24 weeks of treatment (Londborg et al., 2001).

The first step in assessing treatment resistance is to identify various factors that may be interfering with treatment. These factors include psychiatric comorbidity, substance abuse, ongoing trauma exposure, and treatment nonadherence. These factors will be discussed briefly next.

Psychiatric comorbidity rates are high in PTSD (Kessler et al., 1995). Depression, other anxiety disorders, somatoform disorders, sleep disorders, and substance use disorders may worsen treatment outcomes. Substance use disorders are one of the most common co-occurring disorders in PTSD sufferers. Prevalence rates for substance use disorders in civilians with PTSD are as high as 43% with even higher rates seen in combat veterans (Jacobsen, Southwick, & Kosten, 2001). Patients with PTSD and substance use disorders have higher rates of comorbid Axis I and II disorders and have more severe PTSD symptoms, predominantly in avoidance and arousal symptom clusters (Jacobsen et al., 2001). PTSD and substance use comorbidity is associated with higher treatment costs (Brown, Stout, & Mueller, 1999).

Ongoing trauma may interfere with recovery from PTSD. Lifetime rates of trauma exposure are high, in the range of 50% to 90% (Wittchen et al., 2009). Certain population groups are at increased risk of repeated trauma exposure. Soldiers in particular are a high-risk group for ongoing trauma exposure.

Treatment nonadherence can be due to several factors. Many medications used in PTSD have troublesome side effects, including gastrointestinal symptoms, weight gain, sleep disturbance, and sexual dysfunction. Patients may not be able to tolerate side effects, and close monitoring is necessary when medications are started or doses adjusted. Patients should be informed about side effects, and shared decision making may be helpful (Lin et al., 1995).

Proposed Strategies for Managing Treatment-Resistant Posttraumatic Stress Disorder

Strategies for managing treatment-resistant PTSD can be guided by the general approach to the management of treatment-resistant anxiety disorders. This includes increasing the dose and duration of pharmacotherapy, switching to a different treatment, or augmenting with a drug from a different class (Ipser et al., 2006). Alternative agents, augmentation strategies, combination with psychotherapy, and novel treatment approaches will be discussed in the following sections.

Alternative Agents

Given that monotherapy studies of various antidepressants, anticonvulsants, and antipsychotics show evidence of efficacy, a number of these agents can be considered as alternative pharmacotherapy options. Venlafaxine, an SNRI, has been shown in two large RCTs to be superior to placebo and comparable to sertraline (Davidson, Baldwin et al., 2006; Davidson, Rothbaum et al., 2006).

Several other antidepressants have been studied in PTSD and can be considered. Mirtazepine, a serotonergic and noradrenergic agent, has been shown to be superior to placebo and comparable to sertraline in small studies (Chung et al., 2004; Davidson et al., 2003). There have been no recent RCTs for TCAs or MAOIs, but older studies support their use and they remain possible treatment options for patients who do not respond to SSRI or SNRI treatment (Southwick, Yehuda, Giller, & Charney, 1994; Ver Ellen & van Kammen, 1990).

Anticonvulsants act on glutamate and GABA, and they may be effective in treating impulsive behavior, hyperarousal, and flashbacks in patients with PTSD (Berlin, 2007). However, the RCT evidence for anticonvulsants in PTSD is mixed (Davidson, Brady, Mellman, Stein, & Pollack, 2007; Hertzberg et al., 1999; Tucker et al., 2007). Given the important role of glutamate and GABA in PTSD, further trials of anticonvulsant medications are warranted.

Antipsychotics act on the dopaminergic and other systems. There have, however, been few trials of antipsychotics as monotherapy. Two small studies of risperidone monotherapy found risperidone to be superior to placebo in reducing PTSD symptoms (Padala et al., 2006; Reich, Winternitz, Hennen, Watts, & Stanculescu, 2004). However, a recent 6-month RCT found that risperidone compared with placebo did not reduce PTSD symptoms among patients with military-related PTSD with serotonin reuptake inhibitor resistant symptoms (Krystal et al., 2011). An olanzapine monotherapy pilot study failed to show superiority over placebo (Butterfield et al., 2001).

Low-dose cortisol showed positive results in a small placebo-controlled crossover study (Aerni et al., 2004). During a 3-month observation period, low-dose cortisol monotherapy was administered to three patients with PTSD. CAPS ratings after each month showed cortisol-related improvements for reexperiencing symptoms and in one patient for avoidance symptoms. Further work is needed before this intervention can be clinically recommended.

Several other agents have not been shown to be effective as monotherapy in PTSD. The only RCT conducted using benzodiazepine monotherapy for PTSD was negative (Braun, Greenberg, Dasberg, & Lerer, 1990). In a small trial, inositol did not show any effect on PTSD (Kaplan, Amir, Swartz, & Levine, 1996). D-cycloserine was also not effective as monotherapy in a small placebo controlled trial (Heresco-Levy et al., 2002). The $5HT_2$ antagonist cyproheptidine was found to be ineffective (Jacobs-Rebhun et al., 2000).

Augmentation Strategies

Augmentation is another strategy when approaching treatment-resistant PTSD. Augmentation agents include the new-generation antipsychotics, adrenergic blockers, and newer antidepressant agents. A Cochrane review of treatment-resistant anxiety disorders reviewed medication augmentation strategies for treatment-resistant PTSD patients (Ipser et al., 2006). Although there were few studies of PTSD, three out of four trials found significant reductions in symptom severity after the augmentation strategy.

Data from individual augmentation trials are summarized in Table 6.2. The data on augmentation of SSRIs with the atypical antipsychotic agents risperidone and olanzapine are promising (Bartzokis, Lu, Turner, Mintz, & Saunders, 2005; Hamner et al., 2003; Monnelly, Ciraulo, Knapp, & Keane, 2003; Stein, Kline, & Matloff, 2002). However, one of the few trials to assess pharmacotherapy in a nonveteran population found no improvement when risperidone was added to setraline (Rothbaum, Killeen, Davidson, Brady, & Heekin, 2008). Given its antagonistic action at the alpha$_1$ receptor, which has been linked to sleep disruption, prazosin was evaluated for its effects on nightmares and insomnia. There was an overall symptom reduction (Raskind et al., 2003; 2007; Taylor et al., 2008).

Some augmentation agents have been shown to be ineffective in RCTs. An RCT with guanfacine augmentation failed to show superiority over placebo (Neylan et al., 2006). Buproprion has been studied in groups taking other psychotropic medications, but no benefit over placebo has been demonstrated in augmentation trials in PTSD (Becker et al., 2007; Hertzberg, Moore, Feldman, & Beckham, 2001).

Combination with Psychotherapy

Until recently there were no controlled studies of the combination of pharmacotherapy and psychotherapy in PTSD (Bandelow, Seidler-Brandler, Becker, Wedekind, & Rüther, 2007; Black, 2006). A 2010 review that included four trials concluded that there were too few studies to confirm or refute whether combination therapies had better outcomes (Hetrick, Purcell, Garner, & Panslow, 2010). However, some of these preliminary studies were encouraging. A pilot study looking at Cambodian refugees with PTSD compared combination therapy with CBT to sertraline alone and showed that combined treatment offered additional benefit in the range of medium to large effect sizes for PTSD and associated symptoms (Otto et al., 2003). Another small study showed further reduction in PTSD symptom severity when prolonged exposure therapy was added to sertraline (Rothbaum et al., 2006). A pilot RCT of combined TFCBT and sertraline for childhood PTSD symptoms following sexual trauma showed only minimal benefit to adding sertraline to TFCBT (Cohen, Mannarina, Perel, & Staron, 2007). The addition of paroxetine to continued prolonged exposure therapy compared to placebo showed no improvement in individuals who remained symptomatic after initial prolonged exposure therapy (Simon et al., 2008). A RCT assigned adult survivors of the 9/11 World Trade Center attack to 10 weeks of prolonged exposure plus paroxetine (N = 19) or prolonged exposure plus placebo (N = 18). Patients treated with prolonged exposure plus paroxetine had greater improvement in PTSD symptoms, improved response rate, and improved quality of life (Schneier et al., 2011).

D-cycloserine (DCS), a partial NMDA agonist, has also being considered as an adjunct to prolonged exposure therapy. In animal studies, DCS has been shown to improve extinction of fear in rodents when given before or shortly after exposure to fearful cues (Davis, Ressler, Rothbaum, & Richardson, 2006). Subsequent human studies found that exposure therapy combined with DCS resulted in larger reductions of symptoms in patients with acrophobia (Ressler et al., 2004). Similar results have been shown for social anxiety

TABLE 6.2 Posttraumatic Stress Disorder Augmentation Placebo-Controlled Studies

Medication	Study	Population	Comparison Group	N	Duration of Trial (weeks)	Results
Antipsychotics						
Olanzapine	(Stein, Kline, & Matloff, 2002)	Veterans	Placebo	19	8	Decrease in CAPS total, CES-D and PSQI
Risperidone	(Hamner et al., 2003)	Veterans	Placebo	40	5	Decrease in PANSS and CAPSS reexperiencing
Risperidone	(Monnelly, Ciraulo, Knapp, & Keane, 2003)	Veterans	Placebo	15	6	Decrease in OAS-M irritability and PCL-M
Risperidone	(Bartzokis, Lu, Turner, Mintz, & Saunders, 2005)	Veterans	Placebo	73	16	Decrease in CAPS total, arousal, HAM-A, PANSS positive
Risperidone	(Rothbaum et al., 2008)	Civilians	Placebo	20	8	No effect of risperidone was detected at end point on CAPS
Adrenergic blockers						
Prazosin	(Raskind et al., 2003)	Veterans	Placebo	10	20	Prazosin superior to placebo in sleep and overall PTSD symptoms on CGI-I
Prazosin	(Raskind et al., 2007)	Veterans	Placebo	40	8	Prazosin superior to placebo in sleep and overall PTSD symptoms on CGI-I
Prazosin	(Taylor et al., 2008)	Civilians	Placebo	13	7	Prazosin superior to placebo in sleep and PTSD symptoms
Guanfacine	(Neylan et al., 2006)	Veterans	Placebo	63	8	No effect on sleep or PTSD symptoms
Antidepressants						
Buproprion	(Hertzberg, Moore, Feldman, & Beckham, 2001)	Veterans	Placebo	15	12	No superiority over placebo
Buproprion	(Becker et al., 2007)	Civilian and veteran	Placebo	30	8	No superiority over placebo

CAPS, Clinician Administered PTSD Scale; CES-D, Center for Epidemiologic Studies Depression Scale; CGI-I, Clinical Global Impression Improvement; HAM-A, Hamilton Rating Scale for Anxiety; OAS-M, Overt-Aggression Scale-Modified for Outpatients; PANSS, Positive and Negative Syndrome Scale for Schizophrenia; PCL-M, Patient Checklist for PTSD-Military Version; PSQI, Pittsburgh Sleep Quality Inventory.

disorder (Sanjay, Price, & Charney, 2008). There is ongoing work evaluating this approach to PTSD.

Novel Approaches

The psychobiological advances in the understanding of the pathophysiology of PTSD have led to targeted research of several novel agents in the treatment of PTSD. These include corticotrophin-releasing factor antagonists, glutamate modulators, and neuropeptide modulators or agonists related to substance P, neuropeptide Y, oxytocin, orexin, and galanin (Sanjay et al., 2008). These agents show promise in preclinical research.

There is also ongoing work on the psychobiology of PTSD and resilience. Several possible psychobiological factors have been identified as predictors of resilience against extreme stress and PTSD (Charney, 2004). These factors include constrained increase of cortisol by negative feedback loops, enhanced dehydroepiandrasterone release, restrained initial CRH response to acute stress, adaptive changes in CRH_1 and CRH_2 receptors, reduced locus ceruleus-noradrenalin activity, increase in amygdala neuropeptide Y levels, increase in amygdala galanin levels, optimal cortical and subcortical dopamine levels, high-affinity postsynaptic $5HT_1A$ receptors density, resistance to stress-induced down-regulation of benzodiazepine receptors, high level of benzodiazepine receptor density, increased testosterone levels, and short-term increases in estrogen levels (Charney, 2004). These provide useful targets for future studies.

Conclusion

There have been several important advances in our understanding of the psychobiology and management of PTSD. In particular, there is now a range of data pointing to disruptions of particular neurocircuitry and molecular mechanisms in PTSD, and it can be suggested that specific pharmacological and psychotherapeutic interventions are able to reverse these disruptions. Early work on the pharmacotherapy of PTSD largely followed developments in the treatment of depression. However, advances in psychobiology have now provided targets that may be specific for PTSD, and there is significant interest in ongoing D cyclo-serine trials.

Given that many patients do not respond to first-line interventions, many challenges remain for the field. A more complete understanding of the genetic and environmental contributors to PTSD may help predict who responds to particular interventions and may lead to new targets. Much remains to be learned about nonadherence in PTSD and about the adaptation of psychotherapeutic interventions to diverse populations; perhaps more culturally targeted psychotherapies would decrease dropout and improve response. The number of studies in the field remains surprisingly few; additional work is needed in a range of areas, including studies in refractory patients, special populations (e.g., children, elderly, comorbid substance use), work on combined pharmacotherapy and psychotherapy, and large effectiveness studies.

For now, clinicians have at their disposal a number of useful first-line options and several options for treatment refractory patients, including switching, augmentation, and combination.

Disclosure Statement

D.J.S. has received research grants and/or consultancy honoraria from Abbott, Astrazeneca, Eli-Lilly, GlaxoSmithKline, Jazz Pharmaceuticals, Johnson & Johnson, Lundbeck, Orion, Pfizer, Pharmacia, Roche, Servier, Solvay, Sumitomo, Takeda, Tikvah, and Wyeth. K.-A.L. has no conflicts of interest to disclose.

References

Aerni, A., Traber, R., Hock, C., Roozendaal, B., Schelling, G., Papassotiropoulos, A., et al. (2004). Low-dose cortisol for symptoms of posttraumatic stress disorder. *American Journal of Psychiatry*, *161*, 1488–1490.

American Psychiatric Association. (2000). *Diagnostic and statistical manual of mental disorders* (4th ed., Text rev.). Washington, DC: Author.

American Psychiatric Association. (2004). *Treatment of acute stress disorder and posttraumatic stress disorder*. Retrieved December 2010, from http://psychiatryonline.org/guidelines.aspx

Baldwin, D. S., Anderson, I. M., Nutt, D. J., Bandelow, B., Bond, A., Davidson, J. R., et al. (2005). Evidence-based guidelines for the pharmacological treatment of anxiety disorders: Recommendations from the British Association for Psychopharmacology. *Journal of Psychopharmacology*, *19*, 567–596.

Bandelow, B., Seidler-Brandler, U., Becker, A., Wedekind, D., & Rüther, E. (2007). Meta-analysis of randomized controlled comparisons of psychopharmacological and psychological treatments for anxiety disorders. *World Journal of Biological Psychiatry*, *8*, 175–187.

Bartzokis, G., Lu, P., Turner, J., Mintz, J., & Saunders, C. (2005). Adjunctive risperidone in the treatment of chronic combat-related posttraumatic stress disorder. *Biological Psychiatry*, *57*, 474–479.

Becker, M., Hertzberg, M., Moore, S., Dennis, M., Bukenya, D., & Beckham, J. (2007). A placebo-controlled trial of bupropion SR in the treatment of chronic posttraumatic stress disorder. *Journal of Clinical Psychopharmacology*, *27*, 193–197.

Berlin, H. (2007). Antiepileptic drugs for the treatment of post-traumatic stress disorder. *Current Psychiatry Reports*, *9*, 291–300.

Binder, E. B., Bradley, R. G., Liu, W., Epstein, M. P., Deveau, T. C., Mercer, K. B., et al. (2008). Association of FKBP5 polymorphisms and childhood abuse with risk of posttraumatic stress disorder symptoms in adults. *Journal of the American Medical Association*, *299*, 1291–1305.

Bisson, J. (2007). Post-traumatic stress disorder. *Occupational Medicine*, *57*, 399–403.

Bisson, J., & Andrew, M. (2007). Psychological treatment of post-traumatic stress disorder. *Cochrane Database of Systematic Reviews*, CD003388.

Black, D. (2006). Efficacy of combined pharmacotherapy and psychotherapy versus monotherapy in the treatment of anxiety disorders. *CNS Spectrums*, *11*, 29–33.

Brady, K., Pearlstein, T., Asnis, G., Baker, D., Rothbaum, B., Sikes, C., et al. (2000). Efficacy and safety of sertraline treatment of posttraumatic stress disorder. *Journal of the American Medical Association*, *283*, 1837–1844.

Brady, K., Sonne, S., Anton, R., Randall, C., Back, S., & Simpson, K. (2005). Sertraline in the treatment of co-occuring alcohol dependence and posttraumatic stress disorder. *Alcoholism, Clinical and Experimental Research*, *29*, 395–401.

Braun, P., Greenberg, D., Dasberg, H., & Lerer, B. (1990). Core symptoms of posttraumatic stress disorder unimproved by alprazolam treatment. *Journal of Clinical Psychiatry*, *51*, 236–238.

Bremner, J., Randall, P., Scott, T., Bronen, R., Seibyl, J., Southwick, S., et al. (1995). MRI-based measurement of hippocampal volume in patients with combat-related posttraumatic stress disorder. *American Journal of Psychiatry*, *152*, 973–981.

Brewin, C. R., Andrews, B., & Valentine, J. D. (2000). Meta-analysis of risk factors for posttraumatic stress disorder in trauma exposed adults. *Journal of Consulting and Clinical Psychology*, *68*, 748–766.

Broekman, B., Olff, M., & Boer, F. (2007). The genetic background to PTSD. *Neuroscience and Biobehavioural Reviews*, *31*, 348–362.

Brown, P. J., Stout, R. L., & Mueller, T. (1999). Substance use disorder and posttraumatic stress disorder comorbidity: Addiction and psychiatric treatment rates. *Psychology of Addictive Behaviors*, *13*, 115–122.

Butterfield, M., Becker, M., Connor, K., Sutherland, S., Churchill, L., & Davidson, J. (2001). Olanzapine in the treatment of post-traumatic stress disorder: A pilot study. *International Clinical Psychopharmacology*, *16*, 197–203.

Charney, D. S. (2004). Psychobiological mechanisms of resilience and vulnerability: Implications for stressful adaptation to extreme stress. *American Journal of Psychiatry, 161*, 195–216.

Chung, M., Min, K., Jun, Y., Kim, S., Kim, W., & Jun, E. (2004). Efficacy and tolerability of mirtazapine and sertraline in Korean veterans with posttraumatic stress disorder. *Human Psychopharmacology, 19*, 489–494.

Cloitre, M. (2009). Effective psychotherapies for posttraumatic stress disorder: A review and critique. *CNS Spectrums, 14*, 32–43.

Cohen, J., Mannarina, A., Perel, J., & Staron, V. (2007). A pilot randomized controlled trial of combined trauma-focused CBT and sertraline for childhood PTSD symptoms. *Journal of the American Academy of Child and Adolescent Psychiatry, 46*, 811–819.

Committee on Treatment of Posttraumatic Stress Disorder. (2008). *Treatment of posttraumatic stress disorder: An assessment of the evidence*. Washington, DC: National Academies Press.

Connor, K., Sutherland, S., Tupler, L., Malik, M., & Davidson, J. (1999). Fluoxetine in post-traumatic stress disorder: Randomised, double-blind study. *British Journal of Psychiatry, 175*, 17–22.

Davidson, J., Baldwin, D., Stein, D., Kuper, E., Benattia, I., Ahmed, S., et al. (2006). Treatment of posttraumatic stress disorder with venlafaxine extended release: A 6-month randomized, controlled trial. *Archives of General Psychiatry, 63*, 1158–1165.

Davidson, J., Brady, K., Mellman, T., Stein, M., & Pollack, M. (2007). The efficacy and tolerability of tiagabine in adult patients with post-traumatic stress disorder. *Journal of Clinical Psychopharmacology, 27*, 85–88.

Davidson, J., Connor, K. M., Hertzberg, M., Weisler, R., Wilson, W., & Payne, V. (2005). Maintenance therapy with fluoxetine in posttraumatic stress disorder: A placebo-controlled discontinuation study. *Journal of Clinical Psychopharmacology, 25*, 166–169.

Davidson, J., Hughes, D., Blazer, D., & George, L. (1991). Posttraumatic stress disorder in the community: An epidemiological study. *Psychological Medicine, 21*, 713–721.

Davidson, J., Pearlstein, T., Londborg, P., Brady, K., Rothbaum, B., Bell, J., et al. (2001). Efficacy of sertraline in preventing relapse of posttraumatic stress disorder: Results of a 28-week double-blind, placebo-controlled study. *American Journal of Psychiatry, 158*, 1974–1981.

Davidson, J., Rothbaum, B., Tucker, P., Asnin, G., Benattia, I., & Musgnung, M. (2006). Venlafaxine extended release in posttraumatic stress disorder: A sertraline and placebo-controlled study. *Journal of Clinical Psychopharmacology, 26*, 259–267.

Davidson, J., Rothbaum, B., van der Kolk, C., Sikes, C., & Farfel, G. (2001). Multicenter, double-blind comparison of sertraline and placebo in the treatment of posttraumatic stress disorder. *Archives of General Psychiatry, 58*, 485–492.

Davidson, J., Weisler, R., Butterfield, M., Casat, C., Connor, K., Barnett, S., et al. (2003). Mirtazapine vs placebo in posttraumatic stress disorder: A pilot trial. *Biological Psychiatry, 53*(2), 188–191.

Davidson, P., & Parker, K. (2001). Eye movement desensitization and reprocessing (EMDR): A meta-analysis. *Journal of Consulting and Clinical Psychology, 2*, 305–316.

Davis, M., Ressler, K., Rothbaum, B., & Richardson, R. (2006). Effects of D-cycloserine on extinction: Translation from preclinical to clinical work. *Biological Psychiatry, 60*, 369–375.

Duman, R., Nakagawa, S., & Malberg, J. (2001). Regulation of neurogenesis by antidepressant treament. *Neuropsychopharmacology, 25*, 836–844.

Friedman, M., Marmar, C., Baker, D., Sikes, C., & Farfel, G. (2007). Randomized double-blind comparison of sertraline and placebo for post-traumatic stress disorder in a Department of Veterans Affairs setting. *Journal of Clinical Psychiatry, 68*, 711–720.

Geracioti, T. J., Baker, D., Ekhator, N., West, S., Hill, K., Bruce, A., et al. (2001). CSF norepinephrine concentrations in posttraumatic stress disorder. *American Journal of Psychiatry, 158*, 1227–1230.

Gilbertson, M., Shenton, M., Ciszewski, A., Kasai, K., Lasko, N., Orr, S., et al. (2002). Smaller Hippocampal volume predicts pathological vulnerability to psychological trauma. *Nature Neuroscience, 5*, 1242–1247.

Hamner, M., Faldowski, R., Ulmer, H., Frueh, B., Huber, M., & Arana, G. (2003). Adjunctive rispiridone treatment in post-traumatic stress disorder: A preliminary controlled trial of effects of comorbid psychotic symptoms. *International Clinical Psychopharmacology, 18*, 1–8.

Heim, C., & Nemeroff, C. (2009). Neurobiology of posttraumatic stress disorder. *CND Spectrums, 14*, 13–24.

Heresco-Levy, U., Kremer, I., Javitt, D., Goichman, R., Reshef, A., Blanaru, M., et al. (2002). Pilot-controlled trial of D-cycloserine for the treatment of post-traumatic stress disorder. *International Journal of Neuropsychopharmacology, 5*, 301–307.

Hertzberg, M., Butterfield, M., Feldman, M., Beckham, J., Sutherland, S., Connor, K., et al. (1999). A preliminary study of lamotrigine for the treatment of posttraumatic stress disorder. *Biological Psychiatry, 45*, 1226–1229.

Hertzberg, M., Feldman, M., Beckhan, J., Kudler, H., & Davidson, J. (2000). Lack of efficacy for fluoxetine in PTSD: A placebo controlled trial in combat veterans. *Annals of Clinical Psychiatry, 12*, 101–105.

Hertzberg, M., Moore, S., Feldman, M., & Beckham, J. (2001). A preliminary study of bupropion sustained-release for smoking cessation in patients with chronic posttraumatic stress disorder. *Journal of Clinical Psychopharmacology, 21*, 94–98.

Hetrick, S., Purcell, R., Garner, B., & Panslow, R. (2010). Combined pharmacotherapy and psychological therapies for post traumatic stress disorder. *Cochrane Database Systematic Review*, CD007316.

Ipser, J. C., & Stein, D. J. (2011). Evidence-based pharmacotherapy of post-traumatic stress disorder. *International Journal of Neuropsychopharmacology*, 1–16. [Epub ahead of print].

Ipser, J. C., Carey, P., Dhansay, Y., Seedat, S., Fakier, N., & Stein, D. (2006). Pharmacotherapy augmentation strategies in treatment resistant anxiety disorders. *Cochrane Database of Systematic Reviews*, CD005473.

Jacobs-Rebhun, S., Schnurr, P., Friedman, M., Peck, R., Brophy, M., & Fuller, D. (2000). Posttraumatic stress disorder and sleep difficulty. *American Journal of Psychiatry, 157*, 1525–1526.

Jacobsen, L. K., Southwick, S. M., & Kosten, T. R. (2001). Substance use disorders in patients with posttraumatic stress disorder: A review of the literature. *American Journal of Psychiatry*, 1184–1190.

Jensen, J., Jessop, D., Harbuz, M., Mork, A., Sanchez, C., & Mikkelsen, J. (1999). Acute and long term treatments with the selective serotonin reuptake inhibitor citalopram modulate the HPA axis activity at different levels in male rats. *Journal of Neuroendocrinology, 62*, 326–332.

Jezova, D., Tokarev, D., & Rusnak, M. (1995). Endogenous excitatory amino acids are involved in stress-induced adrenocorticotropin and catecholamine release. *Neuroendocrinology, 62*, 326–332.

Kaplan, Z., Amir, M., Swartz, M., & Levine, J. (1996). Inositol treatment of post-traumatic stress disorder. *Anxiety, 2*, 51–52.

Karl, A., Schaefer, M., Malta, L., Drfel, D., Rohleder, N., & Werner, A. (2006). A meta-analysis of structural brain abnormalities in PTSD. *Neuroscience and Biobehavioural Reviews, 30*, 1004–1031.

Kessler, R. (2000). Posttraumatic stress disorder. *The Journal of Clinical Psychiatry, 61*, 4–12.

Kessler, R., Chiu, W., Demler, O., Merikangas, K., & Waters, E. (2005). Prevalence, severity, and comorbidity of 12-month DSM-IV disorders in the National Comorbidity Survey Replication. *Archives General Psychiatry, 62*, 617–627.

Kessler, R., Sonnega, A., Bromet, E., Hughes, M., & Nelson, C. (1995). Posttraumatic stress disorder in the National Comorbidity Survey. *Archives of General Psychiatry, 52*, 1048–1060.

Kroll, J. (2003). Posttraumatic symptoms and the complexity of responses to trauma. *Journal of the American Medical Association, 290*, 667–670.

Krystal, J., Rosenheck, R., Vessichio, J., Jones, K., Vertrees, J., Horney, R., et al. (2011). Adjunctive risperidone treatment for antidepressant-resistant symptoms of chronic military service related PTSD: A randomized trial. *Journal of the American Medical Association, 306*(5), 493–502.

Liberzon, I., & Sripada, C. (2008). The functional neuroanatomy of PTSD: A critical review. *Progress in Brain Research, 167*, 151–169.

Liebschutz, J., Saitz, R., Brower, V., Keane, T., Lloyd-Travaglini, C., Averbuch, T., et al. (2007). PTSD in urban primary care: High prevalence and low physician recognition. *Journal of General Internal Medicine, 22*, 719–793.

Lin, E., von Korff, M., Katon, W., Bush, T. S., Walker, E., & Robinson, P. (1995). The role of the primary care physician in patients' adherence to antidepressent therapy. *Medical Care, 33*, 67–74.

Londborg, P., Hegel, M., Goldstein, S., Goldstein, D., Himmelhoch, J., Maddock, R., et al. (2001). Sertraline treatment of posttraumatic stress disorder: Results of weeks of open-label continuation treatment. *Journal of Clinical Psychiatry, 62*, 325–331.

Maren, S. (2001). Neurobiology of Pavlovian fear conditioning. *Annual Review of Neuroscience, 24*, 897–931.

Marshall, R., Beebe, K., Oldham, M., & Zaninelli, R. (2001). Efficacy and safety of paroxetine treatment for chronic PTSD: A fixed-dose-placebo-controlled study. *American Journal of Psychiatry, 158*, 1982–1988.

Marshall, R., Lewis-Fernandez, R., Blanco, C., Simpson, H., Lin, S., Vermes, D., et al. (2007). A controlled trial of paroxetine for chronic PTSD, dissociation, and interpersonal problems in mostly minority adults. *Depression and Anxiety, 24*, 77–84.

Martenyi, F., Brown, E., & Caldwell, C. (2007). Failed efficacy of fluoxetine in the treatment of posttraumatic stress disorder: Results of a fixed dose, placebo-controlled study. *Journal of Clinical Psychopharmacology, 27*, 166–170.

Martenyi, F., Brown, E., Zhang, H., Koke, S., & Prakash, A. (2002). Fluoxetine v. placebo in prevention of relapse in post-traumatic stress disorder. *British Journal of Psychiatry, 63*, 199–206.

Martenyi, F., Brown, E., Zhang, H., Prakash, A., & Koke, S. (2002). Fluoxetine versus placebo in posttraumatic stress disorder. *Journal of Clinical Psychiatry, 63*, 199–206.

Martin, E. I., Ressler, K. J., Binder, E., & Nemeroff, C. B. (2009). The neurobiology of anxiety disorders: Brain imaging, genetics, and psychoneuroendocrinology. *Psychiatry Clinics of North America, 32*, 549–575.

Matthew, S. J., Price, R. B., & Charney, D. S. (2008). Recent advances in the neurobiology of anxiety disorders: Implications for novel therapeutics. *American Journal of Medical Genetics, 15*, 89–98.

Monnelly, E., Ciraulo, D., Knapp, C., & Keane, T. (2003). Low dose risperidone as adjunctive therapy for irritable aggression in posttraumatic stress disorder. *Journal of Clinical Psychopharmacology, 19*, 377–378.

National Institute for Health and Clinical Excellence. (2005). *Post Traumatic Stress Disorder (PTSD) (CG26)*. Retrieved September 2010, from: http://www.nice.org.uk/CG26

Neylan, T., Lenoci, M., Franklin, K., Metzler, T., Henn-Haase, C., Hierholzer, R., et al. (2006). No improvement of posttraumatic stress disorder symptoms with guanfacine treatment. *American Journal of Psychiatry, 163*, 2186–2188.

Otto, M., Hinton, D., Korbly, N., Chea, A., Gershuny, B., & Pollack, M. (2003). Treatment of pharmacotherapy-refractory posttraumatic stress disorder among Cambodian refugees: A pilot study of combination treatment with cognitive-behavior therapy vs sertraline alone. *Behaviour Research and Therapy, 41*, 1271–1276.

Padala, P., Madison, J., Monnahan, M., Marcil, W., Price, P., Ramaswamy, S., et al. (2006). Risperidone mono-therapy for post-traumatic stress disorder related to sexual assault and domestic abuse in women. *International Clinical Psychiatry, 21*, 275–280.

Peleg, T., & Shalev, A. (2006). Longitudinal studies of PTSD:overview of findings and methods. *CNS Spectrums, 11*, 589–602.

Phelps, E., & LeDoux, J. (2005). Contributions of the amygdala to emotion processing: From animal models to human behaviour. *Neuron, 48*, 175–187.

Raskind, M., Peskind, E., Hoff, D., Hart, K., Holmes, H. A., et al. (2007). A parallel group placebo-controlled study of prazosin for trauma nightmares and sleep disturbance in combat veterans with post-traumatic stress disorder. *Biological Psychiatry, 61*, 928–934.

Raskind, M., Peskind, E., Kanter, E., Petrie, E., Radont, A., Thompson, C., et al. (2003). Reduction of nightmares and other PTSD symptoms in combat veterans by prazosin: A placebo-contolled study. *American Journal of Psychiatry, 160*, 371–373.

Rauch, S., Shin, L., Segal, E., Pitman, R., Carson, M., McMullin, K., et al. (2003). Selectively reduced regional cortical volumes in post-traumatic stress disorder. *NeuroReport, 14*, 913–916.

Ravindra, L. N., & Stein, M. B. (2009). Pharmacotherapy of PTSD: Premises, principles, and priorities. *Brain Research, 1293*, 24–39.

Reich, D., Winternitz, S., Hennen, J., Watts, T., & Stanculescu, C. (2004). A preliminary study of risperidone in the treatment of posttraumatic stress disorder related to childhood abuse in women. *Journal of Clinical Psychiatry, 65*, 1601–1606.

Resnick, H., Kilpatrick, D., Dansky, B., Sanders, B., & Best, C. (1993). Prevalence of civilian trauma and post-traumatic stress disorder in a representative national sample of women. *Journal of Consulting and Clinical Psychology, 61*, 948–991.

Resnick, H., Yehuda, R., Ptiman, R., & Foy, D. (1995). Effect of previous trauma on acute plasma cortisol level following rape. *American Journal of Psychiatry, 152*, 1675–1677.

Ressler, K. J., & Mayberg, H. S. (2007). Targeting abnormal neural circuits in mood and anxiety disorders: From the laboratory to the clinic. *Nature Neuroscience, 10*, 1116–1124.

Ressler, K. J., Rothbaum, B. O., Tannenbaum, L., Anderson, P., Graap, K., Zimand, E., et al. (2004). Cognitive enhancers as adjuncts to psychotherapy. *Archives of General Psychiatry, 61*, 1136–1144.

Rothbaum, B., Cahill, S., Foa, E., Davidson, J., Compton, J., Connor, K., et al. (2006). Augmentation of sertra-line with prolonged exposure in the treatment of posttraumatic stress disorder. *Journal of Traumatic Stress, 19*, 625–638.

Rothbaum, B., Killeen, T., Davidson, J., Brady, K. K., & Heekin, M. (2008). Placebo-controlled trial of risperidone augmentation for selective serotonin reuptake inhibitor-resistant civilian posttraumatic stress disorder. *Journal of Clinical Psychiatry, 69*, 520–525.

Sanjay, M., Price, R., & Charney, D. (2008). Recent advances in the neurobiology of anxiety disorders: Implications for novel therapeutics. *American Journal of Medical Genetics, 148C*, 89–98.

Schneier, F. R., Neria, Y., Pavlicova, M., Hembree, E., Suh, E. J., Amsel, L., et al. (2011). Combined Prolonged Exposure Therapy and paroxetine for PTSD related to the World Trade Center attack: A randomized con-trolled trial. *American Journal of Psychiatry, AiA*, 1–9.

Shalev, A. Y. (2009). Posttraumatic stress disorder and stress-related disorders. *Psychiatric Clinics of North America*, *32*, 687–704.

Shin, L., Rauch, S., & Pitman, R. (2006). Amygdala, medial prefrontal cortex, and hippocampal function in PTSD. *Annals of the New York Academy of Sciences*, *1071*, 67–79.

Simon, N., Connor, K., Lang, A., Rauch, S., Krulewicz, S., LeBeau, R., et al. (2008). Paroxetine CR augmentation for posttraumatic stress disorder refractory to prolonged exposure therapy. *Journal of Clinical Psychiatry*, *69*(3), 400–405.

Southwick, S., Yehuda, R., Giller, E., & Charney, D. I. (1994). Use of tricyclics and monoamine oxidase inhibitors in the treatment of PTSD: A quantitative review. In M. Murburg (Ed.), *Catecholamine function in post-traumatic stress disorder: Emerging concepts* (pp. 293–305). Washington, DC: American Psychiatric Association.

Stein, D., Davidson, J., Seedat, S., & Beebe, K. (2003). Paroxetine in the treatment of posttraumatic stress disorder: Pooled analysis of placebo-controlled studies. *Expert Opinion on Pharmacotherapy*, *4*, 1829–1838.

Stein, D. J., Ipser, J., & McAnda, N. (2009). Pharmacotherapy of posttraumatic stress disorder: A review of meta-analyses and treatment guidelines. *CNS Spectrums*, *14*, 25–31.

Stein, D., Seedat, S., Iversen, A., & Wessly, S. (2007). Post-traumatic stress disorder: Medicine and politics. *Lancet*, *369*, 139–144.

Stein, M., Kline, N., & Matloff, J. (2002). Adjunctive olanzapine for SSRI-resistant combat-related PTSD: A double-blind, placebo-controlled study. *American Journal of Psychiatry*, *159*, 1777–1779.

Taylor, F., Martin, P., Thompson, C., Williams, J., Mellman, T., Gross, C., et al. (2008). Prazosin effects on objective sleep measures and clinical symptoms in civilian trauma posttraumatic stress disorder: A placebo-controlled study. *Biological Psychiatry*, *63*, 629–632.

Tokarev, D., & Jezova, D. (1997). Effect of central administration of the non-NMDA receptor antagonist DNQX on ACTH and corticosterone release before and during immobilisation stress. *Methods and Findings in Experimental and Clinical Pharmacology*, *19*, 323–328.

Tucker, P., Potter-Kimball, R., Wyatt, D., Parker, D., Burgin, C., Jones, D., et al. (2003). Can physiological assessment and side effects tease out differences in PTSD trials? A double-blind comparison of citalopram, sertraline, and placebo. *Psychopharmacology Bulletin*, *37*, 135–149.

Tucker, P., Trautman, R., Wyatt, D., Thompson, J., Wu, S., Capece, J., et al. (2007). Efficacy and safety of topiramate monotherapy in civilian posttraumatic stress disorder: A randomised, double-blind placebo-controlled study. *Journal of Clinical Psychiatry*, *68*, 201–206.

Tucker, P., Zaninelli, R., Yehuda, R., Ruggiero, L., Dillingham, K., & Pitts, C. (2001). Paroxetine in the treatment of chronic posttraumatic stress disorder: Results of a placebo-controlled, flexible dose trial. *Journal of Clinical Psychiatry*, *62*, 860–868.

van der Kolk, B., Dreyfuss, D., Michaels, M., Shera, D., Berkowitz, R., Fisler, R., et al. (1994). Fluoxetine versus placebo in posttraumatic stress disorder. *Journal of Clinical Psychiatry*, *55*, 517–522.

van der Kolk, B., Spinazzola, J., Blaustein, M., Hopper, J., Hopper, E., Korn, D., et al. (2007). A randomized clinical trial of eye movement desensitization and reprocessing (EMDR), fluoxetine, and pill placebo in the treatment of posttraumatic stress disorder: Treatment effects and long-term maintenance. *Journal of Clinical Psychiatry*, *68*, 37–46.

Ver Ellen, P., & van Kammen, D. (1990). The biological findings in post-traumatic stress disorder: A review. *Journal of Applied Social Psychology*, 1789–1821.

Vermetten, E., Vythilingam, M., Southwick, S., Charney, D., & Bremner, J. (2003). Long-term treatment with paroxetine increases verbal declarative memory and hippocampal volume in posttraumatic stress disorder. *Biological Psychiatry*, *54*, 693–702.

Vieweg, W., Julius, D., Fernandez, A., Beatty-Brooks, M., Hettema, J., & Pandurangi, A. (2006). Posttraumatic stress disorder: Clinical features, pathophysiology, and treatment. *American Journal of Medicine*, *119*, 383–390.

Wittchen, H-U., Gloster, A., Beesdo, K., Schonfeld, S., & Perkonigg, A. (2009). Posttraumatic stress disorder: Diagnostic and epidemiological perspectives. *CNS Spectrums*, *14*, 5–12.

Yehuda, R. (2002). Post traumatic stress disorder. *New England Journal of Medicine*, *346*, 108–114.

Yehuda, R., & McFarlane, A. (1995). Conflict between current knowledge about posttraumatic stress disorder and its original conceptual basis. *American Journal of Psychiatry*, *152*, 1705–1713.

Yehuda, R., McFarlanlane, A., & Shaylev, A. (1998). Predicting the development of posttraumatic stress disorder from the cute response to the traumatic event. *Biological Psychiatry*, *44*, 1305–1313.

Zohar, J., Amital, D., Miodownik, C., Kotler, M., Bleich, A., Lane, R., et al. (2002). Double-blind placebo-controlled pilot study of sertraline in military veterans with posttraumatic stress disorder. *Journal of Clinical Psychopharmacology*, *22*, 190–195.

Treatment-Resistant Social Anxiety Disorder

Eric Bui and Mark H. Pollack

Diagnosis and Subtypes

Social anxiety disorder (SAD), also known as social phobia, is a condition characterized by a persistent fear of being embarrassed or humiliated in social or performance situations in which the person is exposed to unfamiliar people or to possible scrutiny by others, with marked anxiety, situationally bound panic attacks, avoidance, and distress (American Psychiatric Association [APA], 2000). According to the *Diagnostic and Statistical Manual of Mental Disorders, fourth edition (DSM-IV)*, SAD is categorized as either generalized with fear/avoidance of multiple social situations or nongeneralized with fear of only a limited number of social situations (APA, 2000). However, this dichotomous approach to subtyping has recently been challenged because it has been suggested that the number of feared social situations was distributed continuously with increased number of feared situations associated with increased functional impairment (Vriends et al., 2007). *DSM-IV* diagnostic criteria are reported in Table 7.1.

Epidemiology

SAD is a common disorder and according to the recent National Comorbidity Survey–Replication, its lifetime and 12-month prevalence in the United States are estimated as 12.1% and 7.1%, respectively (Ruscio et al., 2008). Reported prevalence rates are lower in European countries (Fehm et al., 2005; Alonso and Lepine, 2007), and even lower in non-Westernized countries, although some evidence points to the relevance of this disorder in countries culturally distant (Stein and Stein, 2008). A number of studies also report that women are more often affected by SAD than are men (Kessler et al., 2005).

TABLE 7.1 *DSM-IV* **Diagnostic Criteria for Social Phobia**

A. A marked and persistent fear of one or more social or performance situations in which the person is exposed to unfamiliar people or to possible scrutiny by others. The individual fears that he or she will act in a way (or show anxiety symptoms) that will be humiliating or embarrassing.

Note: In children, there must be evidence of the capacity for age-appropriate social relationships with familiar people and the anxiety must occur in peer settings, not just in interactions with adults.

B. Exposure to the feared social situation almost invariably provokes anxiety, which may take the form of a situationally bound or situationally predisposed Panic Attack.

Note: In children, the anxiety may be expressed by crying, tantrums, freezing, or shrinking from social situations with unfamiliar people.

C. The person recognizes that the fear is excessive or unreasonable.

Note: In children, this feature may be absent.

D. The feared social or performance situations are avoided or else are endured with intense anxiety or distress.

E. The avoidance, anxious anticipation, or distress in the feared social or performance situation(s) interferes significantly with the person's normal routine, occupational (academic) functioning, or social activities or relationships, or there is marked distress about having the phobia.

F. In individuals under age 18 years, the duration is at least 6 months.

G. The fear or avoidance is not due to the direct physiological effects of a substance (e.g., a drug of abuse, a medication) or a general medical condition and is not better accounted for by another mental disorder (e.g., Panic Disorder With or Without Agoraphobia, Separation Anxiety Disorder, Body Dysmorphic Disorder, a Pervasive Developmental Disorder, or Schizoid Personality Disorder).

H. If a general medical condition or another mental disorder is present, the fear in Criterion A is unrelated to it, e.g., the fear is not of Stuttering, trembling in Parkinson's disease, or exhibiting abnormal eating behavior in Anorexia Nervosa or Bulimia Nervosa.

Specify if: Generalized: if the fears include most social situations (also consider the additional diagnosis of Avoidant Personality Disorder)

Source: From APA (2000).

Causes and Etiology

To date, the pathogenesis of SAD has not been fully elucidated. Consistent with the pathophysiology of the fear response and of other anxiety disorders, the amygdala (Stein et al., 2002; Phan et al., 2006; Klumpp et al., 2010), medial prefrontal cortex (Campbell et al., 2007; Blair et al., 2008), hippocampus (Irle et al., 2010), and striatum (Sareen et al., 2007) have been implicated in the pathogenesis of SAD.

Along with the neurotransmitters serotonin and dopamine (Argyropoulos et al., 2004; Hariri et al., 2006; Furmark, 2009), neuropeptides such as oxytocin may also be relevant in the underlying neurobiology of SAD (Bartz and Hollander, 2006). Furthermore, though recent advances in genetics have identified several potential candidates genes that might be associated with social anxiety, including those coding for the β1-adrenergic receptor (ADRB1), catechol-O-methyltransferase (COMT), corticotropin-releasing hormone (CRH), serotonin transporter (5HTTLPR), and glutamic acid decarboxylase 1 (GAD1) (Stein et al., 2004; Smoller et al., 2005; Stein et al., 2005; Smoller et al., 2008), to date, none has been consistently shown to be associated with SAD.

Course of Illness

SAD typically has an early age of onset and chronic course of illness. The National Comorbidity Survey–Replication reported a median age of onset of 13 years for SAD, with the age of first avoidance (12–14 years) 1–2 years later than the age of first fear (10–13 years) (Kessler et al., 2005; Ruscio et al., 2008). According to the same study, only 20%–40% of SAD cases recover within 20 years of onset, and only 40%–60% recover within 40 years (Ruscio et al., 2008).

Consequences of Social Anxiety Disorder

SAD has been reported to result in significant impairment, particularly in terms of social, vocational, and family function (Ruscio et al., 2008). It is associated with poorer outcome in terms of wages, education, and professional attainment as well as increased risk of suicide attempts and utilization of health care resources (Katzelnick et al., 2001). Rates of comorbidity are high, with individuals with SAD experiencing sixfold increased odds for fulfilling criteria for at least one other psychiatric disorder (Ruscio et al., 2008). Comorbid conditions include other anxiety disorders (OR = 5.9 [95% CI: 4.8–7.4]), mood disorders (OR = 4.8 [95% CI: 4.1–5.6]), and substance use disorders (OR = 2.8 [95% CI: 2.3–3.3]).

Pharmacological Treatment

Effective treatments for SAD include both pharmacologic and psychosocial therapeutics. In this section, we will review the pharmacologic interventions for SAD.

Serotonin Reuptake Inhibitors: Selective Serotonin Reuptake Inhibitors and Serotonin-Norepinephrine Reuptake Inhibitors

For over a decade, selective serotonin reuptake inhibitors (SSRIs) have been considered as the first-line pharmacotherapy of generalized SAD because of their efficacy, safety, and favorable side effect profile compared to older agents, as well as their effectiveness in treating commonly comorbid conditions (Hansen et al., 2008; Van Ameringen et al., 2009; Stein et al., 2010).

A number of randomized controlled trials have reported on the efficacy and tolerability of SSRIs in the treatment of SAD, with two, sertraline (Katzelnick et al., 1995; Van Ameringen et al., 2001; Liebowitz et al., 2003) and paroxetine (Stein et al., 1998; Allgulander, 1999; Baldwin et al., 1999; Liebowitz et al., 2002; Lepola et al., 2004), receiving FDA approval for this indication, though all agents in the class are likely effective. Fluvoxamine was the first SSRI studied with regard to its efficacy in SAD (van Vliet et al., 1994; Stein et al., 1999; Davidson et al., 2004; Asakura et al., 2007; Owen, 2008) and, along with citalopram and escitalopram, has been reported to be effective in SAD (Lader et al., 2004; Furmark et al., 2005; Kasper et al., 2005); fluoxetine also appears effective for SAD, though the reported study results are mixed (Kobak et al., 2002; Clark et al., 2003; Davidson et al., 2004).

The serotonin-norepinephrine reuptake inhibitor (SNRI), venlafaxine extended release formulation has demonstrated efficacy for SAD (Rickels et al., 2004; Liebowitz et al., 2005; Stein et al., 2005) and has also been FDA approved for this indication; there are data suggesting the efficacy of the SNRI duloxetine for the treatment of SAD as well (Simon et al., 2010).

There have been a few head-to-head comparisons of SSRI/SNRI agents for SAD (Allgulander et al., 2004; Lader et al., 2004; Liebowitz et al., 2005), with no substantive evidence suggesting the superiority of one agent or class over another. Of interest, a recent meta-analysis of the efficacy and tolerability of second-generation antidepressants in SAD (Hansen et al., 2008) pooling results from 15 randomized controlled trials of an SSRI or SNRI (versus placebo or in head-to-head comparisons) suggested that escitalopram, paroxetine, sertraline, and venlafaxine produced significantly more responders than placebo (evidence also favored fluvoxamine, although the results were not significant) and that there were no differences in terms of efficacy between these four agents in a network meta-analysis. These results were in line with those of previous meta-analyses (van der Linden et al., 2000; Fedoroff and Taylor, 2001; Blanco et al., 2003; Hedges et al., 2007).

Overall, the evidence supports SRIs as first-line pharmacotherapy for SAD. Initial doses for SAD and other anxiety disorders are generally kept low initially to minimize emergent anxiety and increased gradually based on clinical response and side effects to typical therapeutic doses comparable to that used for depression. SRIs used in SAD and initial and therapeutic doses and side effects are listed in Table 7.2.

TABLE 7.2 Pharmacological Agents Used in the Treatment of Social Anxiety Disorder

Name	Usual Initial Dosage (mg)	Dosage Range (mg/day)	Common Side Effects/Limitations
SSRIs			
Sertraline[a]	25	25–200	
Paroxetine[a]	10	10–60	
Paroxetine CR[a]	12.5	12.5–62.5	Nausea, loss of appetite, diarrhea; anxiety or irritability; insomnia
Fluvoxamine	50	50–300	or drowsiness; decreased
Citalopram	10	20–60	libido; headaches or dizziness; serotonergic syndrome
Escitalopram	5	10–20	
Fluoxetine	10	10–80	
SNRIs			
Venlafaxine XR[a]	37.5	75–225	Same as SSRIs plus: Hypertension (venlafaxine) and urinary retention (duloxetine)
Duloxetine	30	60–120	
MAOIs			
Phenelzine	15–30	45–90	Postural hypotension, hypertensive crises, drowsiness, insomnia, weight gain, sexual dysfunction. Tyramine- and sympathomimetic-free diet
Benzodiazepines			
Clonazepam	.25	1–5	Sedation, abuse, psychomotor and memory impairment
Other agents			
Propranolol	10–20 prn	10–80	Depression
Buspirone	5 tid	15–60	Dysphoria

[a]FDA approved for treatment of social anxiety disorder.
MAOIs, monoamine oxidase inhibitors; SNRI, serotonin-norepinephrine reuptake inhibitor; SSRI, selective serotonin reuptake inhibitors.

Monoamine Oxidase Inhibitors and Reversible Inhibitors of Monoamine Oxidase Type A

The use of monoamine oxidase inhibitors (MAOIs) in SAD predates that of the serotonin reuptake inhibitors. Several studies have shown robust efficacy for phenelzine in treating SAD (Gelernter et al., 1991; Liebowitz et al., 1992; Versiani et al., 1992; Heimberg et al., 1998; Liebowitz et al., 1999) and a more recent study replicated these earlier findings (Blanco et al., 2010). Meta-analyses have failed to demonstrate the superiority of MAOIs over SSRIs (van der Linden et al., 2000; Fedoroff and Taylor, 2001; Blanco et al., 2003) for SAD; and given the risk of serious adverse events (including hypertensive crisis) and dietary restrictions associated with the MAOIs, they are generally reserved as second- or third-line agents.

Studies of the reversible inhibitors of monoamine oxidase type A (RIMAs) for SAD have produced mixed findings. Brofaromine was shown to be effective (van Vliet et al., 1992; Fahlen et al., 1995; Lott et al., 1997) but was withdrawn due to safety issues; on the other hand, the RIMA moclobemide failed to show superiority over placebo in short-term studies (Noyes et al., 1997; Schneier et al., 1998).

Benzodiazepines

The effects of benzodiazepines on anxiety are explained by their enhancement of the effect of the inhibitory neurotransmitter gamma-amino-butyric acid (GABA). Clonazepam, bromazepam, and alprazolam have been reported efficacious for the treatment of SAD (Gelernter et al., 1991; Davidson et al., 1993; Versiani et al., 1997; Otto et al., 2000; Seedat and Stein, 2004); however, the number of randomized placebo controlled trials with this class of agents is limited. Their potential for abuse and dependence in predisposed individuals and their lack of effectiveness for the common comorbidity of depression constrains their use as first-line agents for this indication (Van Ameringen et al., 2009).

ß-blockers

β-blockers such as propranolol or atenolol have been recommended on an "as-needed" basis in nongeneralized SAD or "performance anxiety" as they appear to interrupt the escalation of fear in these situations by blocking physiological symptoms of arousal. However, early work failed to support the use of β-blockers in generalized SAD (Liebowitz et al., 1992), and they are believed not to be effective on the emotional and cognitive aspects of SAD. Consistent with this, recent guidelines recommended β-blockers as a therapeutic option only in nongeneralized SAD (Jorstad-Stein and Heimberg, 2009; Stein et al., 2010) or for patients whose SAD is limited to a number of particular situations and marked by symptoms of autonomic nervous system arousal (Westenberg, 2009).

Psychotherapeutic Interventions

Psychotherapies, most notably exposure-based cognitive-behavioral interventions (CBT) administered in individual or group settings, have demonstrated efficacy for the treatment of SAD. CBT usually comprises twelve to sixteen 60- to 90-minute weekly sessions. A recent meta-analysis of results from 30 studies reported that the overall effect size of psychological treatments on social anxiety was 0.70, indicating "a large effect" (Acarturk et al., 2009), although the magnitude of this effect appeared to be less in patients with more severe disease or in studies utilizing a more rigorous control group. In a study comparing the efficacy of group CBT (CBGT) and the MAOI phenelzine for SAD, both interventions were generally comparably efficacious acutely (although phenelzine was superior on some outcome measures) (Heimberg et al., 1998), but CBGT-treated patients were more likely to maintain benefit after treatment discontinuation (Liebowitz et al., 1999).

Few data are available on the efficacy of other psychotherapeutic interventions in SAD. Research on the efficacy of interpersonal therapy, a time-limited intervention based on building interpersonal skills, has yielded conflicting results (Borge et al., 2008; Lipsitz et al., 2008). Although some authors have suggested that a focused type of psychodynamic intervention might be effective (Gabbard, 1992), to date, this therapeutic approach has never been examined in treatment trials. Other novel nonpharmacological interventions have been considered recently, including acceptance and commitment therapy (Dalrymple and Herbert, 2007) and meditation (Koszycki et al., 2007), though further study of these interventions is required before definitive conclusions can be reached regarding their utility.

Treatment Resistance

To date, although the use of SRIs and CBT as first-line treatments for SAD is well established, it is not uncommon for patients to respond incompletely or not at all to these interventions (Davidson, 2006). In clinical trials, roughly one half to two thirds of patients respond to SRIs or CBT (Heimberg et al., 1998; Davidson et al., 2004; Stein and Stein, 2008), though if we consider that less-responsive patients with significant medical or psychiatric comorbidity are usually excluded from these randomized controlled trials, the number of responders in practice is likely lower. However, while at least one third of the treated patients will remain symptomatic and impaired after first-line therapy, to date surprisingly few data are available in the literature on next-step interventions for SAD.

Definition

SAD can be considered as refractory or treatment resistant "when there are residual symptoms or when symptoms do not improve at all after some form of therapeutic intervention" (Pollack et al., 2008). Since no consensus has been reached as to the number or duration of failed therapeutic attempts, it seems reasonable to rely on failure to achieve relevant clinical outcome endpoints such as "the sustained resolution of core anxiety symptoms, functional disability, and psychiatric comorbidities" in defining refractory SAD (Pollack et al., 2008).

Some authors have proposed specific definitions of resolution or remission of SAD on standardized symptoms measures: for example, a cutoff score of 30 (Ballenger, 2001) or 36 (Bandelow et al., 2006) on the Liebowitz Social Anxiety Scale.

Although failing to respond to a first-line psychotherapy would qualify as treatment resistance by the aforementioned definitions, this issue is not commonly addressed in the CBT literature; to the best of our knowledge, no empirical data are available on treating CBT-refractory SAD. This section will therefore mainly address the management of pharmacotherapy refractory SAD, although we will discuss the use of CBT in this context.

General Principles

These principles are derived in part from general approaches to the management of treatment resistance in anxiety disorders (Smoller and Pollack, 1996).

Address Comorbidity

According to results from the recent National Comorbidity Survey–Replication, 62.9% to 90.2% of respondents with lifetime SAD meet criteria for at least one other lifetime disorder with the proportions increasing with the reported number of fears (Ruscio et al., 2008). The most frequent comorbid disorders are other anxiety disorders, depressive disorders, and substance- or alcohol-related disorders (Ruscio et al., 2008). Evidence supports that anxiety with comorbid conditions is more likely to be treatment resistant (Bystritsky, 2006). The presence of comorbid conditions may be associated with treatment resistance by reflecting greater overall severity of illness, requiring additional or focused interventions such as in the case of comorbid substance abuse, or interfere with and/or complicate the treatment of the social anxiety itself (Smoller and Pollack, 1996). To date, few studies have addressed this issue. For example, a study reported that atomoxetine might be efficacious in SAD comorbid with attention-deficit/hyperactivity disorder (Adler et al., 2009). Paroxetine also seems to be efficacious in SAD patients with comorbid alcohol abuse (Book et al., 2008), and escitalopram was found to be effective in SAD patients both with and without depressive symptoms (Stein et al., 2004). Although few data are available on the specific choice of treatment for SAD with comorbid disorders, it is reasonable to select interventions that may address the comorbid condition as well as the SAD; for example, use of an antidepressant for patients with comorbid depression or targeted substance abuse treatment for patients with comorbid drug or alcohol abuse.

Optimization of First-Line Pharmacotherapy

Length of Treatment

Results from studies on SSRIs and SNRIs suggest that some patients might not respond until 12 weeks of treatment (Stein et al., 2002). It seems therefore reasonable to prescribe medication for at least 2 to 3 months at therapeutic doses before considering it ineffective.

Dose

Although one study on escitalopram showed that a higher dose was associated with greater clinical response compared to a lower dose (Lader et al., 2004), two studies on paroxetine and venlafaxine, using fixed-dose design, suggested that the dose–response curve for these agents in SAD might be flat (Liebowitz et al., 2002; Stein et al., 2005). Similarly, another study reported that although increasing the dose of duloxetine was associated with a moderate effect size, the difference was not significant at endpoint (Simon et al., 2010). These conflicting results are in line with those on the optimal dose for SSRI in other anxiety disorders; for example, in a study in panic disorder, increasing dose of SSRIs was not associated with a better outcome at 12 weeks (Simon et al., 2009).

Augmentation

Although there is no systematic data at present demonstrating the relative benefits of augmentation of existing initial treatment compared to switching to an alternate treatment, it may be reasonable to consider augmentation prior to switching for persistent symptoms after 8 to 12 weeks of a first-line agent at adequate dose, particularly in patients who have a history of multiple unsuccessful treatment episodes with first-line agents (e.g., two or more SRIs) (Smoller and Pollack, 1996).

A randomized controlled trial reported a trend (though not reaching significance) toward a better outcome at 10 weeks using paroxetine combined with clonazepam versus paroxetine only (Seedat and Stein, 2004). Another double-blind crossover trial failed to show any difference between paroxetine and paroxetine combined with the β-blocker pindolol (Stein et al., 2001). Open-label studies reported benefit for SRI refractory SAD with augmentation with the atypical antipsychotics aripiprazole (Worthington et al., 2005) and with risperidone (Simon et al., 2006). Finally, buspirone augmentation was reported effective in a series of SAD patients remaining symptomatic despite SSRI therapy (Van Ameringen et al., 1996).

Switching

Serotonin-Norepinephrine Reuptake Inhibitors or Selective Serotonin Reuptake Inhibitors

The paucity of randomized controlled trials on the treatment of refractory SAD or head-to-head comparisons of efficacy between SSRIs and SNRIs in the literature make it difficult to provide guidance on the expected benefits on switching to one SRI after a failed trial on another. One open trial on 29 SAD patients who failed at least one trial with paroxetine reported that after 12 weeks on escitalopram (mean dose = 16.2 mg), half the patients were responders (Pallanti and Quercioli, 2006). Another open trial on 12 SAD patients, nonresponders to SSRIs, reported a significant decrease in symptoms after switching to venlafaxine (Altamura et al., 1999).

Monoamine Oxidase Inhibitors

As noted earlier, meta-analyses have failed to show a superiority of MAOIs over SSRIs (van der Linden et al., 2000; Fedoroff and Taylor, 2001; Blanco et al., 2003). However, one case series reported that 6 out of 7 SAD patients refractory to at least one other treatment improved after switching to phenelzine (Aarre, 2003).

Other Pharmacological Treatments

A variety of *anticonvulsants* have been studied for the treatment of SAD. Gabapentin (Pande et al., 1999) and pregabalin (Pande et al., 2004), α2δ calcium channel antagonists, have both demonstrated some efficacy for SAD in randomized placebo controlled trials ($n = 69$ and $n = 135$, respectively), though the results in the fixed dose pregabalin study were only positive at the highest dose utilized (600 mg/day). Although results from an open-label study of levetiracetam were promising (Simon et al., 2004), two subsequent randomized controlled trials failed to show any efficacy of this agent over placebo (Zhang et al., 2005; Stein et al., 2010). Topiramate (Van Ameringen et al., 2004), valproate (Kinrys et al., 2003) and tiagabine (Dunlop et al., 2007) have also shown positive results in open-label studies, although to date, no randomized controlled trials have confirmed these findings.

There is some evidence suggesting the potential efficacy of *atypical antipsychotics* for the treatment of SAD. Quetiapine has been reported effective for SAD in both an open-label study (Schutters et al., 2005) and in a small (*n* = 15) randomized placebo-controlled trial (Vaishnavi et al., 2007). Similarly, olanzapine was also reported effective in another small (*n* = 12) randomized placebo-controlled trial (Barnett et al., 2002). Although further research needs to be conducted to confirm these preliminary results, atypical antipsychotics may have a role in treatment strategies in SAD, although concerns about significant adverse metabolic and neurologic effects suggest their use should best be reserved for patients failing safer alternatives.

Tricyclic antidepressants have failed to show efficacy for SAD (Benca et al., 1986; Simpson et al., 1998). The noradrenergic and serotonergic antidepressant mirtazapine has been reported to be effective for SAD in open-label studies in adults (Van Veen et al., 2002) and in children (Mrakotsky et al., 2008) as well as in randomized placebo-controlled studies specifically in women (Muehlbacher et al., 2005). However, a recent randomized placebo-controlled trial failed to replicate these results in a sample (*n* = 60), including adults of both sexes (Schutters et al., 2010).

Buspirone monotherapy failed to show efficacy over placebo in a small randomized controlled trial (van Vliet et al., 1997); recently, other studies also failed to support the efficacy of the selective norepinephrine reuptake inhibitor atomoxetine (Ravindran et al., 2009) or an experimental neurokinin-1 antagonist (Tauscher et al., 2010) for SAD.

Augmentation with Cognitive-Behavioral Therapy

A few studies have investigated the efficacy of combining psychotherapy and medication in SAD (Blomhoff et al., 2001; Davidson et al., 2004; Blanco et al., 2010) with mixed results. Blomhoff et al (2001) failed to show a significant superiority of sertraline and CBT over sertraline alone, while in another study, fluoxetine combined with CBT failed to yield any further advantage over either treatment alone (Davidson et al., 2004). On the other hand, a recent study (Blanco et al., 2010) showed that phenelzine and CBT was superior to monotherapy with either intervention. There are no studies examining augmentation with CBT in pharmacotherapy refractory patients (Rodrigues et al., 2010). However, results from such studies in other anxiety disorders (posttraumatic stress disorder (Hinton et al., 2005), panic disorder (Simon et al., 2009), or obsessive-compulsive disorder (Simpson et al., 2008) suggest that augmentation with CBT may be a potentially effective next step strategy.

Conclusion

SAD is prevalent and associated with significant distress and impairment. Effective pharmacologic and psychosocial treatments are available; however, many patients failed to achieve remission after receiving first-line treatment. Although a variety of pharmacologic and psychosocial therapeutics have shown some promise for the treatment of individuals remaining symptomatic after initial therapeutics, there has been a paucity of systematic study addressing this issue. Further research is clearly needed to develop optimal and novel interventions to improve outcomes for individuals suffering with SAD.

Disclosure Statement

E.B. has no conflicts of interest to disclose.

M.H.P. has served on the Advisory Boards and provided consultation to Medavante, Otsuka, and Targia Pharmaceuticals in the last twelve months. He received research grants from Bristol Myers Squibb, Euthymics, Forest Laboratories, Glaxo SmithKline, NCCAM, NIDA, and the NIMH. He holds equity in Medavante, Mensante Corporation, Mindsite, and Targia Pharmaceuticals. He also holds royalty/patent interests in SIGH-A and SAFER interviews.

References

Aarre, T. F. (2003). Phenelzine efficacy in refractory social anxiety disorder: a case series. *Nord J Psychiatry* 57(4): 313–315.

Acarturk, C., P. Cuijpers et al. (2009). Psychological treatment of social anxiety disorder: a meta-analysis. *Psychol Med* 39(2): 241–254.

Adler, L. A., M. Liebowitz et al. (2009). Atomoxetine treatment in adults with attention-deficit/hyperactivity disorder and comorbid social anxiety disorder. *Depress Anxiety* 26(3): 212–221.

Allgulander, C. (1999). Paroxetine in social anxiety disorder: a randomized placebo-controlled study. *Acta Psychiatr Scand* 100(3): 193–198.

Allgulander, C., R. Mangano et al. (2004). Efficacy of venlafaxine ER in patients with social anxiety disorder: a double-blind, placebo-controlled, parallel-group comparison with paroxetine. *Hum Psychopharmacol* 19(6): 387–396.

Alonso, J., & J. P. Lepine (2007). Overview of key data from the European Study of the Epidemiology of Mental Disorders (ESEMeD). *J Clin Psychiatry* 68(Suppl 2): 3–9.

Altamura, A. C., R. Pioli et al. (1999). Venlafaxine in social phobia: a study in selective serotonin reuptake inhibitor non-responders. *Int Clin Psychopharmacol* 14(4): 239–245.

American Psychiatric Association. (2000). *Diagnostic and Statistical Manual of Mental Disorders DSM-IV-TR* (4th edition, Text revision). Washington, DC: American Psychiatric Publishing.

Argyropoulos, S. V., S. D. Hood et al. (2004). Tryptophan depletion reverses the therapeutic effect of selective serotonin reuptake inhibitors in social anxiety disorder. *Biol Psychiatry* 56(7): 503–509.

Asakura, S., O. Tajima et al. (2007). Fluvoxamine treatment of generalized social anxiety disorder in Japan: a randomized double-blind, placebo-controlled study. *Int J Neuropsychopharmacol* 10(2): 263–274.

Baldwin, D., J. Bobes et al. (1999). Paroxetine in social phobia/social anxiety disorder. Randomised, double-blind, placebo-controlled study. Paroxetine Study Group. *Br J Psychiatry* 175: 120–126.

Ballenger, J. C. (2001). Treatment of anxiety disorders to remission. *J Clin Psychiatry* 62(Suppl 120: 5–9.

Bandelow, B., D. S. Baldwin et al. (2006). What is the threshold for symptomatic response and remission for major depressive disorder, panic disorder, social anxiety disorder, and generalized anxiety disorder? *J Clin Psychiatry* 67(9): 1428–1434.

Barnett, S. D., M. L. Kramer et al. (2002). Efficacy of olanzapine in social anxiety disorder: a pilot study. *J Psychopharmacol* 16(4): 365–368.

Bartz, J. A., & E. Hollander (2006). The neuroscience of affiliation: forging links between basic and clinical research on neuropeptides and social behavior. *Horm Behav* 50(4): 518–528.

Benca, R., W. Matuzas et al. (1986). Social phobia, MVP, and response to imipramine. *J Clin Psychopharmacol* 6(1): 50–51.

Blair, K., M. Geraci et al. (2008). Neural response to self- and other referential praise and criticism in generalized social phobia. *Arch Gen Psychiatry* 65(10): 1176–1184.

Blanco, C., R. G. Heimberg et al. (2010). A placebo-controlled trial of phenelzine, cognitive behavioral group therapy, and their combination for social anxiety disorder. *Arch Gen Psychiatry* 67(3): 286–295.

Blanco, C., F. R. Schneier et al. (2003). Pharmacological treatment of social anxiety disorder: a meta-analysis. *Depress Anxiety* 18(1): 29–40.

Blomhoff, S., T. T. Haug et al. (2001). Randomised controlled general practice trial of sertraline, exposure therapy and combined treatment in generalised social phobia. *Br J Psychiatry* 179: 23–30.

Book, S. W., S. E. Thomas et al. (2008). Paroxetine reduces social anxiety in individuals with a co-occurring alcohol use disorder. *J Anxiety Disord* 22(2): 310–318.

Borge, F. M., A. Hoffart et al. (2008). Residential cognitive therapy versus residential interpersonal therapy for social phobia: a randomized clinical trial. *J Anxiety Disord* 22(6): 991–1010.

Bystritsky, A. (2006). Treatment-resistant anxiety disorders. *Mol Psychiatry* 11(9): 805–814.

Campbell, D. W., J. Sareen et al. (2007). Time-varying amygdala response to emotional faces in generalized social phobia. *Biol Psychiatry* 62(5): 455–463.

Clark, D. M., A. Ehlers et al. (2003). Cognitive therapy versus fluoxetine in generalized social phobia: a randomized placebo-controlled trial. *J Consult Clin Psychol* 71(6): 1058–1067.

Dalrymple, K. L., & J. D. Herbert (2007). Acceptance and commitment therapy for generalized social anxiety disorder: a pilot study. *Behav Modif* 31(5): 543–568.

Davidson, J., J. Yaryura-Tobias et al. (2004). Fluvoxamine-controlled release formulation for the treatment of generalized social anxiety disorder. *J Clin Psychopharmacol* 24(2): 118–125.

Davidson, J. R. (2006). Pharmacotherapy of social anxiety disorder: what does the evidence tell us? *J Clin Psychiatry* 67(Suppl 12): 20–26.

Davidson, J. R., E. B. Foa et al. (2004). Fluoxetine, comprehensive cognitive behavioral therapy, and placebo in generalized social phobia. *Arch Gen Psychiatry* 61(10): 1005–1013.

Davidson, J. R., N. Potts et al. (1993). Treatment of social phobia with clonazepam and placebo. *J Clin Psychopharmacol* 13(6): 423–428.

Dunlop, B. W., L. Papp et al. (2007). Tiagabine for social anxiety disorder. *Hum Psychopharmacol* 22(4): 241–244.

Fahlen, T., H. L. Nilsson et al. (1995). Social phobia: the clinical efficacy and tolerability of the monoamine oxidase -A and serotonin uptake inhibitor brofaromine. A double-blind placebo-controlled study. *Acta Psychiatr Scand* 92(5): 351–358.

Fedoroff, I. C., & S. Taylor (2001). Psychological and pharmacological treatments of social phobia: a meta-analysis. *J Clin Psychopharmacol* 21(3): 311–324.

Fehm, L., A. Pelissolo et al. (2005). Size and burden of social phobia in Europe. *Eur Neuropsychopharmacol* 15(4): 453–462.

Furmark, T. (2009). Neurobiological aspects of social anxiety disorder. *Isr J Psychiatry Relat Sci* 46(1): 5–12.

Furmark, T., L. Appel et al. (2005). Cerebral blood flow changes after treatment of social phobia with the neurokinin-1 antagonist GR205171, citalopram, or placebo. *Biol Psychiatry* 58(2): 132–142.

Gabbard, G. O. (1992). Psychodynamics of panic disorder and social phobia. *Bull Menninger Clin* 56(2 Suppl A): A3–A13.

Gelernter, C. S., T. W. Uhde et al. (1991). Cognitive-behavioral and pharmacological treatments of social phobia. A controlled study. *Arch Gen Psychiatry* 48(10): 938–945.

Hansen, R. A., B. N. Gaynes et al. (2008). Efficacy and tolerability of second-generation antidepressants in social anxiety disorder. *Int Clin Psychopharmacol* 23(3): 170–179.

Hariri, A. R., E. M. Drabant et al. (2006). Imaging genetics: perspectives from studies of genetically driven variation in serotonin function and corticolimbic affective processing. *Biol Psychiatry* 59(10): 888–897.

Hedges, D. W., B. L. Brown et al. (2007). The efficacy of selective serotonin reuptake inhibitors in adult social anxiety disorder: a meta-analysis of double-blind, placebo-controlled trials. *J Psychopharmacol* 21(1): 102–111.

Heimberg, R. G., M. R. Liebowitz et al. (1998). Cognitive behavioral group therapy vs phenelzine therapy for social phobia: 12-week outcome. *Arch Gen Psychiatry* 55(12): 1133–1141.

Hinton, D. E., D. Chhean et al. (2005). A randomized controlled trial of cognitive-behavior therapy for Cambodian refugees with treatment-resistant PTSD and panic attacks: a cross-over design. *J Trauma Stress* 18(6): 617–629.

Irle, E., M. Ruhleder et al. (2010). Reduced amygdalar and hippocampal size in adults with generalized social phobia. *J Psychiatry Neurosci* 35(2): 126–131.

Jorstad-Stein, E. C., & R. G. Heimberg (2009). Social phobia: an update on treatment. *Psychiatr Clin North Am* 32(3): 641–663.

Kasper, S., D. J. Stein et al. (2005). Escitalopram in the treatment of social anxiety disorder: randomised, placebo-controlled, flexible-dosage study. *Br J Psychiatry* 186: 222–226.

Katzelnick, D. J., K. A. Kobak et al. (1995). Sertraline for social phobia: a double-blind, placebo-controlled cross-over study. *Am J Psychiatry* 152(9): 1368–1371.

Katzelnick, D. J., K. A. Kobak et al. (2001). Impact of generalized social anxiety disorder in managed care. *Am J Psychiatry* 158(12): 1999–2007.

Kessler, R. C., P. Berglund et al. (2005). Lifetime prevalence and age-of-onset distributions of DSM-IV disorders in the National Comorbidity Survey Replication. *Arch Gen Psychiatry* 62(6): 593–602.

Kinrys, G., M. H. Pollack et al. (2003). Valproic acid for the treatment of social anxiety disorder. *Int Clin Psychopharmacol* 18(3): 169–172.

Klumpp, H., M. Angstadt et al. (2010). Amygdala reactivity to faces at varying intensities of threat in generalized social phobia: an event-related functional MRI study. *Psychiatry Res* 183(2): 167–169.

Kobak, K. A., J. H. Greist et al. (2002). Fluoxetine in social phobia: a double-blind, placebo-controlled pilot study. *J Clin Psychopharmacol* 22(3): 257–262.

Koszycki, D., M. Benger et al. (2007). Randomized trial of a meditation-based stress reduction program and cognitive behavior therapy in generalized social anxiety disorder. *Behav Res Ther* 45(10): 2518–2526.

Lader, M., K. Stender et al. (2004). Efficacy and tolerability of escitalopram in 12- and 24-week treatment of social anxiety disorder: randomised, double-blind, placebo-controlled, fixed-dose study. *Depress Anxiety* 19(4): 241–248.

Lepola, U., B. Bergtholdt et al. (2004). Controlled-release paroxetine in the treatment of patients with social anxiety disorder. *J Clin Psychiatry* 65(2): 222–229.

Liebowitz, M. R., N. A. DeMartinis et al. (2003). Efficacy of sertraline in severe generalized social anxiety disorder: results of a double-blind, placebo-controlled study. *J Clin Psychiatry* 64(7): 785–792.

Liebowitz, M. R., A. J. Gelenberg et al. (2005). Venlafaxine extended release vs placebo and paroxetine in social anxiety disorder. *Arch Gen Psychiatry* 62(2): 190–198.

Liebowitz, M. R., R. G. Heimberg et al. (1999) Cognitive-behavioral group therapy versus phenelzine in social phobia: long-term outcome. *Depress Anxiety* 10(3):89–98.

Liebowitz, M. R., R. M. Mangano et al. (2005). A randomized controlled trial of venlafaxine extended release in generalized social anxiety disorder. *J Clin Psychiatry* 66(2): 238–247.

Liebowitz, M. R., F. Schneier et al. (1992). Phenelzine vs atenolol in social phobia. A placebo-controlled comparison. *Arch Gen Psychiatry* 49(4): 290–300.

Liebowitz, M. R., M. B. Stein et al. (2002). A randomized, double-blind, fixed-dose comparison of paroxetine and placebo in the treatment of generalized social anxiety disorder. *J Clin Psychiatry* 63(1): 66–74.

Lipsitz, J. D., M. Gur et al. (2008). A randomized trial of interpersonal therapy versus supportive therapy for social anxiety disorder. *Depress Anxiety* 25(6): 542–553.

Lott, M., J. H. Greist et al. (1997). Brofaromine for social phobia: a multicenter, placebo-controlled, double-blind study. *J Clin Psychopharmacol* 17(4): 255–260.

Mrakotsky, C., B. Masek et al. (2008). Prospective open-label pilot trial of mirtazapine in children and adolescents with social phobia. *J Anxiety Disord* 22(1): 88–97.

Muehlbacher, M., M. K. Nickel et al. (2005). Mirtazapine treatment of social phobia in women: a randomized, double-blind, placebo-controlled study. *J Clin Psychopharmacol* 25(6): 580–583.

Noyes, R., Jr., G. Moroz et al. (1997). Moclobemide in social phobia: a controlled dose-response trial. *J Clin Psychopharmacol* 17(4): 247–254.

Otto, M. W., M. H. Pollack et al. (2000). A comparison of the efficacy of clonazepam and cognitive-behavioral group therapy for the treatment of social phobia. *J Anxiety Disord* 14(4): 345–358.

Owen, R. T. (2008). Controlled-release fluvoxamine in obsessive-compulsive disorder and social phobia. *Drugs Today (Barc)* 44(12): 887–893.

Pallanti, S., & L. Quercioli (2006). Resistant social anxiety disorder response to Escitalopram. *Clin Pract Epidemiol Ment Health* 2: 35.

Pande, A. C., J. R. Davidson et al. (1999). Treatment of social phobia with gabapentin: a placebo-controlled study. *J Clin Psychopharmacol* 19(4): 341–348.

Pande, A. C., D. E. Feltner et al. (2004). Efficacy of the novel anxiolytic pregabalin in social anxiety disorder: a placebo-controlled, multicenter study. *J Clin Psychopharmacol* 24(2): 141–149.

Phan, K. L., D. A. Fitzgerald et al. (2006). Association between amygdala hyperactivity to harsh faces and severity of social anxiety in generalized social phobia. *Biol Psychiatry* 59(5): 424–429.

Pollack, M. H., M. W. Otto et al. (2008). Novel treatment approaches for refractory anxiety disorders. *Depress Anxiety* 25(6): 467–476.

Ravindran, L. N., D. S. Kim et al. (2009). A randomized controlled trial of atomoxetine in generalized social anxiety disorder. *J Clin Psychopharmacol* 29(6): 561–564.

Rickels, K., R. Mangano et al. (2004). A double-blind, placebo-controlled study of a flexible dose of venlafaxine ER in adult outpatients with generalized social anxiety disorder. *J Clin Psychopharmacol* 24(5): 488–496.

Rodrigues, H., I. Figueira et al. (2010). CBT for pharmacotherapy non-remitters-a systematic review of a next-step strategy. *J Affect Disord* 129: 219–228.

Ruscio, A. M., T. A. Brown et al. (2008). Social fears and social phobia in the USA: results from the National Comorbidity Survey Replication. *Psychol Med* 38(1): 15–28.

Sareen, J., D. W. Campbell et al. (2007). Striatal function in generalized social phobia: a functional magnetic resonance imaging study. *Biol Psychiatry* 61(3): 396–404.

Schneier, F. R., D. Goetz et al. (1998). Placebo-controlled trial of moclobemide in social phobia. *Br J Psychiatry* 172: 70–77.

Schutters, S. I., H. J. Van Megen et al. (2010). Mirtazapine in generalized social anxiety disorder: a randomized, double-blind, placebo-controlled study. *Int Clin Psychopharmacol* 25(5): 302–304.

Schutters, S. I., H. J. van Megen et al. (2005). Efficacy of quetiapine in generalized social anxiety disorder: results from an open-label study. *J Clin Psychiatry* 66(4): 540–542.

Seedat, S., & M. B. Stein (2004). Double-blind, placebo-controlled assessment of combined clonazepam with paroxetine compared with paroxetine monotherapy for generalized social anxiety disorder. *J Clin Psychiatry* 65(2): 244–248.

Simon, N. M., E. A. Hoge et al. (2006). An open-label trial of risperidone augmentation for refractory anxiety disorders. *J Clin Psychiatry* 67(3): 381–385.

Simon, N. M., M. W. Otto et al. (2009). Next-step strategies for panic disorder refractory to initial pharmacotherapy: a 3-phase randomized clinical trial. *J Clin Psychiatry* 70(11): 1563–1570.

Simon, N. M., J. J. Worthington et al. (2004). An open-label study of levetiracetam for the treatment of social anxiety disorder. *J Clin Psychiatry* 65(9): 1219–1222.

Simon, N. M., J. J. Worthington et al. (2010). Duloxetine for the treatment of generalized social anxiety disorder: a preliminary randomized trial of increased dose to optimize response. *CNS Spectr* 15(7): 367–373.

Simpson, H. B., E. B. Foa et al. (2008). A randomized, controlled trial of cognitive-behavioral therapy for augmenting pharmacotherapy in obsessive-compulsive disorder. *Am J Psychiatry* 165(5): 621–630.

Smoller, J. W., & M. H. Pollack (1996). Pharmacologic approaches to treatment-resistant social phobia and generilized anxiety disorder. pgs. 141–170. In: M. H. Pollack, M. W. Otto, & J. F. Rosenbaum, editors. *Challenges in Clinical Pratice*. New York: The Guilford Press.

Simpson, H. B., F. R. Schneier et al. (1998). Imipramine in the treatment of social phobia. *J Clin Psychopharmacol* 18(2): 132–135.

Smoller, J. W., M. P. Paulus et al. (2008). Influence of RGS2 on anxiety-related temperament, personality, and brain function. *Arch Gen Psychiatry* 65(3): 298–308.

Smoller, J. W., L. H. Yamaki et al. (2005). The corticotropin-releasing hormone gene and behavioral inhibition in children at risk for panic disorder. *Biol Psychiatry* 57(12): 1485–1492.

Stein, D. J., D. S. Baldwin et al. (2010). A 2010 evidence-based algorithm for the pharmacotherapy of social anxiety disorder. *Curr Psychiatry Rep* 12(5): 471–477.

Stein, D. J., S. Kasper et al. (2004). Escitalopram in the treatment of social anxiety disorder: analysis of efficacy for different clinical subgroups and symptom dimensions. *Depress Anxiety* 20(4): 175–181.

Stein, D. J., M. B. Stein et al. (2002). Predictors of response to pharmacotherapy in social anxiety disorder: an analysis of 3 placebo-controlled paroxetine trials. *J Clin Psychiatry* 63(2): 152–155.

Stein, M. B., M. D. Fallin et al. (2005). COMT polymorphisms and anxiety-related personality traits. *Neuropsychopharmacology* 30(11): 2092–2102.

Stein, M. B., A. J. Fyer et al. (1999). Fluvoxamine treatment of social phobia (social anxiety disorder): a double-blind, placebo-controlled study. *Am J Psychiatry* 156(5): 756–760.

Stein, M. B., P. R. Goldin et al. (2002). Increased amygdala activation to angry and contemptuous faces in generalized social phobia. *Arch Gen Psychiatry* 59(11): 1027–1034.

Stein, M. B., M. R. Liebowitz et al. (1998). Paroxetine treatment of generalized social phobia (social anxiety disorder): a randomized controlled trial. *JAMA* 280(8): 708–713.

Stein, M. B., M. H. Pollack et al. (2005). Efficacy of low and higher dose extended-release venlafaxine in generalized social anxiety disorder: a 6-month randomized controlled trial. *Psychopharmacology (Berl)* 177(3): 280–288.

Stein, M. B., L. N. Ravindran et al. (2010). Levetiracetam in generalized social anxiety disorder: a double-blind, randomized controlled trial. *J Clin Psychiatry* 71(5): 627–631.

Stein, M. B., J. Sareen et al. (2001). Pindolol potentiation of paroxetine for generalized social phobia: a double-blind, placebo-controlled, crossover study. *Am J Psychiatry* 158(10): 1725–1727.

Stein, M. B., N. J. Schork et al. (2004). A polymorphism of the beta1-adrenergic receptor is associated with low extraversion. *Biol Psychiatry* 56(4): 217–224.

Stein, M. B., & D. J. Stein (2008). Social anxiety disorder. *Lancet* 371(9618): 1115–1125.

Tauscher, J., W. Kielbasa et al. (2010). Development of the 2nd generation neurokinin-1 receptor antagonist LY686017 for social anxiety disorder. *Eur Neuropsychopharmacol* 20(2): 80–87.

The International Multicenter Clinical Trial Group on Moclobemide in Social Phobia. Moclobemide in social phobia. A double-blind, placebo-controlled clinical study. (1997). *Eur Arch Psychiatry Clin Neurosci* 247(2): 71–80.

Vaishnavi, S., S. Alamy et al. (2007). Quetiapine as monotherapy for social anxiety disorder: a placebo-controlled study. *Prog Neuropsychopharmacol Biol Psychiatry* 31(7): 1464–1469.

Van Ameringen, M. A., R. M. Lane et al. (2001). Sertraline treatment of generalized social phobia: a 20-week, double-blind, placebo-controlled study. *Am J Psychiatry* 158(2): 275–281.

Van Ameringen, M., C. Mancini et al. (1996). Buspirone augmentation of selective serotonin reuptake inhibitors (SSRIs) in social phobia. *J Affect Disord* 39(2): 115–121.

Van Ameringen, M., C. Mancini et al. (2004). An open trial of topiramate in the treatment of generalized social phobia. *J Clin Psychiatry* 65(12): 1674–1678.

Van Ameringen, M., C. Mancini et al. (2009). Pharmacotherapy for social anxiety disorder: an update. *Isr J Psychiatry Relat Sci* 46(1): 53–61.

van der Linden, G. J., D. J. Stein et al. (2000). The efficacy of the selective serotonin reuptake inhibitors for social anxiety disorder (social phobia): a meta-analysis of randomized controlled trials. *Int Clin Psychopharmacol* 15(Suppl 2): S15–23.

Van Veen, J. F., I. M. Van Vliet et al. (2002). Mirtazapine in social anxiety disorder: a pilot study. *Int Clin Psychopharmacol* 17(6): 315–317.

van Vliet, I. M., J. A. den Boer et al. (1992). Psychopharmacological treatment of social phobia: clinical and biochemical effects of brofaromine, a selective MAO-A inhibitor. *Eur Neuropsychopharmacol* 2(1): 21–29.

van Vliet, I. M., J. A. den Boer et al. (1994). Psychopharmacological treatment of social phobia: a double blind placebo controlled study with fluvoxamine. *Psychopharmacology (Berl)* 115(1–2): 128–134.

van Vliet, I. M., J. A. den Boer et al. (1997). Clinical effects of buspirone in social phobia: a double-blind placebo-controlled study. *J Clin Psychiatry* 58(4): 164–168.

Versiani, M., A. Nardi et al. (1997). Double-blind placebo controlled trial with bromazepam in social phobia. *J Bras Psiquiatr* 43(3): 167–171.

Versiani, M., A. E. Nardi et al. (1992). Pharmacotherapy of social phobia. A controlled study with moclobemide and phenelzine. *Br J Psychiatry* 161: 353–360.

Vriends, N., E. S. Becker et al. (2007). Subtypes of social phobia: are they of any use? *J Anxiety Disord* 21(1): 59–75.

Westenberg, H. G. (2009). Recent advances in understanding and treating social anxiety disorder. *CNS Spectr* 14(2 Suppl 3): 24–33.

Worthington, J. J., 3rd, G. Kinrys et al. (2005). Aripiprazole as an augmentor of selective serotonin reuptake inhibitors in depression and anxiety disorder patients. *Int Clin Psychopharmacol* 20(1): 9–11.

Zhang, W., K. M. Connor et al. (2005). Levetiracetam in social phobia: a placebo controlled pilot study. *J Psychopharmacol* 19(5): 551–553.

Treatment-Resistant Generalized Anxiety Disorder

Victoria Osman-Hicks, John Potokar, and David J. Nutt

Introduction

Anxiety is a normal reaction to many everyday situations. Generalized anxiety disorder (GAD) represents the extreme end of a continuum of the anxiety spectrum constituting an abnormal state of continuous free-floating anxiety, first classified in 1980 in *DSM-III* (American Psychiatric Association [APA], 1980).

Epidemiology

Anxiety disorders in general are common; the European lifetime prevalence of GAD in the adult population is in the range of 0.1% to 21.7%; removing the outliers, the true lifetime prevalence falls between 0.1% and 6.4% of the population (Leib et al., 2005). The European point prevalence is between 0.8% and 2.1% and the cumulative incidence of GAD at age 34 years is 4.3% (et al., 2005; Beesdo et al., 2010). The highest peak of incidence is in adolescence and early adulthood and the highest peak of prevalence is seen in the 55 and over age group or the young adult age group depending on the cohort, with a 2:1 female-to-male sex ratio (Wittchen et al., 1994; Offord et al., 1996; Carter et al., 2001; Lieb et al., 2005; Beesdo et al., 2010). GAD is the most common anxiety disorder in the elderly age group (Beekman et al., 1998). In the older samples (over 55 years) the past year prevalence is 2.2% to 2.8%—the majority with comorbidity and only 0.53% without (Carter et al., 2001; Mackenzie, et al., 2011).

Comorbidity

GAD is highly comorbid with other psychiatric conditions and can be a primary or secondary disorder. In one study only 6.9% of those with GAD did not have a comorbid disorder (Carter et al., 2001). GAD is recognized to have the highest rates of comorbidity with depressive disorders; up to 70.6% had this combination in a German study (Carter et al., 2001). GAD can predict a higher chance of onset and persistence of depressive episodes

(Kessler, et al., 2008). GAD and depressive episodes follow a similar age of onset slope, both with a peak of incidence in early adulthood or late adolescence (Beesdo et al., 2010). Both conditions have some shared and some discrete risk factors. There is ongoing debate whether depressive disorder and GAD should be classified in a hierarchical manner, as is the current consensus (Zimmerman & Chelminski, 2003).

The second commonest comorbidity is somatoform disorders (48.1%), followed by specific phobias (29.3%), social phobia (28.9%), panic disorder (21.5%), nicotine dependence (14.0%), agoraphobia without panic (11.3%), alcohol abuse or dependence (6.4%), any eating disorder (2.5%), and drug abuse or dependence (1.4%) (Carter et al., 2001).

Lifetime prevalence of comorbid substance misuse disorders is around 2% in the National Epidemiological Survey (Alegria, et al., 2010). Therefore, in this study around half of those with GAD have comorbid substance misuse in this sample. This subgroup is also associated with higher disability and higher vulnerability to other psychopathology, compared to those without substance misuse disorders (Alegria, et al., 2010).

Personality disorders are also highly comorbid; even in an older adult sample, around 25% had both diagnoses (Mackenzie, 2011). Another important comorbidity is sleep disorder (Pollack, 2009).

Increased rates of medical disorders, in general, are also highly associated. There is an increased risk of primary headache seen in one small case-control study, and there appears to be an increase in cardiovascular events in those with coronary heart disease and GAD (Martens et al., 2010; Mercante et al., 2011).

Risk Factors and Heritability

Risk factors for development of GAD include the following in childhood: low socioeconomic status of the parents, dysfunctional family functioning, childhood separation events, maltreatment, conduct problems, more inhibited temperament, reward dependence, internalizing behaviors, parental overprotection, and parental GAD (Moffitt, et al., 2007; Beesdo, 2010). In adulthood, an additional risk factor appears to be a deficit in emotional intelligence (Lizerreti & Extremera, 2011). Adult cohorts demonstrate that the affective states, specifically mania, moderate depressive episodes, and dysthymia, and the anxiety disorders, specifically agoraphobia, panic disorder, and simple phobia, are risk factors for onset of GAD (Kessler, 2002). Simple phobia is the only disorder to increase the risk of persistence of GAD after onset (Kessler, et al., 2002). Heritability estimates in both sexes is around 15%–30% only, which is fairly modest (Kendler, et al., 1992; Hettema, 2001).

Recognition and Diagnosis

GAD is common in primary and secondary care. Despite this, it is often either missed or recognized as another psychiatric disorder; as a result it is untreated or undertreated, causing significant functional impairment (Baldwin et al., 2005). GAD is the second commonest psychiatric condition seen in primary care, after depression, and 7.9%–10% of those that attend the general practitioner for any consultation meet the diagnosis of GAD (Maier et al., 2000; Lieb et al., 2005; Üstün & Sartorius, 2005). Therefore, untreated and unrecognized patients with GAD are costly high primary care consultation users. Help seeking for the specific symptoms of GAD is poor; in an older adult sample only 18% to 28.3% sought help despite an associated increase in medical disorders in general in those with GAD (Mackenzie, 2011).

The flow diagram (see Fig. 8.1), as advocated by the British Association for Psycho-pharmacology, suggests the process the clinician should go through to investigate anxiety-related symptoms (Baldwin et al., 2005). The consultation should be an empathic conversation that allows the patient to discuss important life events and stressors (such as bereavement) which may have precipitated or may maintain the current mental state, along with establishing a diagnosis. Important information to discuss includes illicit drug, alcohol, and caffeine use; personality traits or disorders; and coping strategies. The key message in suspected treatment-resistant patients is to recheck the diagnosis at an early stage and assess for common comorbid disorders.

Impairment and Disability

GAD can cause significant distress and disability without adequate and timely treatment. It is correlated with reduced social function and impairment in several domains of health-related quality of life (Comer, 2011).

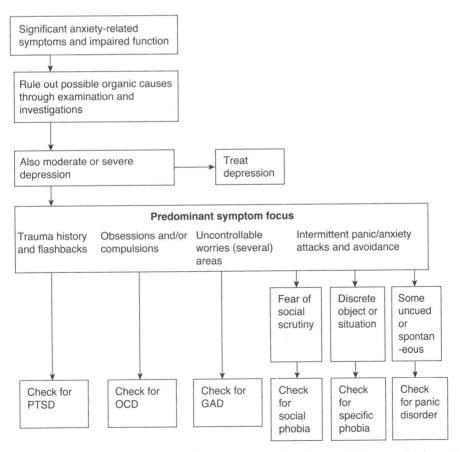

FIGURE 8.1 Scheme for the exploration of a suspected anxiety disorder. GAD, generalized anxiety disorder; OCD, obsessive-compulsive disorder; PTSD, posttraumatic stress disorder. Adapted from BAP guidelines (Baldwin et al., 2005).

Untreated GAD is also associated with higher risk of cardiovascular events in those with preexisting comorbid coronary heart disease, so insufficient GAD treatment can have wider implications to the patient's health (Martens et al., 2010). This chapter will focus on the first-line treatments and more extensively the management of treatment resistance in adults.

First-Line Treatments

First-line treatments involve a patient-centred stepped care approach of (1) explanation, then (2) self-help or group psychoeducation, then (3) drug treatment or cognitive-behavioral therapy (CBT), and then (4) specialist care often involving combination treatments (NICE, 2011). Useful information leaflets to reinforce psychoeducation for patients on their condition and the treatments are available on the homepage of the Royal College of Psychiatrists Web site at http://www.rcpsych.ac.uk.

For the latest guidance for first-line pharmacological treatments, see also the British Association for Psychopharmacology Guidelines (Baldwin et al., 2005) or individual NICE guidelines at http://www.nice.org.

First-Line Pharmacological Treatment

The most common pharmacological approach is a trial of a selective serotonin reuptake inhibitor (SSRI) with meta-analysis evidence of effectiveness in generalized anxiety disorder (GAD) along with a number of other anxiety disorders (Ipser et al., 2009; Baldwin et al., 2011).

In the United Kingdom, the following medications are licensed for GAD (with American trade names in parentheses): escitalopram (Lexapro), paroxetine (Paxil), pregabalin (Lyrica), venlafaxine (Effexor), and duloxetine (Cymbalta). The General Medical Council (United Kingdom) advocates the use of licensed medications in general over unlicensed prescribing. Of the licensed options, escitalopram (Lexapro) brings the best chance of inducing remission (Baldwin et al., 2011).

Of all the medications with placebo-controlled evidence for acute efficacy in GAD, the SSRIs have the best evidence overall for their use from placebo-controlled data, in particular, citalopram (Celexa), escitalopram (Lexapro), fluoxetine (Prozac), paroxetine (Paxil), and sertraline (Zoloft) (Baldwin et al., 2005). Baldwin's meta-analysis demonstrated fluoxetine (Prozac) as the most efficacious medication to induce a response, a 50% reduction in symptoms, with an odds ratio of 0.27 (confidence intervals 0.09–0.81, $p < .05$) (Baldwin et al., 2011). Fluoxetine (Prozac) had a 62.9% chance of bringing about a response and a 60.6% chance of remission. However, this is a cautious recommendation because this is based on only one study of fluoxetine (Prozac) compared with placebo. It was possible that this study was an outlier. There are no head-to head randomized controlled trials (RCTs) of fluoxetine (Prozac) against another active agent. Therefore, it is best to advocate SSRIs in general as the most efficacious agent. The meta-analysis included 27 RCTs and so the evidence base as a whole for pharmacological treatments remains suboptimal (Baldwin et al., 2011).

SSRIs acutely appear to change some of the cognitive bias toward threat interpretation, which has been demonstrated to be greater in those with GAD than those without.

SSRIs appear to reduce the excessive threat interpretation, which is postulated to contribute to the reduction of anxiety levels in those with GAD seen after SSRI treatment (Mogg et al., 2004).

SSRIs with trial evidence in the long term and in relapse prevention are paroxetine (Paxil) and escitalopram (Lexapro) (Baldwin et al., 2005). There is no evidence for fluoxetine (Prozac) or sertraline (Zoloft) in the longer term; this explains why they have not been able to gain a UK license for GAD specifically (Baldwin et al., 2011). There is a paucity of long-term trials for SSRIs, particularly head-to-head trials to inform practice.

One of the few head-to-head studies compared escitalopram (Lexapro) 5, 10, and 20 mg to paroxetine (Paxil) 20 mg and showed the superiority of escitalopram (Lexapro) 20 mg at 12 weeks of treatment (Baldwin et al., 2006). This suggests escitalopram (Lexapro) is a better first-line choice than paroxetine (Paxil). Escitalopram (Lexapro) has been shown in GAD to demonstrate a dose–response relationship in those treated with it; 20 mg is superior to 10 mg, which is superior to 5 mg (Baldwin et al., 2006). Therefore, this study supports the option of increasing the dose in steps to 20 mg to bring about a response or remission. Interestingly adverse side effects do not appear significantly different between the higher doses of escitalopram (Lexapro) (10 and 20 mg), suggesting there is no reason to suggest increasing side effect rates with increasing doses of escitalopram (Lexapro) (Baldwin et al., 2006).

The National Institute of Clinical Excellence (NICE) UK guidance from 2011 recommends for those with GAD the first-line use of sertraline (Zoloft) if the patient chooses a drug treatment (NICE, 2011). This is primarily because of its cost-effectiveness compared to the other SSRIs, despite it being unlicensed for GAD in the United Kingdom and less evidence in longer term efficacy (NICE, 2011). Sertraline (Zoloft) in RCTs appears the most tolerable pharmacotherapy for GAD, with the lowest dropout rate when all high-quality RCTs are meta-analyzed (Baldwin et al., 2011). However, escitalopram (Lexapro) appears the most efficacious licensed medication in terms of remission (Baldwin et al., 2011). A proton pump inhibitor is advised for those prescribed SSRIs at higher risk of gastrointestinal bleeding. A review of the person in a week after prescription of medication, then regularly, is best practice and advised by the NICE (NICE, 2011).

The serotonin and noradrenalin reuptake inhibitors (SNRIs) venlafaxine (Effexor) and duloxetine (Cymbalta) have evidence for acute efficacy in patients; and both are licensed (Baldwin et al., 2005; IPAP, 2011). Duloxetine (Cymbalta) appears superior at bringing about a clinical response, but venlafaxine (Effexor) appears superior at bringing about remission and therefore preventing chronic treatment-resistant cases (Baldwin et al., 2011). Venlafaxine (Effexor) extended-release preparation has been demonstrated in a dosing study to be effective in adults 18 to 65 years old with GAD at a dose of 75 mg/day or more. There is evidence of a dose–response relationship, 150 mg showing a greater reduction in anxiety than 75 mg than 37.5 mg, with 70% of patients responding to 75 mg or 150 mg as a first-line treatment in the short term (Allgulander et al., 2001). In the longer term, ongoing venlafaxine (Effexor) treatment, after a course of 6 months effective treatment, prevents relapse; 9.8% relapsed on venlafaxine (Effexor) compared with 53.7% on placebo (Rickels et al., 2010). This demonstrates the importance of medication for prevention of relapse. For those that relapse off medication, who have previously taken an effective medication, previous medication response predicts subsequent efficacy for that particular medication for that individual, as demonstrated by Rickels et al (2010).

Duloxetine (Cymbalta) (60–120 mg a day) has less discontinuation symptoms on stopping (occurring in one third of patients) than venlafaxine (Effexor) extended release (75–225 mg a day) when compared head to head in those with GAD (Hartford et al., 2007; Carter & McCormack 2009). However, duloxetine (Cymbalta) has extensive cytochrome P450 (CYP) metabolism by CYP1A2 and CYP2D6, so drug interactions are important to consider (Carter & McCormack, 2009).

Another treatment strategy is pregabalin (Lyrica); NICE recommend the use of pregabalin (Lyrica) first line for those who cannot tolerate an SSRI or SNRI (NICE, 2011). Pregabalin (Lyrica) acts by attenuating the release of multiple neurotransmitters in the brain and spinal cord. Pregabalin (Lyrica) (300 mg dose) has been shown to be more efficacious than placebo or alprazolam (a benzodiazepine) in the short term (Rickels et al., 2005). Pregabalin (Lyrica) appears to have a fairly rapid onset of action with significant reduction in symptoms after 1 week (Pande et al., 2003; Rickels et al., 2005). It has been shown to be helpful for both psychic and somatic anxiety in GAD (Rickels et al., 2005). In terms of choice of dosing regimen, there appears to be no advantage of three times a day administration over two divided doses; therefore, twice a day prescription would be advisable as the simplest regimen with the best chance of compliance (Pohl et al., 2005). Pregabalin (Lyrica) is also well tolerated in RCTs, second only to the SSRI sertraline (Zoloft) (Baldwin et al., 2011). In the longer term (6 months), pregabalin (Lyrica) reduces the relapse rate from 65% with placebo to 42% with pregabalin (Lyrica) in those who showed a response to pregabalin (Lyrica) at 8 weeks (Feltner et al., 2008).

Other medications with evidence for acute efficacy in GAD also included the tricyclic antidepressant (TCA) imipramine (imipramine hydrochloride) and the benzodiazepines alprazolam, clonazepam, lorazepam, and diazepam (Baldwin et al., 2005; IPAP, 2011). Despite proven acute efficacy, the use of benzodiazepines is not routinely recommended by the NICE except for short-term courses during crises, mainly because of the potential of tolerance and dependence (NICE, 2011). Imipramine hydrochloride (180 mg/day) coprescription has some benefit in those with GAD having benzodiazepine withdrawal and discontinuation reactions (after long-term use); in particular, imipramine hydrochloride helps to maintain patients off benzodiazepines at 3 months and modestly reduces anxiety levels (Rickels et al., 2000b).

The antipsychotic classes are also no longer recommended by the NICE to be initiated in primary care for GAD, but they can be prescribed in secondary care in the United Kingdom (NICE, 2011). Quetiapine (Seroquel) has positive evidence for acute efficacy as a monotherapy with four high-quality studies, including 2,265 patients demonstrating its superiority over placebo (Depping et al., 2010). The odds ratio was 2.21 (95% confidence interval 1.1 to 4.45) (Depping et al., 2010). However, this Cochrane review demonstrates that the dropout rate in those taking antipsychotic monotherapy over an antidepressant was considerably higher, primarily due to the side effects of sedation and weight gain (Depping et al., 2010). Therefore, despite a similar efficacy to antidepressant medications, antidepressants are clearly better tolerated, suggesting that they are a better first choice. The main benefit in side effect profile of quetiapine (Seroquel) (extended-release preparation) is that it has fewer sexual side effects than the SSRI paroxetine (Paxil) (7.4% on paroxetine [Paxil] 20 mg versus 1.8% on quetiapine [Seroquel] 150 mg), demonstrated in one RCT of 873 patients (Bandelow et al., 2010).

Treatments such as mirtazapine (Remeron); trazodone (trazodone hydrochloride); bupropion hydrochloride and riluzole; the azapirones buspirone hydrochloride and tandospirone; hydroxyzine; the anticonvulsant tiagabine hydrochloride; the typical antipsychotics flupenthixol, sulpiride, and trifluoperazine hydrochloride; and sodium valproate (valproate sodium) all have some evidence for their use in GAD, but to a lesser extent than those previously mentioned (Baldwin et al., 2005; Aliyev & Aliyev, 2007; IPAP, 2011).

1. Buspirone (buspirone hydrochloride) primarily acts as a $5HT_{1A}$ receptor partial agonist with some action on dopamine receptors D_2 and as an alpha 1 and 2 adrenergic receptor antagonist. Buspirone hydrochloride (30 mg/day) reduces anxiety compared with placebo, but not to the same extent as the SNRI venlafaxine (Effexor) (75 or 150 mg/day) in a short-term trial (Davidson et al., 1999). It is licensed for short-term use for anxiety in the United Kingdom.

2. Hydroxyzine is a histamine receptor antagonist. Fifty milligrams per day hydroxyzine has been demonstrated to be equally as acutely efficacious as bromazepam at 6 mg per day (a benzodiazepine) in an RCT of 369 outpatients (Llorca et al., 2002).

3. Mirtazapine (Remeron), a noradrenergic and specific serotonergic antidepressant (NASSA) with $5HT_{2C}$ antagonism, has positive evidence for bringing about response in nearly 80% in an open-label trial at a fixed dose of 30 mg for 12 weeks, but remission is modest at 36.4% only of this small sample (Gambi et al., 2005). Mirtazapine (Remeron) does not have high-quality trials to back its use first line.

4. Trazodone (trazodone hydrochloride), a serotonin antagonist and reuptake inhibitor (SARI) with $5HT_{2A}$ antagonism, is a sedating antidepressant with some anxiolytic properties. Early studies suggested it was similar, possibly a little inferior, to the TCA imipramine hydrochloride with benefit over diazepam from week 3 of treatment at a mean dose of 255 mg (Rickels et al., 1993). Diazepam was superior in the short term for the first 2 weeks (Rickels et al., 1993).

5. Buprorion hydrochloride is an antidepressant acting as a dopamine reuptake inhibitor, norepinephrine reuptake inhibitor. Buprorion hydrochloride has shown some promise in a small open trial of 300 mg/day extended-release preparation compared to escitalopram (Lexapro) 20 mg/day, with evidence that it could be superior (Bystritsky et al., 2005). However, there are no good quality trials to support this finding.

6. Riluzole, a presynaptic glutamate release inhibitor, at a fixed dose of 100 mg/day, has shown some preliminary benefits at reducing anxiety and bringing about remission in around half of patients at week 8 in an open-label study (Matthew et al., 2005). This is an interesting avenue of exploration considering treating glutamate dysregulation or dysfunction in GAD as an alternative neurotransmitter to target. Currently there is insufficient evidence to use it as a first-line treatment.

7. Tiagabine is a selective gamma-aminobutyric acid (GABA) reuptake inhibitor. Tiagabine in meta-analysis appears to be the least effective medication at bringing

about response or remission of those medications with high-quality RCT trials (Baldwin et al., 2011). In head-to-head studies, venlafaxine (Effexor) is superior to tiagabine, in part as there are two unfavorable studies for tiagabine (Baldwin et al., 2011).

8. Flupenthixol, sulpiride, and trifluperazaine (typical antipsychotics). This class of medication was used more commonly in the past, but use is limited by their high rate of extrapyramidal side effects.

9. In terms of mood stabilizers, there is a small preliminary RCT suggesting the benefit of sodium valoproate (valproate sodium) over placebo at bringing about a response in GAD, but there are no other high-quality studies to support its routine use (Aliyev & Aliyev, 2007).

Length of Treatment

Longer term efficacy is seen in patients (in trials) treated with escitalopram (Lexapro), paroxetine (Paxil), venlafaxine (Effexor), and CBT only. The British Association of Psychopharmacology (BAP) advise continuing drug treatment for a further 6 months after initial response at 12 weeks (Baldwin et al., 2005).

Special Prescribing Consideration in the Elderly

There is a paucity of evidence for the pharmacological treatment of GAD in the elderly, with few studies recruiting those over 65 years only.

Pregabalin (Lyrica) has been demonstrated in individuals over 65 years to be safe and efficacious as a first-line treatment for pure GAD. In one placebo-controlled study the anxiolytic effects were seen from 2 weeks for psychic anxiety and from 4 weeks for somatic anxiety (Montgomery et al., 2008). Pregabalin (Lyrica) was administered at a mean dose of 270 mg/day (range 150–600 mg/day) with a 10.7% discontinuation rate (fairly similar to the placebo group). Overall, pregabalin (Lyrica) was found to be safe and well tolerated in the majority, and 64% responded by week 8 of treatment (Montgomery et al., 2008).

Citalopram (Celexa), sertraline (Zoloft), venlafaxine (Effexor), buspirone, paroxetine (Paxil), and trazodone (trazodone hydrochloride) have some positive evidence in elderly populations with GAD (Katz et al., 2002; Lenze et al., 2005; Mokhber et al., 2010). Citalopram (Celexa) was shown to be helpful in a small placebo-controlled study of 17 individuals, although this is too small to make any strong conclusions from (Lenze et al., 2005).

Venlafaxine (Effexor) has more extensive evidence that it is safe and effective acutely in older adult populations (over 60 years), with two thirds having a response to treatment in a pooled analysis of five studies, with only a 15% rate of discontinuation (Katz et al., 2002).

Escitalopram (Lexapro) has shown an equivocal result in an RCT, with no significant benefit over placebo after an intention-to-treat analysis. It is unclear whether the study was underpowered or whether the choice of primary outcome measure (not the usual reduction in anxiety on the Hamilton Anxiety Scale) would change the result (Lenze et al., 2009). This appears to show escitalopram (Lexapro) is less effective in older adults compared to younger adults.

Buspirone hydrochloride has some positive evidence for its role in the elderly. A small single blind trial of buspirone compared to sertraline (Zoloft) in older subjects demonstrated that buspirone and sertraline (Zoloft) both reduced anxiety levels statistically, with buspirone having an effect earlier at weeks 2 and 4, more so than sertraline (Zoloft) (Mokhber et al., 2010). This needs a further large high-quality study to support buspirone's use more widely.

Benzodiazepines, despite widespread use, have limited benefit in the elderly and convey increased risks such as falls. If they are used, shorter acting medications such as lorazepam would be the least harmful at a low dose (Flint, 2005).

Antipsychotics for GAD in those with comorbid dementia should be avoided due to the increased risk of cerebrovascular events.

First-Line Psychological Treatments

There are a range of evidence-based psychological therapies available for GAD. These can be helpful when provided by trained and supervised staff at reducing symptoms severity. This fits with several psychological theoretical models of GAD such as the cognitive, the emotional or experiential, conceptual, and the integrated models of GAD (Dugas et al., 1998; Behar et al., 2009).

The commonest and gold standard psychotherapy offered in the United Kingdom for GAD is CBT, which has the largest evidence base for acute efficacy of all of the psychotherapies for those aged 18 to 75 years (Hunot et al., 2010). CBT for GAD focuses on improving coping mechanisms to reduce anxiety via identifying and challenging unhelpful thoughts and beliefs through self-monitoring, relaxation training and practice, cognitive therapy, and practicing coping strategies.

In terms of the good quality evidence for CBT in GAD, the Cochrane Library Review contains over 20 studies of CBT including 1,060 participants; however, only one study has Grade A methodological quality (Akkerman et al., 2001). Table 8.1 summarizes the evidence from this review for CBT in GAD and in comparison to other psychotherapies. On average, 46% of patients in CBT trials show a response, a modest treatment gain (Hunot et al., 2010).

In terms of recovery, meta-analysis demonstrates that CBT with applied relaxation (AR) seems to offer greater chance of recovery at 6 months follow-up with 50%–60% achieving recovery, compared with 40% or less in pure CBT approaches (Fisher & Durham, 1999).

CBT also has evidence for longer term efficacy in patients (Baldwin et al., 2005; IPAP, 2011). In an 8- to 14-year follow-up after two CBT trials comparing CBT with medication or placebo in primary care, CBT demonstrated benefits over medication in terms of less top-up treatment required over the follow-up and less severe symptomatology in the longer term. However, in the trial cohort as a whole only 30%–40% recovered and 30%–40% went on to have severe symptoms needing secondary care intervention (Durham et al., 2003), thus demonstrating that those with severe symptoms tend to have the worst outcome in the longer term. This highlights the importance of prompt treatment such as CBT for those with mild to moderate GAD.

A challenge for primary care is to find brief and cost-effective psychological strategies for those with mild to moderate symptoms of GAD and to try to prevent chronic and disabling symptoms. This is even more important when we consider the number of appointments those with unrecognized or undertreated GAD use, which is clearly costly to the health service.

TABLE 8.1 First-Line Cognitive-Behavioral Therapy Evidence Base from Cochrane Review (2010)

Comparison	Clinical Response (%)	Reduction in Anxiety	Improvement in Quality of Life (SMD)	Attrition (%)
Any form of CBT vs. control	46% vs. 14%	SMD –1.00 (95% CI –1.24 to –0.77)	0.44 (95% CI 0.06 to 0.82)	16.5% vs. 13.3%
Interpretation	CBT more favorable	CBT more favorable	CBT more favorable	No difference statistically
CT with AM vs. psychodynamic psychotherapy	28% vs. 7%	WMD –13.41 (95% CI –19.09 to –7.74) at 6 months	No data	22% vs. 33%
Interpretation	CT with AM more favorable	At 6-month follow-up CT more favorable		No difference statistically
CBT vs. ST	42% vs. 28%	SMD –0.40 (95% CI –0.66 to –0.14) post treatment SMD –0.42 (95% CI 0.83 to –0.02) at 6 months	SMD 0.30 (95% CI –10.77 to 11.37)	24% vs. 24%
	No difference statistically	Post treatment and at 6 months CBT more favorable	No difference but one study only	No difference
Individual CBT vs. group CBT (vs. control)	RR 0.63 (95% CI 0.51 to 0.76) vs. 0.66 (95% CI 0.54 to 0.82)	SMD –0.98 (95% CI –1.32 to –0.65) vs. –1.02 (95% CI –1.35 to 0.69)	No data	9% vs. 24.2%
	Both similar and better than control	Both similar and better than control		Individual CBT has significantly lower attrition

AM, anxiety management; CBT, cognitive-behavioral therapy; CT, cognitive therapy; ST, supportive therapy; WMD, weighted mean difference,
Source: Adapted from data from Hunot et al. (2010).

Meta-analysis of those who have shorter versus longer courses of psychotherapy seems to show that both CBT interventions (eight sessions or less versus greater than eight sessions) convey benefit over placebo acutely with a similar size clinical response in both (Hunot et al., 2010). In CBT compared with supportive therapy (ST), in those having eight sessions or less, there was no difference in clinical response between CBT and ST, but above eight sessions CBT gained benefit in bringing about a clinical response with no additional benefit from further ST sessions. This suggests ST should be limited to short courses for GAD in most individuals with CBT having a course length of up to or above eight sessions as required for the individual with applied relaxation, as the data are mixed.

Psychodynamic and psychoanalytic therapies are considered for those with GAD but rarely used as a first-line treatment. Cognitive therapy has been shown to be better than a 6-month course of psychoanalytic weekly therapy (Durham et al., 1994). CBT also appears superior to short-course (6 months) psychodynamic psychotherapy in terms of reducing state-trait anxiety, worry, and depressive symptoms after treatment and at 6 months follow-up for all but the latter (Leichsenring et al., 2009). This is not surprising in that CBT focuses the treatment on troublesome worry, mood, and anxiety, and some of the cognitive types of anxiety are weighted more in the instruments they used. However, both treatments brought about significant improvements in anxiety symptoms. At this stage, there is no evidence to suggest psychodynamic therapy should replace CBT as the first-line psychotherapy.

Anxiety management training, a behavioral approach, has been helpful and brought about significant improvement in patients but is not as effective as cognitive therapy (CT) (Durham et al., 1994). Similar results have been found comparing individual behavior therapy (BT) with CBT, showing CBT is superior in those with moderate to severe GAD post treatment and at 18 months follow-up (Butler et al., 1991). CT offers similar results to applied relaxation alone (Ost & Breitholtz, 2000), and CT and BT seem inferior to CBT, suggesting CBT would always be the first-line therapy choice.

Innovative approaches of delivering psychological care have included CBT within a specific package. A recent trial looking at the choice of CBT or medication in a primary care patient group with a range of anxiety disorders showed that a package including Web-based outcome monitoring and a nonexpert care manager promoting adherence was better than usual care (Roy-Byrne et al., 2010). Another approach tested is a palmtop computer program that also prompts patients in between sessions to do CBT homework tasks and practice (Newman et al., 1999). A trial registered but not yet completed also is trying an online CBT program in comparison to sertraline (Zoloft) or placebo to see whether such an intervention would be beneficial in primary care (Christensen et al., 2010).

Special Consideration in the Elderly

CBT appears to be less effective in elderly cohorts compared to younger adults (Hunot et al., 2010). The exact mechanisms behind this are not fully understood. Meta-analysis suggests elderly individuals respond to CBT less than younger adults in terms of gaining less improvement in their anxiety (Hunot et al., 2010). Individual CBT is still efficacious for a proportion of participants; in one study of individuals over 60 years old, 45% respond versus 8% to a minimal contact control; however, the responders did not resume normal levels of function (Stanley et al., 2003). There is insufficient meta-analysis data to understand what effect CBT has on improving quality of life on the whole (Hunot et al., 2010). Another important consideration is that one in four of elderly patients undergoing CBT drop out, which is substantially greater than younger adult cohorts (Hunot et al., 2010).

When CBT is compared to an active control such as a discussion group, there was very limited additional benefit gained from CBT over the discussion group and no clear benefit at 6 months follow-up (Wetherell et al., 2003). Similar results were found with supportive psychotherapy (ST) as a comparator, with no clear superiority in CBT; this is backed up by Cochrane meta-analysis (Mohlman, 2004; Hunot et al., 2010). There is insufficient good quality data in older adults as to the benefits of CT compared with BT and CBT compared with psychodynamic psychotherapy (Hunot et al., 2010). Table 8.2 summarizes the key statistics comparing adult CBT to elderly adult CBT.

Treatment Resistance

There is no consensus as to what defines "treatment-resistant" GAD, but Cochrane collaboration reviews use failure to respond to one first line medication. For the purposes of this chapter, we will use failure of one appropriate first-line treatment (pharmacological or psychological).

TABLE 8.2 First-Line Cognitive-Behavioral Therapy Evidence Base from Cochrane Review Adults Versus Elderly

Comparison	Clinical Response	Reduction in Anxiety	Improvement in Quality of Life (SMD)	Attrition (%)
CBT adults vs. elderly (vs. control)	RR 0.68 (95% CI 0.55 to 0.84) vs. 0.62 (95% CI 0.50 to 0.75)	SMD −1.25 (95% CI −1.57 to −0.93) vs. −0.73 (95% CI −1.07 to 0.40)	No data	9.2% vs. 26.4%
Interpretation	Both age groups were similar and found CBT more favorable than control	Both age groups found CBT more favorable than control, adults greater than elderly		Elderly has significantly higher attrition rate, which was greater than control. Adults had a lower attrition rate, which was lower than control
CBT vs. ST adults vs. elderly	RR 0.80 (95% CI 0.62 to 1.05) vs. 1.07 (95% CI 0.77 to 1.49)	SMD −0.49 (95% CI −0.80 to −0.19) vs. −0.13 (95% CI −0.64 to −0.37)		RR 1.03 (95% CI 0.62 to 1.71) vs. 1.07 (95% CI 0.60 to 1.89)
Interpretation	CBT better for adults and ST better for elderly but nonsignificantly	CBT better than ST for adults and no difference in elderly		No statistical difference in attrition in the two age groups
CT vs. BT (adults vs. elderly)	No data	No data	No data	No data
CBT vs. psychodynamic therapy (adults vs. elderly)	No data	No data	No data	No data

CBT, cognitive behavioral therapy; ST, supportive therapy.
Source: Adapted from data from Hunot et al. (2010).

Pharmacological Treatments

In terms of cases that fail first-line treatments, there appears to be no advantage in general to increasing the dose after initial nonresponse (unless the dose was subtherapeutic) and switching appears more advantageous (NICE, 2004). However, several studies have demonstrated a dose–response relationship in particular for venlafaxine (Effexor) and escitalopram (Lexapro), suggesting these may be exceptions to this general principle so in these medications it is important to try increasing the dose (Allgulander et al., 2001; Baldwin et al., 2006).

An important consideration in treating any disorder is the risks and benefits of additional treatments. For example, an antipsychotic may reduce a specific symptom but may cause significant side effects or harm through precipitating a metabolic syndrome, neuroleptic malignant syndrome, or akathisia, for example. Within the scope of this chapter, we will not list all the potential side effects of each treatment, but the British National Formulary (http://www.bnf.org) or the Maudsley guidelines (Taylor et al., 2009) offer a comprehensive list. The reader should bear in mind the potential contraindications and side effects of treatments.

There is low-level positive evidence for switching from an SSRI to venlafaxine (Effexor) or duloxetine (Cymbalta) or to the TCA imipramine hydrochloride (unlicensed) in resistant patients. One can consider short-term benzodiazepines after SSRI and SNRI failure for cover and then subsequently combining medications (Baldwin et al., 2005).

Pregabalin (Lyrica) augmentation of an SSRI or SNRI was shown to bring about at least a 50% reduction in anxiety in 50% of trial participants in one double-blind RCT (Weaver et al., 2009).

In terms of SSRI augmentation with the atypical antipsychotics, aripiprazole (Abilify) (a partial D2 agonist) has some preliminary evidence of its benefit in GAD in open trials, $n = 59$ (Worthington et al., 2005; Hoge et al., 2008; Lorenz et al., 2010). But it does not have a strong evidence base. In one small trial, 13% discontinued due to side effects, in particular sedation, restlessness, and chest discomfort, although this sample also included those with panic disorder (Hoge et al., 2008). Other important side effects noted by participants with GAD were nausea, weight gain, insomnia, and jitteriness (Lorenz et al., 2010).

Olanzapine (Zyprexa) (up to 20 mg/day, with a mean dose of 8.7 mg/day) has been tested specifically in combination with fluoxetine (Prozac) (20 mg/day) as an augmenter. It can improve response rates to acute fluoxetine (Prozac) treatment but did not bring about remission any more so than placebo in its only RCT, $n = 21$ (Pollack et al., 2006). There are no other studies with olanzapine (Zyprexa) augmentation to support its use. Olanzapine (Zyprexa) also caused significant weight gain (55%), sedation (91%), and gastrointestinal side effects (36%) in those taking with combination treatment (Pollack et al., 2006; Lorenz et al., 2010). The significant weight gain may mean its risk may be greater than its benefit.

Quetiapine (Seroquel) as an augmentation agent has been tested in three small trials, two randomized and controlled, in those with treatment-resistant symptoms of GAD (Lorenz et al., 2010). The first open-label trial looked at flexible dosing paroxetine (Paxil) controlled release with quetiapine (Seroquel) (up to 400 mg/day), $n = 22$, with six completing quetiapine (Seroquel) augmentation (Simon et al., 2006). This showed no statistical or clinical benefit of quetiapine (Seroquel) over placebo augmentation after 8 weeks (Simon et al., 2006). There seems to be no benefit of this combination to bring about a response acutely; however, it is difficult to form any conclusions from just six patients.

In the RCTs, quetiapine (Seroquel) was used to augment a heterogeneous group of usual first-line antidepressants with a flexible dose regimen with a maximum dose of 800 mg/day for 12 weeks (Katzman et al., 2008). The mean dose of quetiapine (Seroquel) was 386 mg/day in a study of 40 patients. There were significant rates of remission of symptoms at week 12 at 72.1% and the medication was well tolerated (Katzman et al., 2008). The second RCT was in a sample of partial and nonresponders using in contrast low-dose quetiapine (Seroquel) (mean dose 50 mg/day) for 8 weeks. This pilot study showed a statistically nonsignificant improvement in symptoms at 8 weeks (60% versus 30%) with a trend to suggest low-dose quetiapine (Seroquel) may be helpful (Altamura et al., 2011). This could represent that there is a trend that quetiapine (Seroquel) may be effective as an anxiolytic, but it is unclear what dose would be best. A large RCT with different dosing regimens for quetiapine (Seroquel) would help to answer this question.

Risperidone (Risperdal) has mixed evidence of reducing GAD symptoms in short-term trials, including two randomized and controlled. The largest RCT so far ($n = 390$) of risperidone (Risperdal) (up to 2 mg/day, mean dose 0.86 mg/day) compared it to placebo augmentation of a heterogeneous group of first-line treatments, including SSRIs, SNRIs, and other antidepressants. The outcome was that risperidone (Risperdal) was not significantly better than placebo overall, although a post-hoc analysis of those with moderate to severe GAD demonstrated a benefit of risperidone (Risperdal) (Pandina et al., 2007).

Two further smaller trials showed some benefit of augmentation with risperidone (Risperdal) (Brawman-Mintzer et al., 2005; Simon et al., 2006) with mean daily treatment doses of 1.1 mg and 1.12 mg. There is currently no convincing evidence in large RCTs of the benefit of adjunctive risperidone (Risperdal).

Ziprasidone hydrochloride augmentation (at a flexible dosing regimen of 20 to 80 mg per day) has some initial pilot randomized controlled evidence that there is a trend that it reduces anxiety symptoms in the short term; but not to a level that reached statistical significance in a small study of 62 participants (Lohoff et al., 2010). There was an over 30% dropout rate in the ziprasidone arm, considerably more so than placebo, suggesting tolerability as with all antipsychotics can be a problem (Lohoff et al., 2010). There is also a small open trial suggesting ziprasidone may be efficacious (Snyderman et al., 2005). There is no evidence for augmentation with asenapine (Saphris), paliperidone (Invega), or clozapine (Lorenz et al., 2010). There is clearly a need for high-quality large augmentation trials to support the use of antipsychotics. Despite this, clinically the use of antipsychotics in treatment-resistant patients appears to be mainstream in the United Kingdom.

Other agents suggested to be beneficial include mirtazapine (Remeron), trazodone hydrochloride, bupropion hydrochloride, buspirone hydrochloride, hydroxyzine, tiagabine, flupenthixol, trifluoperazine HCL, sulpiride, and riluzole; all but buspirone are unlicensed (Baldwin et al., 2005). For a full list of starting and maximum doses in GAD, including speed of dose increments, Table 8.3 suggests what doses can be used in clinical practice.

Novel Pharmacological Treatments

1. Cholecystokinin (CCK) B receptor antagonists. CCK-B receptors are mainly situated in the brain and may transform dopaminergic function, causing anxiolytic effects in rodents (Hughes et al., 1990). In humans, an RCT of one such agent named CI-988 showed no effect at the dose tested; however, it did have poor bioavailability (Adams et al., 1995). A second-generation CCK-B receptor antagonist CI-1015 is being developed as a candidate agent in humans with 10 times the bioavailability of the previous agent CI-988 (Trivedi et al., 1998). Other potential neuropeptide receptors of interest for drug targets include agonists of neuropeptide Y and antagonists of CRF receptors.

2. Opipramol is a tricyclic iminostilbene derivative with D_2, $5HT_2$, and H_1 blockade and affinity nonselectively to sigma 1 and 2 receptors. In an RCT, opipramol showed anxiolytic properties superior to placebo and in a similar range to alprazolam, its active comparator (Möller et al., 2001). Although widely prescribed in Germany, it is unlicensed in the United Kingdom.

3. Deramciclane (5HT2a/2c receptor antagonist). This has shown some potential as an anxiolytic agent in animal studies. In humans, a placebo-controlled RCT has shown that it appears safe and well tolerated at up to 60 mg/day and efficacious over placebo in a significant manner at 60 mg/day (Naukkarinen et al., 2005). This may lead to further research as a new potential drug for GAD.

4. Gepirone ($5HT_{1A}$ agonist, an analog of buspirone). This agent was initially developed as an antidepressant. Gepirone was then tested in those with GAD and was found to be inferior to diazepam with a high dropout rate (58%) (Rickels et al., 1997). The common side effects are headache and nausea. An extended-release preparation was subsequently developed to be better tolerated, but there remains no current positive evidence for its use in GAD. Other potential serotonergic targets are drugs acting on 5HT3 as an antagonist, dual-acting $5HT_{1A}$ and $5HT_{2A}$ and $5HT_{2C}$ receptors.

5. Alpidem, abecarnil, and bretazenil (partial benzodiazapine receptor agonists). In preclinical research these have appeared to be promising anxiolytics. These would have the potential advantage of the anxiolytic effects of traditional benzodiazepines without dependence, sedation, and withdrawal effects. An RCT of abecarnil compared with placebo and diazepam found at 6 weeks abecarnil was not significantly better than placebo and did in fact cause sedation but without discontinuation symptoms (Rickels et al., 2000a). There is no clear evidence at this stage that partial benzodiazepaine receptor agonists may be helpful.

6. Ocinaplon, a $GABA_A$ receptor modulator, is a novel anxiolytic agent still in the early stages of clinical trials. One proof of concept clinical trial demonstrated 270 mg/day ocinaplon was superior to placebo and the medication did not produce the side effects of sedation or dizziness commonly associated with benzodiazepines (Czobar et al., 2010). This is a promising avenue of research and development for GAD.

7. *Passiflora incarnate* (passionflower). This has long been a traditional medicine for anxiety. One small 4-week pilot study found 45 drops/day passiflora had an equivocal effect to oxaxepam 30 mg/day (Akhondzadeh et al., 2002). There is no large-scale trial to support its use beyond this.

8. *Piper methysticum* (kava kava). Kava is a traditional medicine and in Fiji is made into a foul-tasting drink for traditional ceremonies and for celebrations due to its psychoactive properties. Currently there is no evidence for its use in GAD, and in fact it appears that placebo is significantly better in one study (Connor et al., 2006).

9. Ginkgo biloba special extract EGb 761. A small RCT suggests there may be some benefit of this herbal supplement over placebo in the short term (Woelk et al., 2007). There was a 44% response rate (with a p value of .004), demonstrated by a reduction in the Hamilton Anxiety Scale in those taking 480 mg/day (Woelk et al., 2007). This is a very preliminary finding and may support further evaluation of this product.

10. Valerian, another herbal remedy, has been studied but has no benefit in meta-analyses for GAD (Miyasaka et al., 2009).

Psychological Therapies

There is limited evidence for additional benefit of drug treatment and CBT in combination (Baldwin et al., 2005), although in clinical practice this approach is often taken. In practice, expert secondary care CBT is often undertaken sometimes with a wider psychological treatment approach encompassing other comorbidities or maintaining factors.

TABLE 8.3 Doses of Medications for General Anxiety Disorder in Nonelderly Adults

Medication	UK License (Y/N)	Start Dose (mg/day)	Frequency	Maximum Dose (mg)	Dose Increments	Preparations
Citalopram	N	20	OM	60	20 mg per 2 weeks	Tablets and oral drops
Escitalopram	Y	5–10	OM	20	5–10 mg per 1–2 weeks	Tablets and oral drops
Sertraline*	N	25	OM	200	25 mg in first week, then 25–50 mg per 1–2 weeks	Tablets and liquid
Fluoxetine	N	10	OM	60	10–20 mg per 2 weeks	Capsules and liquid
Paroxetine	Y	10–20	OM	50	10–20 mg per 2 weeks	Tablets and liquid
Duloxetine	Y	30	OM	120	30 mg after 1–2 weeks	Capsules only
Venlafaxine	Y	37.5–75	OM	225		Tablet and modified release capsule
Imipramine	N	25	OM	300	25 mg every 4 days, then in 50 mg increments after 100 mg	Tablets
Mirtazapine	N	15	ON	45	15 mg per 1–2 weeks	Tablets and orodispersible tablets
Trazadone	N	50	ON	400	50 mg per 3–4 days	Capsules, tablets, liquid
Bupropion	N	100	OD, then BD	300	150 mg per 6 days	Tablets
Lorazepam	N	2	1 mg BD–0.5 mg QDS	4** to 6	1–2 mg per week	Tablet (0.5 mg = half tablet) IM
Diazepam	N	15	5 mg TDS	30** to 40	5 mg after 4–7 days, then 10 mg weekly	Tablet, oral solution, IM, IV, rectal tube, suppository
Clonazepam	N	2	ON–QDS	6	1–2 mg per week	Tablet
Alprazolam	N	0.75–1.5	0.25–0.5 mg TDS	4	0.5 mg every 3–4 days	Tablet
Buspirone	N	10–15	5 mg BD-TDS	45** to 60	5 mg every 3 days	Tablet

Drug	Recommended	Starting dose	Dose regimen	Maximum dose	Titration	Formulation
Tandospirone	N	15–30	5–10 mg TDS	60	15 mg every 2–4 weeks	Tablet
Pregabalin	Y and EU	150	75 mg BD	600	150 mg per 4–7 days	Capsule
Hydroxyzine	N	50	25 mg BD-QDS	100	50 mg per week	Tablet, syrup
Tiagabine	N	4	2 mg BD	16	2–4 mg per week	Tablet
Flupentixol	N	0.5–3	BD	3	1 mg a week	Tablet
Sulpiride	N	50	ON/OM	200	50 mg after 3–4 days, then 100 mg after 1 week	Tablet, oral solution
Ziprasidone	N	40	20 mg BD	160	20 mg every 2–3 days***	Tablet
Quetiapine	N	25	OM/ON if modified release BD if not	800	25–50 mg increase daily for up to 4 days, then slower***	Tablet or modified release
Risperidone	N	2	OD-BD	6	1 mg a day maximum***	Tablet, orodispersible tablet
Olanzapine	N	2.5	OM/ON	20	2.5 mg steps***	Tablet, orodispersible tablet
Riluzole	N	50	?OM	100	50 mg after 1–3 days	Tablet
Sodium valproate	N	250	OD-TDS	1–2 g, or not greater than 45 g/kg	250 mg weekly***	Tablet

*Recommended by NICE, 2011 for first-line medication.
**Lower dose maximum is British National Formulary advice; upper maximum dose is other sources.
***Very limited evidence for rate of increments in GAD specifically and appropriate maximum dose.
Source: Adapted from IPAP with reference to British National Formulary (http://www.bnf.org; IPAP, 2011).

There is limited positive evidence for the following psychological therapies, but there is no clear evidence that any cause harm, so these could be considered in those that have had conventional psychological approaches already:

1. Meditation therapies (specifically transcendental meditation, muscle biofeedback, and relaxation training) have limited RCT evidence with one old study with a narrative analysis showing that participants all showed a significant reduction in symptoms (using an anxiety scale) after 18 weeks of treatment, with no evidence of harm. However, meditation did not improve sleep, sex life, and marital relations, and there was a high dropout rate of 33% (Raskin et al., 1980).

2. Mindfulness-based cognitive therapy (group therapy) may be an option in treatment-resistant patients. In a nonrandomized controlled trial it has shown to have acute efficacy in non-treatment-resistant population, but there is yet to be a large RCT to support this finding (Evans et al., 2008).

3. Additional interpersonal therapy or experiential therapy components with conventional CBT may be helpful because of the significant comorbidity of GAD with other disorders. The effectiveness of these combination therapies is yet to be fully evaluated to be recommended routinely (Borkovec et al., 2003).

4. Acceptance-based behavioral therapy is based on the experiential theories of GAD and encourages experiential acceptance. At post treatment and 3-month follow-up, one open trial shows this can improve symptoms and quality of life (Roemer & Orsillo, 2007). A subsequent small RCT ($n = 31$) also demonstrated benefit, with 78% no longer meeting the criteria for GAD and 77% achieving high-level function (Roemer et al., 2008). This is showing some promise and needs further evidence because this appears to better than current best evidence-based approach of CBT with applied relaxation. There is no evidence of its merits in the longer term.

5. Well-being therapy (WBT) with CBT is based on the principle that restoring function is as important as gaining a treatment response. One trial of eight sessions of CBT compared with CBT for four sessions and then WBT for four sessions shows combination treatment appeared more efficacious (Fava et al., 2005). This is a very preliminary finding and further work needs to be done. There is also no evidence of its merits in the longer term.

6. Metacognitive therapy based on the metacognitive model of GAD has preliminary non-RCT evidence that it may be beneficial with high rates of recovery (87.5%) post treatment and continued high recovery at 12 months in three quarters of participants (Wells & King, 2006). There is no evidence of its merits in the longer term beyond 12 months.

7. Psychodynamic or analytic approaches, as previously discussed, are in general inferior to CBT for pure GAD but may help with interpersonal and wider psychological issues, particularly in those with comorbidity, which is extremely common.

Figure 8.2 suggests one possible approach to the treatment of a patient who has failed to respond or remit with first-line therapy. The flow diagram considers the steps of pharmaco-therapies and psychotherapies to consider in order. However, in most cases this should be

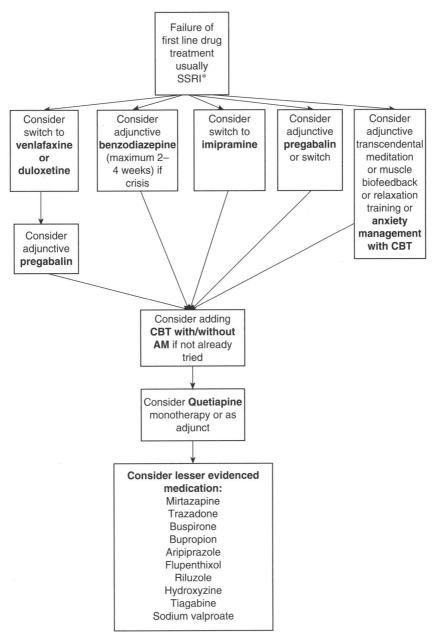

FIGURE 8.2 Augmentation options if generalized anxiety disorder, *3-month course. AM, anxiety management; CBT, cognitive-behavioral therapy; SSRI, selective serotonin reuptake inhibitor.

adapted to take into account the patient's specific wishes and comorbidities and as part of a wider approach considering the patient's psychosocial needs.

Treating Comorbidity

This chapter does not have the scope to consider the treatment strategy of every important comorbidity seen in treatment resistance. Clearly, untreated comorbidities will maintain or exacerbate most cases of GAD and so diagnosis, acknowledgment, and treatment of them may improve the course of GAD and prevent chronic treatment resistance. Finally, we will consider the comorbidity of GAD with insomnia.

Insomnia with General Anxiety Disorder

Generalized anxiety is one of the more common comorbidities in those with insomnia and vice versa, especially in the elderly, and so it is important to consider the evidence for treating the two conditions simultaneously. Treating coexisting insomnia may improve the course of GAD, although this is not clearly established.

Sleep disruption can affect daytime function, specifically causing fatigue, cognitive impairment, incoordination, psychomotor performance, physiological dysfunction, anxiety level, and mood changes, and these factors can lead to accidents (Krystal, 2010). Specific changes in sleep patterns are seen in those with GAD, including initial, middle, and early morning insomnia, increased sleep latency, and decreased total sleep time and quality (Krystal, 2010).

Secondary sleep disturbance from illicit substance use, alcohol misuse, caffeine excess, or poor sleep hygiene should also be considered in the assessment of insomnia, prior to initiating any treatment.

Trials of patients with both insomnia and GAD are not plentiful, and there is no consensus guideline as to how to treat the two conditions most effectively.

Short-term double-blind trials with acute efficacy in comorbid GAD and insomnia have included the following:

1. Zolpidem extended release (ER) 12.5 mg and escitalopram (Lexapro) 10 mg with improvement in subjective total sleep time at 8 weeks compared with placebo, but zolpidem has no inherent anxiolytic effect (Fava et al., 2009).
2. Eszopiclone 3 mg and escitalopram (Lexapro) 10 mg with improvement in reduced sleep latency, increased total sleep time, and reduced anxiety using HAM-A score at 2 months compared with placebo (Pollock et al., 2008a).
3. Zopiclone monotherapy with improvement in sleep parameters with a mild anxiolytic effect is better than the comparator nitrazepam (Agnoli et al., 1989).
4. Agomelatine monotherapy improved sleep compared with placebo (Stein et al., 2008).
5. CBT targeting excessive worry significantly reduced comorbid insomnia, demonstrated in reduced scores on the Insomnia Severity Index (Bélanger et al., 2004).

In the United States, triazolam, temazepam, flurazepam, quazepam (Doral), estazolam, zolpidem, zolpidem CR, esozopiclone, and zaleplon are licensed for use in insomnia (Krystal, 2010). In the United Kingdom, zolpidem and zopiclone are the most commonly prescribed Z-drugs for insomnia. Zolpidem is an imidazopyridine, and zopiclone and its S-enatomer esozopiclone are cyclopyrrolones (Jia et al., 2009). Both improve sleep and insomnia through actions at different GABA$_A$-Rs subtypes and exert different electroencephalogram patterns and slightly different sleep patterns (Jia et al., 2009). Both increase sleep duration and help maintain sleep (Jia et al., 2009). Esozopiclone prolongs non-REM sleep and increases total REM sleep, whereas Zolpidem does not (Jia et al., 2009). On the current evidence there may be a benefit of esozopiclone or zopiclone over zolpidem because of the additional mild anxiolytic effect in GAD in combination with escitalopram (Lexapro) or offering a prompt course of CBT depending on patient preference for those with comorbid insomnia. This will help to improve daytime function and may reduce the chance of the patient developing treatment resistance.

Conclusions

GAD is a highly comorbid and chronic anxiety disorder when left untreated or undertreated. The importance of diagnosis in primary care, secondary care general medicine, and psychiatry is the first barrier for many patients. With diagnosis, psychoeducation and prompt access to evidence-based psychotherapies and pharmacotherapies are key to ensuring patients have the best chance of response and remission. Patients and practitioners do need to remember that GAD can take up to 12 weeks to respond to pharmacotherapy, which is longer than depressive episodes, and so patience is required before a response is seen.

The evidence base of treatment-resistant GAD is lagging behind that of depressive disorder, but we do have five licensed medications in the United Kingdom with evidence that they can bring about remission along with the psychotherapy CBT. There is increasing evidence for second-line treatments along with considering any of the usual first-line therapies not already tried.

Directions for future research include the following:

1. Large head-to-head RCTs of first-line pharmacotherapy agents with the primary outcome being remission of GAD, rather than acute response.
2. Large CBT high-quality trials with long-term follow-up for GAD in non-treatment-resistant individuals particularly looking at therapist factors and expertise (Durham et al., 2005).
3. Large head-to-head pharmacological and psychological therapy trials in treatment-resistant individuals with GAD with long-term follow-up to inform practice.
4. Large high-quality trials with long-term follow-up for GAD in non-treatment-resistant and treatment-resistant elderly subjects for both psychological and pharmacological approaches.
5. Large high-quality trials of treatment (first line and second line) of specific comorbid disorders with GAD, looking at best treatment, for example, in depression and GAD.
6. Developing the basic science of GAD, including neuroendocrinology, translational research, and neuroimaging, in combination with other methods of study (Pollack et al., 2008b).

Disclosure Statement

V.O.-H. has no conflicts of interest to disclose.

J.P. has received an overdose a research grant from Schering-Plough.

D.J.N. is on the advisory boards for Lundbeck, Servier, Pfizer, Reckitt Benkiser, and D&A Pharma. He has also received speaking honoraria from Bristol-Meyers Squibb, Glaxo SmithKlein, and Schering-Plough. He has received grants and clinical trial payments from

P1Vital, the Medical Research Council, and the National Health Service. He has been an expert witness in a number of legal cases relating to psychotropic drugs and has edited and written over 25 books, some of which have been purchased by pharmaceutical companies.

References

Adams J., Pyke R., Costa J., Cutler N., Schweizer E., Wilcox C., Wisselink P., Greiner M., Pierce M., & Pande A. (1995). A double blind placebo controlled study of a CCK B receptor antagonist, CI-988, in patients with generalized anxiety disorder. *Journal of Clinical Psychopharmacology, 15*(6), 428–434.

Agnoli A., Manna V., & Martucci N. (1989). Double blind study on the hypnotic and anti-anxiety effects of zopiclone compared with nitrazepam in the treatment of insomnia. *International Journal of Clinical Pharmacology Research, 9,* 277–281.

Akhondzadeh S., Naghavi H., Vazirian M., Shayeganpour A., Rashidi H., & Khani M. (2002). Passionflower in the treatment of generalized anxiety: A pilot double blind randomized controlled study. *Journal of Clinical Pharmacy and Therapeutics, 26*(5), 363–367.

Akkerman R., Stanley M., Averill P., Novy D., Snyder A., & Diefenbach G. (2001). Recruiting older people with generalized anxiety disorder. *Journal of Mental Health and Ageing, 7*(14), 385–394.

Alegria A., Hasin D., Nunes E., Liu S., Davies C., Grant B., & Blanco C. (2010). Comorbidity of generalized anxiety disorder and substance misuse disorders: Results from the National Epidemiological Survey on alcohol and related conditions. *Journal of Clinical Psychiatry, 71*(9), 1187–1195.

Aliyev N., & Aliyev Z. (2007). Valproate (depakine-chrono) in the acute treatment of outpatients with generalized anxiety disorders without psychiatric co-morbidity: Randomized, double blind placebo controlled study. *European Psychiatry, 23*(2), 109–114.

Allgulander C., Hackett D., & Salinas E. (2001). Venlafaxine extended release (ER) in the treatment of generalised anxiety disorder: Twenty four week placebo controlled dose-ranging study. *British Journal of Psychiatry, 179,* 15–22.

Altamura A., Serati M., Buoli M., & Dell'Osso B. (2011). Augmentative quetiapine in partial/nonresponders with generalized anxiety disorder: A randomised placebo controlled study. *International Clinical Psychopharmacology,* [Epub ahead of print].

American Psychiatric Association. (Ed.). (1980). *Diagnostic and statistical manual of mental disorders* (3rd ed.). Washington, DC: Author.

Baldwin D., Anderson I., Nutt D., Bandelow B., Bond A., Davidson J., den Boer J., Fineberg N., Knapp M., Scott J., & Witchen H-U. (2005). Evidence based guidelines for the pharmacological treatment of anxiety disorders: Recommendations from the British Association for Psychopharmacology. *Journal of Psychopharmacology, 19,* 567–596.

Baldwin D., Huusom AKT., & Mæhlum E. (2006). Escitalopram and paroxetine in the treatment of generalised anxiety disorder: Randomised, placebo-controlled, double-blind study. *British Journal of Psychiatry, 189,* 264–272.

Baldwin D., Woods R., Lawson R., & Taylor D. (2011). Efficacy of drug treatments for generalised anxiety disorder: Systematic review and meta-analysis. *The British Medical Journal, 342,* 1199–1210.

Bandelow B., Chouinard G., Bobes J., Ahokas A., Eggens I., Liu S., & Eriksson H. (2010). Extended-release quetiapine fumarate (Quetiapine XR): A once-daily monotherapy effective in generalized anxiety disorder. Data from a randomized, double-blind, placebo and active controlled study. *International Journal of Neuropsychopharmacology, 13*(3), 305–320.

Bélanger L., Morin C., Langlois F., & Ladouceur R. (2004). Insomnia and generalized anxiety disorders: Effects of cognitive behavioural therapy for GAD on insomnia. *Journal of Anxiety Disorders, 18*(4), 561–571.

Beekman A., Bremmer M., Deeg D., van Balkom A., Smit J., de Beurs E., van Dyck R., & van Tilburg W. (1998). Anxiety disorders in later life: A report from the Longitudinal Aging Study Amsterdam. *International Journal of Geriatric Psychiatry, 13,* 717–726.

Beesdo K., Pine D., Lieb R., & Wittchen H-U. (2010). Incidence and risk patterns of anxiety and depressive disorders and categorization of generalized anxiety disorder. *Archives of General Psychiatry, 67*(1), 47–57.

Behar E., DiMarco I., Hekler E., Mohlman J., & Staples A. (2009). Current theoretical models of generalized anxiety disorder (GAD): Conceptual review and treatment implications. *Journal of Anxiety Disorders, 23*(8), 1011–1123.

Borkovec TD., Newman M., & Castonguay L. (2003). Cognitive behavioural therapy for Generalised Anxiety Disorder with integrations from interpersonal and experiential therapies. *CNS Spectrums, 8,* 382–389.

Brawman-Mintzer O., Knapp R., & Nietert P. (2005). Adjunctive risperidone in generalized anxiety disorder: A double blind, placebo controlled study. *Journal of Clinical Psychiatry, 66*(10), 1321–1325.

Brystritsky A., Kerwin L., Eiduson S., & Vapnik T. (2005). A pilot controlled trial of bupropion vs. escitalopram in generalized anxiety disorder (GAD). *Neuropsychopharmacology, 30*, S101.

Butler G., Fennell M., Robson P., & Gelder M. (1991). Comparison of behaviour therapy with cognitive behaviour therapy in the treatment of generalized anxiety disorder. *Journal of Consulting and Clinical Psychology, 59*(1), 167–175.

Carter N., & McCormack P. (2009). Duloxetine: A review of its use in the treatment of generalized anxiety disorder. *CNS Drugs, 23*(6), 523–541.

Carter R., Wittchen H-U., Pfister H., & Kessler R. (2001). One year prevalence of sub-threshold and threshold DSM-IV generalized anxiety disorder in a nationally representative sample. *Depression and Anxiety, 13*, 78–88.

Christensen H., Guastella A., Mackinnon A., Griffiths K., Eagleson C., Batterham P., Kalia K., Kenardy J., Bennett K., & Hickie I. (2010). Protocol for a randomised controlled trial investigating the effectiveness of an online e-health application compared to attention placebo or sertraline in the treatment of generalised anxiety disorder. *Trials, 11*, 48.

Comer J., Blanco C., Hasin D., Liu S., Grant B., Turner J., & Olfson M. (2011). Health related quality of life across the anxiety disorders: Results from the National Epidemiological Survey on alcohol and related conditions (NESARC). *Journal of Clinical Psychiatry, 72*(1), 43–50.

Connor K., Payne V., & Davidson J. (2006). Kava in generalised anxiety disorder: Three placebo controlled trials. *International Clinical Psychopharmacology, 21*(5), 249–253.

Czobar P., Skolnik P, Beer B., & Lippa A. (2010). A multicenter, placebo controlled, double-blind study of efficacy and safety of Ocinaplon (DOV 273, 547) in generalized anxiety disorder. *CNS Neuroscience and Therapeutics, 16*(2), 63–75.

Davidson J., DuPont R., Hedges D., & Haskins JT. (1999). Efficacy, safety and tolerability of venlafaxine extended release and buspirone in outpatients with generalized anxiety disorder. *Journal of Clinical Psychiatry, 60*(8), 528–535.

Depping A., Komossa K., Kissling W., & Leucht S. (2010). Second generation antipsychotics for anxiety disorders. *Cochrane Database of Systematic Reviews, 8*(12), CD008120.

Dugas M., Gagnon F., Ladouceur R., & Freeston M. (1998). Generalized anxiety disorder: A preliminary test of a conceptual model. *Behaviour Research and Therapy, 36*(2), 215–226.

Durham R., Chambers J., Macdonald R., Power K., & Major K. (2003). Does cognitive behavioural therapy influence the long term outcome of generalized anxiety disorder? An 8–14 year follow up of two clinical trials. *Psychological Medicine, 33*, 499–509.

Durham R., Chambers J., Power K., Sharp D., Macdonald R., Major K., Dow M., & Gumley A. (2005). Long-term outcome of cognitive behaviour therapy clinical trials in central Scotland. *Health Technology Assessment, 9*(42), 1–3.

Durham R., Murphy T., Allan T., Richard K., Treliving L., & Fenton G. (1994). Cognitive therapy, analytic psychotherapy and anxiety management. *British Journal of Psychiatry, 165*, 315–323.

Evans S., Ferrando S., Findler M., Stowell C., Smart C., & Haglin D. (2008). Mindfulness-based cognitive therapy for generalized anxiety disorder. *Journal of Anxiety Disorders, 22*(4), 716–721.

Fava M., Asnis G., Shrivastava R., Lydiard B., Bastani B., Sheehan D., & Roth T. (2009). Zolpidem extended release improves sleep and next day symptoms in co-morbid insomnia and generalized anxiety disorder. *Journal of Clinical Psychopharmacology, 29*(3), 222–230.

Fava G., Ruini C., Rafanelli C., Finos L., Salmaso L., Mangelli L., & Sirigatti S. (2005). Well-being therapy of generalized anxiety disorder. *Psychotherapy and Psychosomatics, 74*(1), 26–30.

Feltner D., Wittchen H-U., Kavoussi R., Brock J., Baldinetti F., & Pande A. (2008). Long term efficacy of pregabalin in generalized anxiety disorder. *International Clinical Psychopharmacology, 23*(1), 18–28.

Fisher P., & Durham R. (1999). Recovery rates in generalized anxiety disorder following psychological therapy: An analysis of clinically significant change in the STAI-T across outcome studies since 1990. *Psychological Medicine, 29*(6), 1425–1434.

Flint A. (2005). Generalised anxiety disorder in elderly patients: epidemiology, diagnosis and treatment options. *Drugs and Ageing, 22*(2), 101–114.

Gambi F., De Berardis D., Campanella D., Carano A., Sepedre G., Salini G., Mezzano D., Cicconetti A., Penna L., Salerno RM., & Ferro FM. (2005). Mirtazapine treatment of generalized anxiety disorder: A fixed dose, open label study. *Journal of Psychopharmacology, 19*(5), 483–487.

Hartford J., Kornstein S., Liebowitz M., Pigott T., Russell J., Detke M., Walker D., Ball S., Dunayevich E., Dinkel J., & Erickson J. (2007). Duloxetine as an SNRI treatment for generalized anxiety disorder: Results from a placebo controlled trial. *International Clinical Psychopharmacology, 22*(3), 167–174.

Hettema J., Prescott C., & Kendler K. (2002). A population based twin study of generalized anxiety disorder in men and women. *Journal of Nervous and Mental Disease, 189*(7), 413–420.

Hoge E., Worthington J., Kaufman R., Delong H., Pollack M., & Simon N. (2008). Aripiprazole as augmentation treatment of refractory generalized anxiety disorder and panic disorder. *CNS Spectrums, 13*(6), 522–527.

Hughes J., Boden P., Costall B., Domeney A., Kelly E., Horwell D., Hunter J., Pinnock R., & Woodruff G. (1990). Development of a class of selective Cholecystokinin B receptor antagonist having potent anxiolytic activity. *Proceedings of the National Academy of Sciences USA, 87*, 6728–6732.

Hunot V., Churchill R., Teixeira V., & Silva de Lima M. (2010). Psychological therapies for generalised anxiety disorder (Review). *Cochrane Database of Systematic Reviews, 4*, CD001848.

IPAP (2011). Cite references, Retrieved 1st February 2011 from http://www.ipap.org

Ipser J C., Carey P., Dhansay Y., Fakier N., Seedat S., & Stein D J. (2009). Pharmacotherapy augmentation strategies in treatment-resistant anxiety disorders. *Cochrane Database of Systematic Reviews, 1*, CD005473.

Jia F., Goldstein P., & Harrison N. (2009). The modulation of synaptic GABA$_A$ receptors in the thalamus by esozopiclone and zolpidem. *Journal of Pharmacology and Experimental Therapeutics, 328*, 1000–1006.

Katz I., Reynolds C., Alexopolous G., & Hackett D. (2002). Venlafaxine ER as a treatment for generalized anxiety disorder in older adults: Pooled analysis of five randomized placebo-controlled clinical trials. *Journal of the American Geriatrics Society, 50*(1), 18–25.

Katzman M., Vermani M., Jacobs L., Marcus M., Kong B., Lessard S., Galarraga W., Struzik L., & Gendron A. (2008). Quetiapine as an adjunctive pharmacotherapy for the treatment of non-remitting generalized anxiety disorder: A flexible dose, open label pilot trial. *Journal of Anxiety Disorders, 22*(8), 1480–1486.

Kendler K., Neale M., Kessler R., Heath A., & Eaves L. (1992). Generalized anxiety disorder in women. A population based twin study. *Archives of General Psychiatry, 49*(4), 267–272.

Kessler R., Andrade L., Bijl R., Offord D., Demler O., & Stein D. (2002). The effects of comorbidity on the onset and persistence of generalized anxiety disorder in the ICPE surveys. International Consortium in Psychiatric Epidemiology. *Psychological Medicine, 32*(7), 1213–1225.

Kessler R., Gruber M., Hettema J., Hwang I., Sampson N., & Yonkers K. (2008). Comorbid major depression and generalized anxiety disorders in the National Comorbidity Survey follow up. *Psychological Medicine, 38*(3), 365–374.

Krystal A. (2010). In vivo evidence of the specificity of effects of GABA-A receptor modulating medications. *Sleep, 33*(7), 859–860.

Leichsenring F., Salzer S., Jaeger U., Kächele H., Kreische R., Leweke F., Rüger U., Winkelbach C., & Leibing E. (2009). Short term psychodynamic psychotherapy and cognitive behavioural therapy in generalised anxiety disorder: A randomized controlled trial. *American Journal of Psychiatry, 166*, 875–881.

Lenze E., Mulsant B., Shear M., Dew M., Miller M., Pollock B., Houck P., Tracey B., & Reynolds C. (2005). Efficacy and tolerability of citalopram in the treatment of late-life anxiety disorders: Results from an eight week randomised controlled trial. *American Journal of Psychiatry, 162*, 146–150.

Lenze E., Rollman B., Shear K., Dew M., Pollock B., Ciliberti C., Costantino M., Snyder S., Shi P., Spitznagel E., Andreescu C., Butters M A., & Reynolds C F., 3rd. (2009). Escitalopram for older adults with generalized anxiety disorder. *Journal of the American Medical Association, 301*(3), 295–303.

Lieb R., Becker E., & Altamura C. (2005). The epidemiology of generalized anxiety disorder in Europe. *European Neurosychopharmacology, 15*, 445–452.

Lizeretti N., & Extremera N. (2011). Emotional intelligence and clinical symptoms in outpatients with generalized anxiety disorder (GAD). *Psychiatric Quarterly.* [Epub ahead of print].

Llorca P-M., Spadone C., Sol O., Danniau A., Bougerol T., Corruble E., Faruch M., Macher J-P., Sermet E., & Servant D. (2002). Efficacy and safety of hydroxyzine in the treatment of generalized anxiety disorder: A 3 month double-blind study. *Journal of Clinical Psychiatry, 63*(11), 1020–1027.

Lohoff F., Etemad B., Mandos L., Gallop R., & Rickels K. (2010). Ziprasidone treatment of refractory generalized anxiety disorder: A placebo controlled, double blind study. *Journal of Clinical Psychopharmacology, 30*(2), 185–189.

Lorenz R., Jackson C., & Saitz M. (2010). Adjunctive use of atypical antipsychotics for treatment resistant generalized anxiety disorder. *Pharmacotherapy, 30*(9), 942–951.

Mackenzie C., Reynolds K., Chou K., Pagura J., & Sareen J. (2011). Prevalence and correlates of generalised anxiety disorder in a national sample of older adults. *American Journal of Geriatric Psychiatry, 19*(4), 305–315.

Maier W., Gaensicke M., Freyberger H., Linz M., Heun R., & Lecrubier Y. (2000). Generalized anxiety disorder (ICD-10) in primary care from a cross-cultural perspective, a valid diagnostic entity? *Acta Psychiatrica Scandinavica, 101*, 29–36.

Martens E., de Jonge P., Na B., Cohen B., Lett H., & Whooley M. (2010). Scared to death? Generalized anxiety disorders and cardiovascular events in patients with stable coronary heart disease. *Archives of General Psychiatry, 67*(7), 750–758.

Matthew S., Amiel J., Coplan J., Fitterling H., Sackeim H., & Gorman J. (2005). Open label trial of riluzole in generalized anxiety disorder. *American Journal of Psychiatry, 162*, 2379–2381.

Mercante J., Peres M., & Bernik M. (2011). Primary headaches in people with generalised anxiety disorder. *Journal of Headache and Pain*. [Epub ahead of print].

Miyasaka L., Atallah Á., & Soares B. (2009). Valerian for anxiety disorders. *Cochrane Database of Systematic Reviews, 1*, CD004515.

Moffitt T., Caspi A., Harrington H., Milne B., Melchior M., Goldberg D., & Poulton R. (2007). Generalised anxiety disorder and depression: Childhood risk factors in a birth cohort followed to age 32. *Psychological Medicine, 37*, 441–452.

Mogg K., Baldwin D., Brodrick P., & Bradley B. (2004). Effect of short term SSRI treatment on cognitive bias in generalised anxiety disorder. *Psychopharmacology, 176*(3–4), 466–470.

Mohlman J. (2004). Psychosocial treatment of late-life generalized anxiety disorder: Current status and future directions. *Clinical Psychology Review, 24*(2), 149–169.

Mokhber N., Azarpahzooh M., Khajehdaulee M., Velayati A., & Hopwood M. (2010). Randomized, single-blind trial of sertraline and buspirone for treatment of elderly patients with generalized anxiety disorder. *Psychiatry and Clinical Neurosciences, 64*(2), 128–133.

Möller H-J., Volz H-P., Reimann I., & Stoll K-D. (2001). Opipramol for the treatment of generalized anxiety disorder: A placebo controlled trial including an alprazolam treated group. *Journal of Clinical Psychopharmacology, 21*(1), 59–65.

Montgomery S., Vhatamra K., Pauer L., Whalen E., & Baldinetti F. (2008). Efficacy and safety of pregabalin in elderly people with generalised anxiety disorder. *British Journal of Psychiatry, 193*, 389–394.

NICE. (2004). *The management of panic disorder and generalised anxiety disorder in primary and secondary care.* London: National Collaborating Centre for Mental Health.

NICE. (2011). *Generalised anxiety disorder and panic disorder (with or without agoraphobia) in adults. Management in primary, secondary and community care.* NICE Clinical Guidance 113. London: National Collaborating Centre for Mental Health and National Collaborating Centre for Primary Care.

Naukkarinen H., Raassina R., Penttinen J., Ahokas A., Jokinen R., Koponen H., Lepola U., Kanerva H., Lehtonen L., Pohjalainen T., Partanen A., Mäki-Ikola O., Rouru J., & Deramciclane Dose-Finding Study Group. (2005). Deramciclane in the treatment of generalized anxiety disorder: A placebo controlled, double blind dose-finding study. *European Neuropsychopharmacology, 15*(6), 617–623.

Newman M., Consoll A., & Barr Taylor C. (1999). A palmtop computer program for the treatment of generalized anxiety disorder. *Behaviour Modification, 23*(4), 597–619.

Offord D., Boyle M., Campbell D., Goering P., Lin E., Wong M., & Racine YA.(1996). One year prevalence of psychiatric disorder in Ontarians 15 to 64 years of age. *Canadian Journal of Psychiatry/Revue Canadienne de Psychiatrie, 41*, 559–563.

Ost L-G., & Breitholtz E. (2000). Applied relaxation vs. cognitive therapy in the treatment of generalized anxiety disorder. *Behaviour Research and Therapy, 38*, 777–790.

Pande A., Crockatt J., Feltner D., Janney C., Smith W., Weisler R., Londborg PD., Bielski RJ., Zimbroff DL., Davidson JR., & Liu-Dumaw M. (2003). Pregabalin in generalized anxiety disorder: A placebo controlled trial. *American Journal of Psychiatry, 160*, 533–540.

Pandina G., Canuso C., Turkoz I., Kujawa M., & Mahmoud R. (2007). Adjunctive risperidone in the treatment of generalized anxiety disorder: A double blind, prospective, placebo-controlled, randomized trial. *Psychopharmacology Bulletin, 40*(3), 41–57.

Pohl R., Felyner D., Fieve R., & Pande A. (2005). Efficacy of pregabalin in the treatment of generalized anxiety disorder: A double-blind, placebo-controlled comparison of BID versus TID dosing. *Journal of Clinical Psychopharmacology, 25*(2), 151–158.

Pollack M. (2009). *Sleep and anxiety: Focus on post traumatic stress disorder and generalised anxiety disorder.* Retrieved April 2011, from http://www.medscape.org/viewarticle/701543_print.

Pollack M., Kinrys G., Krystal A., McCall V., Roth T., Schaefer K., Rubens R., Roach J., Huang H., & Krishnan R. (2008a). Eszopiclone coadministered with escitalopram in patients with insomnia and comorbid generalized anxiety disorder. *Archives of General Psychiatry, 65*(5), 551–562.

Pollack M., Otto M., Roy-Byrne P., Coplan P., Rothbaum B., Simon N., & Gorman J. (2008b). Novel treatment approaches for refractory anciety disorders. *Focus*, *1*(4), 486–495.

Pollack M., Simon N., Zalta A., Worthington J., Hoge E., Mick E., Kinrys G., & Oppenheimer J. (2006). Olanzapine augmentation of fluoxetine for refractory generalised anxiety disorder: A placebo controlled study. *Biological Psychiatry*, *59*, 211–215.

Raskin M., Bali L., & Peeke H. (1980). Muscle biofeedback and transcendental meditation. *Archives of General Psychiatry*, *37*, 93–97.

Rickels K., Demartinis M., & Aufdembrinke B. (2000a). A double blind, placebo controlled trial of abecarnil and diazepam in the treatment of patients with generalized anxiety. *Journal of Clinical Psychopharmacology*, *20*(1), 12–18.

Rickels K., Demartinis M., Garcia-España F., Greenblatt D., Mandos L., & Rynn M. (2000b). Impiramine and buspirone in treatment of patients with generalized anxiety disorder who are discontinuing long term benzodiazepine therapy. *American Journal of Psychiatry*, *157*, 1973–1979.

Rickels K., Downing R., Schweizer E., & Hassman H. (1993). Antidepressants for the treatment of generalized anxiety disorder. A placebo controlled comparison of imipramine, trazodone and diazepam. *Archives of General Psychiatry*, *50*(11), 884–895.

Rickels K., Etemad B., Khalid-Khan S., Lohoff F., Rynn M., & Gallop R. (2010). Time to relapse after 6 and 12 months' treatment of generalized anxiety disorder with venlafaxine extended release. *Archives of General Psychiatry*, *67*(12), 1274–1281.

Rickels K., Pollack M., Feltner D., Lydiard R., Zimbroff D., Bielski R., Tobias K., Brock JD., Zornberg GL., & Pande AC. (2005). Pregabalin for treatment of generalized anxiety disorder: A 4-week, multicenter, double-blind, placebo-controlled trial of pregabalin and alprazolam. *Archives of General Psychiatry*, *62*, 1022–1030.

Rickels K., Schweizer E., DeMartinis N., Mandos L., & Mercer C. (1997). Gepirone and diazepam in generalized anxiety disorder: A placebo controlled trial. *Journal of Clinical Psychopharmacology*, *17*(4), 272–277.

Roemer L., & Orsillo S. (2007). An open trial of an acceptance based behaviour therapy for generalized anxiety disorder. *Behaviour Therapy*, *38*(1), 72–85.

Roemer L., Orsillo S., & Salters-Pedneault K. (2008). Efficacy of an acceptance-based behaviour therpy for genetalized anxiety disorder: Evaluation in a randomised controlled trial. *Journal of Clinical and Consulting Psychology*, *76*(6), 1083–1089.

Roy-Byrne P., Craske MG., Sullivan G., Rose RD., Edlund MJ., Lang AJ., Bystritsky A., Welch SS., Chavira DA., Golinelli D., Campbell-Sills L., Sherbourne CD., & Stein MB. (2010). Delivery of evidence-based treatment for multiple anxiety disorders in primary care: A randomized controlled trial. *Journal of the American Medical Association*, *303*(19), 1921–1928.

Simon N., Connor K., Le Beau R., Hoge E., Worthington J., Zhang W., Davidson J., & Pollack M. (2006). Quetiapine augmentation of paroxetine CR for the treatment of refractory generalized anxiety disorder: Preliminary findings. *Psychopharmacology*, *197*(4), 675–681.

Snyderman S., Rynn M., & Rickels K. (2005). Open label pilot study of ziprasidone for refractory generalized anxiety disorder. *Journal of Clinical Psychopharmacology*, *25*(5), 497–499.

Stanley M., Beck J., Novy D., Averill P., Swann A., Diefenbach G., Gretchen J., & Hopko D. (2003). Cognitive-behavioural treatment for late life generalized anxiety disorder. *Journal of Consulting and Clinical Psychology*, *71*(2), 309–319.

Stein D., Ahokas A., & de Bodinat C. (2008). Efficacy of agomelatine in generalized anxiety disorder: A randomized, double blind, placebo controlled study. *Journal of Clinical Psychopharmacology*, *28*, 561–566.

Taylor D., Paton C., & Kapur S. (2009). *The Maudsley prescribing guidelines*. (10th ed.) London: Informa Healthcare.

Trivedi B., Padia J., Holmes A., Rose S., Wright D., Hinton J., Pritchard M., Eden J., Kneen C., Webdale L., Suman-Chauhan N., Boden P, Singh L., Field M., & Hill D. (1998). Second generation "peptoid" CCK-B receptor antagonists: Identification and development of N-(Adamantyloxycarbonyl)-α-methyl-(R)-tryptophan derivative (CI-1015) with an improved pharmacokinetic profile. *Journal of Medicinal Chemistry*, *41*(1), 38–45.

Üstün T., & Sartorius N. (1995). *Mental illness in general health care, an international study*. Chichester, England: Wiley.

Weaver J., Miceli J., Shiovitz T., Ramey T., & Knapp L. (2009). Adjunctive pregabalin after partial response to SSRI or SNRI in GAD: Results of a double blind placebo controlled trial. *European College of Neuropsychopharmacology*. Istanbul Turkey 12–16th September.

Wells A., & King P. (2006). Meta-cognitive therapy for generalized anxiety disorder: An open trial. *Journal of Behaviour Therapy*, *37*(3), 206–212.

Wetherell J., Gatz M., & Craske M. (2003). Treatment of generalised anxiety in older adults. *Journal of Consulting and Clinical Psychology, 71*(1), 31–40.

Wittchen HU., Zhao S., Kessler RC., & Eaton W. (1994). DSM-III-R generalized anxiety disorder in the National Comorbidity Survey. *Archives of General Psychiatry, 51,* 355–364.

Woelk H. Arnoldt KH, Kieser M, Hoerr R (2007). Gingko biloba special extract EGb761 in generalized anxiety disorder and adjustment disorder with anxious mood: A randomized, double blind, placebo controlled trial. *Journal of Psychiatric Research, 41,* 472–480.

Worthington J., Kinrys G., Wygant L., & Pollack M. (2005). Aripiprazole as an augmentor of selective serotonin reuptake inhibitors in depression and anxiety disorder patients. *International Clinical Psychopharmacology, 20*(1), 9–11.

Zimmerman M., & Chelminski I. (2003). Generalized anxiety disorder in patients with major depression: Is DSM IV's hierarchy correct? *American Journal of Psychiatry, 160,* 504–512.

Treatment-Resistant Obsessive-Compulsive Disorder

Robert Hudak, Priya Gopalan,
and Darin D. Dougherty

Introduction

Once thought to be a rare psychiatric condition, obsessive-compulsive disorder (OCD) was found to occur much more commonly than expected (Karno et al., 1988), and research has determined that the lifetime prevalence of OCD is between 1.9% and 3.3% (Goodman, 1999), making it the fourth most common psychiatric disorder (Rasmussen and Eisen, 1994). The diagnosis of OCD is made in a relatively straightforward manner using *DSM-IV* criteria. A person may have either obsessions or compulsions and at some point during the disorder the person has recognized that the symptoms are excessive or unreasonable, cause marked distress, are time consuming, or significantly interfere with the patient's functioning (American Psychiatric Association [APA], 1994). Obsessions are defined as recurrent and persistent thoughts, impulses, or images that are experienced, at some time during the disturbance, as intrusive and inappropriate and cause marked anxiety or distress. They are recognized by the individual to arise in the person's own mind and to be illogical (at least at some point in the illness). The themes of obsessions can range from common ones such as concerns about dirt, germs, or contamination, or concerns about accidents or disasters, to unusual concerns such as the fear of turning into someone or something else, or assuming unwanted characteristics (Volz and Heyman, 2007). Compulsions are defined as repetitive behaviors (e.g., hand washing, ordering, checking) or mental acts (e.g., praying, counting, repeating words silently) that the person feels driven to perform in response to an obsession, or according to rules that must be applied rigidly (APA, 1994). While compulsions will briefly reduce the anxiety or distress associated with the obsessions, any relief is not long lasting and the obsessions will reoccur. The *DSM* has an additional qualifier for OCD for patients with poor insight. While previous additions of the *DSM* did not recognize that poor insight could occur, *DSM-IV* Field trials showed that 8% of current OCD patients did not recognize their obsessions as being unreasonable, and that 5% never did (Foa and Kozak, 1995).

Unlike most other psychiatric disorders, the clinical characteristics of OCD are mostly identical in adults as well as children (Swedo et al., 1989). One exception is that children may have a higher rate of poor insight. It is unknown at this time whether the presence of poor insight may lead to a higher risk of treatment refractory illness. Eisen et al. (2001) noted that patients with poor insight do indeed respond to behavioral therapy as long as they are willing to participate in appropriate treatment. However, since patients with poor insight may be less willing to seek behavioral therapy, this may be a contributor to treatment resistance if the patient is insisting upon engaging in a pharmacological-only approach.

Treatment Refractory Obsessive-Compulsive Disorder

Due to the potential for severe impairment, the World Health Organization has listed OCD among the 10 medical and psychiatric conditions most likely to cause disability (Murray and Lopez, 1996). Karno et al. (1988) demonstrated that about 36% of patients with OCD had occupational difficulties, and it is estimated that an individual with OCD will lose 3 years of wages due to the illness during the course of their lives. Approximately one quarter of OCD patients experience problems with marital relationships, and patients with OCD are less likely to marry than people without OCD (Goodman, 1999).

Since OCD is a chronic illness that is present throughout the life of the affected individual, the likelihood for a full remission is low among adult patients; only 12% experience complete remission (Eisen et al., 1999). Skoog and Skoog showed that at the 40-year follow-up mark, 20% and 28% of patients achieved full and partial remission, respectively, and a total of 83% showed improvement (1999). A 2-year prospective follow-up of OCD patients noted that 24% of patients obtained either a full or partial remission and that earlier age of onset of OCD, greater severity of symptoms at intake, older age at intake, and being male were all associated with a decreased possibility of remission (Eisen et al., 2010). Insight and the number of comorbid Axis I disorders were not associated with the rate of remission; however, obsessive symptoms of overresponsibility regarding harm had a greater rate of remission. Ferrão et al. (2006) demonstrated that the presence of sexual/religious symptoms, low economic status, and high modification on family function due to OCD were independently associated with treatment refractoriness. There are suggestions that a substantial percentage of patients who are initially labeled refractory may improve symptomatically over time (Ross et al., 2008).

In patients who receive appropriate treatment with selective serotonin reuptake inhibitors (SSRIs), up to 40%–60% of them do not receive a satisfactory response (Walsh and McDougle, 2004; Bloch et al., 2006; Pallanti and Quercioli, 2006). As many as 25% of patients fail to experience any improvement from the initial serotonin reuptake inhibitors (SRIs) trial, but one third of these nonresponders will respond when switched to a different SRI (Bloch et al., 2006). In pediatric OCD, the POTS study showed that complete resolution of OCD symptoms is rare after the use of SRIs or cognitive-behavioral therapy (CBT) (2004). After two consecutive SRI trials, as many as 30%–40% of pediatric patients do not obtain an adequate response (Storch et al., 2008b).

There is little known regarding clinical characteristics between children who have adequate response compared to those who are considered treatment resistant, although it is suggested that more severe obsessions and repeating compulsions, greater baseline academic impairment, and the presence of disruptive behavior disorders are related to treatment resistance (Storch et al., 2008b). Interestingly, that study also showed that treatment responders showed a higher level of depressive symptoms than patients who were treatment resistant, leading the authors to hypothesize that the use of SRIs may improve a patient's insight into the severity of his or her OCD, leading to subsequent distress with regard to the patient's illness (Storch et al., 2006). The Pediatric Obsessive Compulsive Treatment Study (POTS; 2004) showed that youths with decreased severity of symptoms, less OCD-related functional impairment, greater insight, fewer comorbid externalizing symptoms, and lower levels of family accommodation showed greater improvement across treatment conditions. Pediatric patients with a family history of OCD had a marked decrease in response to CBT (Garcia et al., 2010). Forty-one percent of pediatric patients will continue to have OCD as a diagnosis at 9-year follow-up (Micali et al., 2010).

Definition of Treatment Resistance

There is no accepted standard definition of treatment resistance currently in place for OCD (Pallanti et al., 2004). Different authors have used different terms, such as treatment resistance, treatment refractory, treatment failure, and nonresponse. Some authors have defined treatment resistance as patients who have not shown a satisfactory response to at least to two SRIs (Goodman et al., 1998). In some cases, it has been proposed that "treatment resistant" and "treatment refractory" be given different criteria, and that these represented two separate states. In addition to no standard term in wide usage, there is no consensus or a standardized criterion for defining what treatment response in OCD is. This obviously makes defining treatment resistance problematic because it creates difficulties in comparing research studies. Treatment response in OCD medication studies is not generally defined as a remission of OCD symptoms, but instead is defined as a percentage of decline in symptoms. Typically, response is operationalized as either a 25%–30% reduction in the Yale-Brown Obsessive-Compulsive Scale (Y-BOCS) or a decline in symptoms below a threshold of 16, which is the boundary between mild and moderate symptoms (Pittenger et al., 2006). The use of criteria such as a percentage decline in symptoms is problematic, because such patients may still have significant impairment due to their illness (Bloch et al., 2006). In fact, many such patients may still be sick enough to be eligible for entering the same study that they have just concluded. Even patients with a Y-BOCS score below 16 often have clinically significant symptoms. In addition, the Y-BOCS may not be sensitive to subtle changes in measuring symptom severity, such as a decrease in rituals from 5 to 3 hours per day (Pallanti and Quercioli, 2006). The same authors have proposed a staging system for OCD consisting of seven stages ranging from recovery down to refractory, which is defined as no change or worsening with all available therapies (Pallanti and Quercioli, 2006).

The need exists to assess outcome beyond simple significance tests of pre- and post-symptom severity (Boschen et al., 2008). The lack of consistent criteria for nonresponse has prevented the development of a cumulative body of data on a homogeneous sample of patients, creating limits on the generalizability of existing studies and data, which therefore creates obstacles in the development of useful new studies (Pallanti and Quercioli, 2006). Subjective impressions of response to treatment have rarely been considered, and only a small number of studies have been performed in which the patient's quality of life is measured (Pallanti and Quercioli, 2006). Recognizing that the disparity in criteria in various studies makes generalizing information among them problematic, treatment protocols in future studies ideally should contain the same criteria for treatment resistance in order to improve research and clinical applications in this area. Because few patients in community treatment receive adequate behavioral therapy, clinicians should insist upon an adequate course of CBT prior to labeling a patient treatment refractory (Husted and Shapira, 2004). For the practicing mental health clinician, patients' subjective reports as to whether they feel further improvement is needed is vital in making routine, clinical assessments regarding an individual's treatment resistance.

Treatment for Obsessive-Compulsive Disorder

To properly recognize treatment resistance, a review of proper treatment for OCD is essential. It has been shown that the vast majority (>90%) of patients with OCD are not offered adequate pharmacotherapy during psychiatric visits (Hankin et al., 2009). Clinical experience suggests that a very high percentage of patients are not offered, or do not receive, adequate psychotherapy in the form of exposure with response prevention (ERP), and this has been borne out in the literature (Blanco et al., 2006). Typically, the decision on whether to start a medication in OCD is based on severity of the OCD, patient request, and on clinical judgment. However, due to its efficacy in the treatment of OCD, ERP should always be offered as a first-line therapy, either alone or with medications. In particular, for patients without significant comorbid depression or anxiety, ERP may be the only treatment modality that is required, particularly if the symptoms are mild to moderate (March et al., 1997; APA, 2007). Medications are typically offered when the symptoms are moderate to severe in intensity, if the clinician or patient feels that doing adequate ERP will be difficult without medications, or by patient request. A medication trial may reduce the severity of the OCD symptoms enough that the person will eventually be able to successfully enter into a course of ERP. Even though combining ERP and SRIs is not necessary for all patients (Cottraux et al., 2005), combining medications and therapy may lead to improved response rates in many OCD patients. Even in the presence of major depression, ERP should be offered to patients in addition to medications (Foa et al., 1992).

The first-line medications used for OCD should be the selective serotonin reuptake inhibitors (SSRIs), which also include the tricyclic antidepressant clomipramine, which is often called an SRI because it is not selective for serotonin as it also acts on additional receptor sites. In clinical practice, at least two to three SSRIs are given to patients before a trial of clomipramine is used, due to the additional side effects of this medication. Dosing of the SSRIs is vital. While initial doses of these medications will generally follow manufacturer's guidelines, the final doses used are much higher. These increased doses are often required to achieve an antiobsessional response compared to the doses used in major depression (Math and Reddy, 2007). See Table 9.1 for dosage guidelines for SSRIs in the use of OCD.

While patients may often be placed on lower doses of these medications initially, a lack of response at the lower dose does not indicate a treatment resistance to that medication, as

TABLE 9.1 Dosage Guidelines for Selective Serotonin Reuptake Inhibitors (SSRIs) in the Use of Obsessive-Compulsive Disorder

SSRI	Starting and Incremental Dose (mg/day)	Usual Maximum Dose (mg/day)	Occasionally Prescribed Maximum Dose (mg/day)
Citalopram	20	80	120
Clomipramine	25	250	*
Escitalopram	10	40	60
Fluoxetine	20	80	120
Fluvoxamine	50	300	450
Paroxetine	20	60	100
Sertraline	50	200	400

*Combined plasma levels of clomipramine plus desmethylclomipramine 12 hours after the dose should be kept below 500 ng/mL to minimize risk of seizures and cardiac conduction delay.
Source: Adapted from APA Practice Guidelines (2007).

patients will often respond to a higher dose of the same medication (Ninan et al., 2006). Patients often take up to 12 weeks to respond to a particular SSRI (Fineberg et al., 2005). For this reason, a trial of an SSRI can only be considered adequate and therapeutic if the patient has been on the highest dose possible for a minimum of 12 weeks, with the possibility of a further trial of an additional month or longer if the patient starts to show benefit only at the end of the original 12-week trial (March et al., 1997). If a patient still does not show adequate response to an SSRI at the end of a therapeutic trial, a switch to a different SSRI may still work, and this is supported by several studies (APA, 2007).

Summary

A patient should not be considered treatment resistant unless he or she has had the following as part of treatment:

1) Use of an SSRI
2) Use of the SSRI at the maximum dose per APA guidelines or at the highest dose tolerated
3) A trial of the SSRI at the maximum dose for a minimum of 12–16 weeks
4) The addition of adequate ERP by a trained therapist to the SSRI trial

While the research definition of treatment resistance is still not settled, and various definitions are based on criteria such as the percentage of symptom decline or the number of medications failed, the aforementioned guidelines should be followed in clinical practice prior to declaring a patient treatment resistant to a particular medication.

Augmentation of Selective Serotonin Reuptake Inhibitors

When the failure of SSRI treatment occurs, the pharmacological response suggests either switching the SSRI or the use of augmentation. The American Psychiatric Association

Practice Guidelines recommend second-generation antipsychotics as an augmentation strategy to SSRI treatment, whether the SSRI produced a partial response or little to no response, and whether it is used alone or in combination with CBT. A second antipsychotic may be tried if the initial augmenting agent is not successful (APA, 2007). Generally, it is better to use augmentation only after an adequate trial of an SSRI primary medication. In most cases, this means a 3-month trial of the maximum dose of the SSRI (Skapinakis, 2007).

While the number of studies looking at antipsychotics as augmentation agents is not vast, there are several randomized placebo-controlled trials that compare these medicines to placebo. Specifically, pooled data suggests a number needed to treat of 4.5 for a reduction in YBOCS of 35% using this augmentation strategy (Bloch et al., 2006). This reduction is not minor when considering that this is a group of patients who have been otherwise treatment resistant. When considered collectively, there is evidence to suggest that antipsychotics are an effective and reasonable augmentation strategy (Spakinakis, 2007). While the primary pathophysiology behind OCD appears to be serotonergic in nature, there appears to be a dopaminergic component to the illness as well. However, treatment with an antipsychotic alone has been found in several studies to be ineffective (Fineberg et al., 2006).

An important consideration when using antipsychotic agents for augmentation, however, is the potential obsessogenic quality of these medications. There are numerous case reports reporting exacerbation or de novo OC symptoms in patients started on antipsychotic treatment. These studies have been primarily in schizophrenic patients (Husted and Shapira, 2004), but it is still important to keep this data in mind when using antipsychotic medication and to monitor carefully for clinical improvement when starting these agents. Another area that requires further study is the dose–response requirements of antipsychotic agents; results have been mixed as to whether there is a dose-related response to these medications (Ramasubbu et al., 2000).

Mechanism of Action

The 5-HT_{1D} receptor subtype hypothesized to have a role in OCD has been found in animal studies to require high doses and long duration of SRI treatment in order to undergo desensitization (Husted and Shapira, 2004). This is consistent with clinical practice, where the treatment of OCD patients generally requires higher doses of SSRIs and can respond after more than the 6–8 weeks observed in depressive illnesses.

There is, however, data suggesting that dopamine is involved in the disease process of OCD. Animal models show stereotypic movements with dopamine. Multiple studies with rats have demonstrated that using the dopamine (D2/D3) agonist quinpirole causes checking and repetitive behaviors in the animals; while these behaviors are interruptible, they have been difficult to stop altogether (Szechtman, 1998). Neuroimaging studies also implicate dopamine in the mechanism of OCD, though data are limited in this regard due to small sample sizes; in particular, positron emission tomography (PET) imaging has shown increased density of dopamine receptors in the basal ganglia of OCD patients compared to healthy controls (van der Wee et al., 2004). Moreover, a PET study of SRI-refractory patients randomized to risperidone or placebo showed increased activity in the striatum, cingulate gyrus, the prefrontal cortex, especially in the orbital region, and the thalamus, and involvement of both serotonin and dopamine systems (Buchsbaum et al., 2006).

Augmentation with a second-generation antipsychotic is considered a reasonable strategy given this data, but the implications of such a strategy are not yet completely clear. While the dopamine transporter is hypothesized to be involved, the role of specific dopamine receptors still needs to be explored. Most antipsychotics are D2 antagonists, though there is some variability in each medication's affinity to the D2 receptor. Moreover, given that risperidone and olanzapine have high D4 affinity, as well as affinity to the D1 receptor, the role of other dopamine receptors becomes less clear. These agents, in particular, risperidone and olanzapine, have strong 5-HT$_{2A}$ antagonism as well (and in fact, in these two drugs in particular, the affinity to 5-HT2A is stronger than the affinity to D2), so this receptor also has a potential role in the mechanism of the illness (Schotte et al., 1996).

Second-generation antipsychotics are not uniform in their mechanism of action and, in particular, are quite diverse in terms of their receptor profiles. While it can be said as a general statement that most of the second-generation antipsychotics are potent 5HT-2A antagonists with a ratio of 5-HT2A:D2 potency being estimated as being 10:1, other serotinergic receptor subtypes have also been implicated in OCD. In particular, the 5HT-2C receptor agonism has been found to be a potential mechanism in the treatment of OCD (Shapiro, 2003).

Risperidone

Risperidone, a benzisoxazole structure, is a second generation antipsychotic with high affinity and antagonistic effects at the D2 and 5HT$_{2A}$ receptors. The medication as well as its metabolite, 9-hydroxyrisperidone, are antagonists at the α1 and α2 receptor, as well as the H1 receptor (Stahl, 2005). There is some data to suggest that it also has affinity to the D4 receptor, D1 receptor, though the role of these receptors in OCD is unclear (Schotte et al., 1996; Ramasubbu et al., 2000). Similarly, there is also affinity to the D3 receptor (Leysen, 1994).

Of all of the second generation antipsychotics, risperidone has the most evidence for its use as an adjunctive medication in treatment-resistant OCD. There have been several randomized, placebo-controlled studies comparing risperidone to placebo, and while the studies were generally small, evidence indicates that risperidone is superior to placebo as evidenced by improved Y-BOCS (McDougle, 2000; Arias, 2006; Hollander, 2003; Erzegovesi, 2005).

The first such randomized controlled trial was conducted by McDougle et al. with 36 patients. They were first treated in an open-label fashion with SRI monotherapy, which was titrated up such that the patients were on maximum tolerated doses for at least 8 weeks. Risperidone or placebo was then started. Significant reductions in YBOCS occurred at a mean dose of 2.2 mg daily, and the medicine was well-tolerated. (McDougle et al., 2000). A similar trial by Hollander in 2003 showed a similar reduction in YBOCS for the risperidone arm versus placebo, but was unable to show statistical significance due to small sample size; however, four patients with risperidone augmentation improved compared to no patients who received the placebo (Hollander et al., 2003a).

A smaller randomized double-blinded, placebo-controlled study by Li et al. showed that the effects of risperidone augmentation can be rapid, with a YBOCS reduction occurring within 2 weeks of SRI augmentation where the SRI was given at a therapeutic dose for 12 weeks prior (Li et al., 2005). There is also evidence that the response can occur at low doses, as demonstrated by a trial conducted by Erzegovesi et al., where 45 medication-naïve patients were given fluvoxamine, then the twenty patients who were found to be nonresponders were randomized to 0.5 mg risperidone or placebo—of these patients, five patients given risperidone had symptom improvement in 6 weeks compared to two patients in the placebo arm (Erzegovesi et al., 2005). In addition, risperidone augmentation in patients who were treatment resistant to a combination of clomipramine and an SSRI showed clinical improvement as well (Ravizza et al., 1996).

There are also open-label trials showing the effectiveness of risperidone in treating treatment-refractory OCD (McDougle et al., 1995a; Stein et al., 1997; Saxena et al., 1996; Pfanner et al., 2000). One small case series of open-label risperidone addition to fluvoxamine-treated nonresponders showed a significant reduction in YBOCS scores within 4 weeks at a dose of 1 mg daily (McDougle et al., 1995a).

Risperidone has also been found to be effective in the treatment of tics in patients with OCD and a concomitant tic disorder. Patients with OCD versus patients with OCD and tics respond equally well to risperidone augmentation (McDougle et al., 2000). In addition, risperidone is generally well-tolerated in terms of its side effect profile. It also has also been shown to improve comorbid mood and anxiety disorders as noted by a reduction in HAM-D scores (McDougle et al., 2000). This effect also occurs with a shorter duration of treatment with the antipsychotic (Li et al., 2005). Moreover, there is also evidence that risperidone is also an effective treatment for children and adolescents with treatment-resistant OCD, though the data is limited to case reports (Fitzgerald et al., 1999; Thomsen, 2004).

Risperidone augmentation appears to be an appropriate strategy to use in treatment-resistant OCD patients. Given that risperidone dosing in augmentation ranges in most studies between 0.5 mg to 3 mg, it is reasonable to conclude that the use of low doses is an effective strategy to augment SRI therapy in treatment-resistant OCD.

Olanzapine

Olanzapine has extensive receptor activity with antagonism at 5-HT2A and D2, but also at D1, D4, α1, M1 through M5, and H1 (Stahl). There is less data overall about the efficacy of olanzapine in treating treatment-resistant OCD compared to risperidone. While there is a randomized placebo-controlled trial that showed a positive response with olanzapine addition to SRI treatment (Bystritsky et al., 2004), there is also a placebo-controlled study that showed no significant difference in response to olanzapine compared to placebo in terms of reductions in YBOCS scores (Shapira et al., 2004). It is important to note, though, that the positive study by Byritzsky had a dose range for olanzapine of 5–20 mg with a mean daily dose of 11.2 mg, where the negative study by Shapira had a lower mean of 6 mg daily.

There are numerous open-label studies that show the efficacy of olanzapine in treatment-resistant patients (Weiss et al., 1999; Bogetto et al., 2000; Koran et al., 2000; Francobandiera, 2001; Crocq et al., 2002; D'Amico et al., 2003). In a 10-patient case series, 7 out of the 9 patient who completed the trial had some response to treatment (Weiss et al., 1999).

While there are few head-to-head studies comparing second-generation antipsychotics for this illness, there is one study comparing risperidone to olanzapine as an augmenting agent. This trial, in which either risperidone (1–3 mg with a mean dose of 2 mg) or olanzapine (2.5–10 mg with a mean dose of 5 mg) was added to patients who were deemed treatment-resistant after a 16 week trial of an SRI, and there were no significant differences in treatment response (Maina et al., 2008). There were significant differences in the side effect profiles, though, and while both groups experienced side effects, it should be noted that olanzapine caused more weight gain: an average of 2.8 pounds versus 0.77 pounds for risperidone, a difference which is statistically significant By contrast, six patients in the risperidone arm compared to one in the olanzapine arm experienced amenorrhea as a side effect. Given the differences in side effect profiles, treatment should be tailored to the patient's individual characteristics and tolerability.

A recent study found monotherapy of olanzapine for patients with a primary diagnosis of trichotillomania to be superior to placebo in a 25 patient sample trial comparing the medications. In this randomized, 12-week trial, patients on olanzapine (mean dose 10.8 mg daily) had significant reductions in scores for the CGI (Clinical Global Improvement) and the Yale Brown Obsessive Compulsive Scale for Trichotillomania when compared to placebo. There was also an overall reduction in the Massachusetts Hospital Hair-Pulling Scale, though this did not separate from placebo. (Van Ameringen et al., 2010).

Quetiapine

Quetiapine is structurally a dibenzodiazepine and has activity at multiple receptor sites. While it has antagonism at the D2 and D1 dopamine receptors, the D2 antagonism of quetiapine is less than those of risperidone and olanzapine. Quetiapine is also an antagonist of the 5-HT_2 receptor, as well as the 5-HT_6, H1, $\alpha 1$, and $\alpha 2$ receptors (Nasrallah, 2008).

There are three randomized, placebo-controlled trials of quetiapine augmentation of SRI treatment in OCD, which have had mixed results in terms of treatment efficacy. The first of these trials randomized 40 patients to SRI and quetiapine versus SRI and placebo. Treatment resistance was defined as failure of two SRIs after maximum tolerated dose for at least 8 weeks, and the trial duration was 8 weeks. The results of this trial showed a significant reduction in YBOCS score compared to placebo (Denys et al., 2007). Subsequent randomized controlled trials, however, were not able to replicate these findings. One of these trials had limitations in its definition of treatment resistance as failure of an SRI for 3 months, but only required 6 weeks of that time to be at maximum dose, which may have caused a more robust placebo response, contributing to the negative results (Carey et al., 2005). The other negative trial, however, did not have these limitations, and was not only more stringent in its definition of treatment failure, but also had a purer sample diagnostically and had the longest follow-up period of four months (Fineberg et al., 2005). All of these studies showed overall tolerability of quetiapine with little difference in drop-out between the drug and placebo groups. A single-blind study comparing quetiapine to placebo in 27 treatment-refractory patients who had had 3 months of SRI treatment showed positive results in terms of YBOCS reductions (Atmaca et al., 2002). When the data from the randomized trials were pooled together, there was evidence of YBOCS reduction (Fineberg et al., 2006;).

There is one positive study of quetiapine addition to citalopram in non-treatment-resistant OCD patients, in which the patients were randomized to antipsychotic or placebo at the initiation of the SRI (Vulink et al., 2009). There is also a recent, 21-patient open-label trial where quetiapine and clomipramine were compared as augmentation agents in SRI-resistant patients with OCD; the quetiapine group had a better improvement in YBOCS scores compared to the clomipramine group, but this study is limited by the numerous factors including its lack of a placebo arm and non-blinding of its clinical evaluators (Diniz et al., 2010).

Given the limited data available, the small numbers involved with the randomized placebo-controlled trials, and the conflicting nature of the results, it is reasonable based on research data alone to consider quetiapine as an augmenting agent for treatment-resistant OCD, but only as a second-line agent after failed trials of risperidone and olanzapine. Clinically, however, given that olanzapine causes more weight gain on average than quetiapine (Nasrallah, 2008), quetiapine may be a more reasonable second choice after risperidone.

Aripiprazole

The mechanism of aripiprazole is different than the antipsychotics that have been discussed so far. The medication has a complex receptor profile that includes numerous potential actions at the D2 receptor: partial agonism, full agonism, or antagonism (Shapiro et al., 2003; Kessler, 2007). Aripiprazole has also been found to be a partial agonist at the 5-HT$_{2C}$ receptor, which has been implicated in OCD. The drug does show antagonism at the 5-HT$_{2A}$ subtype, consistent with the other second-generation antipsychotics (Shapiro et al., 2003). These mechanistic differences from the other available antipsychotic agents lead to the speculation that aripiprazole may result in improvement in treatment-refractory OCD patients.

Aripiprazole has been examined as a potential augmentation agent for treatment-resistant OCD. Initially, research with animal models with medication showed that aripirazole monotherapy in rats inhibits marble-burying behaviors (the established correlate to OCD symptomatology) without effects to motor activity. This effect is hypothesized to be due to aripiprazole's partial agonism at 5-HT$_{1A}$, as agonists of the 5HT$_{1A}$ receptor alone given to rats has shown similar improvements in inhibiting marble-burying behaviors in a way that 5HT-2A antagonists and D2 agonists did not. The D2 receptor antagonism of aripiprazole is also implicated in that a D2 antagonist did inhibit marble burying as well, which goes along with the hypothesized dopamine involvement in the pathway of OCD (Egashira et al., 2008). There are numerous case reports of patients who have been successfully treated with aripiprazole as an adjunct treatment for an SRI to which they were unresponsive (de Rocha and Correa, 2007; Fornaro et al., 2008; Sarkar et al., 2008; Lai, 2009). Pessina et al. (2009) conducted a small prospective, open-label trial of 12 patients with treatment-resistant OCD; of the 8 completers of the study, 3 had a response to aripiprazole by YBOCS and CGI. In addition, there are indications that aripiprazole may be effective in children and adolescents. There are case reports of improvement in treatment-resistant OCD in both adolescents (Storch et al., 2008a; Lai, 2009) and children (Ozturk and Coskun, 2009).

There is one case series of aripiprazole use as monotherapy for OCD in eight medication-naïve patients. The study duration was 8 weeks (dose 10–30 mg) and a reduction in the mean total YBOCS score was observed; three of the seven people who completed the trial were labeled responders (Connor et al., 2005). There is also a published case report of aripiprazole monotherapy in a patient with comorbid major depressive disorder (Pae, 2009). Similarly, aripiprazole has been found to reduce clozapine-induced obsessive-compulsive symptoms in schizophrenic patients (Englisch et al., 2009).

Aripiprazole has been found to be useful in OCD patients with other comorbidities. Aripiprazole has also been found to be effective in both adults and children with Tourette disorder (da Rocha and Correa, 2007; Winter et al., 2008) and other tic disorders (Lai, 2009) comorbid with OCD, both as monotherapy and as an augmentation agent. A case series of three patients with bipolar disorder found improved YBOCS scores in patients with bipolar disorder who had aripiprazole added to their mood stabilizer (Uguz, 2010).

Ziprasidone

There are few studies and no randomized placebo-controlled trials documenting the effectiveness of ziprasidone in OCD. One case report showed a reduction in YBOCS and CGI in a treatment-resistant patient who was switched from clozapine to ziprasidone (Iglesias Garcia et al., 2006). A retrospective study of quetiapine versus ziprasidone as an adjunct to SRI treatment showed that while both medications reduced YBOCS and CGI scores, quetiapine's clinical response rate was 80% compared to 44.4% of the patients on ziprasidone (Savas et al., 2008).

There is one case report documenting a possible ziprasidone-induced mania in one patient with a primary diagnosis of OCD who was treatment resistant to numerous agents. This patient had no history of major depressive disorder, mania, or hypomania, had been tried on multiple SRIs, and developed manic symptoms within 7 days of ziprasidone initiation for augmentation (Wickham and Varma, 2007).

Given that there are limited data on ziprasidone in treatment-resistant OCD, and what limited information is available shows that its efficacy may be inferior to other agents, it is best to consider this medication as a second line in terms of antipsychotic augmentation.

Clozapine

There are no randomized controlled trials of clozapine in the treatment of OCD. A single open-label study done with clozapine as monotherapy for 10 weeks to treat treatment-resistant OCD was found to be negative, with no significant reduction in YBOCS (McDougle et al., 1995b). There is one case report of a schizophrenic patient on aripiprazole whose comorbid OCD improved with addition of clozapine (Peters and DeHaan, 2009).

Clozapine, of all of the antipsychotics, has been found to be more obsessogenic than other antipsychotics, both for exacerbation of existing symptoms and for de novo induction of obsessions and compulsions (Khullar et al., 2001; Lykouras et al., 2003). The number of case reports involving clozapine-induced OC symptoms is greater than any other antipsychotic (Lykouras et al., 2003). There is no dose dependency to this effect, and there is a delay in the onset of the obsessive symptoms, which may be a result of the slow titration of the medication. While most of these reports involved a primary thought disorder, there were a few cases with other primary Axis I disorders (Lykouras et al., 2003).

The lack of positive studies with clozapine either as monotherapy or as an augmentation strategy in treatment-resistant OCD, combined with the strong potential for exacerbation of OC symptoms, makes clozapine an unlikely choice among antipsychotic agents for refractory OCD patients.

First-Generation Antipsychotics

There are fewer studies on the first-generation antipsychotics as an augmenting treatment of refractory OCD. One of the few randomized placebo-controlled trials of the older antipsychotics was a study done in 1994 by McDougle et al. Sixty-two patients who had failed prior SRI treatment were given 8 weeks of fluvoxamine, of which 7 weeks were at maximum dose. The patients who were treatment-refractory were randomized to either halo-peridol (2–10 mg, mean dose 6.2 mg) or placebo. Eleven of seventeen in the haloperidol group were treatment responders compared to none in the placebo group. Eight patients had a comorbid tic disorder, and all of these patients were responders to haloperidol; of the nine patients without tics, three were responders. This shows haloperidol to be an effective agent in terms of YBOCS reduction but also in the treatment of comorbid tic disorders (McDougle et al., 1994). A 9-week cross-over study of risperidone, haloperidol, and placebo showed an improvement in obsessions, compulsions, total YBOCS, and anxiety symptoms with both haldol and risperidone (Li et al., 2005).

An open-label trial of pimozide in a patient with Tourette syndrome on fluvoxamine showed improvement in OCD and tics with the combination of the medications; this was confirmed by a double-blind sequential discontinuation of each of the medications (Delgado et al., 1990). The use of pimozide as an augmentation agent was further corroborated by an open-label trial of pimozide at a mean dose of 6.5 mg in 17 fluvoxamine-resistant patients (McDougle, 1995a).

Drug–Drug Interactions

When adding second-generation antipsychotics to SRI treatment, it becomes important to consider drug-drug interactions. This is especially important because this strategy requires the combination of an antipsychotic agent with an SRI, and this combination has some well-known interactions. The cytochrome P450 enzyme plays a major role in the metabolism of many psychiatric medications, and it should be considered in the clinical use of combination treatments.

Both paroxetine and fluoxetine are inhibitors of the cytochrome P450 2D6 isoenzyme. Risperidone is metabolized in part through this enzyme, so coadministration of these medications can result in elevated levels of serum risperidone (Matsunaga et al., 2009). This interaction could potentially increase the risk of side effects such as sedation and extrapyramidal symptoms.

Fluvoxamine is an inhibitor of the cytochrome P450 1A2 isoenzyme. Olanzapine is metabolized in large part through this enzyme, so coadministration of these two medications can result in elevated olanzapine levels (Matsunaga et al., 2009). Clozapine, clomipramine, and caffeine are other substrates of the 1A2 isoenzyme. Fluvoxamine is also an inhibitor of the 2C19 isoenzyme, for which diazepam is a substrate.

Citalopram has no known effects on the cytochrome P450 system and is an ideal SRI choice if considering use of augmenting drugs for treatment of OCD (Hemeryck and Belpaire, 2002). For that reason, it may also be an ideal choice for those patients who are on numerous other medications at onset of treatment.

Side Effects

The numerous side effects of the antipsychotics are well established in the literature and encompass multiple domains. A full discussion of the side-effect profiles of these medications is outside the scope of this chapter. It is important to give appropriate informed consent when initiating medication therapy as well as to screen for side effects as appropriate. However, a few of the important adverse effects are listed next and should be kept in mind when discussing antipsychotic augmentation for treatment-resistant OCD with patients.

1. *Metabolic effects.* The metabolic side effects of most of the second-generation antipsychotic medications are well established in the literature. There are more data available that implicate olanzapine and clozapine as causing significant increases in weight, as well as glucose intolerance and dyslipidemia (Nasrallah, 2008; Newcomer, 2005; Haddad and Sharma, 2007). Average weight gain with olanzapine has been found to be as high as 12 kg during the first year of treatment; risperidone and quetiapine tend to have more modest amounts of weight gain (mean of 2–3 kg over the first year of treatment), ziprasidone the least (mean of 1 kg), and aripiprazole-induced weight changes may be dependent on baseline body mass indicators (Nasrallah, 2008). This weight gain has also been observed in children on antipsychotics (Federowicz and Fombonne, 2005). Many of the studies have been done in patients with schizophrenia, which may carry its own risk of metabolic side effects (Nasrallah, 2008). At the same time, these side effects, which have cardiac implications and a likely impact on prognosis and quality of life, need to be clearly outlined to patients in a discussion of the risks and benefits of antipsychotic medications in the context of treatment augmentation.

2. *Movement disorders.* Acute and tardive dyskinesias are commonly found in conventional antipsychotics, in some studies found to be anywhere from 50%–75% (Arana, 2000). Rates of movement disorders are generally found to be comparatively less in patients on second-generation antipsychotics (Barnes and McPhillips, 1998; Leucht et al., 1999; Fineberg et al., 2006; Haddad and Sharma, 2007). Of the second-generation antipsychotics, risperidone has been found to have a higher rate of acute extrapyramidal symptoms compared to the other medications (Haddad and Sharma, 2007). Clozapine, in particular, has been found to have lower rates of tardive dyskinesia (Barnes and McPhillips, 1998). Again, these side effects need to be presented to patients as a part of a risk-benefit discussion, and patients should be assessed for movement disorders during psychiatric assessments.

3. *Hyperprolactinemia.* Both first-generation antipsychotics as well as second-generation antipsychotics have been found to cause hyperprolactinemia. Of the newer agents, risperidone and olanzapine have been found to have a higher rate of prolactin release when compared to quetiapine, aripiprazole, clozapine, and ziprasidone (Madhusoodanan et al., 2010).

Predictors of Response

Clinically, there is some evidence that augmentation with second-generation antipsychotics may be more effective in patients with symmetry, ordering, or hoarding behaviors (Matsunaga et al., 2009). In addition, OCD patients with comorbid tics also may have a better response to antipsychotic augmentation (Bloch et al., 2006; Fineberg et al., 2006). Lack of insight is a notoriously difficult feature of OCD to treat (Ravi Kishore et al., 2004), so the presence of insight may be a positive predictive factor for treatment response (Hollander et al., 2003a;

Fineberg et al., 2006). True SRI resistance could also be an indicator of better response to antipsychotic augmentation in treatment-resistant OCD, and there is possible neurobiological basis to this hypothesis (Fineberg et al., 2006). Unfortunately, data in this area are very limited, and further study is necessary to facilitate a better understand of treatment response.

Additional Augmenting Agents

Buspirone

Buspirone is a partial agonist at the 5-HT 1A receptor, and it is approved for the treatment of generalized anxiety disorder. It was initially reported to show improvements in people with OCD when used as an augmenting agent to fluoxetine (Markovitz et al., 1990; Jenike et al., 1991). In a double-blind trial comparing buspirone augmentation of fluvoxamine to fluvoxamine alone, the results between both groups were similar (McDougle et al., 1993). A double-blind study looking at buspirone augmentation of clomipramine showed no difference in the groups that received augmentation versus those that did not: there were, however, individual patients in that study who benefited from the buspirone augmentation (Pigott et al., 1992). When a double study was performed using buspirone augmentation of fluoxetine, again there was no difference between the treatment group and the control group, but again one patient benefited significantly from the augmentation (Grady et al., 1993). Buspirone was well tolerated in all of the studies. As a result of this mixed data, while buspirone is not generally recommended as a first-line augmentation strategy, the fact that some patients do respond to it, as well as the fact that it is so well tolerated, do make it an option that should be considered for the treatment-resistant patient.

Lithium

Lithium has been commonly used to augment antidepressants for patients with major depression, and it has been studied in OCD. An initial case report showed that lithium may have efficacy as an augmentation agent to clomipramine at a dose of 1,200 mg per day (Rasmussen, 1984). However, double-blind studies were less promising, with one study showing only a mild response in a 2-week trial, and no response in a 4-week trial (McDougle et al., 1991). Another 8-week trial also did not demonstrate an effect with lithium augmentation (Pigott et al., 1991). Although the potential benefit in OCD is low, individual patients, especially those with severe depressive symptoms, may benefit from lithium augmentation (Goodman et al., 1998).

Tryptophan

Tryptophan is an essential amino acid and a precursor or serotonin. A case report showed this supplement to be helpful at a dose of 6 grams per day in a patient taking clomipramine for OCD (Rasmussen, 1984). A case series of seven patients noted that tryptophan improved OCD symptoms at doses ranging from 3 to 9 grams per day, although increased aggressive behavior was noted in two patients who had a history of aggression. The addition of tryptophan after a failed trial of pindolol and an SSRI where the pindolol remained on board had a positive effect on OCD symptoms (Blier and Bergeron, 1996) in a series of 13 patients.

While sale of tryptophan was banned in the United States due to an outbreak of eosinophilia myalgia syndrome in the early 1990s, it is available again for sale.

Anticonvulsants

There are very limited data on the use of anticonvulsants as therapy in OCD. A trial of carbamazepine demonstrated no significant response during an 8-week trial (Joffe and Swinson, 1987). An open-label study involving topiramate as an adjunct to SSRI treatment showed some efficacy (Rubio et al., 2006), although this has not been replicated in a controlled format. Gabapentin has not been shown to be efficacious as an augmentation agent to fluoxetine in the treatment of OCD (Husted and Shapira, 2004). Lamotrigine has not been shown to be effective as an augmentation strategy to fluoxetine (Kumar and Khanna, 2000). As of this time, no anticonvulsants can be recommended for use as augmentation in OCD patients.

Clonazepam

While benzodiazepines and especially clonazepam are often used clinically in OCD treatment either as a first-line agent or as augmentation in treatment refractory patients, there is little evidence to support their use (Goodman et al., 1998; Husted and Shapira, 2004). Since the possibility exists that anxiolytics may interfere with the ability of the trained behavioral therapist to perform the anxiety-provoking ERP therapy, there is little reason to recommend this class of medications.

Inositol

Inositol is a simple polyol second messenger precursor that is available over the counter in the United States. At a dose of 18 grams per day, it was found to be more effective than placebo in the treatment of OCD (Fux et al., 1996). However, as an augmentation agent to SSRIs, it was not found to be more effective than placebo (Fux et al., 1999) suggesting the possibility of this as a primary alternative treatment rather than augmentation. Its most common side effects have been noted to be gastrointestinal distress.

Intravenous Medications

Clomipramine (CMI) is a tricyclic antidepressant that is approved for the treatment of OCD. After ingestion, the first past effect transforms the active compound CMI to a less serotonin-specific metabolite, desmethylclomipramine (DCMI). Since CMI is available in IV formulation, this method would enable higher plasma levels of CMI. IV CMI has been shown to be more effective than placebo in patients who previously did not respond to oral clomipramine (Fallon et al., 1998) and appears to be more efficacious when the drug is pulse-loaded as opposed to gradual dose increases (Koran et al., 1997). Unfortunately, the IV form of CMI is not available in the United States. A strategy to improve the CMI/DCMI ratio in patients taking the oral medication, and therefore replicating the avoidance of the first-pass effect, has been used to improve outcomes in treatment-resistant patients. The addition of fluvoxamine, a potent CYP1A2 inhibitor, will increase the CMI/DCMI ratio by inhibiting the metabolism of CMI. The CMI/fluvoxamine combination is well tolerated, particularly when the total CMI level was below 450 ng/ml (defined as the combined CMI and DCMI levels) (Szegedi et al., 1996). This combination allows an increase in CMI/DCMI ratio in patients. It is recommended that clinicians using this protocol maintain total CMI levels of 450 ng/ml or less, and that the goal CMI/DCMI ratio should be 4:1 or greater (Szegedi et al., 1996).

Another SSRI, citalopram, is available in intravenous form. It has been shown in an open-label study to be well tolerated and to have rapid efficacy in a majority of treatment-resistant patients (Pallanti et al., 2002). This formulation is currently not available in the United States.

Pindolol

Pindolol is a beta-adrenoreceptor/5-HT1A receptor agonist (Walsh and McDougle, 2004) and has been studied as an augmentation agent in many psychiatric illnesses. In an open study (Koran et al., 1996) only one of eight patients responded. However, in a double-blind placebo-controlled study pindolol augmentation to paroxetine was associated with greater improvement compared to placebo in patients who had failed at least two prior SSRI treatments (Dannon et al., 2000). Subjects were treated with 2.5 mg of pindolol three times a day during the duration of that study.

Additional Medications

Venlafaxine

Venlafaxine is a serotonin norepinephrine reuptake inhibitor (SNRI). It is not currently FDA approved for OCD, and the evidence is mixed on its efficacy in OCD. It has been compared to placebo in one small trial where no significant benefit was noted, although the duration of the trial was short and doses used were only up to 225 mg per day (Yaryure-Tobias and Neziroglu, 1996). It has been shown to be helpful in patients who failed SSRI treatment when studied in an open-label format (Hollander et al., 2003b) and has demonstrated comparable efficacy to clomipramine (Albert et al., 2002) and paroxetine (Denys et al., 2003), although both studies lacked a placebo controlled arm. In one study, nonresponders to venlafaxine or paroxetine were switched to the alternate medication, and the group switched to paroxetine did significantly better than the group switched to venlafaxine (Denys et al., 2004b). In this study, the sample sizes were small, and there was no placebo control group. As a result of the aforementioned information, venlafaxine may be considered as an alternative medication if a patient does not respond to an adequate trial of multiple SSRIs or is intolerant of SSRIs. Factors to consider when using venlafaxine include its often severe discontinuation syndrome and a greater potential for toxicity in overdose. This toxicity occurs predominately when it is mixed with alcohol or other drugs and includes prolongation of the QT interval, bundle branch block, and QRS prolongation.

Stimulants

Stimulant medications such as amphetamines (Owley et al., 2002) and caffeine (Koran et al., 2009) have been explored in preliminary reports for treatment-resistant OCD. While such strategies cannot be recommended at this time, further study is warranted for medications of this pharmacological profile.

Glutamatergic Medications

Because of the high rate of treatment resistance with SSRI medications, other avenues of pathology and treatment have been explored. There has been growing evidence that abnormalities of glutamate neurotransmission in the cortico-striato-thalamo-cortical circuitry may contribute to OCD, and that medications that modify glutamate may be efficacious in treatment-resistant OCD (Pittenger et al., 2006). Excessive glutamate activity has been noted in cerebral spinal fluid analysis in 18 OCD patients, who were compared with 21 healthy controls (Chakrabarty et al., 2005). Genetic studies have been conducted that indicate an association between an altered glutamate transporter gene found in early-onset OCD in males but not females, though data are mixed (Arnold et al., 2006; Dickel et al., 2006). There have been suggestions that the effect of SSRIs may be explained via a glutamatergic mechanism (Rosenberg et al., 2000); numerous glutamatergic medications are being explored as a result.

Riluzole

One of the glutamate modulating medications that has received the most attention is riluzole, which is approved in the United States for the treatment of amyotrophic lateral sclerosis. Riluzole is associated with a reduction in synaptic glutamate release and the uptake of glutamate by astrocytes; other effects may include the modulation of acetylcholine and dopamine, as well as the potentiation of glycine and GABA (Pittenger et al., 2006). The medication is generally well tolerated, with the most notable adverse event being a transient rise in liver enzymes in approximately half of those taking it. It is recommended that patients taking riluzole have their liver functions monitored monthly for 3 months, then every 3 months for 1 year with periodic monitoring thereafter (PDR).

Following a successful trial of riluzole in a single patient with OCD and major depression (Coric et al., 2003), a 12-week open-label trial of riluzole in 13 patients diagnosed with treatment-resistant OCD was performed. Seven patients were reported to have significant response (defined as >35% reduction in Y-BOCS score) and five were characterized as treatment responders (defined as >35% reduction in Y-BOCS plus a final score less than 16) (Coric et al., 2005). In that trial, riluzole was given at a dose of 50 mg twice daily and the medication was added to existing pharmacotherapy. Another open-label trial involved six children with treatment-resistant OCD who were given riluzole at an average dose of 101 mg in addition to previously prescribed medication (two children were on no medications at the time of riluzole initiation). Four of the participants had significant decline in OCD symptoms (defined as >30% reduction in Y-BOCS as well as a score of "Much Improved" or "Very Much Improved" on the CGI-I) by the end of the 12-week trial and one of the remaining two subjects responded after an additional 4-week trial (Grant et al., 2007). A second case series of 13 treatment-resistant patients demonstrated a response to riluzole augmentation in 7 people as defined by a reduction of ≥ 35% Y-BOCS. Significantly, three of the responders had prominent hoarding symptoms (Pittenger et al., 2008). The dosing of riluzole was between 100 and 200 mg per day in this series. One of the patients in this case series had previously been reported to have a successful response to riluzole augmentation with her symptoms of pathological skin picking and disordered eating (Sasso et al., 2006). As of now, riluzole augmentation has been successful in about half of adults studied, and it has been successful in children as well. It appears to be a well-tolerated medication, and double-blind placebo-controlled studies are needed to better examine this potentially useful medication.

Memantine

Memantine is a noncompetitive NMDA receptor antagonist that is approved for the treatment of moderate to severe Alzheimer disease. Memantine is thought to confer neuroprotection by limiting the negative effects of glutamatergic neurotoxicity (Aboujaoude et al., 2009). In a case series of 14 treatment-resistant patients using memantine augmentation at 20 mg per day, six patients had a response as defined by a reduction in Y-BOCS score of >25% with minimal side effects (Aboujaoude et al., 2009). A single blind study of 22 patients in intensive residential treatment (IRT) with 22 matched control subjects demonstrated a greater Y-BOCS improvement in the memantine patients. In addition, the case group was significantly more likely to have a >50% decrease in Y-BOCS symptoms (Stewart et al., 2010). Memantine was also shown to be useful in a single case report in an adolescent (Hezel et al., 2009).

D-cycloserine

D-cycloserine (DCS) is a glutamatergic partial N-methyl-d-aspartate (NDMA) that is being studied as an adjunct to ERP. It has been shown to facilitate extinction learning and demonstrated significantly greater decreases in obsession-related distress compared to a placebo group after four sessions of therapy (Kushner et al., 2007). Placebo patients tended to catch up in time, and at the end of the study both groups were equal. A second study showed that when 100 mg given 1 hour prior to ERP patients had a significantly greater response at the midpoint of treatment. Depressive symptoms were significantly better in the DCS group throughout the study (Wilhelm et al., 2008). In pediatric patients, when DCS was given at a 250 mg 4 hours prior to ERP, no response was noted (Storch et al., 2007). When smaller doses (25–50 mg) were given just 1 hour prior to therapy, a numerical though not a statistical difference was noted (Storch et al., 2010). Timing and dosing for DCS administration appear to be important variables, and the possibility exists that DCS could enhance a negative outcome after a poor session. This is a promising medication, and additional studies are ongoing.

Additional compounds are being explored for antiobsessional properties, including beta-lactam antibiotics (Pittenger et al., 2006), which may have glutamatergic properties; N-acetylcysteine, which has been explored as both an augmentation agent in OCD treatment in a case report (Lafleur et al., 2006) and has been explored in a double-blind placebo-controlled format for trichotillomania successfully (Grant et al., 2009); and morphine, which showed some response as well (Koran et al., 2005). While these novel treatments cannot be recommended as routine options at this time, clearly the field of OCD pharmacology is an exciting and expanding one.

Behavioral Treatments for Treatment-Resistant Obsessive-Compulsive Disorder

ERP is a specific type of CBT that is used in the treatment of OCD. ERP has been shown to be the most effective psychotherapy for the treatment of OCD and is superior to other psychotherapies, such as relaxation therapy (Foa et al., 2005). However, even with the efficacy of ERP well studied, only 18% of patients with OCD have been offered an adequate trial of ERP (Blanco et al., 2006). Since ERP is considered a first-line treatment for OCD (March et al., 1997), it should be offered to more individuals. ERP given twice weekly has been shown to work well in augmenting medications in OCD patients who were not considered to be having sufficient response to adequate SSRI therapy (Simpson et al., 2008). Another study suggests that ERP has equal efficacy to ERP plus clomipramine use and that both are better than clomipramine alone (Foa et al., 2005). Obviously, ERP is a useful augmentation strategy in treatment-resistant OCD, but it should be offered to all OCD patients regardless. It has been suggested that the amount of ERP ranges from 13 to 24 hours to determine treatment failure (Rauch et al., 1996). However, some patients will remain refractory even after this amount of appropriate ERP therapy; modifications in the intensity of therapy can be made, which can improve treatment outcomes.

There are different levels or intensities of ERP therapy available for OCD patients. Beyond traditional outpatient therapy, it is possible to refer someone for intensive outpatient therapy, partial hospitalization, residential treatment, or inpatient hospitalization (which is available in the United Kingdom but not in the United States). A complete description of these therapies is beyond the scope of this chapter but can be found elsewhere (Hudak and Dougherty, 2011). While it is recommended that intensive outpatient therapy be made available to any patient who requests it (March et al., 1997), it has been demonstrated that patients may have better response to more frequent sessions (Abramovitz et al., 2003). Patients who are treatment refractory should therefore be offered a higher level of therapy. Severe, treatment-resistant OCD has been shown to respond to inpatient treatment, with the majority of participants obtaining a significant reduction in the severity of their symptoms (Drummond, 1993; Drummond et al., 2007). Additionally, these individuals have maintained their progress as assessed in follow-up evaluations 18 months following discharge (Boschen et al., 2008).

Intensive residential treatment (IRT) was developed to treat patients with severe, treatment refractory OCD who had failed other standard outpatient treatment modalities (Stewart et al., 2005) and as alternatives to other approaches for refractory illness such as neurosurgery or intravenous medications. IRT may be especially useful in treatment of refractory illness if symptoms of contamination obsessions along with overt rituals are present in the absence of depressive symptomology, and such demographic variables such as being employed during treatment, never having been treated previously, female gender, lower initial OCD severity, and higher psychosocial functioning (Buchanan et al., 1996; Stewart et al., 2006). However, IRT should be considered for any severe, treatment-resistant patient prior to recommending treatments such as surgical options.

Neurosurgical Treatments for Intractable Obsessive-Compulsive Disorder

For patients with OCD who have not achieved response with all known conventional treatments, including behavioral therapy and pharmacotherapy, neurosurgical interventions are a viable option. While a full review of neurosurgical treatments for intractable OCD is beyond the scope of this chapter, a brief description of currently used neurosurgical options should be useful to the reader. Before reviewing these treatment options, it is important to state that neurosurgical interventions should be used only in patients with OCD who have failed to respond to all conventional treatments. To ensure that this is the case, a multidisciplinary committee (composed of psychiatrists, neurosurgeons, neurologists, and perhaps ethicists) is recommended in order to review all records of potential candidates. In this manner, the adequacy of past treatments, comorbidities, and medical issues can all be assessed in reviewing a patient's candidacy. Careful and precise patient selection is paramount and, as such, at this time only experienced tertiary care centers are recommended for neurosurgical intervention. Additionally, it is important to note that improvement following neurosurgical intervention may not occur until 3–12 months postoperatively. Lastly, as is the case for any intracranial procedure, there is a slight (1%–2%) risk of seizures or infection following the intracranial procedure.

Neurosurgical interventions for intractable OCD can be divided into two categories, ablative and deep brain stimulation (DBS). Stereotactic ablative procedures have been performed since the mid-1960s, while DBS is a more recent addition to neurosurgical interventions for intractable OCD. Following is a brief description of each of these interventions.

Anterior Capsulotomy

Anterior capsulotomy has originated by Talairach and was further developed by Leksell and colleagues. Initially, under magnetic resonance guidance, an insulated thermoelectrode was introduced to the target, the anterior limb of the internal capsule bilaterally, and the tip was heated to produce a lesion (this procedure is called thermocapsulotomy). The affected fibers connect the prefrontal cortex to subcortical structures, including the dorsomedial thalamus. Beginning in the 1990s, the gamma knife was used to create the lesion at the target; this allowed the procedure to be performed without burr holes. The first publication describing outcome following thremocapsulotomy (Herner, 1961) reported a response rate of about half in patients with OCD or major affective disorders. Subsequently, Bingley et al. (1977) reported a response rate of 71% in a cohort of patients with OCD. A later review (Waziri, 1990) reported that 67% of OCD patients were significantly improved following thermocapsulotomy. With the advent of gamma knife capsulotomy, investigators at the Karolinska Institute found that 48% of patients with OCD responded following thermocapsulotomy or gamma knife capsulotomy and that there was no significant difference between the groups receiving the two procedures (Ruck et al., 2008). Short-term adverse events include headache, confusion, and incontinence. Less frequent, but potentially longer lasting, side effects include weight gain, fatigue, and memory difficulties. There is some initial evidence that these adverse events are less common following gamma knife capsulotomy compared to thermocapsulotomy.

Anterior Cingulotomy

Over 1,000 anterior cingulotomies have been performed at the Massachusetts General Hospital since 1962. Indications have included OCD, affective illness, and intractable pain. Anterior cingulotomy always involves thermoablation; the lesion is too large to be performed with gamma knife procedures. The target is the bilateral dorsal anterior cingulate. Multiple reports, of increasing sophistication, have been published regarding outcome following anterior cingulotomy for intractable OCD. The first (Ballantine et al., 1987), using subjective outcome measures, described significant improvement in 56% of patients with intractable OCD. Analyzing these data using more stringent outcome data resulted in only 33% achieving substantial benefit (Cosgrove, 2000). However, prospective studies were then performed. The most recent showed that 45% of patients with intractable OCD achieved full or partial response following anterior cingulotomy for intractable OCD (Dougherty et al., 2002). Short-term side effects include headache, nausea, and difficulty with urination.

Subcaudate Tractotomy

Subcaudate tractotomy, introduced in 1964, targets the white matter just inferior to the head of the caudate. These fibers connect the orbitofrontal cortex to subcortical structures. By 1973, over 650 patients with major depression, OCD, or other anxiety disorders had undergone the procedure, mostly in the United Kingdom. In 1994, Bridges and colleagues (1994) reviewed 1,300 cases with multiple diagnoses (including anxiety, phobic anxiety, OCD, major depression, and bipolar disorder) and reported that 40%–60% of patients benefited. Short-term effects include somnolence, confusion, and temporary decreases in cognitive function. Subcaudate tractotomy involves thermoablation; no gamma knife subcaudate tractotomies have been reported.

Limbic Leucotomy

Limbic leucotomy is simply the combination of undergoing both anterior cingulotomy and subcaudate tractotomy. The first report of limbic leucotomy for intractable OCD reported significant improvement in 89% of patients; however, the outcome measure was a simple 5-point rating scale (Kelly et al., 1973). Twenty years later, Hay and colleagues (1993) reported significant improvement in 38% of their OCD patients treated with limbic leucotomy. More recently, Kim and colleagues (2002) reported a mean change in YBOCS from 34 to 3 in a small ($n = 12$) cohort. Short-term side effects include headache, confusion, lethargy, perseveration, and lack of sphincter control. In some reports, the lethargy was enduring.

Deep Brain Stimulation

Given that ablative procedures showed improvement in some patients with intractable OCD, in the late 1990s investigators began to explore the use of DBS at ablative targets. DBS does not involve ablation but instead utilizes existing hardware used for movement disorders to implant electrodes at a target with power and control of stimulation parameters delivered by a pacemaker-like device implanted in the chest wall with subcutaneous wires connecting it to the electrode. In this manner, the target area can be affected using a wide range of stimulation parameter options (as opposed to ablation). The first report (Nuttin et al., 1999) involved placement of DBS electrodes at the anterior capsulotomy target in four patients with intractable OCD; three of the four were considered responders. Since then, the worldwide experience with DBS at this target has grown (Greenberg et al., 2008), and DBS at the ventral capsule/ventral striatum (VC/VS) target has received HDE approval from the US FDA for intractable OCD. Additional targets are currently being explored (e.g., subthalamic nucleus;

Mallet et al., 2008) and further studies at the VC/VS target are under way. An important issue that differentiates DBS from the ablative procedures is the need for an experienced psychiatrist to explore the parameter space postoperatively, identify the optimal stimulation parameters, and provide continued long-term follow-up for DBS patients. Side effects have included transient exacerbation of psychiatric symptoms, permanent neurological sequelae, and suicide.

Summary

OCD is one of the more common psychiatric conditions, and knowledge about its treatment has progressed tremendously over the last two decades. While the first medication for OCD treatment was only approved for treatment in the United States in 1989, there are now five FDA-approved medications for OCD as well as two other SSRIs that have been shown to work—a great expansion in the range of treatment options. In addition, knowledge about behavioral therapy has been studied extensively as well, and E/RP has been demonstrated to have significant effects in improvement in OCD symptoms. However, despite the widening of options for OCD pharmacotherapy and the benefit of a specific psychotherapy, many patients with OCD still do not achieve an adequate response of their symptoms. While some of this is attributable to a lack of appropriate treatment being available to some patients, or mental health clinicians not utilizing appropriate treatment guidelines, much of the treatment-resistant nature of OCD is due to the chronic nature of the illness itself. Fortunately, research is ongoing in ways to improve OCD treatment in patients who are treatment resistant. Such research is focusing not just on novel pharmacotherapy but methods for improving psychotherapy protocols as well. Neurosurgery can be used in the most severe and intractable of patients. The setting and intensity level of OCD treatment is also being explored for treatment-resistant patients. As a result, the options for the clinician to treat the severe OCD patients are increasing.

Disclosure Statement

Darin Dougherty has received honoraria and research grants from Medtronic, Eli Lilly, Reed Elsevier, and Cyberonics.
P.G. has no conflicts of interest to disclose.
R.H. has no conflicts of interest to disclose.

References

Aboujaoude E, Barry JJ, Gamel N. Memantine augmentation in treatment-resistant obsessive-compulsive disorder: an open-label trial. *J Clin Psychopharmacol* 2009;29(1):51–55.

Abramowitz JS, Foa EB, Franklin ME. Exposure and ritual prevention for obsessive-compulsive disorder: effects of intensive versus twice-weekly sessions. *J Consult Clin Psychol* 2003;71:394–398.

Albert U, Aguglia E, Maina G, Bogetto F: Venlafaxine versus clomipramine in the treatment of obsessive-compulsive disorder: a preliminary single-blind, 12-week, controlled study. *J Clin Psychiatry* 2002;63:1004–1009.

American Psychiatric Association. Diagnostic and Statistical Manual of Mental Disorders (4th ed.). Washington, DC: American Psychiatric Association, 1994.

American Psychiatric Association. Practice Guidelines for the Treatment of Patients with Obsessive Compulsive Disorder. Washington, DC: American Psychiatric Association, 2007.

Arana GW. An overview of side effects caused by typical antipsychotics. *J Clin Psychiatry* 2000;61(Suppl 8): 5–11.

Arias Horcajadas F, Soto JA, García-Cantalapiedra MJ, Rodríguez Calvin JL, Morales J, Salgado M. Effectiveness and tolerability of addition of risperidone in obsessive-compulsive disorder with poor response to serotonin reuptake inhibitors. *Actas Esp Psiquiatr* 2006;34(3):147–152.

Arnold PD, Sicard T, Burroughs E, Richter MA, Kennedy JL. Glutamate transporter gene SLC1A1 associated with obsessive-compulsive disorder. *Arch Gen Psychiatry* 2006;63(7):769–776.

Atmaca M, Kuloglu M, Tezcan E, Gecici O. Quetiapine augmentation in patients with treatment resistant obsessive-compulsive disorder: a single-blind, placebo-controlled study. *Int Clin Psychopharmacol* 2002;17(3): 115–119.

Ballantine HT Jr, Bouckoms AJ, Thomas EK, Giriunas IE. Treatment of psychiatric illness by stereotactic cingulotomy. *Biol Psychiatry* 1987;22:807–819.

Barnes TR, McPhillips MA. Novel antipsychotics, extrapyramidal side effects and tardive dyskinesia. *Int Clin Psychopharmacol* 1998;13(Suppl 3):S49–S57.

Bingley T, Leksell L, Meyerson BA, Rylander G. Long term results of stereotactic capsulotomy in chronic obsessive-compulsive neurosis. In: Sweet WH, Obrador Alcade S, Martin-Rodriquez JG, eds., Neurological Treatment in Psychiatry, Pain, and Epilepsy: Proceedings of the Fourth World Congress of Psychiatry Surgery, Sept 7–10, Madrid, Spain. Baltimore: University Park Press, 1977; 287–299.

Blanco C, Olfson M, Stein DJ, Simpson HB, Gameroff MJ, Narrow WH. Treatment of Obsessive-Compulsive Disorder by U.S Psychiatrists. *J Clin Psychiatry* 2006;67:6.

Blier P, Bergeron R. Sequential administration of augmentation strategies in treatment-resistant obsessive-compulsive disorder: preliminary findings. *Int Clin Psychopharmacol* 1996;11(1):37–44.

Bloch MH, Landeros-Weisenberger A, Kelmendi B, Coric V, Bracken MB, Leckman JF. A systematic review: antipsychotic augmentation with treatment refractory obsessive-compulsive disorder. *Mol Psychiatry* 2006;11(7):622–632.

Bogetto F, Bellino S, Vaschetto P, Ziero S. Olanzapine augmentation of fluvoxamine-refractory obsessive-compulsive disorder (OCD): a 12-week open trial. *Psychiatry Res* 2000;96(2):91–98.

Boschen MJ, Drummond LM, Pillay A. Treatment of severe, treatment-refractory obsessive-compulsive disorder: a study of inpatient and community treatment. *CNS Spectr* 2008;13(12):1056–1065.

Bridges PK, Bartlett JR, Hale AS, Poynton AM, Malizia AL, Hodgkiss AD. Psychosurgery: stereotactic subcaudate tractotomy. An indispensable treatment. *Br J Psychiatry* 1994;165:599–611.

Buchanan AW, Meng KS, Marks IM. What predicts improvement and compliance during the behavioral treatment of obsessive compulsive disorder? *Anxiety* 1996;2:22–27.

Buchsbaum MS, Hollander E, Pallanti S, Baldini Rossi N, Platholi J, Newmark R, Bloom R, Sood E. Positron emission tomography imaging of risperidone augmentation in serotonin reuptake inhibitor-refractory patients. *Neuropsychobiology* 2006;53(3):157–168.

Bystritsky A, Ackerman DL, Rosen RM, Vapnik T, Gorbis E, Maidment KM, Saxena S. Augmentation of serotonin reuptake inhibitors in refractory obsessive-compulsive disorder using adjunctive olanzapine: a placebo-controlled trial. *J Clin Psychiatry* 2004;65(4):565–568.

Carey PD, Vythilingum B, Seedat S, Muller JE, van Ameringen M, Stein DJ. Quetiapine augmentation of SRIs in treatment refractory obsessive-compulsive disorder: a double-blind, randomised, placebo-controlled study. *BMC Psychiatry* 2005;5:5.

Chakrabarty K, Bhattacharyya S, Khanna S, Christopher R. Glutamatergic dysfunction in OCD. *Neuropsychopharmacology* 2005;30:1735–1740.

Connor KM, Payne VM, Gadde KM, Zhang W, Davidson JR. The use of aripiprazole in obsessive-compulsive disorder: preliminary observations in 8 patients. *J Clin Psychiatry* 2005;66(1):49–51.

Coric V, Taskiran S, Pittenger C, Wasylink S, Mathalon DH, Valentine G, Saksa J, Wu YT, Gueorguieva R, Sanacora G, Malison RT, Krystal JH. Riluzole augmentation in treatment-resistant obsessive-compulsive disorder: an open-label trial. *Biol Psychiatry* 2005;58(5):424–428.

Cosgrove GR. Surgery for psychiatric disorders. *CNS Spect* 2000;5:43–52.

Cottraux J, Bouvard MA, Milliery M. Combining pharmacotherapy with cognitive-behavioral interventions for obsessive-compulsive disorder. *Cogn Behav Ther* 2005;34:185–192.

Crocq MA, Leclercq P, Guillon MS, Bailey PE. Open-label olanzapine in obsessive-compulsive disorder refractory to antidepressant treatment. *Eur Psychiatry* 2002;17(5):296–297.

D'Amico G, Cedro C, Muscatello MR, Pandolfo G, Di Rosa AE, Zoccali R, La Torre D, D'Arrigo C, Spina E. Olanzapine augmentation of paroxetine-refractory obsessive-compulsive disorder. *Prog Neuropsychopharmacol Biol Psychiatry* 2003;27(4):619–623.

Dannon PN, Sasson Y, Hirschmann S, Iancu I, Grunhaus LJ, Zohar J. Pindolol augmentation in treatment-resistant obsessive compulsive disorder: a double-blind placebo controlled trial. *Eur Neuropsychopharmacol* 2000;10(3):165–169.

da Rocha FF, Correa H. Successful augmentation with aripiprazole in clomipramine-refractory obsessive-compulsive disorder. *Prog Neuropsychopharmacol Biol Psychiatry* 2007;31(7):1550–1551.

Delgado PL, Goodman WK, Price LH, Heninger GR, Charney DS. Fluvoxamine/pimozide treatment of concurrent Tourette's and obsessive-compulsive disorder. *Br J Psychiatry* 1990;157:762–765.

Denys D, Fineberg N, Carey PD, Stein DJ. Quetiapine addition in obsessive-compulsive disorder: is treatment outcome affected by type and dose of serotonin reuptake inhibitors? *Biol Psychiatry* 2007;61(3):412–414.

Denys D, de Geus F, van Megen HJ, Westenberg HG. A double-blind, randomized, placebo-controlled trial of quetiapine addition in patients with obsessive-compulsive disorder refractory to serotonin reuptake inhibitors. *J Clin Psychiatry* 2004a;65(8):1040–1048.

Denys D, van Megen HJ, van der Wee N, Westenberg HG. A double-blind switch study of paroxetine and venlafaxine in obsessive-compulsive disorder. *J Clin Psychiatry* 2004b;65:37–43.

Denys D, van der Wee N, van Megen HJ, Westenberg HG. A double-blind comparison of venlafaxine and paroxetine in obsessive-compulsive disorder. *J Clin Psychopharmacol* 2003;23:568–575.

Dickel DE, Veenstra-VanderWeele J, Cox NJ, Wu X, Fischer DJ, Van Etten-Lee M, Himle JA, Leventhal BL, Cook EH Jr, Hanna GL. Association testing of the positional and functional candidate gene SLC1A1/EAAC1 in early-onset obsessive-compulsive disorder. *Arch Gen Psychiatry* 2006;63(7):778–785.

Diniz JB, Shavitt RG, Pereira CA, Hounie AG, Pimentel I, Koran LM, Dainesi SM, Miguel EC. Quetiapine versus clomipramine in the augmentation of selective serotonin reuptake inhibitors for the treatment of obsessive-compulsive disorder: a randomized, open-label trial. *J Psychopharmacol* 2010;24(3):297–307.

Dougherty DD, Baer L, Cosgrove GR, Cassem EH, Price BH, Nierenberg AA, et al. Prospective long-term follow-up of 44 patients who received cingulotomy for treatment-refractory obsessive-compulsive disorder. *Am J Psychiatry* 2002;159:269–275.

Drummond LM. The treatment of severe, chronic, resistant obsessive-compulsive disorder. An evaluation of an in-patient programme using behavioral psychotherapy in combination with other treatments. *Br J Psychiatry* 1993;163:223–229.

Drummond LM, Pillay A, Kolb P, Rani S. Specialised in-patient treatment for severe, chronic, resistant obsessive-compulsive disorder. *Psychiatric Bull* 2007;31:49–52.

Egashira N, Okuno R, Matsushita M, Abe M, Mishima K, Iwasaki K, Nishimura R, Oishi R, Fujiwara M. Aripiprazole inhibits marble-burying behavior via 5-hydroxytryptamine (5-HT)1A receptor-independent mechanisms. *Eur J Pharmacol* 2008;592(1–3):103–108.

Eisen JL, Goodman WK, Keller MB, Warshaw MG, DeMarco LM, Luce DD, Rasmussen SA. Patterns of remission and relapse in obsessive-compulsive disorder: a 2-year prospective study. *J Clin Psychiatry* 1999;60(5):346–351.

Eisen JL, Pinto A, Mancebo MC, Dyck IR, Orlando ME, Rasmussen SA. A 2-year prospective follow-up study of the course of obsessive-compulsive disorder. *J Clin Psychiatry* 2010;71(8):1033–1039.

Eisen JL, Rasmussen SA, Phillips KA, Price LH, Davidson J, Lydiard RB, Ninan P, Piggott T. Insight and treatment outcome in obsessive-compulsive disorder. *Compr Psychiatry* 2001;42(6):494–497.

Englisch S, Esslinger C, Inta D, Weinbrenner A, Peus V, Gutschalk A, Schirmbeck F, Zink M. Clozapine-induced obsessive-compulsive syndromes improve in combination with aripiprazole. *Clin Neuropharmacol* 2009;32(4):227–229.

Erzegovesi S, Guglielmo E, Siliprandi F, Bellodi L. Low-dose risperidone augmentation of fluvoxamine treatment in obsessive-compulsive disorder: a double-blind, placebo-controlled study. *Eur Neuropsychopharmacol* 2005;15(1):69–74.

Fallon BA, Liebowitz MR, Campeas R, Schneier FR, Marshall R, Davies S, Goetz D, Klein DF. Intravenous clomipramine for obsessive-compulsive disorder refractory to oral clomipramine: a placebo-controlled study. *Arch Gen Psychiatry* 1998;55:918–924.

Fedorowicz VJ, Fombonne E. Metabolic side effects of atypical antipsychotics in children: a literature review. *J Psychopharmacol* 2005;19(5):533–550.

Ferrão YA, Shavitt RG, Bedin NR, de Mathis ME, Carlos Lopes A, Fontenelle LF, Torres AR, Miguel EC. Clinical features associated to refractory obsessive-compulsive disorder. *J Affect Disord* 2006;94(1–3):199–209.

Fineberg NA, Gale TM, Sivakumaran T. A review of antipsychotics in the treatment of obsessive compulsive disorder. *J Psychopharmacol* 2006;20(1):97–103.

Fineberg NA, Sivakumaran T, Roberts A, Gale T. Adding quetiapine to SRI in treatment-resistant obsessive-compulsive disorder: a randomized controlled treatment study. *Int Clin Psychopharmacol* 2005;20(4):223–226.

Fitzgerald KD, Stewart CM, Tawile V, Rosenberg DR. Risperidone augmentation of serotonin reuptake inhibitor treatment of pediatric obsessive compulsive disorder. *J Child Adolesc Psychopharmacol* 1999;9(2):115–123.

Foa EB, Kozak MJ. DSM-IV field trial: obsessive-compulsive disorder. *Am J Psychiatry* 1995;152:1.

Foa EB, Kozak MJ, Steketee GS, McCarthy PR. Treatment of depressive and obsessive-compulsive symptoms in OCD by imipramine and behavior therapy. *Br J Clin Psychol* 1992;31(Pt. 3):279–292.

Foa EB, Liebowitz MR, Kozak J, Davies S, Campeas R, Franklin ME, Huppert JD, Kjernisted K, Rowan V, Schmidt AB, Simpson HB, Tu X. (2005). Randomized placebo-controlled trial of ERP, clomipramine, and their combination in the treatment of OCD. *Am J Psychiatry* 2005;162:151–161.

Fornaro M, Gabrielli F, Mattei C, Vinciguerra V, Fornaro P. Aripiprazole augmentation in poor insight obsessive-compulsive disorder: a case report. *Ann Gen Psychiatry* 2008;7:26.

Francobandiera G. Olanzapine augmentation of serotonin uptake inhibitors in obsessive-compulsive disorder: an open study. *Can J Psychiatry* 2001;46(4):356–358.

Fux M, Benjamin J, Belmaker RH. Inositol versus placebo augmentation of serotonin reuptake inhibitors in the treatment of obsessive-compulsive disorder: a double-blind cross-over study. *Int J Neuropsychopharmacol* 1999;2(3):193–195.

Fux M, Levine J, Aviv A, Belmaker RH. Inositol treatment of obsessive-compulsive disorder. *Am J Psychiatry* 1996;153(9):1219–1221.

Garcia AM, Sapyta JJ, Moore PS, Freeman JB, Franklin ME, March JS, Foa EB. Predictors and moderators of treatment outcome in the Pediatric Obsessive Compulsive Treatment Study (POTS I). *J Am Acad Child Adolesc Psychiatry* 2010;49(10):1024–1033.

Goodman WK. Obsessive-compulsive disorder: diagnosis and treatment. *J Clin Psychiatry* 1999;60 (Suppl 18): 27–32.

Goodman WK, Ward HE, Murphy TK. Biological approaches to treatment refractory obsessive-compulsive disorder. *Psychiatr Ann* 1998;28(11):641–649.

Grady TA, Pigott TA, L'Heureux F, Hill JL, Bernstein SE, Murphy DL. Double-blind study of adjuvant buspirone for fluoxetine-treated patients with obsessive-compulsive disorder. *Am J Psychiatry* 1993;150(5):819–821.

Grant JE, Odlaug BL, Kim SW. N-acetylcysteine, a glutamate modulator, in the treatment of trichotillomania: a double-blind, placebo-controlled study. *Arch Gen Psychiatry* 2009;66(7):756–763.

Grant P, Lougee L, Hirschtritt M, Swedo SE. An open-label trial of riluzole, a glutamate antagonist, in children with treatment-resistant obsessive-compulsive disorder. *J Child Adolesc Psychopharmacol* 2007;17(6):761–767.

Greenberg BD, Gabriels LA, Rezai AR, Friehs GM, Okun MS, Shapira NA, Foote KD, Cosyns PR, Kubu CS, Malloy PF, Salloway SP, Giftakis JE, Rise MT, Machado AG, Baker KB, Stypulkowski PH, Goodman WK, Rasmussen SA, Nuttin BJ. Deep brain stimulation of the ventral internal capsule/ventral striatum for obsessive-compulsive disorder: worldwide experience. *Mol Psychiatry* 2008. [Epub ahead of print].

Haddad PM, Sharma SG. Adverse effects of atypical antipsychotics: differential risk and clinical implications. *CNS Drugs* 2007;21(11):911–936.

Hankin CS, Koran LM, Bronstone A, Black DW, Sheehan DV, Hollander E, Dunn JD, Culpepper L, Knispel J, Dougherty DD, Wang Z. Adequacy of pharmacotherapy among Medicaid-enrolled patients newly diagnosed with obsessive-compulsive disorder. *CNS Spectr* 2009;14(12):695–703.

Hay P, Sachdev P, Cumming S, Smith JS, Lee T, Kitchner P, Matheson J. Treatment of obsessive-compulsive disorder by psychosurgery. *Acta Pschiatr Scand* 1993;87:197–207.

Hemeryck A, Belpaire FM. Selective serotonin reuptake inhibitors and cytochrome P-450 mediated drug-drug interactions: an update. *Curr Drug Metab* 2002;3(1):13–37.

Herner T. Treatment of mental disorders with frontal stereotactic thermo-lesions: a follow-up of 116 cases. *Acta Psychiatr Scand* 1961;58(Suppl 36):1–140.

Hezel DM, Beattie K, Stewart SE. Memantine as an augmenting agent for severe pediatric OCD. *Am J Psychiatry* 2009;166(2):237.

Hollander E, Baldini Rossi N, Sood E, Pallanti S. Risperidone augmentation in treatment-resistant obsessive-compulsive disorder: a double-blind, placebo-controlled study. *Int J Neuropsychopharmacol* 2003a;6(4):397–401.

Hollander E, Friedberg J, Wasserman S, Allen A, Birnbaum M, Koran LM. Venlafaxine in treatment-resistant obsessive-compulsive disorder. *J Clin Psychiatry* 2003b;64(5):546–550. *Erratum in: J Clin Psychiatry* 2003; 64(8):972.

Hudak R, Dougherty D, eds. Clinical Obsessive Compulsive Disorders. New York: Cambridge Univeristy Press, 2011

Husted DS, Shapira NA. A review of the treatment for refractory obsessive-compulsive disorder: from medicine to deep brain stimulation. *CNS Spectr* 2004;9(11):833–847.

Iglesias Garcia C, Santamarina Montila S, Alonso Villa MJ. Ziprasidone as coadjuvant treatment in resistant obsessive-compulsive disorder treatment. *Actas Esp Psiquiatr* 2006;34(4):277–279.

Jenike MA, Baer U, Buttolph U. Buspirone augmentation of fluoxetine in patients with obsessive compulsive disorder. *J Clin Psychiatry* 1991;52:13–14.

Joffe RT, Swinson RP. Carbamazepine in obsessive-compulsive disorder. *Biol Psychiatry* 1987;22(9):1169–1171.

Karno M, Golding JM, Sorenson SB, Burnham MA. The epidemiology of obsessive-compulsive disorder in five US communities. *Arch Gen Psychiatry* 1988;45:1094–1099.

Kelly D, Richardson A, Mitchell-Heggs N, Greenup J, Chen C, Hafner RJ. Stereotactic limbic leucotomy: a preliminary report on forty patients. *Br J Psychiatry* 1973;123:141–148.

Kessler RM. Aripiprazole: what is the role of dopamine D(2) receptor partial agonism? *Am J Psychiatry* 2007; 164(9):1310–1312.

Khullar A, Chue P, Tibbo P. Quetiapine and obsessive-compulsive symptoms (OCS): case report and review of atypical antipsychotic-induced OCS. *J Psychiatry Neurosci* 2001;26(1):55–59.

Kim MC, Lee TK, Choi CR. Review of long-term results of stereotactic psychosurgery. *Neurol Med Chir (Tokyo)* 2002;42:365–371.

Koran LM, Aboujaoude E, Bullock KD, Franz B, Gamel N, Elliott M. Double-blind treatment with oral morphine in treatment-resistant obsessive-compulsive disorder. *J Clin Psychiatry* 2005;66(3):353–359.

Koran LM, Aboujaoude E, Gamel NN. Double-blind study of dextroamphetamine versus caffeine augmentation for treatment-resistant obsessive-compulsive disorder. *J Clin Psychiatry* 2009;70(11):1530–1535.

Koran LM, Mueller K, Maloney A. Will pindolol augment the response to a serotonin reuptake inhibitor in obsessive-compulsive disorder? *J Clin Psychopharmacol* 1996;16(3):253–254.

Koran LM, Ringold AL, Elliott MA. Olanzapine augmentation for treatment-resistant obsessive-compulsive disorder. *J Clin Psychiatry* 2000;61(7):514–517.

Koran LM, Sallee FR, Pallanti S. Rapid benefit of intravenous pulse loading of clomipramine in obsessive-compulsive disorder. *Am J Psychiatry* 1997;154:396–401.

Kumar TC, Khanna S. Lamotrigine augmentation of serotonin re-uptake inhibitors in obsessive-compulsive disorder. *Aust NZ J Psychiatry* 2000;34(3):527–528.

Kushner MG, Kim SW, Donahue C, Thuras P, Adson D, Kotlyar M, McCabe J, Peterson J, Foa EB. D-cycloserine augmented exposure therapy for obsessive-compulsive disorder. *Biol Psychiatry* 2007;62(8):835–838.

Lafleur DL, Pittenger C, Kelmendi B, Gardner T, Wasylink S, Malison RT, Sanacora G, Krystal JH, Coric V. N-acetylcysteine augmentation in serotonin reuptake inhibitor refractory obsessive-compulsive disorder. *Psychopharmacology (Berl)* 2006;184(2):254–256.

Lai CH. Aripiprazole treatment in an adolescent patient with chronic motor tic disorder and treatment-resistant obsessive-compulsive disorder. *Int J Neuropsychopharmacol* 2009;12(9):1291–1293.

Leucht S, Pitschel-Walz G, Abraham D, Kissling W. Efficacy and extrapyramidal side-effects of the new antipsychotics olanzapine, quetiapine, risperidone, and sertindole compared to conventional antipsychotics and placebo. A meta-analysis of randomized controlled trials. *Schizophr Res* 1999;35(1):51–68.

Leysen JE, Janssen PM, Megens AA, Schotte A. Risperidone: a novel antipsychotic with balanced serotonin-dopamine antagonism, receptor occupancy profile, and pharmacologic activity. *J Clin Psychiatry* 1994;55 (Suppl):5–12.

Li X, May RS, Tolbert LC, Jackson WT, Flournoy JM, Baxter LR. Risperidone and haloperidol augmentation of serotonin reuptake inhibitors in refractory obsessive-compulsive disorder: a crossover study. *J Clin Psychiatry* 2005;66(6):736–743.

Lykouras L, Alevizos B, Michalopoulou P, Rabavilas A. Obsessive-compulsive symptoms induced by atypical antipsychotics. A review of the reported cases. *Prog Neuropsychopharmacol Biol Psychiatry* 2003;27(3):333–346.

Madhusoodanan S, Parida S, Jimenez C. Hyperprolactinemia associated with psychotropics—a review. *Hum Psychopharmacol* 2010;25(4):281–297.

Maina G, Pessina E, Albert U, Bogetto F. 8-week, single-blind, randomized trial comparing risperidone versus olanzapine augmentation of serotonin reuptake inhibitors in treatment-resistant obsessive-compulsive disorder. *Eur Neuropsychopharmacol* 2008;18(5):364–372.

Mallet L, Polosan M, Jaafari N, Baup N, Welter ML, Fontaine D, du Montcel ST, Yelnik J, Chéreau I, Arbus C, Raoul S, Aouizerate B, Damier P, Chabardès S, Czernecki V, Ardouin C, Krebs MO, Bardinet E, Chaynes P, Burbaud P, Cornu P, Derost P, Bougerol T, Bataille B, Mattei V, Dormont D, Devaux B, Vérin M, Houeto JL,

Pollak P, Benabid AL, Agid Y, Krack P, Millet B, Pelissolo A; STOC Study Group. Subthalamic nucleus stimulation in severe obsessive-compulsive disorder. *N Eng J Med* 2008;359:2121–2134.

March JS, Frances A, Carpenter D, Kahn DA. The Expert Consensus Guideline Series: treatment of obsessive-compulsive disorder. *J Clin Psychiatry* 1997; 58(Suppl 4):3–72.

Markovitz PJ, Stagno SJ, Calabrese JR. Buspirone augmentation of fluoxetine in obsessive-compulsive disorder. *Am J Psychiatry* 1990;147:798–800.

Math SB, Reddy CJ. Issues in the pharmacological treatment of obsessive-compulsive disorder. *J Clin Pract* 2007;61(7):1188–1197.

Matsunaga H, Nagata T, Hayashida K, Ohya K, Kiriike N, Stein DJ. A long-term trial of the effectiveness and safety of atypical antipsychotic agents in augmenting SSRI-refractory obsessive-compulsive disorder. *J Clin Psychiatry* 2009;70(6):863–868.

McDougle CJ, Barr LC, Goodman WK, Pelton GH, Aronson SC, Anand A, Price LH. Lack of efficacy of clozapine monotherapy in refractory obsessive-compulsive disorder. *Am J Psychiatry* 1995b;152(12):1812–1814.

McDougle CJ, Epperson CN, Pelton GH, Wasylink S, Price LH. A double-blind, placebo-controlled study of risperidone addition in serotonin reuptake inhibitor-refractory obsessive-compulsive disorder. *Arch Gen Psychiatry* 2000;57(8):794–801.

McDougle CJ, Fleischmann RL, Epperson CN, Wasylink S, Leckman JF, Price LH. Risperidone addition in fluvoxamine-refractory obsessive-compulsive disorder: three cases. *J Clin Psychiatry* 1995a;56(11):526–528.

McDougle CJ, Goodman WK, Leckman JF, Holzer JC, Barr LC, McCance-Katz E, Heninger GR, Price LH. Limited therapeutic effect of addition of buspirone in fluvoxamine-refractory obsessive-compulsive disorder. *Am J Psychiatry* 1993;150(4):647–649.

McDougle CJ, Goodman WK, Leckman JF, Lee NC, Heninger GR, Price LH. Haloperidol addition in fluvoxamine-refractory obsessive-compulsive disorder. A double-blind, placebo-controlled study in patients with and without tics. *Arch Gen Psychiatry* 1994;51(4):302–308.

McDougle, CJ, Price, LH, Goodman WK, Charney DS, Heninger GR. A controlled trial of lithium augmentation in fluvoxamine-refractory obsessive-compulsive disorder: lack of efficacy. *J Clin Psychopharmacol* 1991;11(3):175–184.

Micali N, Heyman I, Perez M, Hilton K, Nakatani E, Turner C, Mataix-Cols D. Long-term outcomes of obsessive-compulsive disorder: follow-up of 142 children and adolescents. *Br J Psychiatry* 2010;197:128–134.

Murray CJ, Lopez AD. The Global Burden of Disease. Cambridge, MA: Harvard University Press, 1996.

Nasrallah HA. Atypical antipsychotic-induced metabolic side effects: insights from receptor-binding profiles. *Mol Psychiatry* 2008;13(1):27–35.

Newcomer JW. Second-generation (atypical) antipsychotics and metabolic effects: a comprehensive literature review. *CNS Drugs* 2005;19(Suppl 1):1–93.

Ninan PT, Koran LM, Kiev A, Davidson JR, Rasmussen SA, Zajecka JM, Robinson DG, Crits-Christoph P, Mandel FS, Austin C. High-dose sertraline strategy for nonresponders to acute treatment for obsessive-compulsive disorder: a multicenter double-blind trial. *J Clin Psychiatry* 2006;67:15–22.

Nuttin B, Cosyns P, Demeulemeester H, Gybels J, Meyerson B. Electrical stimulation in anterior limbs of internal capsule in patients with obsessive-compulsive disorder. *Lancet* 1999;354:1526.

Owley T, Owley S, Leventhal B, Cook EH Jr. Case series: adderall augmentation of serotonin reuptake inhibitors in childhood-onset obsessive compulsive disorder. *J Child Adolesc Psychopharmacol* 2002;12(2):165–171.

Oztürk M, Coskun M. Successful aripiprazole augmentation in a child with drug-resistant obsessive-compulsive disorder. *J Clin Psychopharmacol* 2009;29(6):607–609.

Pae CU. Potential utility of aripiprazole monotherapy for the treatment of major depressive disorder comorbid with obsessive-compulsive disorder. *Psychiatry Clin Neurosci* 2009;63(4):593.

Pallanti S, Hollander E, Goodman WK. A qualitative analysis of nonresponse: management of treatment-refractory obsessive-compulsive disorder. *J Clin Psychiatry* 2004;65(Suppl 14):6–10.

Pallanti S, Quercioli L. Treatment-refractory obsessive-compulsive disorder: methodological issues, operational definitions and therapeutic lines. *Prog Neuropsychopharmacol Biol Psychiatry* 2006;30(3):400–412.

Pallanti S, Quercioli L, Koran LM. Citalopram intravenous infusion in resistant obsessive-compulsive disorder: an open trial. *J Clin Psychiatry* 2002;63:796–801.

Pediatric OCD Treatment Study (POTS) Team. Cognitive Behavior Therapy, sertraline, and their combination for children and adolescents with obsessive compulsive disorder. *JAMA* 2004;292:1969–1976.

Pessina E, Albert U, Bogetto F, Maina G. Aripiprazole augmentation of serotonin reuptake inhibitors in treatment-resistant obsessive-compulsive disorder: a 12-week open-label preliminary study. *Int Clin Psychopharmacol* 2009;24(5):265–269.

Peters B, de Haan L. Remission of schizophrenia psychosis and strong reduction of obsessive-compulsive disorder after adding clozapine to aripiprazole. *Prog Neuropsychopharmacol Biol Psychiatry* 2009;33(8): 1576–1577.

Pfanner C, Marazziti D, Dell'Osso L, Presta S, Gemignani A, Milanfranchi A, Cassano GB. Risperidone augmentation in refractory obsessive-compulsive disorder: an open-label study. *Int Clin Psychopharmacol* 2000;15(5):297–301.

Coric V, Milanovic S, Wasylink S, Patel P, Malison R, Krystal JH. Beneficial effects of the antiglutamatergic agent riluzole in a patient diagnosed with obsessive-compulsive disorder and major depressive disorder. *Psychopharmacology (Berl)* 2003;167(2):219–220.

Pigott TA, L'Heureux F, Hill JL, Bihari K, Bernstein SE, Murphy DL. A double-blind study of adjuvant buspirone hydrochloride in clomipramine-treated patients with obsessive-compulsive disorder. *J Clin Psychopharmacol* 1992;12(1):11–18.

Pigott TA, Pato MT, L'Heureux F, Hill JL, Grover GN, Bernstein SE, Murphy DL. A controlled comparison of adjuvant lithium carbonate or thyroid hormone in clomipramine-treated patients with obsessive-compulsive disorder. *J Clin Psychopharmacol* 1991;11(4):242–248.

Pittenger C, Kelmendi B, Wasylink S, Bloch MH, Coric V. Riluzole augmentation in treatment-refractory obsessive-compulsive disorder: a series of 13 cases, with long-term follow-up. *J Clin Psychopharmacol* 2008; 28(3):363–367.

Pittenger C, Krystal JH, Coric V. Glutamate-modulating drugs as novel pharmacotherapeutic agents in the treatment of obsessive-compulsive disorder. *NeuroRx* 2006;3(1):69–81.

Ramasubbu R, Ravindran A, Lapierre Y. Serotonin and dopamine antagonism in obsessive-compulsive disorder: effect of atypical antipsychotic drugs. *Pharmacopsychiatry* 2000;33(6):236–238.

Rasmussen SA. Lithium and tryptophan augmentation in clomipramine-resistant obsessive-compulsive disorder. *Am J Psychiatry* 1984;141:1283–1285.

Rasmussen SA, Eisen JL. Epidemiology and differential diagnosis of obsessive-compulsive disorder. *J Clin Psychiatry* 1994;55(Suppl 10):5–14.

Rauch SL, Baer L, Jenike MA. Management of treatment resistant obsessive-compulsive disorder: practical considerations and strategies. In: Pollack MH, Otto MW, Rosenbaum JF, eds. Challenges in Psychiatric Treatment: Pharmacologic and Psychosocial Perspectives. New York: The Guilford Press, 1996: 504.

Ravi Kishore V, Samar R, Janardhan Reddy YC, Chandrasekhar CR, Thennarasu K. Clinical characteristics and treatment response in poor and good insight obsessive-compulsive disorder. *Eur Psychiatry* 2004;19(4): 202–208.

Ravizza L, Barzega G, Bellino S, Bogetto F, Maina G. Therapeutic effect and safety of adjunctive risperidone in refractory obsessive-compulsive disorder (OCD). *Psychopharmacol Bull* 1996;32(4):677–682.

Rosenberg DR, MacMaster FP, Keshavan MS, Fitzgerald KD, Stewart CM, Moore GJ. Decrease in caudate glutamatergic concentrations in pediatric obsessive-compulsive disorder patients taking paroxetine. *J Am Acad Child Adolesc Psychiatry* 2000;39(9):1096–103.

Ross S, Fallon BA, Petkova E, Feinstein S, Liebowitz MR. Long-term follow-up study of patients with refractory obsessive-compulsive disorder. *J Neuropsychiatry Clin Neurosci* 2008;20(4):450–457.

Rubio G, Jiménez-Arriero MA, Martínez-Gras I, Manzanares J, Palomo T. The effects of topiramate adjunctive treatment added to antidepressants in patients with resistant obsessive-compulsive disorder. *J Clin Psychopharmacol* 2006;26(3):341–344.

Ruck C, Karlsson A, Steele JD, Edman G, Meyerson BA, Ericson K, Nyman H, Asberg M, Svanborg P. Capsulotomy for obsessive-compulsive disorder: long-term follow-up of 25 patients. *Arch Gen Psychiatry* 2008;65: 914–921.

Sadock BJ, Saddock VA. Kaplan and Sadock's Synopsis of Psychiatry, 10th ed. Philadelphia, PA: Lippincott Williams & Wilkins.

Sarkar R, Klein J, Krüger S. Aripiprazole augmentation in treatment-refractory obsessive-compulsive disorder. *Psychopharmacology (Berl)* 2008;197(4):687–688.

Sasso DA, Kalanithi PS, Trueblood KV, Pittenger C, Kelmendi B, Wayslink S, Malison RT, Krystal JH, Coric V. Beneficial effects of the glutamate-modulating agent riluzole on disordered eating and pathological skin-picking behaviors. *J Clin Psychopharmacol* 2006;26:685–687.

Saxena S, Wang D, Bystritsky A, Baxter LR Jr. Risperidone augmentation of SRI treatment for refractory obsessive-compulsive disorder. *J Clin Psychiatry* 1996 Jul;57(7):303–306.

Savas HA, Yumru M, Ozen ME. Quetiapine and ziprasidone as adjuncts in treatment-resistant obsessive-compulsive disorder: a retrospective comparative study. *Clin Drug Investig* 2008;28(7):439–442.

Schotte A, Janssen PF, Gommeren W, Luyten WH, Van Gompel P, Lesage AS, De Loore K, Leysen JE. Risperidone compared with new and reference antipsychotic drugs: in vitro and in vivo receptor binding. *Psychopharmacology (Berl)* 1996;124(1–2):57–73.

Shapira NA, Ward HE, Mandoki M, Murphy TK, Yang MC, Blier P, Goodman WK. A double-blind, placebo-controlled trial of olanzapine addition in fluoxetine-refractory obsessive-compulsive disorder. *Biol Psychiatry* 2004;55(5):553–555.

Shapiro DA, Renock S, Arrington E, Chiodo LA, Liu LX, Sibley DR, Roth BL, Mailman R. Aripiprazole, a novel atypical antipsychotic drug with a unique and robust pharmacology. *Neuropsychopharmacology* 2003;28(8):1400–1411.

Simpson HB, Foa EB, Liebowitz MR, Ledley DR, Huppert JD, Cahill S, Vermes D, Schmidt AB, Hembree E, Franklin M, Campeas R, Hahn CG, Petkova E. A randomized, controlled trial of cognitive behavioral therapy for augmenting pharmacotherapy in obsessive compulsive disorder. *Am J Psychiatry* 2008;165:621–630.

Skapinakis P, Papatheodorou T, Mavreas V. Antipsychotic augmentation of serotonergic antidepressants in treatment-resistant obsessive-compulsive disorder: a meta-analysis of the randomized controlled trials. *Eur Neuropsychopharmacol* 2007;17(2):79–93.

Skoog G, Skoog I. A 40-year follow-up of patients with obsessive-compulsive disorder [see comments]. *Arch Gen Psychiatry* 1999;56(2):121–127.

Stahl, S. Describing an atypical antipsychotic: receptor binding and its role in pathophysiology. *J Clin Psychiatr Prim Care Comp* 2005;5(Suppl 3):9–13.

Stein DJ, Bouwer C, Hawkridge S, Emsley RA. Risperidone augmentation of serotonin reuptake inhibitors in obsessive-compulsive and related disorders. *J Clin Psychiatry* 1997;58(3):119–122.

Stewart SE, Jenike EA, Hezel DM, Stack DE, Dodman NH, Shuster L, Jenike MA. A single-blinded case-control study of memantine in severe obsessive-compulsive disorder. *J Clin Psychopharmacol* 2010;30(1):34–39.

Stewart SE, Stack DE, Farrell C, Pauls DL, Jenike MA. Effectiveness of intensive residential treatment (IRT) for severe, refractory obsessive-compulsive disorder. *J Psychiatr Res* 2005;39(6):603–609.

Stewart SE, Yen CH, Stack DE, Jenike MA. Outcome predictors for severe obsessive-compulsive patients in intensive residential treatment. *J Psychiatr Res* 2006;40(6):511–519.

Storch EA, Lehmkuhl H, Geffken GR, Touchton A, Murphy TK. Aripiprazole augmentation of incomplete treatment response in an adolescent male with obsessive-compulsive disorder. *Depress Anxiety* 2008a;25(2): 172–174.

Storch EA, Merlo LJ, Bengtson M, Murphy TK, Lewis MH, Yang MC, Jacob ML, Larson M, Hirsh A, Fernandez M, Geffken GR, Goodman WK. D-cycloserine does not enhance exposure-response prevention therapy in obsessive-compulsive disorder. *Int Clin Psychopharmacol* 2007;22(4):230–237.

Storch EA, Merlo LJ, Larson MJ, Marien WE, Geffken GR, Jacob ML, Goodman WK, Murphy TK. Clinical features associated with treatment-resistant pediatric obsessive-compulsive disorder. *Compr Psychiatry* 2008b; 49(1):35–42.

Storch EA, Murphy TK, Goodman WK, Geffken GR, Lewin AB, Henin A, Micco JA, Sprich S, Wilhelm S, Bengtson M, Geller DA. A preliminary study of D-cycloserine augmentation of cognitive-behavioral therapy in pediatric obsessive-compulsive disorder. *Biol Psychiatry* 2010;68(11):1073–1076.

Swedo SE, Rapoport JL, Leonard H, Lenane M, Cheslow D. Obsessive compulsive disorder in children and adolescents: clinical phenomenology of 70 consecutive cases. *Arch Gen Psychiatry* 1989;46:335–341.

Szechtman H, Sulis W, Eilam D. Quinpirole induces compulsive checking behavior in rats: a potential animal model of obsessive-compulsive disorder (OCD). *Behav Neurosci* 1998;112(6):1475–1485.

Szegedi A, Wetzel H, Leal M, Härtter S, Hiemke C. Combination treatment with clomipramine and fluvoxamine: drug monitoring, safety, and tolerability data. *J Clin Psychiatry* 1996;57(6):257–264.

Thomsen PH. Risperidone augmentation in the treatment of severe adolescent OCD in SSRI-refractory cases: a case-series. *Ann Clin Psychiatry* 2004;16(4):201–207.

Uguz F. Successful treatment of comorbid obsessive-compulsive disorder with aripiprazole in three patients with bipolar disorder. *Gen Hosp Psychiatry* 2010;32(5):556–558.

Van Ameringen M, Mancini C, Patterson B, Bennett M, Oakman J. A randomized, double-blind, placebo-controlled trial of olanzapine in the treatment of trichotillomania. *J Clin Psychiatry* 2010;71(10):1336–1343.

van der Wee NJ, Stevens H, Hardeman JA, Mandl RC, Denys DA, van Megen HJ, Kahn RS, Westenberg HM. Enhanced dopamine transporter density in psychotropic-naive patients with obsessive-compulsive disorder shown by [123I]{beta}-CIT SPECT. *Am J Psychiatry* 2004;161(12):2201–2206.

Volz C, Heyman I. Case series: transformation obsession in young people with obsessive-compulsive disorder (OCD). *J Am Acad Child Adolesc Psychiatry* 2007;46:6.

Vulink NC, Denys D, Fluitman SB, Meinardi JC, Westenberg HG. Quetiapine augments the effect of citalopram in non-refractory obsessive-compulsive disorder: a randomized, double-blind, placebo-controlled study of 76 patients. *J Clin Psychiatry* 2009;70(7):1001–1008.

Walsh KH, McDougle CJ. Pharmacological augmentation strategies for treatment-resistant obsessive-compulsive disorder. *Expert Opin Pharmacother* 2004;5(10):2059–2067.

Waziri R. Psychosurgery for anxiety and obsessive-compulsive disorders. In: Burrows M, Roth GD, eds. Handbook of Anxiety: The Treatment of Anxiety. Amsterdam: Elsevier, 1990: 519–535.

Weiss EL, Potenza MN, McDougle CJ, Epperson CN. Olanzapine addition in obsessive-compulsive disorder refractory to selective serotonin reuptake inhibitors: an open-label case series. *J Clin Psychiatry* 1999;60(8): 524–527.

Wickham R, Varma A. Ziprasidone-associated mania in a case of obssessive-compulsive disorder. *CNS Spectr* 2007;12(8):578–579.

Wilhelm S, Buhlmann U, Tolin DF, Meunier SA, Pearlson GD, Reese HE, Cannistraro P, Jenike MA, Rauch SL. Augmentation of behavior therapy with D-cycloserine for obsessive-compulsive disorder. *Am J Psychiatry* 2008;165(3):335–341.

Winter C, Heinz A, Kupsch A, Ströhle A. Aripiprazole in a case presenting with tourette syndrome and obsessive-compulsive disorder. *J Clin Psychopharmacol* 2008;28(4):452–454.

Yaryura-Tobias JA, Neziroglu FA. Venlafaxine in obsessive-compulsive disorder. *Arch Gen Psychiatry* 1996; 53:653–654.

Anorexia and Bulimia Nervosa

Enrica Marzola, Mary Ellen Trunko,
Emily Grenesko-Stevens, and Walter H. Kaye

Introduction

Eating disorders (EDs) are complex and difficult-to-treat illnesses that are often chronic and disabling and are characterized by aberrant patterns of feeding behavior. There are two main disorders: anorexia nervosa (AN) and bulimia nervosa (BN; First, Spitzer, Gibbon, & Williams, 2002). In addition, there is a third category defined as eating disorder not otherwise specified (EDNOS) that encompasses a range of disordered eating that does not meet the full criteria of AN or BN (*DSM-IV*; First et al., 2002). In the service of "simplification," this chapter will focus on AN and BN exclusively.

Individuals affected by AN (Table 10.1) exhibit an egosyntonic resistance to eating coupled with severe weight loss due to a relentless pursuit of thinness and restrictive eating. They are paradoxically obsessed with thoughts about food, despite a reduction in food intake. Even if emaciated, they perceive themselves as fat due to serious body image distortion. Two subtypes of eating-related behaviors in AN have been defined. The first, restricting-type anorexics (R-AN), lose weight purely by dieting and exercising without binge eating or purging. The second, binge-eating/purging-type anorexics (BN-AN), also restrict their food intake and exercise to lose weight, but they also periodically engage in binge eating and/or purging behaviors (*DSM-IV*; APA, 2000).

Individuals affected by BN (Table 10.2) exhibit irregular eating, including fasting and binging episodes. A binge episode is defined as eating an excessive amount of food in a discrete time period until abdominal discomfort or possibly pain. These binges are accompanied by a feeling of loss of control and sometimes dissociation. As a consequence, recurrent and inappropriate compensatory behaviors occur like vomiting, abuse of laxatives or diuretics, and excessive exercising. Similar to individuals with AN, individuals with BN are highly influenced by their weight and body shape. EDNOS is a broad diagnostic category, including clinical features not meeting narrowly defined diagnoses (Table 10.3).

In writing this chapter, several issues must be emphasized. First, compared to other behavioral disorders, there have been relatively few treatment trials in AN and BN. In part,

TABLE 10.1 *DSM IV-TR* **Criteria for Anorexia Nervosa**

1. Refusal to maintain body weight at or above a minimally normal weight for age and height: Weight loss leading to maintenance of body weight <85% of that expected or failure to make expected weight gain during period of growth, leading to body weight less than 85% of that expected.
2. Intense fear of gaining weight or becoming fat, even though under weight.
3. Disturbance in the way one's body weight or shape are experienced, undue influence of body weight or shape on self evaluation, or denial of the seriousness of the current low body weight.
4. Amenorrhea (at least three consecutive cycles) in postmenarchal girls and women. Amenorrhea is defined as periods occurring only following hormone (e.g., estrogen) administration.

Subtypes:
• Restricting type: During the current episode of anorexia nervosa, the person has not regularly engaged in binge-eating or purging behavior (self-induced vomiting or misuse of laxatives, diuretics, or enemas).
• Binge-eating–purging type: During the current episode of anorexia nervosa, the person has regularly engaged in binge-eating or purging behavior (self-induced vomiting or the misuse of laxatives, diuretics, or enemas).

this may be because the prevailing notion has been that these are disorders caused by psychosocial factors. Whatever the explanation, there has been little in the way of attempts to test rigorous, structured psychotherapies or systematically assess medications. Importantly, individuals with these disorders, particularly AN, tend to be resistant to treatment and deny having an illness. Thus, obtaining the cooperation of patients in treatment trials has been a struggle and AN has been a frustrating disorder to treat. There are no proven treatments that reverse core AN symptoms. Still, there has been encouraging progress in developing family-based treatments for adolescents with AN that are effective in normalizing weight and eating in many, but not all, patients. In comparison, there has been a fair amount of progress made in developing treatments for BN, with a considerable number of individuals reporting

TABLE 10.2 *DSM IV-TR* **Criteria for Bulimia Nervosa**

1. Recurrent episodes of binge eating characterized by both:
   – Eating, in a discrete period of time (e.g., within any 2-hour period), an amount of food that is definitely larger than most people would eat during a similar period of time and under similar circumstances
   – A sense of lack of control over eating during the episode, defined by a feeling that one cannot stop eating or control what or how much one is eating

2. Recurrent inappropriate compensatory behavior to prevent weight gain:
   – Self-induced vomiting
   – Misuse of laxatives, diuretics, enemas, or other medications
   – Fasting
   – Excessive exercise

3. The binge eating and inappropriate compensatory behavior both occur, on average, at least twice a week for 3 months.
4. Self-evaluation is unduly influenced by body shape and weight.
5. The disturbance does not occur exclusively during episodes of anorexia nervosa.

Subtypes:
• Purging type: During the current episode of bulimia nervosa, the person has regularly engaged in self-induced vomiting or the misuse of laxatives, diuretics, or enemas.
• Nonpurging type: During the current episode of bulimia nervosa, the person has used inappropriate compensatory behavior but has not regularly engaged in self-induced vomiting or misused laxatives, diuretics, or enemas.

TABLE 10.3 *DSM IV-TR* Criteria for Eating Disorder Not Otherwise Specified

Eating disorder not otherwise specified includes disorders of eating that do not meet the criteria for any specific eating disorder.

1. For female patients, all of the criteria for anorexia nervosa are met except that the patient has regular menses.
2. All of the criteria for anorexia nervosa are met except that, despite significant weight loss, the patient's current weight is in the normal range.
3. All of the criteria for bulimia nervosa are met except that the binge eating and inappropriate compensatory mechanisms occur less than twice a week or for less than 3 months.
4. The patient has normal body weight and regularly uses inappropriate compensatory behavior after eating small amounts of food (e.g., self-induced vomiting after consuming two cookies).
5. Repeatedly chewing and spitting out, but not swallowing, large amounts of food.

Binge-eating disorder is recurrent episodes of binge eating in the absence of regular inappropriate compensatory behavior characteristic of bulimia nervosa.

a substantial reduction in symptoms with talk therapies and with medication. Still, success is often considered to be a reduction in symptoms, rather than abstinence from binge and purge behaviors. In summary, because many to most with AN and BN continue to have some core symptoms after treatment, they might be considered to have some degree of treatment "resistance." Thus, this chapter will review the current state of the art for treatment and describe options for therapy.

Overview of Anorexia Nervosa and Bulimia Nervosa

Improvements in the understanding and treatment of EDs are of immense clinical and public health importance (NICE, 2004) since these are often chronic, relapsing illnesses (Herzog, Keller, Lavori, Kenny, & Sacks, 1992; Keel, Mitchell, Miller, Davis, & Crow, 1999; Klein & Walsh, 2003) with substantial and costly medical morbidity (McKenzie & Joyce, 1992). Importantly, for AN, there is no proven treatment that reverses symptoms (NICE, 2004); consequently, it has the highest death rate of any psychiatric illness (Sullivan, 1995).

EDs are disorders of unknown etiology that most commonly begin during adolescence in women. Causes of EDs are often considered to be complex with contributions from cultural pressures (Strober, 1995), as dieting and the pursuit of thinness are common in industrialized countries. Yet AN and BN affect only an estimated 0.3% to 0.7% and 1.5% to 2.5%, respectively, of females in the general population (Hoek et al., 1995).

Individuals with EDs often go to great lengths to keep their disorder a secret to avoid treatment and maintain the pathological behavior meant to control their weight and body image (Vitousek, Watson, & Wilson, 1998). Unwillingness to seek treatment is a hallmark of these disorders and has relevant effects on AN and BN treatment outcome. In fact, a substantial number of ill individuals do not seek treatment (Hudson, Hiripi, Pope, & Kessler, 2007). Illness often becomes apparent only when patients become emaciated from gradually losing weight or, in the purging subtypes (BN-AN and BN), when patients become physiologically unstable from excessive self-induced loss of fluids or electrolytes.

Subtypes of Eating Disorders

AN and BN are subdivided by eating behavior and psychopathological characteristics (American Psychiatric Association, 2000; Garner, Garfinkel, & O'Shaughnessy, 1985; Halmi & Falk, 1982; Herzog & Copeland, 1985; Strober, Salkin, Burroughs, & Morrell, 1982). AN is characterized by severe emaciation (American Psychiatric Association, 1994). Two types of consummatory behavior are seen in AN. Restricting-type anorexics (R-AN) lose weight purely by restricted dieting and have no history of binge eating or purging. Binge-eating/purging-type anorexics (BN-AN) also restrict their food intake to lose weight but have a periodic disinhibition of restraint and engage in binge eating and/or purging. Individuals with BN do not become emaciated and are able to maintain an average body weight (ABW) above 85% (American Psychiatric Association, 1994). There has been much conjecture regarding the processes underlying pathological eating, but little is understood of their biology (Schweiger & Fichter, 1997; Vitousek & Manke, 1994). Similar to AN, individuals with BN-AN and BN have a seemingly relentless drive to restrain food intake, an extreme fear of weight gain, and a distorted view of their body shape. In contrast to AN, however, BN-AN and BN suffer recurring disinhibition of dietary restraint, resulting in cycles of binge eating and compensatory actions such as self-induced vomiting. Transitions between AN and BN occur frequently, and these disorders are often cross-transmitted in families (Kendler et al., 1991; Lilenfeld et al., 1998; Strober, Freeman, Lampert, Diamond, & Kaye, 2000; Walters & Kendler, 1995). Consequently it has been argued that AN and BN share some risk and liability factors. In summary, similarities and differences of symptoms in AN and BN are a complex, and to some extent, controversial issue (Cassin & von Ranson, 2005; Kaye, Strober, & Jimerson, 2008; Lilenfeld, Wonderlich, Riso, Crosby, & Mitchell, 2006). Our pilot data suggested that it would be best to focus on appetite, reward, and inhibition/disinhibition as discussed in the following sections.

Distinguishing State and Trait in Anorexia Nervosa and Bulimia Nervosa

When malnourished and emaciated, individuals with AN, and to a lesser degree BN, have alterations of brain and peripheral organ function that are arguably more severe than in any other psychiatric disorder. For example, they suffer from enlarged ventricles and sulci widening (Ellison & Fong, 1998); altered brain metabolism in frontal, cingulate, temporal, and parietal regions (Kaye, Wagner, Frank, & UF, 2006); and widespread neuropeptide, hormonal, and autonomic disturbances (Boyar et al., 1974; Jimerson & Wolfe, 2006; Kaye et al., 2008). Determining whether such symptoms are a consequence or a potential cause of pathological feeding behavior or malnutrition is a major methodological problem in the field. It is difficult to study ED prospectively due to the young age of onset and difficulty in premorbid identification of people who will develop ED. Neurobiological studies during the acute illness are confounded by the effects of malnutrition. The fact that behaviors and physiological alterations persist after recovery suggests these are traits that cause the disorder, although it cannot be ruled out that these are scars and a permanent consequence of lengthy malnutrition.

Vulnerabilities that Create a Risk for Developing Anorexia Nervosa and Bulimia Nervosa

Recent studies show that certain childhood temperament and personality traits (Anderluh, Tchanturia, Rabe-Hesketh, & Treasure, 2003; Fairburn, Cooper, Doll, & Welch, 1999; Lilenfeld et al., 2006; Stice, 2002), such as negative emotionality, harm avoidance, perfectionism, inhibition, drive for thinness, altered interoceptive awareness, and obsessive-compulsive personality, create a vulnerability for developing AN and BN. Malnutrition tends to exaggerate these premorbid behavioral traits (Pollice, Kaye, Greeno, & Weltzin, 1997) after the onset of the illness, with the addition of other symptoms that maintain or accelerate the disease process, including exaggerated emotional dysregulation and obsessionality (Godart et al., 2007; Kaye, Bulik et al., 2004).

The process of recovery in AN is poorly understood and, in most cases, protracted. Still, approximately 50% to 70% of affected individuals will eventually have complete or moderate resolution of the illness, often in the early to mid-20s (Steinhausen, 2002; Strober, Freeman, & Morrell, 1997; Wagner et al., 2006). It is important to emphasize that temperament and personality traits such as negative emotionality, harm avoidance and perfectionism, and obsessional behaviors (particularly symmetry, exactness, and order) persist after recovery from both AN and BN (Casper, 1990; Srinivasagam et al., 1995; Steinhausen, 2002; Strober, 1980; Wagner et al., 2006) and are similar to the symptoms described premorbidly in childhood. Compared to the ill state, symptoms in recovered (REC) AN and BN individuals tend to be mild to moderate, including elevated scores on core ED measures. Interestingly, REC AN and BN tend to be more alike than different on many of these measures, although there are some differences on factors related to impulse control or stimuli seeking, such as novelty seeking (Lilenfeld et al., 2006; Strober, Freeman, & Morrell, 1997; Wagner et al., 2006).

Pathogenesis

Pathogenesis of EDs is complex and, to date, only partially understood. It is presumed to be influenced by developmental, social, and biological processes. Certainly, cultural attitudes toward standards of physical attractiveness have relevance, but it is unlikely that the preeminent influences in pathogenesis are sociocultural. Dieting behavior and a drive toward thinness are unusually common in industrialized countries throughout the world, yet AN affects less than 1% of women in the general population. Moreover, this syndrome has a relatively stereotypic clinical presentation, sex distribution, and age of onset, supporting the plausibility of intrinsic biological vulnerabilities (Duvvuri & Kaye, 2009).

The disparity between the high prevalence of pressures for thinness and the low prevalence of EDs combined with the stereotypic presentation, premorbid vulnerabilities, developmentally specific age of onset, and gender distribution underscore the possibility of biological contributions to vulnerabilities. Substantial evidence shows that genes contribute significantly to neurobiological vulnerabilities, accounting for approximately 50% to 80% of the risk (Berrettini, 2000; Bulik et al., 2006; Kendler et al., 1991) for developing AN and BN

(Kaye, Strober, & Jimerson, 2004; Steinglass & Walsh, 2004; Treasure & Campbell, 1994). The transmitted liability to AN and BN may be mediated by a more diffused phenotype of continuous, heritable behavioral traits related to disordered eating regulation (Bulik et al., 2005; Klump, McGue, & Iacono, 2000; Rutherford, McGuffin, Katz, & Murray, 1993; Wade, Martin, & Tiggemann, 1998), often resulting in subthreshold forms of ED in families (Lilenfeld et al., 1998; Strober et al., 2000).

The role of biological factors in the etiology of EDs has been proposed for years (Treasure & Campbell, 1994). There is growing consensus about neurobiological vulnerabilities being crucial factors in the pathogenesis of AN and BN, and there is support that monoamine (dopamine [DA] and serotonin [5-HT]) dysfunctions in particular may play an important role in pathogenesis. The rationale for these hypotheses was the considerable evidence that 5-HT disturbances could contribute to appetite dysregulation (Blundell, 1984; Leibowitz & Shor-Posner, 1986), anxious and obsessional behaviors, and behavioral inhibition and dysinhibition (Cloninger, 1987; Higley & Linnoila, 1997; Lucki, 1998; Mann, 1999; Soubrie, 1986). In addition, altered DA dysfunction could contribute (Haber, Kim, Mailly, & Calzavara, 2006; Phillips, Drevets, & Lane, 2003; Yin & Knowlton, 2006) to altered reward and affect, decision making, and executive control, as well as stereotypic motor activity (Yin & Knowlton, 2006) and decreased food ingestion (Halford, Cooper, & Dovey, 2004) in AN. These possibilities are supported by considerable evidence showing that disturbances of 5-HT and DA function occur when people are ill with ED and persist after recovery from AN and BN (see Kaye, Fudge, & Paulus, 2009).

Treatment

Anorexia Nervosa

The treatment of AN has unique challenges not found in other psychiatric disorders. In addition to effectively treating mood and cognitive disturbances, it is critical to provide weight restoration, since malnutrition itself can exacerbate symptoms and can be life threatening.

However, individuals with AN tend to be resistant to engaging in treatment, so that cooperation and motivation are often severely compromised. Moreover, the process of weight gain is relatively slow. Individuals with AN tend to want to eat small quantities of food (a few hundred calories per day). In contrast, weight gain on the order of 1 to 2 pounds per week tends to require 3,000 to 4,000 calories per day or more. Moreover, AN patients who sometimes need to gain 30 lb may require such large daily caloric amounts sustained over many months. Consequently, because of resistance to treatment and the high caloric need, many individuals with AN are treated in inpatient, residential, or day treatment programs that focus on weight restoration. However, as the etiology of AN is poorly understood, treatment programs tend to use a wide variety of theoretical approaches with little in the way of data supporting the superiority of any particular approach. Moreover, there is relatively little empirical support for treatment interventions in AN, and advances have been slow (Agras, Walsh, Fairburn, Wilson, & Kraemer, 2004). Controlled trials tend to show that compliance with treatment is poor, and relapse is high (Halmi et al., 2005). Moreover, many individuals have a chronic, relapsing course. However, these facts do not diminish the need for such costly and repeated treatments, as AN has the highest mortality rate of any psychiatric disorder, and malnutrition can result in costly and disabling, chronic medical problems. Even periodic and partially successful nutritional restoration may be important for preventing morbidity and death. Nonetheless, there is an urgent need to research and develop more cost-effective treatments and to candidly recognize the substantial limitations to conventional approaches.

Treatment approaches can be subdivided based on therapeutic need into three phases: acute stabilization, weight restoration, and relapse prevention.

Acute Stabilization

Acute stabilization is typically required for unstable vital signs, cardiac monitoring during management of severe electrolyte abnormalities, management of refeeding syndrome at very low weights, and rapid weight loss. Although an adjusted ideal body weight below 75% is usually associated with increased risk of medical complications, patients without acute medical instability are typically not admitted on presentation to the emergency room. Medical hospitalizations tend to be short and focused on medical stabilization, such as normalization of cardiovascular function, but not weight restoration.

Weight Restoration

For emaciated patients, it is generally believed that hospitalization in psychiatric units experienced in the treatment of ED applying interdisciplinary approaches, including supportive nursing care and behavioral techniques, is helpful in weight restoration (American Psychiatric Association Workgroup on Eating Disorders, 2006). A recent article, however, called into question the efficacy of specialized treatments for AN (Gowers et al., 2007). In a randomized trial of 167 adolescents conducted over 2 years, they sought to determine whether specialized ED care, either inpatient or outpatient, offered any advantage over a general outpatient setting. They found that patients in each group improved over 2 years and that specialized units, whether in inpatient or outpatient settings, did not offer any advantage over general outpatient treatment in terms of weight restoration. Importantly, at study completion, only 33% recovered fully and 27% still met AN criteria. Overall, inpatient treatment was predictive of poorer outcomes, and treatment failures from the outpatient setting did very poorly in the inpatient setting. This study supports the use of outpatient settings for weight restoration and limiting the use of expensive inpatient hospitalization to acutely stabilize patients. Furthermore, the lack of an advantage for specialized ED units within the centralized UK health care system might result from a high degree of adherence to evidence-based guidelines, even in treatment programs that are not specialized in EDs. In a far more heterogeneous US health care milieu, the significant discrepancies in implementing evidence-based practices for AN treatment provide specialized ED centers with the important opportunity to offer and promote treatments supported by controlled trials.

Relapse Prevention

Relapse prevention has been studied in a controlled manner in the original Maudsley family study in adolescents (Russell, Szmukler, Dare, & Eisler, 1987) and in a comparison between cognitive-behavioral therapy (CBT) and nutritional counseling for adults (Pike, Walsh, Vitousek, Wilson, & Bauer, 2003). In the Maudsley study, family therapy was more effective than individual supportive psychotherapy (SPT) at 1 year follow-up of 80 weight-restored adolescents. This benefit did not hold for adolescents ill for more than 3 years or for treatment of adults. In the latter study, although CBT was associated more frequently with "good outcome" (44% versus 7%) compared to nutritional counseling, less than a fifth of the participants maintained recovery at 1 year in the CBT treatment arm.

Medications

There are currently no FDA-approved medications for any phase of AN treatment. In the acute phase of treatment, as the focus is on inpatient medical stabilization, deferring psychotropics until the weight restoration phase avoids the complicating impact of side effects that emerge early. Even during the weight restoration phase, the role of medications in the treatment of low-weight patients with AN has typically been limited (Attia, Wolk, Cooper, Glasofer, & Walsh, 2005; Bulik, Berkman, Brownley, Sedway, & Lohr, 2007; Jimerson, Wolfe, Brotman, & Metzger, 1996). In contrast to the effectiveness of antidepressant medications in patients with BN, several studies have failed to demonstrate a beneficial effect for the addition of selective serotonin reuptake inhibitors (SSRIs) in the inpatient treatment of malnourished AN patients (Attia, Haiman, Walsh, & Flater, 1998; Ferguson, La Via, Crossan, & Kaye, 1999; Strober, Pataki, Freeman, & DeAntonio, 1999). Initial interest in the possible benefit of neuroleptics in the treatment of AN was based on clinical observations of weight gain with these medications. However, results from randomized, double-blind controlled trials with pimozide and sulpiride failed to demonstrate accelerated weight gain (Vandereycken, 1984; Vandereycken & Pierloot, 1982). Prompted in part by observations of weight gain in other patient groups associated with the use of atypical antipsychotics, a recent controlled trial of olanzapine showed some efficacy in AN (Bissada, Tasca, Barber, & Bradwejn, 2008). In a placebo-controlled trial in a day hospital setting, 34 patients with AN on 2.5 to 10 mg of olanzapine showed improved weight gain and obsessional symptoms. Previously, promising results had also emerged from case reports, open, and small controlled trials of olanzapine (Barbarich et al., 2004; Boachie, Goldfield, & Spettigue, 2003; Bosanac, Burrows, & Norman, 2003; Brambilla et al., 2007; Dennis, Le Grange, & Bremer, 2006; Ercan, Copkunol, Cykoethlu, & Varan, 2003; Hansen, 1999; Jensen & Mejlhede, 2000; La Via, Gray, & Kaye, 2000; Malina et al., 2003; Mehler et al., 2001; Mondraty et al., 2005; Powers, Santana, & Bannon, 2002; Wang, Chou, & Shiah, 2006), quetiapine (Bosanac et al., 2007; Mehler-Wex, Romanos, Kirchheiner, & Schulze, 2008; Powers, Bannon, Eubanks, & McCormick, 2007), and risperidone (Fisman et al., 1996; Newman-Toker, 2000). Although the side-effect profile from long-term use in this population is largely unknown, clinicians and patients should be aware of risks of insulin resistance, obesity, and hyperlipidemia from extensive experience in the treatment of psychotic illnesses in other psychiatric populations. It is important to periodically monitor lipid profiles and blood glucose levels to accurately assess the risk-benefit ratio in each patient with AN.

Upon weight restoration, patients who have achieved weight restoration often have persisting psychological symptomatology accompanied by a significant risk of recurrence of low-weight episodes. Medication use, particularly of fluoxetine, has prevented relapse in some but not all individuals studied. A clinically based, prospective longitudinal follow-up study failed to show significant benefit of fluoxetine treatment in comparison to historical controls (Strober, Freeman, DeAntonio, Lampert, & Diamond, 1997). Subsequently, a double-blind, placebo-controlled trial in weight-restored restricting-type patients demonstrated that fluoxetine treatment was associated with reduced relapse rate and reductions in depression, anxiety, and obsessions and compulsions (Kaye et al., 2001). However, a recent study of both restricting and binge-eating/purging-type AN failed to demonstrate a difference in time to relapse in weight-restored patients with AN who were receiving cognitive-behavioral therapy (CBT), and were randomly assigned to adjunctive treatment with fluoxetine or placebo (Walsh et al., 2006). Although there is no systematic supporting data, it is our clinical impression that after weight restoration, restricting-type AN respond better than binge-eating/purging-type AN to fluoxetine, which is consistent with differences between the groups in serotonin transporter function (Bailer et al., 2007).

Psychotherapy

A wide variety of psychotherapeutic approaches are currently in use to try to help patients and their families cope with AN. However, few are evidence based and fewer yet show efficacy. Studies have focused mostly on the weight restoration phase, more so in the outpatient compared to the inpatient setting, and less so during relapse prevention.

Little is known about the relative merit of therapies for weight restoration in the inpatient setting. This is particularly problematic because a significant portion of AN treatment occurs in inpatient settings. The one controlled study that assessed inpatient therapy by randomizing adolescents requiring hospitalization to family therapy versus family group psychoeducation found no difference in weight restoration between the groups (Geist, Heinmaa, Stephens, Davis, & Katzman, 2000). The family therapy encouraged parents to take an "active role" in treatment, while psychoeducation involved delivery of information about the illness, such as clinical course and reasons for treatment. At study completion after 4 months of treatment, both groups averaged above 90% ideal body weight. Future studies will need to assess not only the contribution of different types of therapy to treatment efficacy while controlling for inpatient milieu but also assess how different inpatient settings can enhance outcomes while controlling for type of therapy.

To assess weight restoration in the outpatient setting, controlled studies have included both individual and family therapies (Guarda, 2008). Individual therapies with proven efficacy in other psychiatric disorders have been adapted for adults with AN. These include CBT (Ball & Mitchell, 2004; Halmi et al., 2005; McIntosh et al., 2005; Pike et al., 2003), interpersonal therapy (IPT; McIntosh et al., 2005), supportive psychotherapy (SPTI; Eisler et al., 1997; Russell et al., 1987), psychoanalytic (Dare, Eisler, Russell, Treasure, & Dodge, 2001), and psychodynamic (Robin et al., 1999) therapies. We first discuss those studies that compare across individual therapies and then the remainder that included group therapies or medications as comparators. In a comparison between individual therapies, 82% of treatment completers in a variant of SPT with clinical management, termed specialist supportive clinical management (SSCM; McIntosh et al., 2006), were much improved or had minimal symptoms compared to 42% for CBT and 17% for IPT (McIntosh et al., 2005). This was contrary to the central hypothesis of their study that specialized psychotherapies would result in better outcomes. The flexibility offered by SSCM in combining clinical management and supportive psychotherapy in response to patients' presentations may have contributed to its success in this study. In another study, focal psychoanalytic psychotherapy showed modest benefit over a low-contact "routine" treatment over 1 year (Dare et al., 2001).

Among studies that compared individual to group therapies, CBT was as effective as a behavioral family therapy in outcome variables such as nutritional status and eating behaviors (Ball & Mitchell, 2004), while ego-oriented psychotherapy, a psychodynamic therapy, was less effective in weight gain and resumption of menses compared to behavioral family systems therapy in adolescents at study completion (Robin et al., 1999). In a comparison of individual therapy and medication, CBT was no different than fluoxetine or a CBT/fluoxetine combination in predicting treatment completion (Halmi et al., 2005). The lone controlled study of individual therapy in adolescents used family therapy as a comparator and found that SPT did better than Maudsley family therapy (discussed later) when the age of onset was above 18 years of age, and this effect was sustained at 5-year follow-up (Eisler et al., 1997; Russell et al., 1987).

Despite the frustration in treating AN, there is some cause for optimism. Family therapy for weight restoration, an approach developed at the Maudsley Hospital in England, has shown significant promise for treating adolescents. In Maudsley therapy, the family is explicitly trained in regaining parental control over the adolescent patient's eating behavior to achieve weight gain (Russell et al., 1987). Once weight and eating behavior are normalized, control is gradually returned to the adolescent while moving the focus to rebuilding relationships within the family and pursuing developmental milestones. In a study comparing Maudsley family therapies, where families were treated either conjointly or in separate sessions, two-thirds of 40 underweight adolescents with AN were weight restored regardless of therapy arm (Eisler & Dare, 2000). Remarkably, 75% of those patients maintained recovery after 5 years (Eisler, Simic, Russell, & Dare, 2007). Surprisingly, a recent study found that a shorter 10-session version of Maudsley therapy was as effective as the original 20-session version (Lock, Agras, Bryson, & Kraemer, 2005) However, patients with either high levels of eating-related obsessionality/compulsiveness or those from a single-parent/divorced family did better in the longer form of the treatment compared to the shorter version. The lack of a control or of other types of active treatment groups limits insight into the efficacy of Maudsley therapy. An NIH-funded trial of Maudsley therapy versus systemic family therapy, currently under way at multiple sites, including ours, is designed to answer such questions.

One of the practical limitations is that few psychiatry clinics provide the intensive outpatient programs necessary to monitor such patients during weight restoration. Upon weight restoration, a relapse prevention plan is needed to monitor and return the patient to treatment as needed.

New Treatment Approaches

There are additional reasons to be optimistic about the future of treatment for adolescent AN. As noted earlier, there is growing awareness that AN is a highly heritable disorder with a powerful neurobiological predisposition (Kaye et al., 2009) and that certain childhood temperaments and personality traits increase susceptibility during adolescence (Kaye et al., 2009; Lilenfeld et al., 2006). Moreover, there is a better understanding of altered feeding behavior and energy metabolism (Kaye, Gwirtsman, Obarzanek, & George, 1988; Wagner et al., 2008), which can aid in more effective nutritional restoration. Such advances allow for the development of psychoeducational tools and new medication strategies that can be useful adjunctive treatments (Bissada et al., 2008).

Other therapies are also emerging in the treatment of EDs. For example, dialectical behavior therapy (DBT) (Linehan et al., 2002), originally designed to treat patients with borderline personality disorder, has now been adapted for patients who have EDs (Palmer et al., 2003; Wisniewski & Kelly, 2003). DBT for patients with EDs combines standard cognitive-behavioral techniques for emotion regulation and reality testing with concepts of mindfulness, distress tolerance, and acceptance, for better tolerance of emotional dysregulation and resulting reduction in ED symptoms.

Another developing therapy is the cognitive remediation approach, which focuses on altered aspects of cognitive functioning in AN (Tchanturia & Davies, 2007; Treasure, Tchanturia, & Schmidt, 2005). Cognitive remediation includes exercises to decrease rigidity using structured tasks that train different aspects of cognitive flexibility and emphasize strategies to move between detail and a focus on the gestalt using field independence/dependence tasks (Davies & Tchanturia, 2005). Treatment starts with simple tasks to illustrate how rigid, detailed thinking may be counterproductive for some purposes. For example, people with AN may find it difficult to switch between perspectives and so may fail to grasp the essence of visual illusions.

Greater awareness has also been paid to the stress that adolescent AN imparts on family members of the patient. The Carers program developed by Sepulveda, Macdonald, and Treasure (2008) addresses the ability of the caregivers of the patient with AN to support and take care of themselves. In the Carers program, families gain greater understanding about natural tendencies and reactions to patients with EDs, and they learn how to channel that energy into effective management strategies. Light-hearted animal metaphors are used to describe these interactions, and families are encouraged to reflect on their own responses to the person with AN.

Even though advances have been made in the model of treatment for adolescent AN, access is often limited to academic medical centers, and many families find themselves without a local therapist who is knowledgeable about these innovative treatments. They may struggle with nonstandardized treatment approaches or be limited to medical inpatient options with limited therapy. Moreover, there may not be providers in the local community with sufficient expertise in the medical and pharmacologic evaluation and treatment of AN.

To address this gap in treatment delivery, we have developed a 1-week, intensive family-based evaluation and treatment program for adolescent AN based on the most promising and innovative treatments available today (intensive family therapy [IFT]). While this program is weighted toward a Maudsley-Based approach for refeeding, it also includes a range of other treatment strategies. Outcomes on the first 19 cases from a retrospective chart review was done at 52 days to 738 days (mean = 281) post treatment. Admission body mass index (BMI) ranged from 13.4 to 20.8 (mean = 17.0, SD = 2.2). Follow-up BMI ranged from 16.3 to 28.5 (mean = 20.0, SD = 2.7). All but one patient reported a sustained gain in BMI post treatment (mean = 3.1, SD = 3.0). These data provide further support for the notion that short-term family-based therapy may be useful for weight restoration and maintenance in some individuals with AN.

Conclusions

For adolescents with recidivist AN, residential or inpatient admissions have been the standard treatment. The average cost of treatment using the highest remission/recovery thresholds (weight greater than 95% of expected and Eating Disorder Examination [EDE] scores within 1 SD of normal) is estimated at $83,736 (Lock, Couturier, & Agras, 2008). However, it has been shown that patients tend to relapse after they leave structured settings (Gowers, Norton, Halek, & Crisp, 1994). Moreover, many insurance companies do not cover the costs of these prolonged and recurring treatments, which places enormous financial burdens on the family (Kaye, Kaplan, & Zucker, 1996). In addition, because of the cost, many people with AN do not access treatment. While for some individuals inpatient or residential stays for weight restoration may be necessary, or even life-saving, there is little in the way of data from controlled trials showing that such treatment reduces chronicity or symptoms. It is important to emphasize that just getting people with AN to a normal body weight is not enough to "cure" this disorder. That is because behaviors and symptoms, such as an anxious, obsessional focus on weight loss, and physiological disturbances, such as increased metabolism, often persist after weight restoration. Even after successful treatment, it is common that individuals with AN remain anxious, obsessional, and perfectionistic, with continued body image distortions.

Recent data suggest improved outcome for adolescents if families understand the chronicity of such phenomena, and are given the tools necessary to manage their child with AN at home. It is important to note that this treatment program may be particularly effective for some, but not all, families. That is, a successful outcome may be related to having a family that is motivated and has the time, energy, stability, and communication ability to attend such treatment, and the persistence needed to employ these tactics at home. Furthermore, our clinical anecdotes suggest that this intensive program works best with younger adolescents who may be more amenable to parental direction.

In summary, higher levels of care are often warranted for the treatment of AN because of the need for renourishment and weight restoration. Such programs should rely on best-practices and evidence-based management, and have experience in both family-based therapies and pharmacological approaches. As we gain new knowledge about the powerful neurobiology contributing to the cause of AN (Kaye et al., 2009), we are starting to make substantial progress in understanding and providing more effective treatments for this frustrating and difficult illness, for which success has been modest in the past (Bulik et al., 2007). Examples include the efficacy of Maudsley family therapy in restoring and maintaining weight in adolescents, as well as a role for olanzapine in weight restoration.

Bulimia Nervosa

Medications

Numerous controlled trials in the 1980s and early 1990s established antidepressants as more effective than placebo in the treatment of BN (Kaye & Walsh, 2002). Efficacy has been shown across a variety of antidepressant medication classes, including tricyclics, monoamine oxidase inhibitors, and more recently, SSRIs. Success most commonly was measured by decrease in frequency of binging and purging episodes, and though studies varied widely, many achieved reductions of 50%–75% in one or both areas (American Psychiatric Association, 2006).

Despite significant progress in the field, however, it is important for the clinician to realize that most patients who responded to medication continued to binge and purge at a frequency that would meet criteria for a diagnosis of BN at the end of the studies. Only a minority of patients attained remission of binge/purge symptoms (Nakash-Eisikovits, Dierberger, & Westen, 2002).

With their relatively benign side-effect profiles, SSRIs are considered first-line pharmacological treatment of BN (American Psychiatric Association, 2006; NICE, 2004). The SSRI fluoxetine is the only medication that specifically has an indication for BN that was approved by the US Food and Drug Administration. The indication was granted in 1996, after large, multicenter, controlled trials convincingly demonstrated fluoxetine was more effective than placebo in treatment of BN. It was found that a relatively high dose of 60 mg/day was superior to 20 mg/day (Fluoxetine Bulimia Nervosa Collaborative Study Group, 1992), and that a starting dose of 60 mg/day generally was well tolerated in this patient population (Goldstein, Wilson, Thompson, Potvin, & Rampey, 1995).

While it is presumed that any of the SSRIs would be useful in treatment of BN, trials with those other than fluoxetine have been scant. Nonetheless, study drug has proven superior to placebo, except in the case of fluvoxamine, where results have been mixed. While two small controlled trials have shown efficacy (Fichter, Kruger, Rief, Holland, & Dohne, 1996; Milano, Siano, Petrella, & Capasso, 2005), in a much larger randomized trial involving 267 patients in the United Kingdom, the investigators reported that fluvoxamine performed no better than placebo for short- or long-term (1 year) treatment of outpatients with BN. It was noted that the dose range of 50–300 mg may have been too low to show treatment effect with this illness, but adverse events were a problem for many patients, and titration to higher doses may not have been tolerated (Schmidt, Cooper, & Essers, 2004). Overall, therefore, little evidence exists for use of fluvoxamine as an SSRI of choice in BN.

Recent results with sertraline are promising, though only one small randomized trial, with 20 patients, has been reported. Interestingly, significant improvement versus placebo occurred on only 100 mg/day, in contrast with the relatively high doses required for fluoxetine (Milano, Petrella, Sabatino, & Capasso, 2004). The reason for this finding is unknown, but replication on a larger scale would be beneficial, given some patients in clinical practice do have significant side effects on 60 mg or more of fluoxetine.

Only one randomized, controlled trial has compared various SSRIs head to head. The 6-week study, with 91 patients, was designed to explore a genetic basis for drug response. No such basis was discovered, but the authors reported that fluoxetine, fluvoxamine, citalopram, and paroxetine all performed superiorly to placebo. It is noteworthy that this study involved inpatients, a relatively unusual treatment environment for BN (Erzegovesi, Riboldi, & DiBella, 2004).

Bupropion is another antidepressant worth mention. Though it was found effective in reducing BN symptoms in one small controlled study, 4 out of 69 patients taking the drug experienced seizures (Horne et al., 1988). It should be noted that no study has attempted to replicate these findings. Thus, it remains conjectural whether BN patients might be at increased risk for seizures with this drug, but most clinicians in the EDs field avoid its use.

Although antidepressants initially were proposed for treatment of BN because of frequent accompanying mood symptoms, these medications also have shown efficacy in bulimic patients without comorbid anxiety and depressive disorders, and thus they appear to target independently symptoms of binging, purging, and preoccupation with shape and weight (Goldstein, Wilson, Ascroft, & al-Banna, 1999). This result, along with generally a more rapid onset of action and, for fluoxetine, a higher dosage requirement than is seen with treatment of depression, suggests that antidepressant action in BN may occur by an unknown mechanism, perhaps relating in part to underlying neural control of appetite (Kaye & Walsh, 2002). Such possibilities have led to case reports and small trials of novel medications, most notably topiramate and ondansetron.

The anticonvulsant topiramate has been linked to appetite suppression and weight loss (Appolinario & McElroy, 2004). Results from the first randomized, double-blind, placebo-controlled trials of topiramate in BN have been promising (Hedges, Reimherr, & Hoopes, 2003; Hoopes, Reimherr, & Hedges, 2003). In 2003, a 10-week trial of 69 patients began with a dose of 25 mg/day and titrated to a maximum of 400 mg/day (median 100 mg/day). Topiramate was more effective than placebo in decreasing frequency of binge/purge behaviors (to a similar degree as seen in antidepressant trials) and in improving other psychological measures. The authors stated that adverse events generally were mild to moderate, resolved with time or dose reduction, and did not usually lead to withdrawal from the study. Another 10-week controlled trial, conducted in Germany in 2004, had similar findings with regard to reductions in binge/purge behaviors and side effects, and also reported a decrease in weight for the topiramate group. There was an unusually low dropout rate among the 60 participants, possibly because the study enrolled only women with moderate cases of bulimia, or because the medication was titrated slowly and doses were relatively low (25 mg/day to 250 mg/day; Nickel et al., 2005). Despite the report of few intolerable side effects in these small studies, adverse reactions to topiramate are common in clinical psychiatric practice, and it should be considered for use in BN only when other medications have been ineffective (American Psychiatric Association, 2006). Additional concerns include lack of data on longer term safety and efficacy, as well as the physical and emotional complications likely to result if its use leads to weight loss in the normal- or low-weight BN patient. Larger, multi-center trials are needed.

Another novel agent proposed for treatment of bulimia is the antiemetic ondansetron, a drug that acts on the serotonergic system. Ondansetron was found to be more effective than placebo in reducing binge eating and vomiting in a 4-week randomized trial of 25 patients with severe, chronic BN (Faris et al., 2000). More information regarding potential side effects, likelihood of compliance with multiple daily dosing, cost-effectiveness, and impact of the drug on psychological features of BN is necessary to assess the clinical utility of ondansetron for BN.

Finally, with BN, as is the case with many other psychiatric disorders, few controlled trials have studied long-term efficacy of pharmacotherapy. Where such attempts have been made, interpretation of results often has been clouded by significant dropout rates. In the largest trial, the 150 responders (≥50% decrease in weekly vomiting episodes) to an 8-week course of fluoxetine 60 mg/day were randomized to continued drug treatment or placebo for a 1-year follow-up period (Romano, Halmi, Sarkar, Koke, & Lee, 2002). Findings did include a lower rate of "relapse" for the fluoxetine group, but the authors noted a worsening on all measures of efficacy over time. Considering the vast majority of these patients still were binging and purging after the first 8 weeks, and therefore were in need not only of "maintenance" but also further treatment of symptoms, pharmacotherapy alone may not produce an adequate treatment for many patients.

Psychotherapy

Accumulated research (Hay, Bacaltchuk, & Stefano, 2006) suggests that the gold standard for psychotherapy is a structured and manual-based form of CBT specifically developed for BN (CBT-BN) by Fairburn and colleagues (Fairburn, Marcus, & Wilson, 1993). It is focused on symptoms, maladaptive cognitions, and the direct process of change rather than underlying psychological issues (Wonderlich, Mitchell, Swan-Kremier, Peterson, & Crow, 2002). Used in an outpatient setting with either individuals or groups of patients, CBT-BN was designed as a three-phase approach delivered in 15–20 sessions over 4–5 months. The first phase aims to educate about BN and encourage normalized eating patterns. The second phase focuses on identifying cognitive distortions and utilizing behavioral strategies to reduce tendency toward dietary restraint. The third phase emphasizes maintenance and relapse prevention.

More than 50 randomized, controlled trials have tested the psychotherapeutic treatment of BN with more than 20 of these on CBT (Hay et al., 2006). Studies conducted with CBT have shown a decrease in the frequency of binge eating and purging episodes averaging 60%–80%, with a cessation rate of 30%–50% (Fairburn, 2002). These outcome rates for CBT-BN are significantly higher than those seen in various comparison treatments (e.g., behavior therapy, nutritional counseling, focal psychotherapy, hypnobehavioral therapy, stress management training, psychodynamically oriented psychotherapy, supportive psychotherapy, and various forms of exposure with response prevention) or wait lists for treatment. In interpreting results of these studies, it should be considered that dropout rates were as high as 30% (Clausen, 2004), even though study patients likely had relatively higher levels of motivation and fewer psychiatric comorbidities than many BN patients who present for treatment in clinical practice (Becker, 2003).

Early behavior change has been shown to predict the best treatment outcome and maintenance at follow-up (Agras et al., 2000; Fairburn, 2006). Of important note is that even with full recovery from pathological eating behaviors, a substantial number of patients display residual features, including weight-related concerns, dysphoric affect, social discomfort, and personality traits indicative of perfectionism (Stein et al., 2002; Walsh et al., 2000).

For patients with poor initial response to CBT, IPT may be beneficial as a second-level treatment (Wilson, 1996). IPT also is a manual-based treatment involving 12–20 individual sessions over 3–5 months. IPT for EDs was devised based on compelling evidence that eating-disordered individuals typically have interpersonal factors contributing to the development and maintenance of their illness. Discussion of food and weight issues is minimized with the premise that improved interpersonal functioning will result in a reduction of ED symptomatology. The patient gains insight as the therapist consistently highlights the link between symptoms and interpersonal deficits, which may include role disputes, role transitions, and grief. Fairburn et al (1993) and Jacobs-Pilipski, Welch, and Wilfley (2002) compared CBT, IPT, and behavior therapy and found that while IPT appeared to have been less effective overall than CBT when patients were assessed at the end of the treatment period, those treated with IPT and CBT had similar results at long-term follow-up (mean of 5.8 years). Similarly, a second multicenter study found that CBT produced results more rapidly and showed greater efficacy at the end of the 20-week treatment while the effects of IPT were delayed until follow-up (Agras et al., 2000).

Developments in the area of CBT-based self-help and guided self-help (GSH) manuals for BN have suggested these programs may be effective alternatives for patients who otherwise do not have access to treatment (American Psychiatric Association, 2006). While relatively few patients make a full and lasting recovery from GSH alone, it is recommended as a possible first step (when CBT-BN is not feasible) in the management of patients with less severe BN (NICE, 2004). To date, most controlled studies of GSH have occurred at/or in conjunction with EDs treatment centers. For many patients with EDs, however, lack of access to specialty care remains a barrier to treatment, and attempts to broaden dissemination of effective therapies is an emerging area of research. As patients with BN often initially present to primary care providers, three recent randomized, controlled trials have examined whether GSH treatment may be delivered effectively by nonspecialists in primary care settings.

In 2003, a study in the United Kingdom comparing CBT-based GSH provided by general practitioners (GPs) with outpatient care received at ED specialty clinics concluded there was no significant difference in outcome between the two patient groups, and the findings supported the idea that BN can be treated in general practice (Durand & King, 2003). This trial has been criticized on the grounds that the specialty care was far below standard, since the mean number of sessions attended by patients during the 6-month trial was less than five, and therefore drawing conclusions would be difficult given this questionable comparison condition (Fairburn, 2006). Another point is of practical relevance. Following completion of the trial, only 11 of the 32 participating GPs said they would be willing to use the approach again, the main reported difficulty being lack of time—despite the fact that all but two of them were treating just one study patient. Given therapy for BN may last for months or more, the absolute number of patients who could receive treatment exclusively in a primary care setting appears quite limited.

The following year, Walsh and Fairburn reported very different results in a trial conducted in two primary care clinics in the northeastern United States (Walsh, Fairburn, Mickley, Sysko, & Parides, 2004). The comparison was among various treatment options that might be available in this setting (fluoxetine alone, placebo alone, GSH plus fluoxetine, and GSH plus placebo). Fluoxetine was superior to placebo, though rates of remission were low (consistent with results of prior medication trials), and the authors concluded that GSH provided no apparent benefit. Most striking was the fact that two thirds of the 91 patients did not complete the trial, compared with the 20%–35% dropout rate usually seen when BN patients receive GSH interventions at specialty clinics. Of note, providers received only very brief training prior to participation, physician follow-up included 15-minute medication appointments, and GSH occurred in 30-minute sessions with nursing staff—a model, the authors believed, that more closely resembled true field conditions in the typical busy primary care practice (Fairburn, 2006).

Most recently, in a trial with 109 patients, investigators in Australia compared GSH delivered by GPs with a waiting-list control group and reported very favorable results, stating they found decreases in binge/purge symptoms and overall remission rates of the treatment group comparable to those of standard CBT-BN delivered in specialty treatment settings. Perhaps the most important aspect of this study involved the nature of the providers and the extent of services delivered. The GPs were recruited by advertisement, and 13 of the 16 who agreed to participate "had a special interest in EDs in general practice." They received more extensive training than in either study mentioned earlier, apparently treated multiple patients over time, had access to at least occasional expert supervision, and saw the patients on a relatively frequent basis (Banasiak, Paxton, & Hay, 2005).

The aforementioned data appear to support two significant findings. First, where primary care physicians have the available time and interest to receive additional training in GSH techniques and closely follow individuals with BN, a subset of these patients might be manageable in primary care. And secondly, fluoxetine 60 mg/day appears to be a potential treatment option for BN patients seen in primary care, and while it rarely will produce remission, this may be a useful intervention for patients who are awaiting or unable to receive specialty care.

Another treatment modality to consider is therapy involving family members of the adult BN patient (Benninghoven, Schneider, Strack, Reich, & Cierpka, 2003). Despite the paucity of research in this area, it is recommended that family therapy be considered as an adjunct whenever feasible, especially for college-age or other patients still living with parents, older patients with ongoing conflicted interactions with parents, and married/partnered patients experiencing relationship difficulties (American Psychiatric Association, 2006). This may be particularly helpful for those from families that lack cohesion or have difficulty expressing emotion (Bailey, 1991). Clinicians also should be mindful of potential deleterious effects on children of patients with BN. Mothers with active EDs may be more prone to use food for nonnutritive purposes (e.g., as a rewarding stimulus) and to exhibit high levels of concern over their children's weight (Agras, Hammer, & McNicholas, 1999), increasing the risk of development of EDs in offspring.

Treatment Combining Psychotherapy and Medication

At least six controlled trials have assessed direct comparisons of outcome for patients treated with psychotherapy, pharmacotherapy, or a combination (American Psychiatric Association, 2006; Kaye, Strober, & Jimerson, 2004). In general, results showed a greater decrease in the frequency of binge/purge episodes with CBT than with antidepressant medication when each was utilized alone. With treatments used in combination, the results to date have been mixed but slightly favor the addition of medication to psychotherapy for many patients (Steinglass & Walsh, 2004). For example, one well-designed trial by Mitchell and Peterson (2005) found that adding an antidepressant to CBT conferred a modest advantage in symptom reduction (Wilson, Fairburn, Agras, Walsh, & Kraemer, 2002). The potential benefits of medication may be greatest for patients who fail to achieve an early reduction in binging and purging with evidenced-based psychotherapy such as CBT or IPT, or for those who appear to have a depressive syndrome independent of BN (Mitchell & Peterson, 2005; Walsh, 2002). Antidepressants also may be recommended when psychotherapy has been only partially successful. Interestingly, a recent meta-analysis reported that combining an antidepressant with psychotherapy significantly reduced the acceptability of psychological treatment, rendering antidepressants as relatively more acceptable to the patient (Bacaltchuk et al., 2000). The clinical relevance of this finding is uncertain, but it may indicate that a subset of BN patients prefer the perceived simplicity of taking medication to the more time- and effort-intensive nature of psychotherapy. Though more research is needed on combined treatment, there is a general consensus within the clinical community that an approach including both psycho-therapy and medication is worth considering for many patients (American Psychiatric Association, 2006).

Practical Issues—How to Understand and Deal with Bulimia Nervosa

While reviewing treatment options for BN is important, it is also relevant to provide some understanding of the unique symptoms of this disorder and frustrations patients, their fami-lies, and providers encounter when seeking and engaging in treatment.

Early in the course of illness, symptoms of BN may be highly reinforcing for the patient. Many have difficulties with communication and relationships, and binge eating can become a reliable source of comfort, providing a means of coping with dysphoric mood states and interpersonal stress (Becker, 2003; Wilson et al., 2002). But extreme fear of weight gain often drives compensatory purging and an existence dominated by relentless calorie counting and obsessive thoughts about food, weight, and shape. The endless binge/purge cycle fosters shame, secrecy and social isolation, and by the time a patient seeks treatment, the disorder may have taken over her life. Despite this frequently intense level of suffering, BN patients nearly always present with some degree of ambivalence for treatment (Guarda & Heinberg, 2004), an observation that is baffling to many providers. It is helpful to recognize that symptoms may serve as a coping mechanism, albeit a dysfunctional one, and are unlikely to abate without development of new skills and behaviors to take their place (Binford et al., 2005).

For BN patients who initially present to primary care providers, responding to their concerns with compassion and understanding is key to forging a therapeutic alliance. With those unwilling or unable to pursue a specialty treatment program, discussing the elements of healthy eating and exercise can be a place to start. For instance, eating in a healthy way includes all food groups and avoids extreme notions, such as attempting to remove all fat from the diet. Discussing exercise regimens in detail also is important, as some bulimic patients may "purge" with workouts lasting several hours in length. For patients prone to denial and resis-tance, it is helpful to avoid power struggles. This can be accomplished by asking the patient to identify her own goals and then giving suggestions about how they might be achieved.

An important consideration in treatment relates to bulimic patients' overwhelming fear of "fatness", which leads many to strive for an unnaturally low weight. Acceptance of a healthy body weight is crucial to recovery, because attempts to lose weight usually will trigger bulimic symptoms (Hsu, 2004). A classic pattern in BN involves restricting calories for long periods over the course of a day in an attempt to control or lose weight, followed by strong cravings to binge and subsequently purge, only to lead to further restricting. The link between physiological and emotional deprivation and binge eating has been well established (Hetherington, Altemus, Nelson, Bernat, & Gold, 1994), and explaining the factors leading to overwhelming urges to binge can reassure the patient of a rational basis for her symptoms (Hsu, 2004). Improvement of nutritional status impacts both physical and psychological well-being, so a return to eating meals and snacks spaced regularly throughout the day is a vital step in recovery (Wilson, Fairburn, & Agras, 1997). Referral to a registered dietitian who specializes in EDs can facilitate this process.

For patients ready to pursue more intensive treatment, referral to a qualified ED specialist can help with further assessment and determination of appropriate level of care. The National Eating Disorders Association (http://www.edap.org) is an excellent resource for information. In addition, http://www.edreferral.com is a Web site listing therapists and programs throughout the United States. Insured individuals can gather information about providers within their network.

Conclusions

In light of the fact that bulimia nervosa was defined as a diagnostic entity only a few decades ago, researchers and clinicians alike have made great strides in developing and implementing treatments helpful to many patients. Nonetheless, our current established treatments, both psychological and pharmacological, led to a remission rate of perhaps 50% at best over the long term, and a substantial number of patients remain chronically ill (Kaye & Walsh, 2002). To improve success rates with currently available evidenced-based psychotherapies, future studies should examine the reasons for substantial dropout rates from therapy, as well as conditions surrounding subsequent relapse, including impact of features of the disorder that may persist despite remission of binge/purge behaviors by end of treatment (Becker, 2003). Strategies for improving amount and quality of method-specific training received by treatment providers may be another factor important to effective delivery of CBT and IPT (Mussell et al., 2000). Additionally, efforts are under way to test enhancements of the CBT-BN curriculum itself, including greater emphasis on body image disturbances, low self-esteem, perfectionism, and interpersonal difficulties (Fairburn, 2006). The American Psychiatric Association has called for well-conducted studies of alternative or integrated psychotherapeutic treatment approaches for nonresponders, as well as more trials including the complex BN patients with comorbid psychiatric conditions often seen in clinical practice (American Psychiatric Association, 2006).

The number and size of pharmacotherapeutic trials for treatment of the disorder has slowed in recent years, which is unfortunate, as few notable developments in medication management have occurred in the decade since the FDA approved fluoxetine for use in adult patients with BN. As is the case with psychotherapy, there is some evidence that early response to medication predicts positive outcome (Walsh et al., 2006). Therefore, studies investigating antidepressant switching and augmentation strategies, which are nearly nonexistent for treatment of BN (Becker, 2003), are sorely needed. Exploration of medication classes other than antidepressants forms the core of more recent research efforts, but controlled trials have been small and relatively few. This in part may relate to the limited state of knowledge on physiological processes underlying binge/purge behavior. Elucidation of the biological aspects of EDs holds the promise of new drug targets, such as mechanisms of hunger, satiety, and taste perception (American Psychiatric Association, 2006).

Disclosure Statement

E.M. has no conflicts of interest to disclose.

M.E.T. has no conflicts of interest to disclose.

E.G.-S. has no conflicts of interest to disclose.

W.H.K. has received an investigator grant from AstraZeneca and serves as a consultant to Denver Eating Disorder Center.

References

Agras, W., Brandt, H., Bulik, C., Dolan-Sewell, R., Fairburn, C., Halmi, K., Wilfley, D. (2004). Report of the National Institutes of Health workshop on overcoming barriers to treatment research in anorexia nervosa. *International Journal of Eating Disorders, 35*(4), 509–521.

Agras, W. S., Crow, S. J., Halmi, K. A., Mitchell, J. E., Wilson, G. T., & Kraemer, H. C. (2000). Outcome predictors for the cognitive behavior treatment of bulimia nervosa: Data from a multisite study. *American Journal of Psychiatry, 157*(8), 1302–1308.

Agras, W. S., Hammer, L., & McNicholas, F. (1999). A prospective study of the influences of eating-disordered mothers on their children. *International Journal of Eating Disorders, 25*, 253–262.

Agras, W. S., Walsh, B. T., Fairburn, C. G., Wilson, G. T., & Kraemer, H. C. (2000). A multicenter comparison of cognitive-behavioral therapy and interpersonal psychotherapy for bulimia nervosa. *Archives of General Psychiatry, 57*(5), 459–466.

American Psychiatric Association. (1994). *Diagnostic and statistical manual of mental disorders* (4th ed.). Washington, DC: Author.

American Psychiatric Association. (2000). *Diagnostic and statistical manual of mental disorders* (4th ed., Text rev.). Washington, DC: Author.

American Psychiatric Association. (2006). *Practice guideline for the treatment of patients with eating disorders* (3rd ed.). Washington, DC: Author.

American Psychiatric Association Workgroup on Eating Disorders. (2006). Practice guideline for the treatment of patients with eating disorders, 3rd edition. *American Journal of Psychiatry, 163*, 1–54.

Anderluh, M. B., Tchanturia, K., Rabe-Hesketh, S., & Treasure, J. (2003). Childhood obsessive-compulsive personality traits in adult women with eating disorders: Defining a broader eating disorder phenotype. *American Journal of Psychiatry, 160*(2), 242–247.

Appolinario, J., & McElroy, S. L. (2004). Pharmacological approaches in the treatment of binge eating disorder. *Current Drug Targets, 5*(3), 301–307.

Attia, E., Haiman, C., Walsh, B. T., & Flater, S. R. (1998). Does fluoxetine augment the inpatient treatment of anorexia nervosa? *American Journal of Psychiatry, 155*(4), 548–551.

Attia, E., Wolk, S., Cooper, T., Glasofer, D., & Walsh, B. (2005). Plasma tryptophan during weight restoration in patients with anorexia nervosa. *Biological Psychiatry, 57*, 674–678.

Bacaltchuk, J., Trefiglio, R. P., Oliveira, I. R., Hay, P., Lima, M. S., & Mari, J. J. (2000). Combination of antidepressants and psychological treatments for bulimia nervosa: A systematic review. *Acta Psychiatrica Scandinavica, 101*(4), 256–264.

Bailer, U. F., Frank, G., Henry, S., Price, J., Meltzer, C. C., Becker, C., Kaye, W. H. (2007). Serotonin transporter binding after recovery from eating disorders. *Psychopharmacology, 195*(3), 315–324.

Bailey, C. (1991). Family structure and eating disorders: The family environment scale and bulimic-like symptoms. *Youth and Society, 23*(2), 251–272.

Ball, J., & Mitchell, P. (2004). A randomized controlled study of cognitive behavior therapy and behavioral family therapy for anorexia nervosa patients. *Eating Disorders, 12*, 303–314.

Banasiak, S., Paxton, S., & Hay, P. (2005). Guided self-help for bulimia nervosa in primary care: A randomized controlled trial. *Psychological Medicine, 35*, 1–12.

Barbarich, N., McConaha, C., Gaskill, J., LaVia, M., Frank, G. K., Brooks, S., Kaye, W. H. (2004). An open trial of olanzapine in anorexia nervosa. *Journal of Clinical Psychiatry, 65*, 1480–1482.

Becker, A. (2003). Outpatient management of eating disorders in adults. *Current Womens Health Report, 3*(3), 221–229.

Benninghoven, D., Schneider, H., Strack, M., Reich, G., & Cierpka, A. (2003). Family representations in relationship episodes of patients with a diagnosis of bulimia nervosa. *Psychology and Psychotherapy, 76*, 323–336.

Berrettini, W. (2000). Genetics of psychiatric disease. *Annual Review of Medicine, 51*, 465–479.

Binford, R. B., Mussell, M. P., Crosby, R. D., Peterson, C. B., Crow, S. J., & Mitchell, J. E. (2005). Coping strategies in bulimia nervosa treatment: impact on outcome in group cognitive-behavioral therapy. *Journal of Consulting and Clinical Psychology, 73*(6), 1089–1096.

Bissada, H., Tasca, G., Barber, A., & Bradwejn, J. (2008). Olanzapine in the treatment of low body weight and obsessive thinking in women with anorexia nervosa: A randomized, double-blind, placebo-controlled trial. *American Journal of Psychology, 165*(10), 1281–1288.

Blundell, J. E. (1984). Serotonin and appetite. *Neuropharmacology, 23*(12B), 1537–1551.

Boachie, A., Goldfield, G., & Spettigue, W. (2003). Olanzapine use as an adjunctive treatment for hospitalized children with anorexia nervosa: Case reports. *International Journal of Eating Disorders, 33*, 98–103.

Bosanac, P., Burrows, G., & Norman, T. (2003). Olanzapine in anorexia nervosa. *Australian and New Zealand Journal of Medicine, 37*(4), 494.

Bosanac, P., Kurlender, S., Norman, T., Hallasm, K., Wesnes, K., Manktelow, T., & Burrows, G. (2007). An open-label study of quetiapine in anorexia nervosa. *Human Psychopharmacology, 22*, 223–230.

Boyar, R. K., J, Finkelstein, J., Kapen, S., Weiner, H., Weitzman, E., & Hellman, L. (1974). Anorexia nervosa. Immaturity of the 24-hour luteinizing hormone secretory pattern. *New England Journal of Medicine, 291*(17), 861–865.

Brambilla, F., Garcia, C. F., S, Daga, G. F., A, Santonastaso, P., Ramaciotti, C., Bondi, E., Monteleone, P. (2007). Olanzapine therapy in anorexia nervosa: Psychobiological effects. *International Clinical Psychopharmacology, 22*, 197–204.

Bulik, C., Bacanu, S., Klump, K., Fichter, M., Halmi, K., Keel, P., Devlin, B. (2005). Selection of eating-disorder phenotypes for linkage analysis. *American Journal of Medical Genetics B, Neuropsychiatric Genetics, 139*(1), 81–87.

Bulik, C., Berkman, N., Brownley, K., Sedway, J., & Lohr, K. (2007). Anorexia nervosa treatment: A systematic review of randomized controlled trials. *International Journal of Eating Disorders, 40*, 310–320.

Bulik, C., Sullivan, P. F., Tozzi, F., Furberg, H., Lichtenstein, P., & Pedersen, N. L. (2006). Prevalence, heritability and prospective risk factors for anorexia nervosa. *Archives of General Psychiatry, 63*(3), 305–312.

Casper, R. C. (1990). Personality features of women with good outcome from restricting anorexia nervosa. *Psychosomatic Medicine, 52*(2), 156–170.

Cassin, S., & von Ranson, K. (2005). Personality and eating disorders: A decade in review. *Clinical Psychology Review, 25*(7), 895–916.

Clausen, L. (2004). Review of studies evaluating psychotherapy in bulimia nervosa: The influence of research methods. *Scandinavian Journal of Psychology, 45*(3), 247–252.

Cloninger, C. R. (1987). A systematic method for clinical description and classification of personality variants. A proposal. *Archives of General Psychiatry, 44*(6), 573–588.

Dare, C., Eisler, I., Russell, G., Treasure, J., & Dodge, L. (2001). Psychological therapies for adults with anorexia nervosa. Randomised controlled trial of out-patient treatments. *British Journal of Psychiatry, 178*, 216–221.

Davies, H., & Tchanturia, K. (2005). Cognitive remediation therapy as an intervention for acute anorexia nervosa: A case report. *European Eating Disorders Review, 13*, 311–316.

Dennis, K., Le Grange, D., & Bremer, J. (2006). Olanzapine use in adolescent anorexia nervosa. *Eating and Weight Disorders, 11*, e53–e56.

Durand, M. A., & King, M. (2003). Specialist treatment versus self-help for bulimia nervosa: A randomized controlled trial in general practice. *British Journal of General Practice, 53*(490), 371–377.

Duvvuri, V., & Kaye, W. (2009). Anorexia nervosa. *Focus, 7*(4), 455–462.

Eisler, I., & Dare, C. (2000). Family therapy for adolescent anorexia nervosa: The results of a controlled comparison of two family interventions. *Journal of Child Psychology and Psychiatry, 41*(6), 727–736.

Eisler, I., Dare, C., Russell, G. F., Szmukler, G., Le Grange, D., & Dodge, E. (1997). Family and individual therapy in anorexia nervosa. A 5-year follow-up. *Archives of General Psychiatry, 54*, 1025–1030.

Eisler, I., Simic, M., Russell, G., & Dare, C. (2007). A randomised controlled treatment trial of two forms of family therapy in adolescent anorexia nervosa: A five year follow-up. *Journal of Child Psychology and Psychiatry, 48*(6), 552–560.

Ellison, A. R., & Fong, J. (1998). Neuroimaging in eating disorders. In H. W. Hoek, J. L. Treasure, & M. A. Katzman (Eds.), *Neurobiology in the treatment of eating disorders* (pp. 255–269). Chichester, England: Wiley.

Ercan, E., Copkunol, H., Cykoethlu, S., & Varan, A. (2003). Olanzapine treatment of an adolescent girl with anorexia nervosa. *Human Psychopharmacology*, 18(5), 401–403.

Erzegovesi, S., Riboldi, C., & DiBella, D. (2004). Bulimia nervosa, 5-HTTLPR polymorphism and treatment response to four SSRIs: A single-blind study. *Journal of Clinical Psychopharmacology*, 24(6), 680–682.

Fairburn, C. G. (2002). Cognitive-behavioral therapy for bulimia nervosa. In C. G. Fairburn & K. D. Brownell (Eds.), *Eating disorders and obesity: A comprehensive handbook* (2nd ed., pp. 302–307). New York: The Guilford Press.

Fairburn, C. G. (2006). Treatment of bulimia nervosa. In S. Wonderlich, J. Mitchell, M. de Zwaan, & H. Steiger (Eds.), *Annual review of eating disorders, part 2* (pp. 145–156). Oxford, England: Radcliffe.

Fairburn, C. G., Cooper, J. R., Doll, H. A., & Welch, S. L. (1999). Risk factors for anorexia nervosa: Three integrated case-control comparisons. *Archives of General Psychiatry*, 56(5), 468–476.

Fairburn, C. G., Marcus, M. D., & Wilson, G. T. (1993). Cognitive-behavioral therapy for binge eating and bulimia nervosa: A comprehensive treatment manual. In C. G. Fairburn & G. T. Wilson (Eds.), *Binge eating: Nature, assessment, and treatment* (pp. 361–404). New York: The Guilford Press.

Faris, P. L., Kim, S. W., Meller, W. H., Goodale, R. L., Oakman, S. A., Hofbauer, R. D., Hartman, B. K. (2000). Effect of decreasing afferent vagal activity with ondansetron on symptoms of bulimia nervosa: A randomised, double-blind trial. *Lancet*, 355(9206), 792–797.

Ferguson, C. P., La Via, M. C., Crossan, P. J., & Kaye, W. H. (1999). Are serotonin selective reuptake inhibitors effective in underweight anorexia nervosa? *International Journal of Eating Disorders*, 25(1), 11–17.

Fichter, M. M., Kruger, R., Rief, W., Holland, R., & Dohne, J. (1996). Fluvoxamine in prevention of relapse in bulimia nervosa: Effects on eating-specific psychopathology. *Journal of Clinical Psychopharmacology*, 16(1), 9–18.

First, M., Spitzer, R., Gibbon, M., & Williams, J. (2002). Structured clinical interview for DSM-IV-TR axis I disorders, research version, patient edition (SCID-I/P). New York: Biometrics Research.

Fisman, S., Steele, M., Short, J., Byrne, T., Short, J., & Lavalle, C. (1996). Case study: Anorexia nervosa and autistic disorder in an adolescent girl. *Journal of the Academy of Child and Adolescent Psychiatry*, 35, 937–940.

Fluoxetine Bulimia Nervosa Collaborative Study Group. (1992). Fluoxetine in the treatment of bulimia nervosa. A multicenter, placebo-controlled, double-blind trial. *Archives of General Psychiatry*, 49(2), 139–147.

Garner, D. M., Garfinkel, P. E., & O'Shaughnessy, M. (1985). The validity of the distinction between bulimia with and without anorexia nervosa. *American Journal of Psychiatry*, 142(5), 581–587.

Geist, R., Heinmaa, M., Stephens, D., Davis, R., & Katzman, D. K. (2000). Comparison of family therapy and family group psychoeducation in adolescents with anorexia nervosa. *Canadian Journal of Psychiatry*, 45, 173–178.

Godart, N., Perdereau, F., Rein, Z., Berthoz, S., Wallier, J., Jeammet, P., & Flament, M. (2007). Comorbidity studies of eating disorders and mood disorders. Critical review of the literature. *Journal of Affective Disorders*, 97(1–3), 37–49.

Goldstein, D. J., Wilson, M. G., Ascroft, R. C., & al-Banna, M. (1999). Effectiveness of fluoxetine therapy in bulimia nervosa regardless of comorbid depression. *International Journal of Eating Disorders*, 25(1), 19–27.

Goldstein, D. J., Wilson, M. G., Thompson, V. L., Potvin, J. H., & Rampey, A. H., Jr. (1995). Long-term fluoxetine treatment of bulimia nervosa. Fluoxetine Bulimia Nervosa Research Group. *British Journal of Psychiatry*, 166(5), 660–666.

Gowers, S., Clark, A., Roberts, C., Griffiths, A., Edwards, V., Bryan, C., Barrett, B. (2007). Clinical effectiveness of treatments for anorexia nervosa in adolescents. *British Journal of Psychiatry*, 191, 427–435.

Gowers, S., Norton, K., Halek, C., & Crisp, A. H. (1994). Outcome of outpatient psychotherapy in a random allocation treatment study of anorexia nervosa. *International Journal of Eating Disorders*, 15, 165–177.

Guarda, A. (2008). Treatment of anorexia nervosa: Insights and obstacles. *Physiology and Behavior*, 94(1), 113–120.

Guarda, A. S., & Heinberg, L. J. (2004). Inpatient and partial hospital approaches to the treatment of eating disorders. In J. K. Thompson (Ed.), *Handbook of eating disorders and obesity* (pp. 297–320). Hoboken, NJ: Wiley.

Haber, S. N., Kim, K., Mailly, P., & Calzavara, R. (2006). Reward-related cortical inputs define a large striatal region in primates that interface with associative cortical connections, providing a substrate for incentive-based learning. *Journal of Neuroscience*, 26(32), 8368–8376.

Halford, J., Cooper, G., & Dovey, T. (2004). The pharmacology of human appetite expression. *Current Drug Targets*, 5, 221–240.

Halmi, K. A., & Falk, J. R. (1982). Anorexia nervosa. A study of outcome discriminators in exclusive dieters and bulimics. *Journal of the American Academy of Child Psychiatry*, 21(4), 369–375.

Halmi, K., Agras, W. S., Crow, S., Mitchell, J., Wilson, G., Bryson, S., & Kraemer, H. C. (2005). Predictors of treatment acceptance and completion in anorexia nervosa. *Archives of General Psychiatry*, 62, 776–781.

Hansen, L. (1999). Olanzapine in the treatment of anorexia nervosa. *British Journal of Psychiatry, 175,* 592.

Hay, P., Bacaltchuk, J., & Stefano, S. (2004). Psychotherapy for bulimia nervosa and binging. *The Cochrane Database of Systematic Reviews, 3* CD000562.

Hedges, D., Reimherr, F., & Hoopes, S. (2003). Treatment of bulimia nervosa with topiramate in a randomized, double-blinded, placebo-controlled trial, part 2: Improvement in psychiatric measures. *Journal of Clinical Psychiatry, 64*(12), 1449–1454.

Herzog, D. B., & Copeland, P. M. (1985). Eating disorders. *New England Journal of Medicine, 313*(5), 295–303.

Herzog, D. B., Keller, M. B., Lavori, P. W., Kenny, G. M., & Sacks, N. R. (1992). The prevalence of personality disorders in 210 women with eating disorders. *Journal of Clinical Psychiatry, 53*(5), 147–152.

Hetherington, M. M., Altemus, M., Nelson, M. L., Bernat, A. S., & Gold, P. W. (1994). Eating behavior in bulimia nervosa: Multiple meal analysis. *American Journal of Clinical Nutrition, 60,* 864–873.

Higley, J. D., & Linnoila, M. (1997). Low central nervous system serotonergic activity is traitlike and correlates with impulsive behavior. A nonhuman primate model investigating genetic and environmental influences on neurotransmission. *Annals of the New York Academy of Science, 836,* 39–56.

Hoek, H. W., Bartelds, A. I., Bosveld, J. J., van der Graaf, Y., Limpens, V. E., Maiwald, M., & Spaaij, C. J. (1995). Impact of urbanization on detection rates of eating disorders. *American Journal of Psychiatry, 152*(9), 1272–1278.

Hoopes, S., Reimherr, F., & Hedges, D. (2003). Treatment of bulimia nervosa with topiramate in a randomized, double-blind placebo-controlled trial, part 1: Improvement in binge and purge measures. *Journal of Clinical Psychiatry, 64*(11), 1335–1341.

Horne, R. L., Ferguson, J. M., Pope, H. G., Jr., Hudson, J. I., Lineberry, C. G., Ascher, J., & Cato, A. (1988). Treatment of bulimia with bupropion: A multicenter controlled trial. *Journal of Clinical Psychiatry, 49*(7), 262–266.

Hsu, L. K. (2004). Eating disorders: Practical interventions. *Journal of the American Medical Womens Association, 59*(2), 113–124.

Hudson, J., Hiripi, E., Pope, H., & Kessler, R. (2007). The prevalence and correlates of eating disorders in the National Comorbidity Survey Replication. *Biological Psychiatry, 61,* 348–358.

Jacobs-Pilipski, M. J., Welch, R. R., & Wilfley, D. E. (2002). Interpersonal psychotherapy for anorexia nervosa, bulimia nervosa, and binge eating disorder. In T. Brewerton (Ed.), *Clinical handbook of eating disorders: An integrated approach* (pp. 449–471). New York: Marcell Dekker.

Jensen, V. S., & Mejlhede, A. (2000). Anorexia nervosa: Treatment with olanzapine. *British Journal of Psychiatry, 177,* 87.

Jimerson, D., & Wolfe, B. (2006). Psychobiology of eating disorders. In S. Wonderlich, J. E. Mitchell, M. de Zwaan, & H. Steiger (Eds.), *Annual review of eating disorders: Part 2* (pp. 1–15). Oxford, England: Radcliffe.

Jimerson, D. C., Wolfe, B. E., Brotman, A. W., & Metzger, E. D. (1996). Medications in the treatment of eating disorders. *Psychiatric Clinics of North America, 19*(4), 739–754.

Kaye, W., Bulik, C., Thornton, L., Barbarich, N., Masters, K., Fichter, M., Berrettini, W. H. (2004). Comorbidity of anxiety disorders with anorexia and bulimia nervosa. *American Journal of Psychiatry, 161,* 2215–2221.

Kaye, W., Fudge, J., & Paulus, M. (2009). New insight into symptoms and neurocircuit function of anorexia nervosa. *Nature Reviews Neuroscience, 10*(8), 573–584.

Kaye, W., Gwirtsman, H., Obarzanek, E., & George, D. (1988). Relative importance of calorie intake needed to gain weight and level of physical activity in anorexia nervosa. *American Journal of Clinical Nutrition, 47,* 989–994.

Kaye, W., Kaplan, A., & Zucker, M. (1996). Treating eating-disorder patients in a managed care environment. Contemporary American issues and a Canadian response. *Psychiatric Clinics of North America, 19*(4), 793–810.

Kaye, W. H., Nagata, T., Weltzin, T. E., Hsu, L. K., Sokol, M. S., McConaha, C., Deep, D. (2001). Double-blind placebo-controlled administration of fluoxetine in restricting- and restricting-purging-type anorexia nervosa. *Biological Psychiatry, 49*(7), 644–652.

Kaye, W., Strober, M., & Jimerson, D. (2004). The neurobiology of eating disorders. In D. S. Charney & E. J. Nestler (Eds.), *The neurobiology of mental illness* (pp. 1112–1128). New York: Oxford University Press.

Kaye, W., Strober, M., & Jimerson, D. (2008). The neurobiology of eating disorders. In D. Charney & E. Nestler (Eds.), *The neurobiology of mental illness* (3rd ed.). New York: Oxford University Press.

Kaye, W., Wagner, A., Frank, G., & UF, B. (2006). Review of brain imaging in anorexia and bulimia nervosa. In J. Mitchell, S. Wonderlich, H. Steiger, & M. deZwaan (Eds.), *Annual review of eating disorders, Part 2* (pp. 113–130). Abingdon, England: Radcliffe.

Kaye, W. H., & Walsh, B. T. (2002). Psychopharmacology of eating disorders. In K. Davis, D. Charney, J. Coyle, & C. Nemeroff (Eds.), *Neuropsychopharmacology. The fifth generation of progress* (pp. 1675–1683). Philadelphia, PA: Lippincott Williams & Wilkins.

Keel, P. K., Mitchell, J. E., Miller, K. B., Davis, T. L., & Crow, S. J. (1999). Long-term outcome of bulimia nervosa. *Archives of General Psychiatry, 56*(1), 63–69.

Kendler, K. S., MacLean, C., Neale, M., Kessler, R., Heath, A., & Eaves, L. (1991). The genetic epidemiology of bulimia nervosa. *American Journal of Psychiatry, 148*(12), 1627–1637.

Klein, D., & Walsh, B. (2003). Eating disorders. *International Review of Psychiatry, 15*, 205–216.

Klump, K. L., McGue, M., & Iacono, W. G. (2000). Age differences in genetic and environmental influences on eating attitudes and behaviors in preadolescent and adolescent female twins. *Journal of Abnormal Psychology, 109*(2), 239–251.

La Via, M. C., Gray, N., & Kaye, W. H. (2000). Case reports of olanzapine treatment of anorexia nervosa. *International Journal of Eating Disorders, 27*(3), 363–366.

Leibowitz, S. F., & Shor-Posner, G. (1986). Brain serotonin and eating behavior. *Appetite, 7*(Suppl), 1–14.

Lilenfeld, L. R., Kaye, W. H., Greeno, C. G., Merikangas, K. R., Plotnicov, K., Pollice, C., Nagy, L. (1998). A controlled family study of anorexia nervosa and bulimia nervosa: Psychiatric disorders in first-degree relatives and effects of proband comorbidity. *Archives of General Psychiatry, 55*(7), 603–610.

Lilenfeld, L., Wonderlich, S., Riso, L. P., Crosby, R., & Mitchell, J. (2006). Eating disorders and personality: A methodological and empirical review. *Clinical Psychology Review, 26*(3), 299–320.

Linehan, M., Dimeff, L., Reynolds, S., Comtois, K., Welch, S., Heagerty, P., & Kivlahan, D. (2002). Dialectical behavior therapy versus comprehensive validation therapy plus 12-step for the treatment of opioid dependent women meeting criteria for borderline personality disorder. *Drug and Alcohol Dependency, 67*(1), 13–26.

Lock, J., Agras, W., Bryson, S., & Kraemer, H. (2005). A comparison of short- and long-term family therapy for adolescent anorexia nervosa. *Journal of the Academy of Child and Adolescent Psychiatry, 44*(7), 632–639.

Lock, J., Couturier, J., & Agras, W. (2008). Costs of remission and recovery using family therapy for adolescent anorexia nervosa: A descriptive report. *Eating Disorders, 16*(4), 322–330.

Lucki, I. (1998). The spectrum of behaviors influenced by serotonin. *Biological Psychiatry, 44*(3), 151–162.

Malina, A., Gaskill, J., McConaha, C., Frank, G. K., LaVia, M., Scholar, L., & Kaye, W. H. (2003). Olanzapine treatment of anorexia nervosa: A restrospective study. *International Journal of Eating Disorders, 33*(2), 234–237.

Mann, J. J. (1999). Role of the serotonergic system in the pathogenesis of major depression and suicidal behavior. *Neuropsychopharmacology, 21*(2 Suppl), 99S–105S.

McIntosh, V., Jordan, J., Carter, F., Luty, S., McKenzie, J., Bulik, C., Joyce, P. (2005). Three psychotherapies for anorexia nervosa: A randomized control trial. *American Journal of Psychiatry, 162*, 741–747.

McIntosh, V., Jordan, J., Luty, S., Carter, F., McKenzie, J., & Bulik, C. J., PR. (2006). Specialist supportive clinical management for anorexia nervosa. *International Journal of Eating Disorders, 39*(8), 625–632.

McKenzie, J. M., & Joyce, P. R. (1992). Hospitalization for anorexia nervosa. *International Journal of Eating Disorders, 11*(3), 235–241.

Mehler, C., Wewetzer, C., Schulze, U., Warnke, A., Theisen, F., & Dittmann, R. W. (2001). Olanzapine in children and adolescents with chronic anorexia nervosa. A study of five cases. *European Child and Adolescent Psychiatry, 10*(2), 151–157.

Mehler-Wex, C., Romanos, M., Kirchheiner, J., & Schulze, U. (2008). Atypical antipsychotics in severe anorexia nervosa in children and adolescents-review and case reports. *European Eating Disorder Review, 16*, 100–108.

Milano, W., Petrella, C., Sabatino, C., & Capasso, A. (2004). Treatment of bulimia nervosa with sertraline: A randomized controlled trial. *Advances in Therapy, 21*(4), 232–237.

Milano, W., Siano, C., Petrella, C., & Capasso, A. (2005). Treatment of bulimia nervosa with fluvoxamine: A randomized controlled trial. *Advances in Therapy, 22*(3), 278–283.

Mitchell, J. E., & Peterson, C. B. (2005). Treatment planning. In J. Mitchell & C. Peterson (Eds.), *Assessment of eating disorders* (pp. 221–233). New York: The Guilford Press.

Mondraty, N., Birmingham, C., Touyz, S. W., Sundakov, V., Chapman, L., & Beaumont, P. (2005). Randomized controlled trial of olanzapine in the treatment of cognitions in anorexia nervosa. *Australasian Psychiatry, 13*, 72–75.

Mussell, M., Crosby, R., Crow, S., Knopke, A., Peterson, C., Wonderlich, S., & Mitchell, J. (2000). Utilization of empirically supported psychotherapy treatments for individuals with eating disorders: A survey of psychologists. *International Journal of Eating Disorders, 27*, 230–237.

Nakash-Eisikovits, O., Dierberger, A., & Westen, D. (2002). A multidimensional meta-analysis of pharmacotherapy for bulimia nervosa: Summarizing the range of outcome in controlled clinical trials. *Harvard Review of Psychiatry, 10*(4), 193–211.

Newman-Toker, J. (2000). Risperidone in anorexia nervosa. *Journal of the American Academy of Child and Adolescent Psychiatry, 39*(8), 941–942.

NICE. (2004). *Core interventions in the treatment and management of anorexia nervosa, bulimia nervosa and related eating disorders.* (Clinical Guideline 9). London: National Collaborating Centre for Medical Health.

Nickel, C., Tritt, K., Muehlbacher, M., Pedrosa, G., Mitterlehner, F., Kaplan, P., Nickel, M. (2005). Topiramate treatment in bulimia nervosa patients: A randomized, double-blind placebo-controlled trial. *International Journal of Eating Disorders, 38*(4), 295–300.

Palmer, R., Birchall, H., Damani, S., Gatward, N., McGrain, L., & Parker, L. (2003). A dialectical behavior therapy program for people with an eating disorder and borderline personality disorder-description and outcome. *International Journal of Eating Disorders, 33*(3), 281–286.

Phillips, M., Drevets, W. R., SL, & Lane, R. (2003). Neurobiology of emotion perception I: The neural basis of normal emotion perception *Biological Psychiatry, 54*(5), 504–514.

Pike, K., Walsh, B., Vitousek, K., Wilson, G., & Bauer, J. (2003). Cognitive behavior therapy in the posthospitalization treatment of anorexia nervosa. *American Journal of Psychiatry, 160*(11), 2046–2049.

Pollice, C., Kaye, W. H., Greeno, C. G., & Weltzin, T. E. (1997). Relationship of depression, anxiety, and obsessionality to state of illness in anorexia nervosa. *International Journal of Eating Disorders, 21*(4), 367–376.

Powers, P., Bannon, Y., Eubanks, R., & McCormick, T. (2007). Quetiapine in anorexia nervosa patients: An open label outpatient pilot study. *International Journal of Eating Disorders, 40*, 21–26.

Powers, P. S., Santana, C. A., & Bannon, Y. S. (2002). Olanzapine in the treatment of anorexia nervosa: An open label trial. *International Journal of Eating Disorders, 32*, 146–154.

Robin, A. L., Siegel, P. T., Moye, A. W., Gilroy, M., Dennis, A., & Sikand, A. (1999). A controlled comparison of family versus individual therapy for adolescents with anorexia nervosa. *Journal of the American Academy of Child and Adolescent Psychiatry, 38*(12), 1482–1489.

Romano, S. J., Halmi, K. A., Sarkar, N. P., Koke, S. C., & Lee, J. S. (2002). A placebo-controlled study of fluoxetine in continued treatment of bulimia nervosa after successful acute fluoxetine treatment. *American Journal of Psychiatry, 159*, 96–102.

Russell, G. F., Szmukler, G. I., Dare, C., & Eisler, I. (1987). An evaluation of family therapy in anorexia nervosa and bulimia nervosa. *Archives of General Psychiatry, 44*(12), 1047–1056.

Rutherford, J., McGuffin, P., Katz, R. J., & Murray, R. M. (1993). Genetic influences on eating attitudes in a normal female twin population. *Psychological Medicine, 23*(2), 425–436.

Schmidt, U., Cooper, P., & Essers, H. (2004). Fluvoxamine and graded psychotherapy in the treatment of bulimia nervosa: A randomized, double-blind, placebo-controlled multicenter study of short-term and long-term pharmacotherapy combined with a stepped care approach to psychotherapy. *Journal of Clinical Psychopharmacology, 24*(5), 549–552.

Schweiger, U., & Fichter, M. (1997). Eating disorders: Clinical presentation, classification and etiologic models. In D. C. Jimerson & W. H. Kaye (Eds.), *Balliere's clinical psychiatry* (pp. 199–216). London: Balliere's Tindall.

Sepulveda, A., Macdonald, P., & Treasure, J. (2008). Feasibility and acceptability of DVD and telephone coaching-based skills training for carers of people with an eating disorder. *International Journal of Eating Disorders, 41*(4), 318–325.

Soubrie, P. (1986). Reconciling the role of central serotonin neurons in human and animal behavior. *Behavioral and Brain Science, 9*, 319–335.

Srinivasagam, N. M., Kaye, W. H., Plotnicov, K. H., Greeno, C., Weltzin, T. E., & Rao, R. (1995). Persistent perfectionism, symmetry, and exactness after long-term recovery from anorexia nervosa. *American Journal of Psychiatry, 152*(11), 1630–1634.

Stein, D., Kaye, W., Matsunaga, H., Orbach, I., Har-Even, D., Frank, G., Rao, R. (2002). Eating related concerns, moods, and personality traits in recovered bulimia nervosa patients: A replication study. *International Journal of Eating Disorders, 32*(2), 225–229.

Steinglass, J. E., & Walsh, T. (2004). Psychopharmacology of anorexia nervosa, bulimia nervosa, and binge eating disorder. In T. D. Brewerton (Ed.), *Clinical handbook of eating disorders: An integrated approach* (pp. 489–508). New York: Marcel Dekker.

Steinhausen, H. C. (2002). The outcome of anorexia nervosa in the 20th century. *American Journal of Psychiatry, 159*(8), 1284–1293.

Stice, E. (2002). Risk and maintenance factors for eating pathology: A meta-analytic review. *Pychopharmacology Bulletin, 128*, 825–848.

Strober, M. (1980). Personality and symptomatological features in young, nonchronic anorexia nervosa patients. *Journal of Psychosomatic Research, 24*(6), 353–359.

Strober, M. (1995). Family-genetic perspectives on anorexia nervosa and bulimia nervosa. In K. Brownell & C. Fairburn (Eds.), *Eating disorders and obesity-A comprehensive handbook* (pp. 212–218). New York: The Guilford Press.

Strober, M., Freeman, R., & Morrell, W. (1997). The long-term course of severe anorexia nervosa in adolescents: Survival analysis of recovery, relapse, and outcome predictors over 10– 15 years in a prospective study. *International Journal of Eating Disorders, 22*(4), 339–360.

Strober, M., Freeman, R., DeAntonio, M., Lampert, C., & Diamond, J. (1997). Does adjunctive fluoxetine influence the post-hospital course of restrictor-type anorexia nervosa? A 24-month prospective, longitudinal followup and comparison with historical controls. *Psychopharmacology Bulletin, 33*(3), 425–431.

Strober, M., Freeman, R., Lampert, C., Diamond, J., & Kaye, W. (2000). Controlled family study of anorexia nervosa and bulimia nervosa: Evidence of shared liability and transmission of partial syndromes. *American Journal of Psychiatry, 157*(3), 393–401.

Strober, M., Pataki, C., Freeman, R., & DeAntonio, M. (1999). No effect of adjunctive fluoxetine on eating behavior or weight phobia during the inpatient treatment of anorexia nervosa: An historical case- control study. *Journal of Child and Adolescent Psychopharmacology, 9*(3), 195–201.

Strober, M., Salkin, B., Burroughs, J., & Morrell, W. (1982). Validity of the bulimia-restricter distinction in anorexia nervosa. Parental personality characteristics and family psychiatric morbidity. *Journal of Nervous and Mental Disease, 170*(6), 345–351.

Sullivan, P. F. (1995). Mortality in anorexia nervosa. *American Journal of Psychiatry, 152*(7), 1073–1074.

Tchanturia, K., & Davies, H. C., I. (2007). Cognitive remediation therapy for patients with anorexia nervosa: Preliminary findings. *Annals of General Psypchiatry, 6*, 14.

Treasure, J., & Campbell, I. (1994). The case for biology in the aetiology of anorexia nervosa. *Psychological Medicine, 24*(1), 3–8.

Treasure, J., Tchanturia, K., & Schmidt, U. (2005). Developing a model of the treatment of eating disorder: Using neuroscience research to examine the how rather than the what of change. *Counseling and Psychotherapy Research, 5*(3), 1–12.

Vandereycken, W. (1984). Neuroleptics in the short-term treatment of anorexia nervosa. A double- blind placebo-controlled study with sulpiride. *British Journal of Psychiatry, 144*, 288–292.

Vandereycken, W., & Pierloot, R. (1982). Pimozide combined with behavior therapy in the short-term treatment of anorexia nervosa. A double-blind placebo-controlled cross-over study. *Acta Psychiatrica Scandinavica, 66*(6), 445–450.

Vitousek, K., & Manke, F. (1994). Personality variables and disorders in anorexia nervosa and bulimia nervosa. *Journal of Abnormal Psychology, 103*(1), 137–147.

Vitousek, K., Watson, S., & Wilson, G. (1998). Enhancing motivation for change in treatment-resistant eating disorders. *Clinical Psychology Review, 18*(4), 391–420.

Wade, T., Martin, N. G., & Tiggemann, M. (1998). Genetic and environmental risk factors for the weight and shape concerns characteristic of bulimia nervosa. *Psychological Medicine, 28*(4), 761–771.

Wagner, A., Aizenstein, H., Frank, G. K., Figurski, J., May, J. C., Putnam, K., Kaye, W. H. (2008). Altered insula response to a taste stimulus in individuals recovered from restricting-type anorexia nervosa. *Neuropsychopharmacology, 33*(3), 513–523.

Wagner, A., Barbarich, N., Frank, G., Bailer, U., Weissfeld, L., Henry, S., Wonderlich, S. (2006). Personality traits after recovery from eating disorders: Do subtypes differ? *International Journal of Eating Disorders, 39*(4), 276–284.

Walsh, B. (2002). *Pharmacological treatment of anorexia nervosa and bulimia nervosa.* New York: The Guilford Press.

Walsh, B., Kaplan, A., Attia, E., Olmsted, M., Parides, M., Carter, J., Rocket, W. (2006). Fluoxetine after weight restoration in anorexia nervosa: A randomized controlled trial. *Journal of the American Medical Association, 295*, 2605–2612.

Walsh, B. T., Agras, W. S., Devlin, M. J., Fairburn, C. G., Wilson, G. T., Kahn, C., & Chally, M. K. (2000). Fluoxetine for bulimia nervosa following poor response to psychotherapy. *American Journal of Psychiatry, 157*(8), 1332–1334.

Walsh, B. T., Fairburn, C. G., Mickley, D., Sysko, R., & Parides, M. K. (2004). Treatment of bulimia nervosa in a primary care setting. *American Journal of Psychology, 161*(3), 556–561.

Walters, E. E., & Kendler, K. S. (1995). Anorexia nervosa and anorexic-like syndromes in a population-based female twin sample. *American Journal of Psychiatry, 152*(1), 64–71.

Wang, T., Chou, Y., & Shiah, I. (2006). Combined treatment of olanzapine and mirtazapine in anorexia nervosa associated with major depression. *Progress in Neuropsychopharmacology and Biological Psychiatry, 30*, 306–309.

Wilson, G. (1996). Treatment of bulimia nervosa: When CBT fails. *Behavioral Research Therapy, 34*(3), 197–212.

Wilson, T. G., Fairburn, C. G., & Agras, W. S. (1997). Cognitive behavioral therapy for bulimia nervosa. In D. M. Garner & P. E. Garfinkel (Eds.), *Handbook of treatment for eating disorders* (2nd ed., pp. 67–93). New York: The Guilford Press.

Wilson, G., Fairburn, C., Agras, W., Walsh, B., & Kraemer, H. C. (2002). Cognitive-behavioral therapy for bulimia nervosa: Time course and mechanisms of change. *Journal of Consulting and Clinical Psychology, 70*(2), 267–274.

Wisniewski, L., & Kelly, E. (2003). The application of dialectical behavior therapy to the treatment of eating disorders. *Cognitive and Behavioral Practice, 10*(2), 131–138.

Wonderlich, S., Mitchell, J. E., Swan-Kremier, L., Peterson, C. B., & Crow, S. (2002). An overview of cognitive-behavioral approaches to eating disorders. In T. D. Brewerton (Ed.), *Clinical handbook of eating disorders: An integrated approach* (pp. 403–424). New York: Marcel Dekker.

Yin, H., & Knowlton, B. (2006). The role of the basal ganglia in habit formation. *Nature Neuroscience Review, 7*(6), 464–476.

Management of Treatment-Resistant Schizophrenia

Jacob S. Ballon and Jeffrey A. Lieberman

Introduction

Schizophrenia is a serious mental illness responsible for significant morbidity, decrease in quality of life, and loss of productivity. It is the eighth leading cause of disability-associated life years (DALY) lost (Rossler, Salize, van Os, & Riecher-Rossler, 2005) and is responsible for nearly 1.1% of overall DALY losses according to the World Health Organization (Brundtland, 2001). Although there are several treatments for schizophrenia, many continue to suffer from the wide range of symptoms that are associated with the disorder. Current medications target positive symptoms, that is, hallucinations and delusions, but are not particularly effective for negative symptoms, that is, apathy, social dysfunction, flat affect, or cognitive symptoms, such as deficits in executive function and working memory.

The ultimate goal of treatment for any illness is not just the remission of symptoms but a full functional recovery from that illness. Treatment of schizophrenia needs to be undertaken with this goal in mind. The recovery model of schizophrenia treatment actively considers the importance of not just clinical symptoms but also social and occupational domains. Improvements in these areas are crucial to achieving a functional remission and ultimately increased autonomy. These functional gains should be thought to maintain stability in similar terms, that is, time frame and level of improvement, just as one would consider lack of hallucinations for a clinical remission only significant if it was a consistent finding over the course of several months or years (Harvey & Bellack, 2009). Treating patients with the recovery model in mind generally requires a collaborative approach including occupational therapy, job training, and community integration. People with schizophrenia should be treated with optimism, and attempts to decrease internalized stigma are also crucial to helping people set goals (Warner, 2009).

Persistent negative symptoms yield the greatest functional deficit for people with schizophrenia. While negative symptoms remain recalcitrant to medication, research has

shown that increased participation in the community, such as through various forms of rehabilitation like social skills training, can show an improvement in these symptoms (Halford,
Harrison, Kalyansundaram, Moutrey, & Simpson, 1995). Additionally, psychotherapeutic
interventions, such as with body-oriented psychotherapy, have demonstrated modest benefits in improving negative symptoms (Rohricht & Priebe, 2006). Despite these findings,
there remains a gulf between treatment success and the overall armamentarium for working
on these problems.

While there are no definitive treatments for negative symptoms, positive symptoms of
schizophrenia generally respond well to various approaches, including psychopharmacologic,
nonpharmacological somatic, and psychotherapeutic. Although many patients benefit from
these interventions, there are those who continue to experience persistent hallucinations.
Even more difficult to target therapeutically are delusions, which can take years to remit, and
often are with people indefinitely. There are patients who do not have a remittance of positive
symptoms, even with clozapine, which is considered the antipsychotic of choice for patients
with refractory psychotic symptoms.

There are various definitions for what makes a case "refractory" (Meltzer, 1990).
Resolution of positive symptoms has traditionally been considered the benchmark of treatment response. At least 30% of patients can be considered treatment refractory by rigorous
methods of determining refractoriness, though it may actually be closer to 50%–60%
(Borgio, Bressan, Barbosa Neto, & Daltio, 2007; Elkis & Meltzer, 2007). The varying numbers reflect different appreciations for the difficulty in resolving negative and cognitive symptoms. Treatment refractoriness has been defined by the International Psychopharmacology
Algorithm Project (IPAP) as (1) no period of good functioning in previous 5 years; (2) prior
nonresponse to at least two antipsychotic drugs of two different chemical classes for at least
4–6 weeks each at doses ≥400 mg equivalents of chlorpromazine or 5 mg/day risperidone;
(3) moderate to severe psychopathology, especially positive symptoms, such as conceptual
disorganization, suspiciousness, delusions, or hallucinatory behavior (IPAP, 2008). The aforementioned criteria focus on positive symptoms, but the IPAP also considers continued negative or cognitive symptoms, violence, suicidality, and recurrent mood symptoms as elements
of treatment refractoriness.

Schizophrenia is a chronic and disabling disorder, for which treatment is difficult and
often incomplete. Regardless of how one conceptualizes recovery or remission from schizophrenia, many people who have this illness continue to experience significant morbidity
despite treatment. There are many choices that can be made to enhance treatment beyond
monotherapy with an antipsychotic. This chapter will focus on those treatment options,
including modalities such as brain stimulation, psychotherapy, and polypharmacy with multiple antipsychotics or with other adjunctive agents.

Prognostic Factors for Treatment Response

Schizophrenia is an illness that presents with substantial variability between people, and thus
the search for prognostic factors is an ongoing research endeavour. Factors noticeable early in
the illness may yield long-term clues for overall success in treatment (Bachmann, Bottmer, &
Schroder, 2008). Several features that are important in determining the future course for an

individual patient include demographics such as age of onset and gender, method of disease onset, and quality and variability of symptoms. The duration of untreated psychosis and initial response to treatment portend future illness trajectory. Some factors, such as substance abuse, are uncertain whether the association correlates with a better or worse prognosis. The way that people understand their illness, and the role it plays in their life, also influences outcome through internalized stigma. There are also effects of internalized stigma on treatment adherence and dedication toward working on recovery. As the number of potential prognostic markers increases, so does the search for biomarkers to help allow for earlier determination of proximal factors, and ways to measure the effects of disease-modifying treatments.

Rates of treatment refractoriness remain high in schizophrenia, despite advances in treatment. Antipsychotic monotherapy is likewise becoming increasingly rare. In a study from 2002, a community population was shown to have a rate of concomitant pharmacotherapy of over 50% (Buchanan, Kreyenbuhl, Zito, & Lehman, 2002). In a more recent study of a community sample of people with schizophrenia or schizoaffective disorder, 42.5% of patients were receiving at least two antipsychotic medications, and 70% received an adjunctive psychotropic medication to go with the antipsychotic. Only 25% of patients in the sample were on monotherapy with an antipsychotic (Pickar, Vinik, & Bartko, 2008).

Finding the ideal medication for an individual patient can be difficult. Many patients need to try several different medications before finding the right one, and the amount of time on any individual antipsychotic can be short. The CATIE and CUtLASS studies provide prospective analyses of treatment effectiveness (Jones et al., 2006; Siris, 2000). These studies assessed the outcomes of second-generation antipsychotic (SGA) medications in comparison with first-generation antipsychotic (FGA) medications. The CATIE study looked at the time to discontinuation of medication as the primary outcome measure. The study demonstrated that close to 75% of patients switched or discontinued their initial study medication before the conclusion of the study at 18 months duration. Most discontinuations for lack of efficacy came within the first 6 months of treatment. This indicates that the initial choice of antipsychotic is complex, and many are unsatisfied with their initial medication. Subjects who were randomly switched to a new medication, however, had an earlier time to discontinuation than those who were randomized to their current medication (Altamura et al., 2011; Kuehn, 2011). The CUtLASS study focused on quality of life for a primary outcome measure. The results demonstrated that there was a similar effect on quality of life for patients switched to either FGAs or SGAs (Jones et al., 2006).

Switching antipsychotic medications is a difficult but necessary part of treating patients with schizophrenia. There is little data, however, to guide those decisions. This becomes especially difficult in situations in which there is moderate effectiveness from the medication on core clinical symptoms, but side effects are intolerable or unacceptable. Further clinical comparative effectiveness trials are needed to better appreciate the complexity and help determine the best strategies for changing medications safely (Takeuchi, 2008).

There are many reasons for changing medications. A recent study found that while nearly 30% of patients changed medication over the course of 1-year follow-up, there were several distinct risk factors for medication change. In addition to lack of efficacy, akathisia, anxiety, and preexisting depression were major factors for predicting likelihood of medication switch (Nyhuis, 2010). These changes in medication are also associated with increased risk of acute care services and hospitalization, as well as increased health care costs overall (Faries, 2009).

Antipsychotic medications typically show initial antipsychotic effects quickly. Positive symptoms begin to diminish within the first few days of treatment initiation. When efficacy is not seen quickly, it can mean that the particular medication is not appropriate for that patient. When benefits are not seen within the first 2 weeks of an adequate dose of antipsychotic, there is a greater risk of long-term deficit (Kinon, 2010). The art of psychopharmacology balances the need for an adequate duration and dose of medication, with the awareness that changing when needed may be the best course (Glick, 2009).

There are several other correlates of treatment response, many of which are seen differently over the course of the illness. Adherence to treatment is a difficult matter for both clinicians and patients. Poor adherence to medication is associated with worsened long-term functional outcome, increased hospitalizations, more suicide attempts, and decreased life satisfaction (Ascher-Svanum et al., 2006; Dixon et al., 2010). People who are able to adhere to a medication regimen at an adequate dosage are more likely to benefit from treatment, though strategies to enhance treatment adherence are often difficult (Hafner, Hambrecht, Loffler, Munk-Jorgensen, & Riecher-Rossler, 1998).

Stigma related to mental illness has direct impacts on patients on multiple levels. Adherence to treatment is influenced by stigma, and thus treatment course can be influenced by stigma as well. Internalized stigma can lead people to be reticent to seek treatment, to feel worse about their prognosis, and to feel that they have less self-worth. These delays can lead to a longer duration of untreated psychosis (DUP) and a more difficult illness to treat at initial presentation (Bottas, Cooke, & Richter, 2005). Psychosocial treatment efficacy is also impacted by internalized stigma (Tsang, 2008). Likewise, targeting these feelings with psychotherapy can further enhance treatment and functional outcomes (Poyurovsky, Fuchs, & Weizman, 1999).

Stigma felt prior to the onset of treatment also can delay initial access to medication and necessary services. The onset of illness presents with many variables that can influence the prognosis (Lieberman et al., 1993). More severe symptoms at time of initial diagnosis are associated with worsened future course of illness. The mode of onset and the DUP correlate with outcome, with a longer DUP and insidious onset portending a more severe course (Buckley, Miller, Lehrer, & Castle, 2009; McGlashan, 1999). Although the mechanism is not fully understood, there are plastic changes in the brain that occur the longer a person has unopposed psychosis (Thompson et al., 2001). People with a faster recovery time in the initial episode of psychosis demonstrated better treatment outcomes in the first 2 years of illness. Likewise, a slow and insidious initial progression to schizophrenia heralds a worsened prognosis for further illness than a rapid initial episode (Davidson & McGlashan, 1997).

One area that can confound the initial diagnosis of schizophrenia is substance use. Some people use substances prior to diagnosis and formal treatment in an effort to help mollify symptoms of their undiagnosed mental illness. Substance use also provides a conundrum for determining future risk. Cannabis use has been associated with earlier onset of illness and greater likelihood to convert from a putatively prodromal phase of illness to a more severe diagnosis (Compton et al., 2009). Drug use itself, however, has only equivocally been associated with outcome. One theory for this unexpected outcome may be due to the bias for people who are able to procure drugs being of a higher cognitive function than those who are unable to do so. This confound may limit the predictive validity of drug use in schizophrenia (Shaner et al., 1993). Despite that confound, chronic substance abuse, particularly with stimulants, can cause persistent psychotic symptoms and interfere with treatment adherence. In doing so, that can worsen prognosis and interfere with clinical understanding of how the patient is progressing. While the drugs themselves are damaging, the ability to find and purchase drugs may skew for people at a different level of functioning.

Differing symptom patterns lead to differences in treatment effectiveness. Positive symptoms are generally more responsive to antipsychotic medication. If these are the most disabling symptoms for a person, that person has a greater chance of achieving remittance or recovery. Prominent negative symptoms, however, yield more difficult-to-treat outcomes. Patients with negative symptoms were less likely to be able to demonstrate the typical improvements in social functioning that came with sustained employment (Eisen & Rasmussen, 1993).

Deficits in cognition have been shown to correlate with a worse functional outcome (Bowie, 2008). In a study of 78 patients with schizophrenia, those with poorer performance on neuropsychological testing were more likely to have a decreased functional capacity as measured by the UCSD Performance-Based Skills Assessment (UPSA) (Bowie, 2006). Simply having a deficit in processing speed has been shown to have a poorer prognosis for overall outcome on the Disability Assessment Schedule, and it may be a mediator that can explain overall worse performance in other neuropsychological tests (Sanchez et al., 2009). Deficits in processing speed and working memory also show a worse prognosis for social cognition (Bowie et al., 2008). Newer treatments using techniques from studies of cognitive remediation are showing some initial progress in changing the course of cognitive decline in schizophrenia (Medalia, 2009).

In addition to deficits in cognition predicting worse outcome, higher levels of negative symptoms are linked with poorer prognosis (Ongur & Goff, 2005). In a study from Israel, it was shown that when premorbid symptoms were taken into account, the greatest predictor of future outcome was from negative symptoms (Brill et al., 2009). A similar finding from New York prospectively showed that in first-episode patients, those with greater negative symptoms had a more severe course 2 years after initial hospitalization (Haim, Rabinowitz, & Bromet, 2006).

There may be genetic factors to predict treatment refractoriness. For example, there is research looking at the CNR1 gene, which encodes the CB1 cannabinoid receptor. Cannabis usage, particularly in high doses, is known to be a risk factor for schizophrenia (Andreasson, Allebeck, Engstrom, & Rydberg, 1987). Usage of cannabis has been shown to worsen positive and negative symptoms and decrease cognitive performance. CNR1 is located on chromosome 6.14–6.15, a genetic locus that has been associated with schizophrenia, and several single-nucleotide polymorphisms (SNPs) have been associated with increased risk of disorganized schizophrenia. In a study of 59 treatment-refractory patients, Hamdani et al, looked at the 1359 G/A polymorphism and its role in treatment refractoriness measured by changes in Positive and Negative Syndrome Scale (PANSS) scores. Those with the G allele were more likely to be refractory to antipsychotic treatments, up to 76% for those with GG genotype, while those with the AA genotype had a refractoriness rate of 5% (Hamdani et al., 2008).

Imaging has been able to help provide some interesting insights for biological bases of treatment response (Mitelman & Buchsbaum, 2007). Results have been shown with many different imaging modalities, including both functional and structural. Several studies have shown that in those with a worse clinical outcome, they have larger and more asymmetrical ventricles than those with a better outcome. Additionally, cerebellar and temporal cortical abnormalities have been correlated with worsened severity on social and positive symptoms, respectively. Chronically hospitalized patients and those with other markers of poor outcome have been shown to have decreased gray matter compared with healthy controls, but initial studies did not show statistically significant differences from other people with schizophrenia (Mitelman & Buchsbaum, 2007).

More recent findings have implicated more posterior cortical regions for gray matter changes in those with a more refractory course. Positron emission tomography (PET) imaging has shown that those who have functional changes in the posterior cortical regions of the brain are more likely to have a refractory course than those who show other changes. For those with this finding, there is decreased metabolic performance in the cingulate, striatum, and the temporal lobe. Deficits in white matter have also shown a similar pattern of localization in more posterior regions in refractory patients. Additionally, decreased interhemispheric connectivity has been shown, despite treatment-resistant patients overall having a larger splenium in the corpus callosum than in other patients. Given the overall decreased intracranial volume seen in schizophrenia, the increased size of the splenium was surprising, and it provides further support for neurodevelopmental theories of schizophrenia (Sun, Maller, Daskalakis, Furtado, & Fitzgerald, 2009).

Comorbidities

Schizophrenia often is experienced in conjunction with other mental illness. Although there may be comorbid mood symptoms, often there is not sufficient symptomatology to merit a diagnosis for schizoaffective disorder. Anxiety symptoms are also often prominent, and many people with schizophrenia have obsessions and compulsions of a similar degree to those with obsessive-compulsive disorder. Substance abuse, discussed earlier, is quite common in people with schizophrenia and has implications for overall outcomes.

The most severe outcome for any mental illness is suicide. People with schizophrenia are at a significantly higher risk for suicide than the general population. In a 30-year cohort study, nearly 7% of the studied sample died from suicide (Carlborg, 2008). The greatest predictive factor for suicide fatality is previous suicide attempt (Carlborg, 2010). While there have been some studies implicating different rates of suicide between the sexes, that was not shown in this cohort. Other putative risk factors that were not seen included drug use, family history of mental illness or suicide, or previous episodes of compulsory treatment (Reutfors, 2009).

While suicide may be a tragic outcome for some people with schizophrenia, many others will have persistent or intermittent mood symptoms of varying severities. Schizoaffective disorder is intended to capture this comorbidity, but many patients fall outside of these diagnostic criteria yet still have difficulty with mood, leading some to question the validity of schizoaffective disorder as a diagnostic entity (Cheniaux, 2008). Comorbid depression is seen in nearly half of people with schizophrenia (Buckley et al., 2009). The MUFUSSAD study followed a first episode cohort in Munich, Germany over 15 years. Those who presented at diagnosis with mood symptoms, demonstrated a better prognosis, in terms of overall psychopathology, than those who did not (Moller, 2010). These findings are in contrast to other studies that have shown that those with depression are more prone to relapse (Johnson, 1988).

Anxiety disorders are also common comorbidities to schizophrenia. All of the anxiety disorders overlap with schizophrenia. Approximately 25% of people with schizophrenia also show signs of obsessive-compulsive disorder (Buckley et al., 2009). Research is ongoing to better delineate the biological mechanism linking these two disorders. Other anxiety disorders, such as generalized anxiety disorder, panic disorder, and posttraumatic stress disorder are also seen in higher numbers in schizophrenia. Each of these disorders is seen in nearly 10% of people with schizophrenia (Achim et al., 2011). Taken together, the rate of anxiety disorders and the impact that these have on overall prognosis is significant.

Further complicating schizophrenia treatment, nearly half of people with schizophrenia also have a co-occurring substance use disorder (Volkow, 2009). These "dual-diagnosis" patients often present unique challenges for treatment. Neglecting necessary interventions, including behavioral strategies of treating either disorder, may make the other worse, thus necessitating intensive treatment for both disorders (Goldsmith & Garlapati, 2004). There are numerous social and legal consequences of substance use that also become problematic when this occurs.

Treatment Strategies

Many people with schizophrenia respond well to antipsychotic medication, yet many require several trials of medication to find the best fit. For patients who do not respond to initial treatments, there are several strategies to guide further care. Treatment algorithms, such as the TMAP (Moore, Buchanan et al., 2007) and the IPAP (2008) provide guidelines that can help to provide initial tactics that one can try after the first approaches are unsuccessful. Clozapine, which will be discussed in further detail, remains the primary medication for treatment-resistant schizophrenia. The art of psychopharmacology, either through pragmatic polypharmacy or by extending medications to unconventional doses, has little data but is often used out of necessity. There is also an increasing evidence base for new adjunctive medications to be used in conjunction with antipsychotics. Nonpharmacological treatments, including brain stimulation and different forms of psychotherapy, will also be discussed both on their own and in conjunction with pharmacotherapy.

The Texas Medication Algorithm Project (TMAP) provides a rudimentary structure for organizing treatment strategies for several mental illnesses, including schizophrenia (Moore, Buchanan, et al., 2007). In the most recent update to the TMAP algorithm, the authors identified four primary recommendations. The first recommendation is to prescribe medications differently in the first episode of treatment compared with chronic treatment, as first-episode patients are more susceptible to the side effects of antidopaminergic medications. Second, although SGA medications are considered first line, FGA medications are a reasonable second option. Previously, the recommendation was to have two failed trials of an SGA before going to an FGA. The third recommendation was to consider clozapine treatment after two antipsychotic medications fail to lead to sufficient symptom improvement. Previously, the recommendation had been to use clozapine after three previous medications fail to lead to remission. The final recommendation, for treatment refractory schizophrenia specifically, is that clozapine should be augmented with either another antipsychotic or consideration of brain stimulation (ECT or rTMS) if unsuccessful as monotherapy (Moore, Covell, Essock, & Miller, 2007).

Clozapine has been the treatment of choice in treatment refractory schizophrenia for over 20 years (Essali, Al-Haj Haasan, Li, & Rathbone, 2009; Kane, Honigfeld, Singer, & Meltzer, 1988). Clozapine was first discovered decades earlier; however, limited understanding of the risks and complications initially limited its use. In the United States, it was only available on a compassionate use basis for those with severe tardive dyskinesia, significant treatment resistance, or sensitivity to extrapyramidal side effects (Crilly, 2007). Although some would argue for use earlier in the treatment algorithm, clozapine is generally considered only for use in refractory patients. Particularly for those who do not immediately respond to a first-line second-generation antipsychotic, there are calls for earlier consideration of clozapine (Agid, Remington, Kapur, Arenovich, & Zipursky, 2007).

The rationale for reserving clozapine to refractory patients is primarily based on its side-effect profile. All patients prescribed clozapine must be entered into a national registry for monitoring. Adherence to the prescribed regimen is also essential, as missing the medication for as few as 2 days requires retitration (Novartis, 2010).While management strategies are available for many of these side effects, some of the side effects can be potentially fatal. The most serious risk from using clozapine is agranulocytosis. Other black box warnings include seizures, myocarditis, hypotension, and the ubiquitous warning for all antipsychotics of the increased risk of mortality in the elderly. For seizure prophylaxis, higher doses of clozapine are typically accompanied by an antiepileptic agent such as valproic acid. Pulmonary embolism and severe constipation are also dangerous risks for patients on clozapine. To prevent bowel perforation from severe constipation, clozapine should typically be dosed along with stool softeners or other laxatives. Less serious, but nevertheless difficult side effects include sialorrhea and fatigue.

Rates of agranulocytosis dropped significantly with the aggressive hematologic monitoring and slow dose titrations that have become the standard practice when using clozapine (Crilly, 2007). Full dosing and monitoring instructions are available in the package insert and through the clozapine registry. The greatest risk of agranulocytosis occurs during the first 3 months of treatment. Genetic markers of risk continue to be an ongoing area of research, after it was shown that in a small group of Ashkenazi Jews, there was an association with different HLA haplotypes and developing agranulocytosis (Lieberman et al., 1990). These findings have also been shown in non-Ashkenazi Caucasian samples as well (Dettling, 2001). In an analysis of over 11,000 patients from 1990 to 1991, the first years of clozapine's widespread use, it was shown that just under 1% of patients developed agranulocytosis. This was consistent with previous reports of agranulocytosis rates of approximately 1%–2%. In that cohort, there were two patient deaths attributed to hematologic adverse events (Alvir, Lieberman, Safferman, Schwimmer, & Schaaf, 1993).

There are strategies to try if there is a decrease in blood count. While sometimes successful in being able to increase blood counts sufficiently to remain on clozapine, agranulocytosis still remains a reason that patients usually have to stop taking clozapine. When agranulocytosis or other significant drops in blood counts occur, consultation should be made quickly with a hematologist to discuss possible options and management. In some cases, particularly for benign ethnic neutropenia, lithium is able to increase white blood cell production. While it is insufficient to use as a long-term treatment for agranulocytosis, and can even potentially mask a developing case of agranulocytosis, (Blier, Slater, Measham, Koch, & Wiviott, 1998), the ability to increase white blood cell count is usually enhanced with lithium (Silverstone, 1998). In more potentially serious cases, granulocyte colony stimulating factor (G-CSF) may be considered (Rajagopal, Graham, & Haut, 2007). While not a definitive treatment, it can be an effective tool for maintaining someone on clozapine necessitating a discontinuation, and several cases of successful use are reported in the literature, as are some unsuccessful cases (Majczenko & Stewart, 2008; Mathewson & Lindenmayer, 2007).

Metabolic side effects present significant difficulty in using clozapine. Weight gain, dyslipidemia, and risk for diabetes are all seen frequently with clozapine use (Wirshing et al., 2002). It is important to encourage active participation from the patient's primary care provider with respect to managing many of these metabolic effects. This is of greater importance if clozapine has demonstrated that it is uniquely suited to ameliorating their psychotic symptoms. Fortunately, treatments are available for many of the metabolic side effects, though it would still be preferable to have medications that were effective in treating psychosis without these risks. Long-term consequences of metabolic side effects can impact overall life expectancy if not properly managed. Antipsychotic side effects may be a factor in the shortened life expectancy seen in schizophrenia (Hennekens, 2005).

While clozapine may provide the greatest risk for metabolic side effects, these must be considered with all antipsychotic medications. Olanzapine, risperidone, and quetiapine are generally considered to be the higher risk agents for weight gain, while ziprasidone and aripiprazole generally are of lower risk (Allison, 1999). It is important to consider that the newest antipsychotics to the market, lurasidone, iloperidone, and asenapine, have demonstrated relative safety on metabolic parameters, but as they are new to the market, it may not be fully known to what extent they will be metabolically active. Given the increased risk for smoking among schizophrenia patients, and the increased likelihood of sedentary lifestyle, metabolic side effects may be a significant driver behind treatment decisions (Nasrallah, 2004).

When clozapine does not provide adequate symptom relief, it is often considered for use in combination before it is discontinued. Sometimes the addition of another agent can help to lower the dose of clozapine and potentially help by lowering the side-effect burden. While this strategy may have merit, especially after limited success with other treatments, there are limited data to support this practice. The most common reports in the literature describe combining clozapine with aripiprazole. In a small ($n = 24$), retrospective chart review, it was shown that addition of aripiprazole was associated with lower clozapine dose, and that 18 of 24 patients lost weight, with an average loss of 5 kg (Karunakaran, Tungaraza, & Harborne, 2007). In a double-blinded study, the addition of aripiprazole to clozapine was not shown to have benefits on the primary outcome measure of the Brief Psychiatric Rating Scale (BPRS), but it did show benefits of secondary measures, including the Schedule for the Assessment of Negative Symptoms (SANS). No differences were seen in glucose levels, though prolactin was lower in the aripiprazole group compared with placebo

(Chang et al., 2008). Although case reports have suggested benefits from aripiprazole, further studies need to be done to establish its efficacy as an adjunctive agent to clozapine. Risperidone has also shown only limited benefit when added to clozapine (Freudenreich, Henderson, Walsh, Culhane, & Goff, 2007). Clozapine may also be effective when combined with medications that are not otherwise considered antipsychotics on their own.

Polypharmacy that includes medications other than antipsychotics are also a frequently employed strategy to enhance efficacy. As antipsychotic medications may not necessarily provide enough benefit on their own, many look to medications with other primary indications to help bridge the gap. Several agents have been studied in conjunction with antipsychotics for treatment-resistant schizophrenia. Several reports recently have indicated benefit for adding lamotrigine to antipsychotic treatment. Lamotrigine decreases glutamate release and increases GABA release, and when given with clozapine, has shown enhanced diminution of locomotor activity in rats treated with phencyclidine—a common animal measure of potential antipsychotic efficacy. Topiramate is similar mechanistically to lamotrigine and also effects glutamate transmission. In a recent meta-analysis of lamotrigine, the data from a few small trials, all of which were negative, were aggregated for enhanced power to detect a difference between placebo augmentation and lamotrigine augmentation in people who remained with residual symptoms despite treatment with clozapine (Goff, 2009; Goff et al., 2007; Zoccali et al., 2007). In the meta-analysis it was shown that there was a potential benefit with the addition of lamotrigine in these patients. Benefit was only shown as an augmenting agent to clozapine, leading to speculation that the glutamatergic properties of lamotrigine may be uniquely suited to working with clozapine. Longer and more definitive trials are still needed to confirm the benefit of lamotrigine augmentation (Tiihonen, Wahlbeck, & Kiviniemi, 2009). Looking at topiramate, in a small crossover trial of 36 patients receiving varying atypical antipsychotics, a positive effect was seen based on change in PANSS score. Further work needs to be done with topiramate to fully establish efficacy (Tiihonen et al., 2005). Modafinil has demonstrated a limited effect in treating refractory negative symptoms. Although it did not reach statistical significance on the primary outcome measure of the SANS, it was well tolerated without positive symptom exacerbation (Pierre, Peloian, Wirshing, Wirshing, & Marder, 2007). Valproate has also never been established as an effective adjunctive agent in long-term treatment of schizophrenia, though benefits in short-term potentiation of treatment have been seen in one study (Schwarz, Volz, Li, & Leucht, 2008).

Though mood stabilizers have been shown to have some benefit as adjunctive agents, there is no evidence to support using them as monotherapy. The lack of efficacy of lithium, valproic acid, and other mood stabilizers as monotherapy treatment for schizophrenia lends credence to the argument that despite sharing some genetic determinants, and general responsiveness to dopamine antagonists (Murray, 2004), schizophrenia and bipolar disorder are mechanistically separate illnesses. In a Cochrane review, lithium was found to be ineffective as a monotherapy agent in schizophrenia. This meta-analysis looked at over 20 studies and more than 600 patients. There may be some benefit for patients with affective symptoms for lithium as an adjunctive agent, but that has not been fully demonstrated in clinical trials (Leucht, Kissling, & McGrath, 2007).

Antidepressants, particularly selective serotonin reuptake antagonists (SSRIs), are frequently used in people with schizophrenia. Given the phenotypic similarity between negative symptoms and major depression, many assume that these medications will show benefit. At the very least, they are well tolerated and not likely to worsen problems. Many patients also have concurrent mood symptoms for which an SSRI is an appropriate treatment. For example, citalopram was recently shown in a placebo-controlled trial to have a benefit in comorbid subsyndromal depression symptoms in schizophrenia (Zisook et al., 2009). However, there is scant evidence that their use helps with negative symptoms. Most trials have been small, and when compiled in meta-analyses, do not hold up a benefit. In a recent Cochrane review, it was found that there is some, but not firm evidence, that SSRIs are of benefit in negative symptoms, and it was suggested that larger, pragmatic trials be conducted to address this question (Rummel, Kissling, & Leucht, 2006).

Adherence to a medication regimen is essential for successful pharmacotherapy. Patients who are unable to maintain their medication regimen are at a greater risk of relapse, hospitalization, and poor functional outcomes (Dixon et al., 2010). Disruptions in treatment make further episodes often more difficult to remit, and they put patients at a greater chance of developing refractory symptoms. Many patients have difficulty in organizing and managing a daily medication regimen. While simplifying the regimen to using daily instead of multiple daily doses is a start, for many patients, a depot medication is often the most parsimonious treatment. Before starting treatment with a long-acting injectable medication, patients must be able to demonstrate that they can tolerate the medication orally, as the potential consequences of a serious side effect could otherwise be felt for several weeks. The switch from oral to depot medication is generally well tolerated (Faries, 2009). There are currently depot preparations for three second-generation antipsychotics: risperidone (Bai et al., 2006; Taylor, Young, Mace, & Patel, 2004), paliperidone (Carlborg, 2008; Tsang, 2008), and olanzapine (Citrome, 2009; Medalia, 2009). Others are currently in development. These join FGAs haloperidol and fluphenazine as appropriate choices for maintenance therapy. A current large-scale pragmatic clinical trial is under way to compare haloperidol and paliperidone long-acting injectables (Clinicaltrials.gov, 2011).

Using an unconventional dose of an antipsychotic is a reasonable strategy for management in some patients. One must be certain that poor adherence is not behind the inefficacy of a standard dose before deciding to go above the typical threshold. The mechanism for such treatment is often unclear, as dopamine receptors are typically fully saturated well before reaching the maximum for standard doses, but individuality in treatment response can be difficult to predict. Many case reports are available for successful high-dose treatment with different antipsychotic medications. In a small ($n = 40$) double-blind study comparing high-dose olanzapine with clozapine, it was shown both groups showed similar and robust improvement on the PANSS. Seventy-one percent of the olanzapine subjects were taking over 35 mg/day. Metabolic complications were prominent in both groups, though the olanzapine subjects gained considerably more weight (Meltzer et al., 2008). In a double-blind trial of high-dose olanzapine (maximum dose 30 mg) versus clozapine in young, treatment-resistant subjects, clozapine demonstrated an enhanced effect (Kumra et al., 2008a). In an open-label follow-up, clozapine was beneficial in 7 out of 10 patients who did not have an adequate response to olanzapine. Both groups, as is often seen in young people, were exquisitely sensitive to metabolic complications, showing greater weight gain and changes in glucose than is typically seen in older patients (Kumra et al., 2008b).

Increasingly, nonpharmacologic treatments are gaining attention and demonstrating compelling data for their use. Multimodal treatment with medication and psychotherapy is the standard of care in most other psychiatric disorders, and schizophrenia need not be an exception (Rathod, Kingdon, Weiden, & Turkington, 2008). Several models of psychotherapy continue to demonstrate efficacy for the treatment of core schizophrenia symptoms, including hallucinations. Cognitive-behavioral therapy (CBT) is the most thoroughly studied treatment modality, and it has data to support its usage in several domains of illness, including both positive and negative symptoms (Sensky et al., 2000). Beck first reported a case in 1952 of a patient who demonstrated enhanced insight and functional improvement through CBT (Beck, 1952). Additionally, CBT can be helpful in enhancing patient adherence to the overall treatment regimen and patient insight. A recent post-hoc analysis demonstrated a benefit of CBT on suicidal ideation as well (Bateman, Hansen, Turkington, & Kingdon, 2007). Although the benefits may wane after treatment stops, they are profound improvements in the short term, and some benefits such as with insight, can be seen even 1 year after treatment (Rathod, Kingdon, Smith, & Turkington, 2005). The benefits of CBT are more likely to persist than other more benign comparison interventions, such as "befriending" or general supportive care, in which subjects are given the same social benefits of having a therapist to see, but without a specific or targeted intervention (Sensky et al., 2000).

CBT was used recently in a study looking at insight. In this study, subjects were randomly assigned to CBT or treatment as usual. The CBT group was able to better relabel psychotic symptoms and to understand their need for treatment. There was no difference between the groups with respect to overall insight into having an illness (Rathod et al., 2005). Although improvements can be seen with respect to insight, delusions remain difficult to address. However, general psychopathology has been shown to improve, as measured by PANSS, even in patients who are refractory to clozapine treatment. An initial benefit was seen in quality of life as well, though that did not persist at a 6-month follow-up. General psychopathology improvements did maintain after 6 months, however, in comparison to a befriending comparator group (Barretto et al., 2009).

The treatment decisions for patients who are refractory to initial medication trials are complex and challenging. Many patients require close monitoring, and a team approach is often essential. In the most severe cases, an assertive community treatment (ACT) approach can be the most effective. In an ACT model of care, patients are seen at least weekly in their community by social workers and other professionals. Each member of the treatment team interacts with each of the team's patients. This helps minimize burnout while maximizing the ability to help. Patients are seen frequently with an emphasis on helping to manage their needs in their own community without needing to resort to hospitalization when there are urgent issues. Because providers are able to see patients in this manner, crises can be more effectively averted before escalating and causing a rupture in the treatment course. In the ACCESS Trial, Lambert et al (2010) demonstrated that compared with regular treatment in the community, the assertive model significantly helped to keep patients engaged and in treatment over a 1-year period. ACT patients were five times more likely to continue taking their medication over the period of the study. More of the ACT patients were able to live independently and to have a job. Further research to determine the minimum effective length of treatment in the ACT model needs to be done to better know how to deliver this type of intervention to the most people (Lambert et al., 2010).

Brain stimulation techniques are the treatment of choice for mood disorders. These methods, including electroconvulsive therapy (ECT) and especially transcranial magnetic stimulation (rTMS), are becoming safer and easier to administer. ECT has been used to treat schizophrenia for decades, though there are limited data to support its use (Tang & Ungvari, 2002). A Cochrane systematic review recently concluded that ECT could be effective in those patients who do not respond to treatment with antipsychotic medications, particularly those who need especially rapid treatment. The number needed to treat for ECT in this study was six when all the data were compiled (Tharyan & Adams, 2005). ECT has been shown to be better than sham treatment, though benefits from ECT have not been shown to be persistent after treatment is concluded, necessitating maintenance treatment for continued positive effect.

rTMS has been approved by the FDA for treatment of major depressive disorder, but it currently does not have an indication for treatment of schizophrenia. Unlike ECT, there is greater ability to specify treatment location with rTMS. It is also more easily tolerated and only rarely induces a seizure when properly administered. Treatment for depression typically involves rapid TMS, which enhances excitability in the brain. Researched treatments for schizophrenia have been of both the rapid- and slow-wave variety. Treatments targeting auditory hallucinations have largely been targeted at temporoparietal cortex, while treatments targeting negative symptoms have largely been rapid wave rTMS aimed at the prefrontal cortex. As in depression, the prefrontal cortex has been an initial target of the magnet. Initial studies were small, and often confounded by difficulties with blinding the sham treatment (Fitzgerald & Daskalakis, 2008). Decreased auditory hallucinations were found in a recent randomized, sham-controlled trial of rTMS in the bilateral temporoparietal area. This study showed the same findings of improvement on auditory hallucinations, but not general improvements in psychopathology (Vercammen et al., 2009). In a meta-analysis of several small studies, rTMS was shown to be beneficial in alleviating treatment-resistant auditory hallucinations, though the benefit was not seen in overall measures of positive symptoms. Overall, the safety profile of rTMS was reassuring, and treatment was not limited by complications (Aleman, Sommer, & Kahn, 2007).

rTMS has been studied for treatment of negative symptoms, though with limited success (Mogg et al., 2007). In a meta-analysis, rTMS was seen to have a benefit on negative symptoms in initial, uncontrolled studies, but the effect diminished for controlled trials. While these results are encouraging, they prompt further work that will need to be done before this therapy can be used more widely. Given that medications do not treat this cluster of symptoms, however, the progress is exciting. Indeed, research will need to focus on stimulating other areas besides the prefrontal cortex because negative symptoms may arise from other parts of the brain, including the anterior cingulate, cerebellum, occipital cortex, and posterior cortical parietal cortex (Freitas, Fregni, & Pascual-Leone, 2009).

Just as negative symptoms are generally refractory to nearly all methods of treatment we have, cognitive symptoms are also similarly difficult to target. A recent study has demonstrated some benefit from deep rTMS on this target as well (Levkovitz, 2011). Using a special coil that allows for deeper penetration into the brain structures, and for targeting the deeper layers of dorsolateral prefrontal cortex, this small study demonstrates that there may be potential for further improvements by aiming for these structures.

Conclusion

Schizophrenia remains a severe mental illness with substantial morbidity that begins in late adolescence and often lasts throughout a person's life. Many techniques have been developed, yet there is a continued need to innovate and develop better and more complete treatments. People with schizophrenia, despite the severity of the illness, have an amazing capacity for attaining significant levels of functioning in the community. The goal of treatment should always be for full recovery. Setting the bar at this level gives patients, family members, providers, and all affected hope that with this diagnosis there still can be great hope for a meaningful quality of life. Although some require extensive and creative means to achieve these goals, and many fall short, the potential exists for people with schizophrenia to live independently, work regular jobs, and have significant social relationships. The best treatments are those that utilize multiple modalities, including developing a strong treatment alliance, psychotherapeutic methods, psychopharmacology, community building, and community integration. For those who do not recover with the first few attempts at treatment, this chapter has provided some ideas for how to take the next step in care.

Disclosure Statement

J.S.B. has no conflicts of interest to disclose.

J.A.L. serves on the Advisory Board of Alkermes, Bioline, Intracellular Therapies, Pierre Fabre and PsychoGenics. He does not receive direct financial compensation or salary support for participation in research, consulting, or advisory board activities. He receives grant support from Allon, F. Hoffman-La Roche LTD, GlaxoSmithKline, Eli Lilly, Merck, Novartis, Pfizer, Psychogenics, Sepracor (Sunovion) and Targacept; and he holds a patent from Repligen.

References

Achim, A. M., Maziade, M., Raymond, E., Olivier, D., Merette, C., & Roy, M. A. (2011). How prevalent are anxiety disorders in schizophrenia? A meta-analysis and critical review on a significant association. *Schizophrenia Bulletin, 37*(4), 811–821.

Agid, O., Remington, G., Kapur, S., Arenovich, T., & Zipursky, R. B. (2007). Early use of clozapine for poorly responding first-episode psychosis. *Journal of Clinical Psychopharmacology, 27*(4), 369–373.

Aleman, A., Sommer, I. E., & Kahn, R. S. (2007). Efficacy of slow repetitive transcranial magnetic stimulation in the treatment of resistant auditory hallucinations in schizophrenia: A meta-analysis. *Journal of Clinical Psychiatry, 68*(3), 416–421.

Allison, D. B. (1999). Antipsychotic-induced weight gain: A comprehensive research synthesis. *American Journal of Psychiatry, 156*(11), 1686.

Altamura, A. C., Serati, M., Albano, A., Paoli, R. A., Glick, I. D., & Dell'osso, B. (2011). An epidemiologic and clinical overview of medical and psychopathological comorbidities in major psychoses. *European Archives of Psychiatry and Clinical Neuroscience, 261*(7), 489–508.

Alvir, J. M., Lieberman, J. A., Safferman, A. Z., Schwimmer, J. L., & Schaaf, J. A. (1993). Clozapine-induced agranulocytosis. Incidence and risk factors in the United States. *New England Journal of Medicine, 329*(3), 162–167.

Andreasson, S., Allebeck, P., Engstrom, A., & Rydberg, U. (1987). Cannabis and schizophrenia. A longitudinal study of Swedish conscripts. *Lancet, 2*(8574), 1483–1486.

Ascher-Svanum, H., Faries, D. E., Zhu, B., Ernst, F. R., Swartz, M. S., & Swanson, J. W. (2006). Medication adherence and long-term functional outcomes in the treatment of schizophrenia in usual care. *Journal of Clinical Psychiatry, 67*(3), 453–460.

Bachmann, S., Bottmer, C., & Schroder, J. (2008). One-year outcome and its prediction in first-episode schizophrenia—a naturalistic study. *Psychopathology, 41*(2), 115–123.

Bai, Y. M., Chen, T. T., Wu, B., Hung, C. H., Lin, W. K., Hu, T. M., et al. (2006). A comparative efficacy and safety study of long-acting risperidone injection and risperidone oral tablets among hospitalized patients: 12-week randomized, single-blind study. *Pharmacopsychiatry, 39*(4), 135–141.

Barretto, E. M., Kayo, M., Avrichir, B. S., Sa, A. R., Camargo, M. G., Napolitano, I. C., et al. (2009). A preliminary controlled trial of cognitive behavioral therapy in clozapine-resistant schizophrenia. *Journal of Nervous and Mental Disease, 197*(11), 865–868.

Bateman, K., Hansen, L., Turkington, D., & Kingdon, D. (2007). Cognitive behavioral therapy reduces suicidal ideation in schizophrenia: Results from a randomized controlled trial. *Suicide and Life-Threatening Behavior, 37*(3), 284–290.

Beck, A. T. (1952). Successful outpatient psychotherapy of a chronic schizophrenic with a delusion based on borrowed guilt. *Psychiatry, 15*(3), 305–312.

Blier, P., Slater, S., Measham, T., Koch, M., & Wiviott, G. (1998). Lithium and clozapine-induced neutropenia/agranulocytosis. *International Clinical Psychopharmacology, 13*(3), 137–140.

Borgio, J. G., Bressan, R. A., Barbosa Neto, J. B., & Daltio, C. S. (2007). Refractory schizophrenia: A neglected clinical problem. *Revista Brasileira de Psiquiatria, 29*(3), 292–293.

Bottas, A., Cooke, R. G., & Richter, M. A. (2005). Comorbidity and pathophysiology of obsessive-compulsive disorder in schizophrenia: Is there evidence for a schizo-obsessive subtype of schizophrenia? *Journal of Psychiatry and Neuroscience, 30*(3), 187–193.

Bowie, C. R. (2006). Determinants of real-world functional performance in schizophrenia subjects: Correlations with cognition, functional capacity, and symptoms. *American Journal of Psychiatry, 163*(3), 418–425.

Bowie, C. R. (2008). Predicting schizophrenia patients' real-world behavior with specific neuropsychological and functional capacity measures. *Biological Psychiatry, 63*(5), 505.

Bowie, C. R., Leung, W. W., Reichenberg, A., McClure, M. M., Patterson, T. L., Heaton, R. K., et al. (2008). Predicting schizophrenia patients' real-world behavior with specific neuropsychological and functional capacity measures. *Biological Psychiatry, 63*(5), 505–511.

Brill, N., Levine, S. Z., Reichenberg, A., Lubin, G., Weiser, M., & Rabinowitz, J. (2009). Pathways to functional outcomes in schizophrenia: The role of premorbid functioning, negative symptoms and intelligence. *Schizophrenia research, 110*(1–3), 40–46.

Brundtland, G. H. (2001). From the World Health Organization. Mental health: New understanding, new hope. *Journal of the American Medical Association, 286*(19), 2391.

Buchanan, R. W., Kreyenbuhl, J., Zito, J. M., & Lehman, A. (2002). Relationship of the use of adjunctive pharmacological agents to symptoms and level of function in schizophrenia. *American Journal of Psychiatry, 159*(6), 1035–1043.

Buckley, P. F., Miller, B. J., Lehrer, D. S., & Castle, D. J. (2009). Psychiatric comorbidities and schizophrenia. *Schizophrenia Bulletin, 35*(2), 383–402.

Carlborg, A. (2008). Long-term suicide risk in schizophrenia spectrum psychoses: Survival analysis by gender. *Archives of Suicide Research, 12*(4), 347–351.

Carlborg, A. (2010). Attempted suicide predicts suicide risk in schizophrenia spectrum psychosis. *Nordic Journal of Psychiatry, 64*(1), 68–72.

Chang, J. S., Ahn, Y. M., Park, H. J., Lee, K. Y., Kim, S. H., Kang, U. G., et al. (2008). Aripiprazole augmentation in clozapine-treated patients with refractory schizophrenia: An 8-week, randomized, double-blind, placebo-controlled trial. *Journal of Clinical Psychiatry, 69*(5), 720–731.

Cheniaux, E. (2008). Does schizoaffective disorder really exist? A systematic review of the studies that compared schizoaffective disorder with schizophrenia or mood disorders. *Journal of Affective Disorders, 106*(3), 209.

Citrome, L. (2009). Olanzapine pamoate: A stick in time? A review of the efficacy and safety profile of a new depot formulation of a second-generation antipsychotic. *International Journal of Clinical Practice, 63*(1), 140–150.

Clinicaltrials.gov. (2011, March 21). *A comparison of long-acting injectable medications for schizophrenia (ACLAIMS)*. Retrieved May 2011, from http://clinicaltrials.gov/ct2/show/NCT01136772.

Compton, M. T., Kelley, M. E., Ramsay, C. E., Pringle, M., Goulding, S. M., Esterberg, M. L., et al. (2009). Association of pre-onset cannabis, alcohol, and tobacco use with age at onset of prodrome and age at onset of psychosis in first-episode patients. *American Journal of Psychiatry*, *166*(11), 1251–1257.

Crilly, J. (2007). The history of clozapine and its emergence in the US market: A review and analysis. *History of Psychiatry*, *18*(1), 39–60.

Davidson, L., & McGlashan, T. H. (1997). The varied outcomes of schizophrenia. *Canadian Journal of Psychiatry*, *42*(1), 34–43.

Dettling, M. (2001). Genetic determinants of clozapine-induced agranulocytosis: Recent results of HLA subtyping in a non-Jewish Caucasian sample. *Archives of General Psychiatry*, *58*(1), 93–94.

Dixon, L. B., Dickerson, F., Bellack, A. S., Bennett, M., Dickinson, D., Goldberg, R. W., et al. (2010).The 2009 schizophrenia PORT psychosocial treatment recommendations and summary statements. *Schizophrenia Bulletinetin*, *36*(1), 48–70.

Eisen, J. L., & Rasmussen, S. A. (1993). Obsessive compulsive disorder with psychotic features. [Comparative Study]. *The Journal of Clinical Psychiatry*, *54*(10), 373–379.

Elkis, H., & Meltzer, H. Y. (2007). Esquizofrenia refratária [Refractory schizophrenia]. *Revista Brasileira de Psiquiatria*, *29*(Suppl 2), S41–S47.

Essali, A., Al-Haj Haasan, N., Li, C., & Rathbone, J. (2009). Clozapine versus typical neuroleptic medication for schizophrenia. *Cochrane Database of Systematic Reviews*, *1*, CD000059.

Faries, D. E. (2009). Clinical and economic ramifications of switching antipsychotics in the treatment of schizophrenia. *BMC Psychiatry*, *9*(1), 54.

Fitzgerald, P. B., & Daskalakis, Z. J. (2008). A review of repetitive transcranial magnetic stimulation use in the treatment of schizophrenia. *Canadian Journal of Psychiatry*, *53*(9), 567–576.

Freitas, C., Fregni, F., & Pascual-Leone, A. (2009). Meta-analysis of the effects of repetitive transcranial magnetic stimulation (rTMS) on negative and positive symptoms in schizophrenia. *Schizophrenia Research*, *108*(1–3), 11–24.

Freudenreich, O., Henderson, D. C., Walsh, J. P., Culhane, M. A., & Goff, D. C. (2007). Risperidone augmentation for schizophrenia partially responsive to clozapine: A double-blind, placebo-controlled trial. *Schizophrenia Research*, *92*(1–3), 90–94.

Glick, I. D. Balon, R., Ballon, J.S., Rovine, D. (2009). Teaching pearls from the lost art of psychopharmacology. *Journal of Psychiatric Practice*, *15*(5), 423–426.

Goff, D. C. (2009). Review: Lamotrigine may be an effective treatment for clozapine resistant schizophrenia. *Evid Based Ment Health*, *12*(4), 111.

Goff, D. C., Keefe, R., Citrome, L., Davy, K., Krystal, J. H., Large, C., et al. (2007). Lamotrigine as add-on therapy in schizophrenia: results of 2 placebo-controlled trials. *Journal of Clinical Psychopharmacology*, *27*(6), 582–589.

Goldsmith, R. J., & Garlapati, V. (2004). Behavioral interventions for dual-diagnosis patients. [Review]. *Psychiatric Clinics of North America*, *27*(4), 709–725.

Hafner, H., Hambrecht, M., Loffler, W., Munk-Jorgensen, P., & Riecher-Rossler, A. (1998). Is schizophrenia a disorder of all ages? A comparison of first episodes and early course across the life-cycle. *Psychological Medicine*, *28*(2), 351–365.

Haim, R., Rabinowitz, J., & Bromet, E. (2006). The relationship of premorbid functioning to illness course in schizophrenia and psychotic mood disorders during two years following first hospitalization. *Journal of Nervous and Mental Disease*, *194*(10), 791–795.

Halford, W. K., Harrison, C., Kalyansundaram, Moutrey, C., & Simpson, S. (1995). Preliminary results from a psychoeducational program to rehabilitate chronic patients. *Psychiatric Services*, *46*(11), 1189–1191.

Hamdani, N., Tabeze, J. P., Ramoz, N., Ades, J., Hamon, M., Sarfati, Y., et al. (2008). The CNR1 gene as a pharmacogenetic factor for antipsychotics rather than a susceptibility gene for schizophrenia. *European Neuropsychopharmacology*, *18*(1), 34–40.

Harvey, P. D., & Bellack, A. S. (2009). Toward a terminology for functional recovery in schizophrenia: Is functional remission a viable concept? *Schizophrenia Bulletin*, *35*(2), 300–306.

Hennekens, C. H. (2005). Schizophrenia and increased risks of cardiovascular disease. *American Heart Journal*, *150*(6), 1115.

IPAP. (2008, December 22). *Treatment resistant schizophrenia*. Retrieved January, 2012, http://www.ipap.org/pdf/schiz/IPAP_Schiz_bundle.zip.

Johnson, D. A. (1988). The significance of depression in the prediction of relapse in chronic schizophrenia. *British Journal of Psychiatry*, *152*, 320–323.

Jones, P. B., Barnes, T. R., Davies, L., Dunn, G., Lloyd, H., Hayhurst, K. P., et al. (2006). Randomized controlled trial of the effect on Quality of Life of second- vs first-generation antipsychotic drugs in schizophrenia: Cost Utility of the Latest Antipsychotic Drugs in Schizophrenia Study (CUtLASS 1). *Archives of General Psychiatry, 63*(10), 1079–1087.

Kane, J., Honigfeld, G., Singer, J., & Meltzer, H. (1988). Clozapine for the treatment-resistant schizophrenic. A double-blind comparison with chlorpromazine. *Archives of General Psychiatry, 45*(9), 789–796.

Karunakaran, K., Tungaraza, T. E., & Harborne, G. C. (2007). Is clozapine-aripiprazole combination a useful regime in the management of treatment-resistant schizophrenia? *Journal of Psychopharmacology, 21*(4), 453–456.

Kinon, B. J. (2010). Early response to antipsychotic drug therapy as a clinical marker of subsequent response in the treatment of schizophrenia. *Neuropsychopharmacology, 35*(2), 581.

Kuehn, B. M. (2011). Scientists probe oxytocin therapy for social deficits in autism, schizophrenia. [News]. *Journal of the American Medical Association, 305*(7), 659–661.

Kumra, S., Kranzler, H., Gerbino-Rosen, G., Kester, H. M., De Thomas, C., Kafantaris, V., et al. (2008a). Clozapine and "high-dose" olanzapine in refractory early-onset schizophrenia: A 12-week randomized and double-blind comparison. *Biological Psychiatry, 63*(5), 524–529.

Kumra, S., Kranzler, H., Gerbino-Rosen, G., Kester, H. M., DeThomas, C., Cullen, K., et al. (2008b). Clozapine versus "high-dose" olanzapine in refractory early-onset schizophrenia: An open-label extension study. *Journal of Child and Adolescent Psychopharmacology, 18*(4), 307–316.

Lambert, M., Bock, T., Schottle, D., Golks, D., Meister, K., Rietschel, L., et al. (2010). Assertive community treatment as part of integrated care versus standard care: a 12-month trial in patients with first- and multiple-episode schizophrenia spectrum disorders treated with quetiapine immediate release (ACCESS Trial). *Journal of Clinical Psychiatry, 71*(10), 1313–1323.

Leucht, S., Kissling, W., & McGrath, J. (2007). Lithium for schizophrenia. [Review]. *Cochrane Database of Systematic Reviews, 3*, CD003834.

Lieberman, J., Jody, D., Geisler, S., Alvir, J., Loebel, A., Szymanski, S., et al. (1993). Time course and biologic correlates of treatment response in first-episode schizophrenia. *Archives of General Psychiatry, 50*(5), 369–376.

Lieberman, J. A., Yunis, J., Egea, E., Canoso, R. T., Kane, J. M., & Yunis, E. J. (1990). HLA-B38, DR4, DQw3 and clozapine-induced agranulocytosis in Jewish patients with schizophrenia. *Archives of General Psychiatry, 47*(10), 945–948.

Levkovitz, Y. (2011). Deep transcranial magnetic stimulation add-on for treatment of negative symptoms and cognitive deficits of schizophrenia: A feasibility study. *International Journal of Neuropsychopharmacology, 14*(07), 991–996.

Majczenko, T. G., & Stewart, J. T. (2008). Failure of filgrastim to prevent severe clozapine-induced agranulocytosis. *Southern Medical Journal, 101*(6), 639–640.

Mathewson, K. A., & Lindenmayer, J. P. (2007). Clozapine and granulocyte colony-stimulating factor: Potential for long-term combination treatment for clozapine-induced neutropenia. *Journal of Clinical Psychopharmacology, 27*(6), 714–715.

McGlashan, T. H. (1999). Duration of untreated psychosis in first-episode schizophrenia: Marker or determinant of course? *Biological Psychiatry, 46*(7), 899–907.

Medalia, A. (2009). Cognitive remediation in schizophrenia. *Neuropsychology Review, 19*(3), 353–364.

Meltzer, H. Y. (1990). Defining treatment refractoriness in schizophrenia. *Schizophrenia Bulletin, 16*(4), 563–565.

Meltzer, H. Y., Bobo, W. V., Roy, A., Jayathilake, K., Chen, Y., Ertugrul, A., et al. (2008). A randomized, double-blind comparison of clozapine and high-dose olanzapine in treatment-resistant patients with schizophrenia. *Journal of Clinical Psychiatry, 69*(2), 274–285.

Mitelman, S. A., & Buchsbaum, M. S. (2007). Very poor outcome schizophrenia: Clinical and neuroimaging aspects. *International Review of Psychiatry, 19*(4), 345–357.

Mogg, A., Purvis, R., Eranti, S., Contell, F., Taylor, J. P., Nicholson, T., et al. (2007). Repetitive transcranial magnetic stimulation for negative symptoms of schizophrenia: A randomized controlled pilot study. *Schizophrenia Research, 93*(1–3), 221–228.

Moller, H-J. (2010). The Munich 15-year follow-up study (MUFUSSAD) on first-hospitalized patients with schizophrenic or affective disorders: Comparison of psychopathological and psychosocial course and outcome and prediction of chronicity. *European Archives of Psychiatry and Clinical Neuroscience, 260*(5), 367–384.

Moore, T. A., Buchanan, R. W., Buckley, P. F., Chiles, J. A., Conley, R. R., Crismon, M. L., et al. (2007). The Texas Medication Algorithm Project antipsychotic algorithm for schizophrenia: 2006 update. *Journal of Clinical Psychiatry, 68*(11), 1751–1762.

Moore, T. A., Covell, N. H., Essock, S. M., & Miller, A. L. (2007). Real-world antipsychotic treatment practices. *Psychiatric Clinics of North America, 30*(3), 401–416.

Murray, R. M. (2004). A developmental model for similarities and dissimilarities between schizophrenia and bipolar disorder. *Schizophrenia Research, 71*(2–3), 405.

Nasrallah, H. A. (2004). Atypical antipsychotics and metabolic dysregulation evaluating the risk/benefit equation and improving the standard of care. *Journal of Clinical Psychopharmacology, 24*(5), S7–S14.

Novartis. (2010, January). *Clozaril prescribing information.* East Hanover, NJ: Author.

Nyhuis, A. W. (2010). Predictors of switching antipsychotic medications in the treatment of schizophrenia. *BMC psychiatry, 10*(1), 75.

Ongur, D., & Goff, D. C. (2005). Obsessive-compulsive symptoms in schizophrenia: Associated clinical features, cognitive function and medication status. [Research Support, N.I.H., Extramural Research Support, US Gov't, P.H.S. Review]. *Schizophrenia Research, 75*(2–3), 349–362.

Pickar, D., Vinik, J., & Bartko, J. J. (2008). Pharmacotherapy of schizophrenic patients: Preponderance of off-label drug use. *PLoS One, 3*(9), e3150.

Pierre, J. M., Peloian, J. H., Wirshing, D. A., Wirshing, W. C., & Marder, S. R. (2007). A randomized, double-blind, placebo-controlled trial of modafinil for negative symptoms in schizophrenia. *Journal of Clinical Psychiatry, 68*(5), 705–710.

Poyurovsky, M., Fuchs, C., & Weizman, A. (1999). Obsessive-compulsive disorder in patients with first-episode schizophrenia. *American Journal of Psychiatry, 156*(12), 1998–2000.

Rajagopal, G., Graham, J. G., & Haut, F. F. (2007). Prevention of clozapine-induced granulocytopenia/agranulo-cytosis with granulocyte-colony stimulating factor (G-CSF) in an intellectually disabled patient with schizophrenia. *Journal of Intellectual Disability Research, 51*(Pt 1), 82–85.

Rathod, S., Kingdon, D., Smith, P., & Turkington, D. (2005). Insight into schizophrenia: The effects of cognitive behavioural therapy on the components of insight and association with sociodemographics—data on a previously published randomised controlled trial. *Schizophrenia Research, 74*(2–3), 211–219.

Rathod, S., Kingdon, D., Weiden, P., & Turkington, D. (2008). Cognitive-behavioral therapy for medication-resistant schizophrenia: A review. *Journal of Psychiatric Practice, 14*(1), 22–33.

Reutfors, J. (2009). Risk factors for suicide in schizophrenia: Findings from a Swedish population-based case-control study. *Schizophrenia Research, 108*(1–3), 231.

Rohricht, F., & Priebe, S. (2006). Effect of body-oriented psychological therapy on negative symptoms in schizophrenia: A randomized controlled trial. *Psychological Medicine, 36*(5), 669–678.

Rossler, W., Salize, H. J., van Os, J., & Riecher-Rossler, A. (2005). Size of burden of schizophrenia and psychotic disorders. *European Neuropsychopharmacology, 15*(4), 399–409.

Rummel, C., Kissling, W., & Leucht, S. (2006). Antidepressants for the negative symptoms of schizophrenia. [Meta-Analysis Review]. *Cochrane Database of Systematic Reviews, 3*, CD005581.

Sanchez, P., Ojeda, N., Pena, J., Elizagarate, E., Yoller, A. B., Gutierrez, M., et al. (2009). Predictors of longitudinal changes in schizophrenia: The role of processing speed. *Journal of Clinical Psychiatry, 70*(6), 888–896.

Schwarz, C., Volz, A., Li, C., & Leucht, S. (2008). Valproate for schizophrenia. *Cochrane Database of Systematic Revies, 3*, CD004028.

Sensky, T., Turkington, D., Kingdon, D., Scott, J. L., Scott, J., Siddle, R., et al. (2000). A randomized controlled trial of cognitive-behavioral therapy for persistent symptoms in schizophrenia resistant to medication. *Archives of General Psychiatry, 57*(2), 165–172.

Shaner, A., Khalsa, M. E., Roberts, L., Wilkins, J., Anglin, D., & Hsieh, S. C. (1993). Unrecognized cocaine use among schizophrenic patients. *American Journal of Psychiatry, 150*(5), 758–762.

Silverstone, P. H. (1998). Prevention of clozapine-induced neutropenia by pretreatment with lithium. *Journal of Clinical Psychopharmacology, 18*(1), 86–88.

Siris, S. G. (2000). Depression in schizophrenia: Perspective in the era of "Atypical" antipsychotic agents. *American Journal of Psychiatry, 157*(9), 1379–1389.

Sun, J., Maller, J. J., Daskalakis, Z. J., Furtado, C. C., & Fitzgerald, P. B. (2009). Morphology of the corpus callosum in treatment-resistant schizophrenia and major depression. *Acta Psychiatrica Scandinavica, 120*(4), 265–273.

Takeuchi, H. (2008). A randomized, open-label comparison of 2 switching strategies to aripiprazole treatment in patients with schizophrenia add-on, wait, and tapering of previous antipsychotics versus add-on and simultaneous tapering. *Journal of Clinical Psychopharmacology, 28*(5), 540–543.

Tang, W. K., & Ungvari, G. S. (2002). Efficacy of electroconvulsive therapy combined with antipsychotic medication in treatment-resistant schizophrenia: A prospective, open trial. *Journal of ECT, 18*(2), 90–94.

Taylor, D. M., Young, C. L., Mace, S., & Patel, M. X. (2004). Early clinical experience with risperidone long-acting injection: A prospective, 6-month follow-up of 100 patients. *Journal of Clinical Psychiatry, 65*(8), 1076–1083.

Tharyan, P., & Adams, C. E. (2005). Electroconvulsive therapy for schizophrenia. *Cochrane Database of Systematic Reviews, 2*, CD000076.

Thompson, P. M., Vidal, C., Giedd, J. N., Gochman, P., Blumenthal, J., Nicolson, R., et al. (2001). Mapping adolescent brain change reveals dynamic wave of accelerated gray matter loss in very early-onset schizophrenia. *Proceedings of the National Academy of Sciences of the United States of America, 98*(20), 11650–11655.

Tiihonen, J., Halonen, P., Wahlbeck, K., Repo-Tiihonen, E., Hyvarinen, S., Eronen, M., et al. (2005). Topiramate add-on in treatment-resistant schizophrenia: A randomized, double-blind, placebo-controlled, crossover trial. *Journal of Clinical Psychiatry, 66*(8), 1012–1015.

Tiihonen, J., Wahlbeck, K., & Kiviniemi, V. (2009). The efficacy of lamotrigine in clozapine-resistant schizophrenia: A systematic review and meta-analysis. *Schizophrenia Research, 109*(1–3), 10–14.

Tsang, H. W. H. (2008). Self-stigma of people with schizophrenia as predictor of their adherence to psychosocial treatment. *Psychiatric Rehabilitation Journal, 32*(2), 95–104.

Vercammen, A., Knegtering, H., Bruggeman, R., Westenbroek, H. M., Jenner, J. A., Slooff, C. J., et al. (2009). Effects of bilateral repetitive transcranial magnetic stimulation on treatment resistant auditory-verbal hallucinations in schizophrenia: A randomized controlled trial. *Schizophrenia Research, 114*(1–3), 172–179.

Volkow, N. D. (2009). Substance use disorders in schizophrenia—clinical implications of comorbidity. *Schizophrenia Bulletin, 35*(3), 469–472.

Warner, R. (2009). Recovery from schizophrenia and the recovery model. *Current Opinion in Psychiatry, 22*(4), 374–380.

Wirshing, D. A., Boyd, J. A., Meng, L. R., Ballon, J. S., Marder, S. R., & Wirshing, W. C. (2002). The effects of novel antipsychotics on glucose and lipid levels. *Journal of Clinical Psychiatry, 63*(10), 856–865.

Zisook, S., Kasckow, J. W., Golshan, S., Fellows, I., Solorzano, E., Lehman, D., et al. (2009). Citalopram augmentation for subsyndromal symptoms of depression in middle-aged and older outpatients with schizophrenia and schizoaffective disorder: A randomized controlled trial. *Journal of Clinical Psychiatry, 70*(4), 562–571.

Zoccali, R., Muscatello, M. R., Bruno, A., Cambria, R., Mico, U., Spina, E., et al. (2007). The effect of lamotrigine augmentation of clozapine in a sample of treatment-resistant schizophrenic patients: A double-blind, placebo-controlled study. *Schizophrenia Research, 93*(1–3), 109–116.

Management of Treatment-Resistant Substance and Alcohol Abuse

Kathleen T. Brady

Introduction

Alcohol and drug dependence are associated with dramatic costs to society, including lost productivity, social disorder, and increased health care utilization. Studies have estimated that drug dependence costs the United States approximately $67 billion annually in health care costs, crime, lost work productivity, and numerous social problems (Nunes & Levin, 2004; Rice, Kelman, & Miller, 1991). Among the general public, there are a number of negative misperceptions concerning the treatment of addictions. Almost everyone knows at least one person who has been through a treatment program for addictions and relapsed after the end of treatment. Because of this, there is a tendency to conclude that treatment for addictions does not work. However, individuals who are in successful recovery from addictions are not likely to call attention to this fact because of the stigma related to addictive disorders. Considering the prevalence of addictions, it is likely that each one of us interacts daily with numerous individuals who are in successful recovery, but high-profile treatment failures are the ones most likely to make a lasting impression in the public perception of addictions treatment. Successful treatment of addictions leads to substantial improvements in a number of areas, including reduction of alcohol and other drug use, increased personal health and social function, and reduction in threats to public health and safety. Success rates vary according to the type of drug and the population being treated, but 1-year, postdischarge follow-up studies generally find that approximately 40% to 60% of discharged patients have maintained continuous abstinence. Typically, an additional 15% to 30% are not completely abstinent but have not resumed compulsive substance use during this period, indicating reasonable efficacy for the existing treatments for addictions (Finney & Moos, 1992; Gerstein & Harwood, 1990; Hubbard, Craddock, & Anderson, 2003; Institute of Medicine, 1995; McLellan et al., 1995).

According to *DSM-IV-TR*, addictions are by definition "chronic and relapsing disorders" (American Psychiatric Association [APA], 2000), so the expectation of a permanent cure after one treatment episode without adequate continuing care is unrealistic for many individuals with addictions, just as it is for individuals with other chronic disorders. As with other chronic disorders, the only realistic expectation for treatment is patient improvement rather than cure, and continuing care is often essential to maintaining the improvement. Despite this fact, addictions are often viewed as acute conditions; and as such, acute-care procedures, such as detoxification, are sometimes considered appropriate and definitive treatments. Access to a full continuum of care, including residential and long-term continuing care options, is essential for an optimally functioning treatment system. Because of insurance restrictions and other funding limitations, many patients receive only detoxification or acute stabilization with no support for continuing care (McLellan & McKay, 1998; Weisner & Schmidt, 1993). Expensive inpatient facilities do not necessarily provide the most cost-effective answer for long-term management of addictions. Access to supervised living settings, vocational rehabilitation, and other nonmedical, psychosocial support systems can be critical elements in maintaining abstinence, but they may not available or accessible for many individuals. A recent study of the national substance abuse treatment system revealed a lack of medical and other highly trained staff and high staff turnover, which calls into question the ability of the addiction treatment infrastructure to adopt or support effective new therapies, interventions, and medications emerging from research (McLellan, Carise, & Kleber, 2003). These issues are of concern in addressing the area of treatment resistance. In many cases, although efficacious treatments exist, they may not be available to those who need them. In some circumstances what may appear to be a "treatment-resistant" individual is, in fact, a person who does not have access to the treatments that could be efficacious.

Addictions are similar to other chronic medical disorders, such as Type II diabetes and hypertension, in which a confluence of genetic, biological, behavioral, and environmental factors interact to determine the course and severity of the illness. The fact that there is a "volitional" component to addictions has led to the view that addictions are bad behaviors, better managed in the criminal justice system than in the health care system. However, in many chronic disease states there is a volitional component and behavioral choices are critical in determining the effect of treatment. For example, in the case of diabetes and hypertension, behavioral choices such as poor diet, smoking, and lack of exercise play a part in the onset, course, and severity of the disorder. The successful treatment of many chronic medical disorders is dependent on behavioral change and compliance with medications and other treatment recommendations. In a review of over 70 treatment outcome studies for chronic medical disorders, patient compliance was regarded as the most significant determinant of treatment outcome (O'Brien & McLellan, 1996). Similarly, compliance with treatment is an important aspect of successful treatment of addictions and a major factor in treatment resistance.

Assessing and Addressing Specific Issues in Treatment Resistance

Patient Compliance

Studies of treatment response in the area of addictions have shown that patients who comply with the recommended regimen of education, counseling, and medication generally have favorable outcomes during treatment and lasting posttreatment benefits (McLellan, Lewis, O'Brien, & Kleber, 2000). Individual factors such as low socioeconomic status, comorbid psychiatric conditions, and lack of family or social supports for continuing abstinence are all variables associated with lack of compliance in the treatment of addictions. As such, patient compliance is a critical issue in treatment resistance.

The patient's acceptance of a problem and his or her willingness to engage in treatment are important predictors of compliance with recommended treatment. Unfortunately, denial of problems associated with substance use is a core feature of addictions and many individuals with substance use disorders (SUDs) have low motivation to stop using substances. Motivational interviewing (MI) is a patient-centered counseling approach that is specifically designed to enhance motivation to change among individuals who are not ready to change. MI is based on the stages of change model in which the temporal, motivational, and developmental aspects of the process of change are delineated (Prochaska & DiClements, 1992). In moving from recognition of a problem to beginning to take action, individuals move through precontemplation, contemplation, action, and maintenance stages. MI is designed to help build an individual's motivation for change and commitment to change. By employing an empathic interviewing style incorporating a number of strategies, including attempting to elicit self-motivational statements, weighing the pros and cons of changing, and making a change plan, MI can be used to address noncompliance in a nonjudgmental manner. Reflective listening is used to help patients clarify their ambivalence and diffuse resistance (Miller & Rollnick, 1991). MI has been shown to be efficacious across a wide variety of health behavior change areas.

Involving family members or close friends in the treatment plan can also be important in addressing noncompliance. An involved family can encourage the treatment efforts, mobilize social support, and monitor the patient's progress and compliance with medications and subsequent appointments.

Patient compliance is especially important to insuring the effectiveness of medications in the treatment of substance dependence. Although the general area of pharmacotherapy for drug addiction is still developing, there are a number of medications with proven efficacy in relapse prevention in opioid, nicotine, and alcohol dependence. It is important to bear in mind that the use of psychotropic medications is sometimes discouraged in addiction treatment settings in a way that can undermine treatment. Individuals in recovery often have complex and conflicting feelings and attitudes and may see the need for medications as a sign of defectiveness or failure. It is important to discuss the individual's feelings about taking medications, address and minimize medication side effects, and emphasize the need for medication adherence in a proactive manner.

In a number of studies that have looked at interventions designed to improve compliance with treatment across a number of chronic illnesses, almost all of the interventions that were effective for long-term care were complex, including combinations of reminders, self-monitoring, reinforcement, counseling, more convenient care, manual telephone follow-up, and supportive care. In these studies, even the most effective interventions led to only modest improvements in adherence and treatment outcomes (Haynes, Ackloo, Sahota, McDonald, & Yao, 2008). Clearly, more attention to the area of treatment compliance in addictions and other chronic illnesses is of critical importance. Studies applying some of the technologic advances in communication and information processing, such as smart phones and other "real-time" communications devices, would be of particular interest in this regard.

Psychiatric Comorbidity

Individuals with SUDs often have co-occurring psychiatric disorders, which can complicate treatment and result in treatment resistance if undetected. Several large-scale, epidemiologic studies provide data on the prevalence rates of psychiatric disorders in the general population, such as the Epidemiologic Catchment Area (Regier et al., 1990), National Comorbidity Survey (NCS; Kessler, Sonnega, Bromet, Hughes, & Nelson, 1995), and the National Epidemiologic Survey on Alcohol and Related Conditions (NESARC; Grant et al., 2005). As can be seen in Table 12.1, rates of co-occurring mood and anxiety disorders are high among individuals with SUDs in the general population. Rates of these co-occurring disorders tend to be higher among women than men. In the NCS, 72.4% of women diagnosed with alcohol abuse and 86.0% of women diagnosed with alcohol dependence had a lifetime co-occurring mental disorder. Women are also more likely than men to have multiple comorbidities (i.e., three or more co-occurring psychiatric diagnoses in addition to the SUD). The most common psychiatric disorders seen in individuals presenting for treatment of SUDs are affective and anxiety disorders, attention-deficit disorder, and personality disorders. Eating disorders, such as anorexia nervosa, bulimia nervosa, and binge eating disorder, are estimated to be two to three times higher in women than men, and are particularly common among women with SUDs (Grant et al., 2005).

Diagnosis is one of the most difficult challenges in the area of co-occurring psychiatric and SUDs. It is clear that substance use and withdrawal can mimic nearly every psychiatric disorder. Substances of abuse have profound effects on neurotransmitter systems involved in the pathophysiology of anxiety disorders and, with chronic use, may unmask a vulnerability or lead to organic changes that manifest as a psychiatric disorder. The best way to differentiate substance-induced, transient psychiatric symptoms from a psychiatric disorder that warrants treatment is through observation of symptoms during a period of abstinence. Transient substance-related states will improve with time. The duration of abstinence necessary for accurate diagnosis remains controversial and is likely to be based on both the diagnosis being

TABLE 12.1 Rates of Co-Occurring Mood and Anxiety Disorders among Men and Women in the General Population with Substance Use Disorders

	Men	Women
Mood disorders		
Major depression	9.0% to 30.1%	30.1% to 48.5%
Dysthymia	3.6% to 11.2%	10.1% to 20.9%
Bipolar disorders	0.3% to 3.8%	3.8% to 6.8%
Anxiety disorders		
Panic disorder	1.6% to 3.6%	7.3% to 12.0%
Social phobia	10.8% to 19.3%	24.1% to 30.3%
Simple/specific phobia	5.9% to 13.9%	28.2% to 30.7%
Generalized anxiety disorder	2.6% to 8.6%	8.4% to 15.7%

assessed and the substance used. For example, long half-life drugs (e.g., some benzodiazepines) may require several weeks of abstinence for withdrawal symptoms to subside, but shorter acting substances (e.g., alcohol, cocaine, short half-life benzodiazepines) require shorter periods of abstinence to make valid diagnoses. A family history of the psychiatric disorder, the onset of symptoms before the onset of the SUD, and sustained psychiatric symptoms during lengthy periods of abstinence in the past all suggest a psychiatric disorder that warrants treatment.

Appropriate treatment for psychiatric disorders in individuals with SUDs can improve outcomes for both disorders, so careful assessment of psychiatric comorbidity is particularly important in the treatment-resistant individual. A number of studies have found that individuals with co-occurring psychiatric disorders and SUDs have a more complex course of illness with higher health service utilization, including more emergency room visits and hospitalizations, more suicide attempts, and greater medication noncompliance (Strakowski, DelBello, Fleck, & Arndt, 2000).

Research investigating pharmacotherapeutic treatments for co-occurring substance use and psychiatric disorders is progressing rapidly. The appropriate use of medications is becoming increasingly important as data accumulate to suggest that medication treatment of a psychiatric disorder may improve the substance-related outcomes. A recent meta-analysis of studies of the treatment of depression in patients with SUDs found that antidepressant medications had a beneficial effect on depression and substance-related outcomes but was not a stand-alone treatment. Those patients who demonstrated the greatest improvement in the symptoms of depression had the greatest improvement in substance use outcomes (Nunes & Levin, 2004). Buspirone treatment can improve retention in treatment and decrease alcohol use in anxious alcoholics (Kranzler, 1996). Finally, several recent studies have demonstrated that in individuals with co-occurring posttraumatic stress disorder (PTSD) and SUDs, improvement in PTSD symptoms is associated with decreased substance use, whereas decreased substance use does not necessarily lead to improvement in PTSD symptoms (Back, Brady, Sonne, & Verduin, 2006; Hien et al., 2010).

There are several considerations in choosing specific medications. In general, one should use the medications with demonstrated efficacy in the treatment of the psychiatric disorder in question. However, medications that have significant abuse potential, such as benzodiazepines, barbiturates, and stimulants should be avoided. Exceptions to this rule include the use of sedatives during detoxification and in the acute management of anxiety symptoms while other medications begin to take effect. Benzodiazepines may be considered as adjunctive medication during the early treatment phase when activation or latency of onset of the antidepressants is an issue. If a benzodiazepine is prescribed to a patient with a co-occurring SUD, close monitoring for relapse and limited amounts of medication should be given. They should be considered for chronic treatment only when other pharmacological and nonpharmacological treatment options have been exhausted. When the use of a benzodiazepine is indicated, a benzodiazepine with a low abuse potential such as oxazepam and chlordiazepoxide should be considered. Prescribers should also be aware of any toxic interactions between substances of abuse and specific psychotropic medications. For instance, disulfiram inhibits dopamine-beta-hydroxylase and may therefore exacerbate psychosis in individuals with schizophrenia. Finally, because individuals with comorbidity may be particularly susceptible to inadvertent or intentional overdose, the safety profile of the agent should be kept in mind. Fortunately, the newer antidepressant and anxiolytic agents have a more favorable therapeutic window as compared to the tricyclic and monoamine oxidase inhibitor antidepressant agents.

While the use of medications to treat psychiatric disorders in individuals with co-occurring SUDs is gaining broader acceptance, there has been little investigation of the addition of medications specifically targeting substance use to treatment regimens for individuals with co-occurring disorders. Pharmacotherapies specifically targeting SUDs are discussed in more detail later, but several studies investigating the use of these agents in individuals with mood and anxiety disorders have shown promise. In a study of 254 outpatients with alcohol dependence and comorbid psychiatric disorders (primarily PTSD, major depressive disorder, and dysthymia), Petrakis and colleagues (2005) found that patients treated with naltrexone or disulfiram, as compared to placebo, had more consecutive weeks of abstinence and fewer drinking days per week. In comparison to naltrexone-treated participants, disulfiram-treated participants reported less craving from pre- to posttreatment. No clear advantage of combining disulfiram and naltrexone was observed. In a recent study of individuals with co-occurring major depressive disorder and alcohol dependence, Pettinati and colleagues (2010) found that individuals randomized to receive the combination of naltrexone and sertraline had better alcohol-related outcomes and a trend toward decreased depression as compared to individuals who received either medication alone or placebo. These studies suggest that, where possible, adding a medication targeting addiction to the treatment regimen for individuals with co-occurring psychiatric and SUDs can improve treatment outcome.

It is also important to maximize the use of nonpharmacologic treatments. Learning strategies to self-regulate mood and anxiety symptoms can interrupt the cycle of using external agents to combat intolerable subjective states and help individuals to acquire alternative coping strategies. Among psychosocial treatments, cognitive-behavioral therapies are among the most effective for both psychiatric disorders and SUDs. There are now controlled trials of therapies specifically targeting co-occurring SUDs and PTSD and bipolar disorder and a number of preliminary studies in other co-occurring disorders.

Psychosocial Issues

It is important to keep in mind that by the time they present for treatment, most individuals with addictions have problems in multiple life areas that may need to be addressed so that they can derive maximal benefit from addiction-specific treatments. Many have medical problems, marital problems, and financial stressors, including unemployment, and may live in neighborhoods with high levels of crime and drug abuse. Some may be involved in abusive relationships and/or be living with other individuals with active SUDs. Because we know that stress and environmental cues related to substances of abuse are associated with continued vulnerability to relapse, it is important to assess these issues in treatment-resistant cases (Brady & Sinha, 2005). In one study comparing standard methadone services to methadone services enhanced by onsite access to medical/psychiatric, employment, and family therapy, those receiving enhanced services showed significantly better outcomes across a number of functional domains (McLellan, Arndt, Metzger, Woody, & O'Brien, 1993). Case management strategies providing advocacy and coordination of services or residential services, both described later, may be the best solution for individuals whose treatment resistance appears to be related to problems in multiple areas or a nonsupportive living situation.

Approaches to Treatment Resistance
Pharmacotherapy of Addictive Disorders

As advances in knowledge about the neurobiology of addictions grow, the role of medications in the treatment of addictions has become increasingly prominent. Because much of the addiction treatment system has "grown up" outside of traditional medicine, medications are sometimes not considered in treatment planning. In addition, there are still many treatment programs that do not have the necessary medical personnel to evaluate for appropriateness of medication treatment and prescribe as needed (McLellan et al., 2003). In an area where medication treatment is often overlooked entirely, the efficacy of combined medication treatment is profoundly underinvestigated and far from routine practice.

As the development of addictions medications becomes more sophisticated, therapeutic options will increase. For several disorders (i.e., nicotine, opiate and alcohol dependence), there are now multiple medications with established efficacy with differing mechanisms of action. As such, there is clear rationale for the use of some medications in combination with cases of treatment resistance but few controlled trials. In cases of treatment resistance where medications have not been tried, an obvious first step is the addition of a medication for which there is proven efficacy or a medication with some evidence for efficacy in the literature. In cases where one medication has been tried, combination therapy can be a reasonable next step.

In general, there is much variability in the response to medications for the treatment of addictions. Exploration of genetic predictors of pharmacologic response has been an active and fruitful area. No one medication is likely to be safe and efficacious for all individuals. Exploration of genetics-based methods to predict therapeutic response in subgroups of substance-dependent individuals is within reach and should impact treatment choices and the assessment of treatment resistance in the near future (Berritini & Lerman, 2005). It must be noted that pharmacotherapeutic treatment should always be used in conjunction with psychosocial treatment in the management of patients with addictions. Medication options for specific SUDs are briefly reviewed in the following sections.

Nicotine

There are a number of medications with proven efficacy in smoking cessation. The 2008 Public Health Service Clinical Practice Guidelines for nicotine dependence found that five nicotine replacement therapies and two nonnicotine replacement (buproprion SR and varenicline) medications all increased abstinence rates relative to placebo (Fiore et al., 2008).

Nicotine replacement therapy comes in a variety of formulations, including nicotine gum, lozenge, nasal spray and inhaler, and nicotine patch for transdermal administration. In general, nicotine replacement therapy increases smoking cessation rates two- to threefold over behavioral counseling alone (Fiore et al., 2008). Transdermal nicotine replacement is most commonly used and, although effective, only 20%–30% of smokers are able to quit with this form of treatment alone. Dose, duration, and formulation of nicotine replacement can be adjusted to address treatment resistance. The 21 mg patch has been the standard dose for individuals smoking over 10 cigarettes per day, but some studies have reported better outcomes with a 44 mg patch in heavy smokers (Jorenby et al., 1995; Paoletti et al., 1996). With regard to optimal duration of treatment, although meta-analysis and clinical trials (Berritini & Berman, 2005) provide little evidence for improved outcomes beyond 8 weeks of treatment, at least one study showed lower relapse rates with a longer duration of treatment (52 weeks) (Pomerleau et al., 2003). So, while there is not strong support for higher dose or longer duration nicotine replacement therapy overall, the optimal dosage and duration of treatment for subgroups of smokers remain to be determined, and there is some rationale for using higher dose and longer duration of treatment in treatment-resistant individuals. While nicotine lozenge, gum, and nasal spray are not used as commonly as the patch, they may be more effective in some patients as either alone or in combination with the patch. Nicotine nasal spray provides rapid increases in plasma nicotine; and in terms of subjective effect, the nasal spray may most closely mimic cigarette smoking. As such, this could be used as an adjunct to transdermal replacement in high-risk situations for some treatment-resistant patients. Nicotine gum provides oral stimulation that may be of benefit in some patients, but careful instruction concerning appropriate use is essential. Encouraging smokers to sample various delivery systems and to choose the one that is best for them may help in improved utilization and quit rates. There is some suggestion that nicotine replacement therapies are less efficacious in women as compared to men (Cepeda-Benito, Reynoso, & Erath, 2004).

Buproprion SR, an antidepressant medication, has demonstrated efficacy in smoking cessation. A Cochrane Review of 19 buproprion SR trials indicates that it doubles quit rates as compared to placebo, and pooled analyses show quit rates similar to nicotine replacement therapy (Hughes, Stead, & Lancaster, 2004). Bupropion has demonstrated particular efficacy in the treatment of women (Collins et al., 2004; Gonzales et al., 2002), African Americans (Ahluwalia, Harris, Catley, Okuyemi, & Mayo, 2002), and smokers with higher levels of nicotine dependence (Dale et al., 2001). Buproprion SR can decrease the weight gain associated with quitting smoking, which can be an important barrier to quitting (Hays et al., 2001). Varenicline is a partial agonist at the neuronal nicotinic acetylcholine receptor with demonstrated efficacy in smoking cessation. Controlled trials comparing varenicline to placebo and buproprion SR demonstrated that the odds of quitting smoking with 1 mg BID of varenicline were almost quadrupled compared to placebo and almost doubled compared to buproprion SR 150 mg BID at 12 weeks (Gonzales et al., 2006; Jorenby et al., 2006). A number of troubling psychiatric side effects have been reported with varenicline treatment, including nightmares, disinhibition, and suicidal ideation.

Combination therapy in the treatment of nicotine dependence is an underinvestigated area. As the agents described earlier have differing mechanisms of action and/or different pharmacokinetic profiles, there is good rationale for combination therapy in treatment-resistant patients. A number of studies suggest that combination nicotine replacement therapy is more effective than monotherapy (Fiore et al., 2008; Piper et al., 2009). In particular, combining short-acting nicotine replacement therapy (gum, lozenge, inhaler, or nasal spray) with the transdermal patch gives the benefit of a steady plasma level of nicotine supplied by the patch and the ability to supplement with short-acting formulations as needed for coping with high-risk situations and transient urges to smoke. In a recent randomized, placebo-controlled trial comparing five smoking cessation therapies, including buproprion and nicotine replacement therapy alone and in combination, nicotine patch plus lozenge produced the greatest benefit relative to placebo for smoking cessation (Piper et al., 2009). In one study in which patients were encouraged to use combinations of one or more long-acting medications (patch/buproprion) with one or more short-acting nicotine replacement therapies, a higher number of medications predicted greater abstinence at 4 weeks, but not at 6 months (Steinberg, Foulds, Richardson, Burke, & Shah, 2006). The efficacy of combined varenicline and either nicotine replacement therapy or buproprion has not been studied; however, varenicline's mechanism of action as a partial nicotinic agonist could prevent the binding of nicotine from the nicotine replacement therapy and therefore interfere with the mechanism of action. In addition, pharmacokinetic studies of combined nicotine patch and varenicline demonstrated a greater number of patients discontinuing medications because of adverse events as compared to either treatment alone, so this combination is not recommended at present (http://media.pfizer.com/files/products/uspi_chantix.pdf).

Alcohol

A growing body of evidence suggests that pharmacotherapy, in conjunction with psychosocial interventions, is the best treatment option for individuals with alcohol dependence. Alcohol use disorders are extremely heterogeneous, and there is a great deal of variability in individual response to pharmacotherapeutic treatments for relapse prevention. Although the area remains somewhat controversial, here are at least two subtypes of alcohol dependence that are widely recognized (Cloninger, 1987). Type A alcoholism is characterized by a later onset of alcohol dependence (>25 years) and low familial loading. Type B is early-onset alcohol dependence (<25 years), characterized by high familial loading and a broad range of impulse control problems. The key question is distinguishing these two types of alcohol dependence is age of onset. This typology is of importance in a discussion of pharmacotherapeutic treatments and treatment resistance because age of onset of alcohol dependence has proven to be important in predicting treatment response to some of the agents to be discussed.

There are currently four FDA-approved agents for relapse prevention in alcohol dependence: disulfiram, acamprosate, oral naltrexone, and the once-monthly injectable, extended-release naltrexone. Disulfiram alters normal metabolism of ingested alcohol to produce mildly toxic acetaldehyde, resulting in an aversive reaction characterized by vomiting, flushing, headache, and anxiety. Clinical studies do not clearly support the efficacy of disulfiram for the treatment of alcoholism in comparison to placebo; however, none of the larger studies investigating the use of disulfiram used systematic techniques to enhance compliance (Garbutt, West, Carey, Lohr, & Crews, 1999). One advantage of disulfiram is that it fosters complete abstinence, and studies suggest that it can be effective in some patients if combined with monitored dosing ingestion to insure compliance.

Naltrexone is a mu receptor opiate antagonist that has demonstrated efficacy in decreasing alcohol "craving," drinks consumed per occasion, drinking days, and lower rates of relapse as compared to placebo in alcohol-dependent patients (Bouza, Angeles, Munoz, & Amate, 2004). However, the naltrexone data are somewhat inconsistent with only 13 of the 19 most recent clinical trials demonstrating a clear benefit of naltrexone on alcohol-related outcomes.

While the relatively small effect size for naltrexone is one determinant of the inconsistency in results of naltrexone trials, recent evidence suggests that genetic variability also plays a role in the variable response to naltrexone as a functional polymorphism of the μ-opioid receptor gene (OPRM1) and appears to predict positive response to naltrexone with regard to relapse prevention (Anton et al., 2008). Family histories of alcohol dependence and strong cravings or urges to use alcohol have also been associated with good clinical response to naltrexone (Monterosso et al., 2001). While 50 mg/day is the most commonly used dose for alcohol relapse prevention, women appear to be more sensitive to naltrexone-induced nausea, and dose reduction may be important to improving compliance. Alternatively, studies have demonstrated that 100 mg/day is well tolerated by many individuals, so dose escalation should be considered in any individual who is tolerating the medication well but has suboptimal outcomes.

The extended-release formulation of naltrexone may be preferable to oral naltrexone for a number of reasons. By maintain relatively constant plasma levels through slow but regular release of naltrexone, depot naltrexone may be associated with fewer side effects and relatively greater exposure to the therapeutic dose of the drug. In addition, depot naltrexone is useful in addressing problems with medication compliance. In a large controlled trial, one extended-release formulation of naltrexone (Vivitrol 380 mg) was associated with significantly less drinking as compared to placebo for men, but not women (Garbutt et al., 2005). Reasons for this gender difference are not clear, but it must be taken into consideration when considering the use of Vivitrol for treatment-resistant patients.

Acamprosate is a partial NMDA-agonist that has demonstrated reductions in drinking days and increased length of abstinence in alcohol-dependent individuals in several long-term, double-blind, placebo-controlled trials conducted in Europe (Mann, Lehert, & Morgan, 2004). As with naltrexone, the data have been inconsistent and there have been several recent negative trials in the United States (Johnson, 2008). Again, the reasons for this variability in effectiveness are not entirely clear, but the small effect size, coupled with the severity of alcohol dependence, shorter period of sobriety before starting the trial, and the lack of social support for individuals in the US studies may explain the lack of demonstrated efficacy. Because of these inconsistent results and small effect size, acamprosate treatment would not be recommended for the treatment-resistant patient.

There are several other agents under investigation that have shown considerable promise in the treatment of alcohol dependence. Topiramate, an anticonvulsant agent that works through the GABA system, has been shown in two large, placebo-controlled trials to reduce heavy drinking and increase abstinence (Johnson et al., 2007). Baclofen is another GABA-ergic agent, which may be particularly useful in patients with alcoholic liver disease because it is excreted primarily through the kidneys (Addolorato et al., 2007). Ondansetron is a 5-HT3 antagonist that appears to be efficacious in early onset alcohol dependence (Johnson, 2008).

Because the biological basis of alcohol dependence is multifactorial, the idea of combination medication therapy is appealing but understudied. The combination of naltrexone and acamprosate has been studied because their differing proposed mechanisms of action should allow this combination to address several of the neurobiologic systems involved in alcohol dependence. However, in the recently completed COMBINE study, the group who received naltrexone and acamprosate did not have better outcomes than those who received naltrexone alone, so there are no data to support this combination in the treatment-resistant patient (Anton et al., 2006). However, there are still many other medication combinations that make sense mechanistically but have not been studied in clinical trials. Preliminary clinical evidence suggests that the combination of ondansetron and naltrexone may result in added or synergistic therapeutic effects on alcohol drinking, but larger confirmatory studies are needed (Johnson, 2010). Other combination therapies can certainly be considered in the treatment-resistant patient, but it must be kept in mind that these combinations create the potential for reduced compliance, heightened or new treatment-emergent adverse events, or even decreased efficacy if the medications counteract one another. Clearly, this is an area that warrants further systematic investigation.

Opioid Dependence

Opioid agonists, partial agonists, and antagonists are the three primary types of medications available for the treatment of opioid dependence. Agonist medications, such as methadone hydrochloride, may be prescribed in the short term for detoxification protocol or as a maintenance regimen. The long-term effects of detoxification alone, without continuing treatment, are uniformly poor, so if an individual has a poor outcome following opiate detoxification, maintenance therapy should be considered (Mattick & Hall, 1996).

The goal of maintenance treatment is to provide a prescribed opioid agonist (either methadone or buprenorphine) to deter and ideally eliminate use of illicit opioids. Methadone is a mu opioid agonist. As a maintenance medication, methadone's oral route of administration, slow onset of action, and long half-life have been effective in reducing illicit opiate use, crime, and the spread of infectious diseases, as was validated by a National Institutes of Health Consensus Conference (1998). When moderate daily methadone doses (40 to 50 mg) were compared to high daily methadone doses (80 to 100 mg), there was significantly lower illicit opioid use in the high-dose group (Strain, Bigelow, Liebson, & Stitzer, 1999). Similar findings have been reported in regard to treatment retention, with one study showing that patients receiving 80 mg per day of methadone were twice as likely to remain in treatment as those receiving 60 to 79 mg, and four times as likely to remain in treatment when compared to patients receiving less than 60 mg methadone per day. The lowest effective dose of methadone is now widely accepted to be approximately 50 mg, with an optimum average dose for most patients of approximately 80 mg (± 20 mg), although some patients require a dose higher than this range. In cases where higher doses are used, methadone serum levels are obtained to guide dosing. One of the major issues in treatment resistance for individuals in methadone maintenance is underdosing of methadone.

Barriers to patients entering licensed methadone treatment programs include state and federal regulations for program admittance, limited number of programs, the need for daily appointments at the clinic to get the medication, and the social stigma associated with methadone treatment centers. Buprenorphine hydrochloride is a partial mu-agonist that is administered sublingually and is active for approximately 24 to 36 hours (Bickel & Amass, 1995). Unlike methadone, which must be prescribed in the context of a licensed methadone treatment program, buprenorphine can be prescribed in an office-based practice if physicians receive training and obtain a waiver to prescribe buprenorphine. Large double-blind, placebo-controlled trials of buprenorphine have shown reductions in opiate use comparable to methadone treatment but with fewer withdrawal symptoms on discontinuation

(O'Connor et al., 1998). The combination of buprenorphine plus naloxone hydrochloride (suboxone), designed to reduce injection use of the compound, is now available for prescription in primary care settings. One recent study investigated a "stepped care" approach to opiate agonist therapy in which heroin-dependent individuals were randomized to traditional methadone maintenance or suboxone with escalation to methadone maintenance as needed (Kakko et al., 2007). Among completers, 46% of those who were started in suboxone remained on suboxone with increasing negative urine drug screens in both groups. This suggests that suboxone can be a reasonable alternative to methadone maintenance, even in heroin-dependent individuals. Suboxone may be the preferable agonist therapy for the growing group of individuals who are addicted to prescription opiates because it can be prescribed in general outpatient services and thus its use is less disruptive to daily life schedules.

Opioid antagonists, such as naltrexone, block the actions of heroin through competitive binding for 48 to 72 hours. Compliance with naltrexone in opiate-dependent individuals is often poor and, in general, it is not considered a first-line treatment. However, in select populations where consequences of relapse are dramatic, such as a medical professional whose licensure is at risk if relapse occurs, naltrexone may be the treatment of choice. Naltrexone in combination with social or criminal justice sanctions is routinely used in the monitored treatment of physicians, nurses, and other professionals. As such, naltrexone should be considered in the treatment of any treatment-resistant individual who is interested in staying free of any opioid effects. Naltrexone can be used as a maintenance medication, or as an "insurance policy" for usage as needed in situations where the patient is likely to be confronted with relapse risks.

As mentioned earlier, a long-acting preparation of naltrexone has been developed and tested in the treatment of alcohol dependence. The potential applicability of this agent to the treatment of opiate-dependent individuals is clear. The FDA recently approved Vivitrol for the treatment of opioid dependence, but there are few controlled studies. One issue that must be kept in mind with the use of either form of naltrexone is that individuals who are physically dependent on opiates will experience precipitated withdrawal with naltrexone administration, so a test dose of a shorter acting opioid agonist (naloxone) should be administered to test for physical dependence before initiating naltrexone therapy, in particular, the long-acting form of naltrexone. While more research is warranted, long-acting naltrexone is an option to be considered in the opiate-dependent individual, particularly if medication compliance is an issue.

Stimulant Dependence

The search for a pharmacotherapeutic treatment for cocaine dependence has been extremely active over the last 20 years with controlled trials of antidepressants, anticonvulsants, dopamine agonists and antagonists, and many other agents. Unfortunately, many trials are flawed by large dropout rates and medication noncompliance, and there are no medications with clearly demonstrated efficacy in the treatment of cocaine or amphetamine dependence to date.

However, some of the agents tested have shown promise and could be considered for use in the treatment-resistant stimulant-dependent individual. Modafinil is a mild stimulant and glutamatergic agent that is FDA approved for the treatment of narcolepsy. In a single-site placebo-controlled trial, Dackis and colleagues found that modafinil-treated cocaine-dependent subjects submitted significantly more cocaine negative urines and were rated as more improved than the placebo-treated subjects (Dackis, Kampman, Lynch, Pettinati, & O'Brien, 2005). In a larger multisite trial, modafinil was not superior to placebo in promoting cocaine abstinence in the whole study group; however, in the subjects who were not dependent on both alcohol and cocaine (cocaine-dependent only), modafinil was superior to placebo (Anderson et al., 2009). Several other trials of modafinil are ongoing, but the medication is well tolerated and may be useful in reducing cocaine withdrawal symptoms and helping some cocaine-dependent individuals to attain abstinence. There have also been several promising studies with topiramate, an anticonvulsant agent that impacts glutamatergic neurotransmission and has shown promise in the treatment of alcohol dependence (see earlier discussion). In one placebo-controlled trial, topiramate-treated subjects were more likely to achieve 3 weeks of continuous abstinence and were more likely to be rated as clinically improved (Kampman et al., 2004). In addition to its effects on alcohol metabolism, disulfiram blocks the enzymatic degradation of both cocaine and dopamine. It has been hypothesized that increased dopamine levels may help improve hedonic tone in cocaine-dependent individuals, and the increased cocaine levels have been shown to increase cocaine-related anxiety and dysphoria in individuals pretreated with disulfiram (Hameedi et al., 1995). Regardless of the mechanism, four clinical trials to date have demonstrated that disulfiram reduces cocaine use in cocaine-dependent patients (Carroll et al., 2004; George et al., 2000). As such, disulfiram should definitely be considered in treatment-resistant cocaine dependence as long as the individual is willing to remain alcohol free and understands the potential for increased toxicity if he or she uses cocaine.

There are a number of other promising pharmacotherapeutic treatments for stimulant dependence under investigation. Agents that modulate GABA-ergic and glutamatergic systems, such as vigabatrin and N-acetylcysteine, have shown excellent effects in animal models of cocaine dependence and are currently being tested in clinical trials. Human studies of a vaccine that promotes the development of cocaine-specific antibodies have been promising (Martell, Mitchell, Poling, Gonsai, & Kosten, 2005; Martell et al., 2009).

Mood and anxiety disorders are extremely prevalent in cocaine-dependent individuals. In particular, the rates of PTSD in cocaine-dependent individuals are high and several studies have demonstrated that improvement in PTSD symptoms is often associated with decreased substance use. As discussed earlier, the index of suspicion for psychiatric comorbidity should be high when evaluating treatment-resistant cocaine-dependent patients.

Marijuana

As with the stimulants, there are no medications with clearly demonstrated efficacy for the treatment of marijuana dependence. However, a number of marketed medications have been investigated and some of these have shown promise. As such, in the treatment-resistant marijuana-dependent individuals, there is some justification for judicious and well-documented augmentation of psychosocial treatment with a medication trial.

Many individuals with marijuana dependence experience withdrawal symptoms, characterized by depressed mood, anxiety, irritability, and sleep disturbance, which can contribute to relapse (Budney, Vandrey, Hughes, Moore, & Bahrenburg, 2007). Studies have demonstrated that dronabinol, a synthetic formulation of THC, which is the active constituent in marijuana, can suppress symptoms of marijuana withdrawal (Budney et al., 2007; Haney et al., 2008). Unfortunately, studies investigating the relapse prevention potential of dronabinol (Haney et al., 2008; Levin et al., 2011) have not demonstrated a positive effect. As such, short-term, tapering agonist therapy may be useful in helping an individual to attain abstinence from marijuana by relieving withdrawal symptoms that could lead to continued use, but there is no evidence to suggest that continuing a marijuana-dependent individual on agonist therapy will help in achieving long-term abstinence. As with stimulant dependence, many marijuana-dependent individuals have psychiatric comorbidity. In treatment-resistant cases, it is particularly important to carefully assess and treat co-occurring psychiatric disorders.

Case Management

Case management is a set of social service functions that help individuals with SUDs access resources necessary for recovery, including assessment, planning, linking, monitoring, and advocacy (Vanderplasschen, Rapp, Wolf, & Broekaert, 2004). SUD patients frequently receive services from multiple agencies and providers and case management provides coordination from a single point. Case management services are expected to (1) coordinate outpatient substance abuse treatment, mental health treatment if needed, medical care, and social services; (2) utilize psychosocial rehabilitation and social skills training to increase psychosocial functioning; and (3) broker resources to expand employment, financial, and social support (Alexander, Pollack, Nahra, Wells, & Lemak, 2007). The number of randomized and controlled trials examining case management is relatively small, and the literature is difficult to interpret because there is much variability in the level and type of services available (Vanderplasschen, Wolf, Rapp, & Broekaert, 2007). Nevertheless, case management is associated with improved retention in treatment (Laken & Ager, 1996; Mejta, Bokos, Mickenberg, Maslar, & Senay, 1997), improved use of medical care (Saleh et al., 2002), and improved employment (Siegal et al., 1996) reduced use of inpatient services, improved quality of life, and high customer satisfaction (Vanderplasschen et al., 2007). Case management has been used most intensively in the treatment of substance abusers with comorbid severe and persistent mental illnesses. However, case management is likely to be extremely helpful in the treatment-resistant individual who has multiple life problems that appear to be interfering with recovery. Unfortunately, case management is costly and time intensive and resources to provide case management are rarely available in the public substance use treatment system.

Residential Treatment

After a relatively brief period of intensive services or detoxification, many individuals with addictions are not ready for independent living in the community. Residential treatment should also be considered for individuals whose current living arrangements do not support their sobriety. Transitional residential community care is available in many areas of the country to address this need. These programs, commonly called community residential treatment facilities (CRFs) or halfway houses, differ based on philosophy and the number and type of health, mental health, treatment, rehabilitative, and vocational services available to residents. Psychosocial model CRFs provide primarily psychological services such as individual and group therapy, living and social skills training, and self-help groups without regularly scheduled medical or psychiatric care. Supportive rehabilitative CRFs offer work training or therapy and more specialized services such as recreational and occupational therapy in addition to the services listed previously. Intensive treatment model CRFs also supply medical/ psychiatric services, couples/family counseling, nutrition counseling, spiritual counseling, and medications (Moos, Pettit, & Gruber, 1995). In an analysis of approximately 2,800 individuals assessed at admission and discharge from a representative sample of 88 CRFs, the length of stay averaged approximately 42 days, and greater lengths of stay were associated with lower inpatient readmission rates (Moos & King, 1997). In a later study, CRFs with a more structured treatment approach had better retention rates and substance abuse outcomes as compared to programs with a more generic approach (Moos, Finney, Ouimette, & Suchinsky, 1999). While there is a great deal of variability in CRFs, structured, abstinence-oriented residential programs should definitely be considered for the treatment-resistant individual. In particular, these programs are indicated for individuals who have relapsed repeatedly following detoxification and short-stay inpatient programs. As with case management, accessibility of CRFs in the public system is very limited. However, the Veterans Administration Medical Centers have an excellent system of community residential facilities.

Therapeutic community (TC) is a specific type of residential program in which the purposeful use of the community is the primary method for facilitating change. Goals for TC treatment are global changes in identity and lifestyle involving abstinence from substances, employment, cessation of antisocial behavior, and prosocial values (De Leon, 1995). Traditional TCs typically have a 15- to 24-month stay, have clear rules and expectations, and provide a great deal of structure. Oxford House is a TC initiative with over 1,200 residential facilities across the United States. Each house is a rented, financially self-supported multibedroom home for same-sex occupants. Residents live without professional treatment staff and are free to choose which, if any, type of treatment they desire in the context of a supportive abstinent communal setting. There are few systematic studies of TCs; however, one study of 150 substance-dependent individuals randomized following inpatient treatment to either an Oxford House or treatment as usual showed promising results (Jason et al., 2007). Persons living in an Oxford House had significantly lower substance use, higher monthly income, and lower incarceration rates at 12 months. At 24 months, residents with a ≥6-month stay had a 16% relapse rate as compared to 46% in those with less than a 6-month stay. Both, however, were lower than the 65% rate of relapse in the treatment-as-usual group. These results are particularly impressive because most patients who enter TCs have histories of multiple substance use treatments and significant psychosocial dysfunction. It is important to note that there is no required professional involvement in the management and day-to-day function of Oxford Houses and many TCs, so there is a great deal of variability in the quality of the therapeutic environment. Patients must carefully evaluate their "fit" within the particular TC under consideration.

Contingency Management

Skinnerian operant conditioning principles provide the theoretical underpinning for contingency management. Using contingency management, the consequences for continued substance abuse are altered, by introducing incentives (e.g., methadone dose increases, money, vouchers for valued items) to reduce attractiveness of illicit drug use and increase attractiveness of abstinence and prosocial behaviors (Stitzer, Bigelow, & Gross, 1989).

A meta-analysis of contingency management studies conducted in methadone maintenance populations found it to be more effective than usual care in reducing illicit opiate abuse (Griffith, Rowan-Szal, Roark, & Simpson, 2000) and more effective than standard treatment in cocaine-dependent individuals (Higgins et al., 1994; Silverman et al., 1996). Contingency management demonstrated greatest improvements when using the most powerful incentives (increases in methadone dose and methadone take-home privileges), an immediate reinforcement schedule targeting a single drug (e.g., illicit opiates, cocaine, and alcohol), and frequent urine drug screens to verify abstinence. Recent studies have demonstrated the successful use of low-cost contingency management strategies in community treatment settings (Petry et al., 2005). In addition, a number of studies have demonstrated that contingency management combined with medications appears to augment the efficacy of the medication treatment, particularly in the early phases of treatment during the initiation of abstinence (Kampman, 2010). While the use of contingency management should be considered in any treatment-resistant individual, training and experience in developing a contingency management strategy to fit a specific individual or program is essential.

Conclusions

Substance use disorders continue to be a significant public health problem in the United States and throughout the world. While there are many treatment options available and even more under development, the full continuum of treatment is not available to most people because of underfunding of the public treatment system and limits on insurance coverage of treatment for addictions. Despite increasing knowledge about the neurobiology of addictions and consequent development of efficacious pharmacotherapies, medications are vastly underutilized, particularly in the treatment of alcohol dependence. Psychiatric comorbidity is underdiagnosed and psychosocial issues are often difficult to address, both contributing to treatment resistance. Efforts focused on improving compliance, reducing the stigma associated with SUDs, and improving access to treatment would go a long way toward addressing much of the treatment resistance in addictions.

Disclosure Statement

K.T.B. has served as a consultant for Pfizer, Cephalon, and Ovation Pharmaceutical Companies.

References

Addolorato, G., Leggio, L., Ferrulli, A., Cardone, S., Vonghia, L., Mirijello, A., Gasbarrini, G. (2007). Effectiveness and safety of baclofen for maintenance of alcohol abstinence in alcohol-dependent patients with liver cirrhosis: Randomised, double-blind controlled study. *Lancet, 370*(9603), 1915–1922.

Ahluwalia, J. S., Harris, K. J., Catley, D., Okuyemi, K. S., & Mayo, M. S. (2002). Sustained-release bupropion for smoking cessation in African Americans: A randomized controlled trial. *Journal of the American Medical Association, 288*(4), 468–474.

Alexander, J. A., Pollack, H., Nahra, T., Wells, R., & Lemak, C. H. (2007). Case management and client access to health and social services in outpatient substance abuse treatment. *Journal of Behavioral Health Services and Research, 34*(3), 221–236.

American Psychiatric Association. (2000). *Diagnostic and statistical manual of mental disorders* (4th ed., text rev.) Washington, DC: Author.

Anderson, A. L., Reid, M. S., Li, S. H., Holmes, T., Shemanski, L., Slee, A., Elkashef, A. M. (2009). Modafinil for the treatment of cocaine dependence. *Drug and Alcohol Dependency, 104*(1–2), 133–139.

Anton, R. F., O'Malley, S. S., Ciraulo, D. A., Cisler, R. A., Couper, D., Donovan, D. M., Zweben, A. (2006). Combined pharmacotherapies and behavioral interventions for alcohol dependence: The COMBINE study: A randomized controlled trial. *Journal of the American Medical Association, 295*(17), 2003–2017.

Anton, R. F., Oroszi, G., O'Malley, S., Couper, D., Swift, R., Pettinati, H., & Goldman, D. (2008). An evaluation of mu-opioid receptor (OPRM1) as a predictor of naltrexone response in the treatment of alcohol dependence: Results from the Combined Pharmacotherapies and Behavioral Interventions for Alcohol Dependence (COMBINE) study. *Archives of General Psychiatry, 65*(2), 135–144.

Back, S. E., Brady, K. T., Sonne, S. C., & Verduin, M. L. (2006). Symptom improvement in co-occurring PTSD and alcohol dependence. *Journal of Nervous and Mental Disease, 194*(9), 690–696.

Berrettini, W. H., & Lerman, C. E. (2005). Pharmacotherapy and pharmacogenetics of nicotine dependence. *American Journal of Psychiatry, 162*(8), 1441–1451. doi: 10.1176/appi.ajp.162.8.1441

Bickel, W. K., & Amass, L. (1995). Buprenorphine treatment of opioid dependence. *Eperimental and Clinical Psychopharmacology, 3*(4), 477–489.

Bouza, C., Angeles, M., Munoz, A., & Amate, J. M. (2004). Efficacy and safety of naltrexone and acamprosate in the treatment of alcohol dependence: A systematic review. *Addiction, 99*(7), 811–828.

Brady, K. T., & Sinha, R. (2005). Co-occurring mental and substance use disorders: the neurobiological effects of chronic stress. *American Journal of Psychiatry, 162*(8), 1483–1493.

Budney, A. J., Vandrey, R. G., Hughes, J. R., Moore, B. A., & Bahrenburg, B. (2007). Oral delta-9-tetrahydrocannabinol suppresses cannabis withdrawal symptoms. *Drug and Alcohol Dependency, 86*(1), 22–29.

Carroll, K. M., Fenton, L. R., Ball, S. A., Nich, C., Frankforter, T. L., Shi, J., & Rounsaville, B. J. (2004). Efficacy of disulfiram and cognitive behavior therapy in cocaine-dependent outpatients: A randomized placebo-controlled trial. *Archives of General Psychiatry, 61*(3), 264–272.

Cepeda-Benito, A., Reynoso, J. T., & Erath, S. (2004). Meta-analysis of the efficacy of nicotine replacement therapy for smoking cessation: Differences between men and women. *Journal of Consulting and Clinical Psychology, 72*(4), 712–722.

Cloninger, C. R. (1987). Neurogenetic adaptive mechanisms in alcoholism. *Science, 236*, 410–416.

Collins, B. N., Wileyto, E. P., Patterson, F., Rukstalis, M., Audrain-McGovern, J., Kaufmann, V., Lerman, C. (2004). Gender differences in smoking cessation in a placebo-controlled trial of bupropion with behavioral counseling. *Nicotine and Tobacco Research, 6*(1), 27–37.

Dackis, C. A., Kampman, K. M., Lynch, K. G., Pettinati, H. M., & O'Brien, C. P. (2005). A double-blind, placebo-controlled trial of modafinil for cocaine dependence. *Neuropsychopharmacology, 30*(1), 205–211.

Dale, L. C., Glover, E. D., Sachs, D. P., Schroeder, D. R., Offord, K. P., Croghan, I. T., & Hurt, R. D. (2001). Bupropion for smoking cessation: Predictors of successful outcome. *Chest, 119*(5), 1357–1364.

De Leon, G. (1995). Therapeutic communities for addictions: A theoretical framework. *International Journal of Addiction, 30*(12), 1603–1645.

Finney, J. W., & Moos, R. H. (1992). The long-term course of treated alcoholism: II. Predictors and correlates of 10-year functioning and mortality. *Journal of Studies on Alcohol and Drugs, 53*(2), 142–153.

Fiore, M. C., Jaen, C. R., Baker, T. B., Bailey, W. C., Benowitz, N. L., Curry, S. J., Wewers, M. E. (2008). *Treating tobacco use and dependence: 2008 Update*. Washington, DC: US Department of Health and Human Services, Public Health Service.

Garbutt, J. C., Kranzler, H. R., O'Malley, S. S., Gastfriend, D. R., Pettinati, H. M., Silverman, B. L., Ehrich, E. W. (2005). Efficacy and tolerability of long-acting injectable naltrexone for alcohol dependence: A randomized controlled trial. *Journal of the American Medical Association, 293*(13), 1617–1625.

Garbutt, J. C., West, S. L., Carey, T. S., Lohr, K. N., & Crews, F. T. (1999). Pharmacological treatment of alcohol dependence: A review of the evidence. *Journal of the American Medical Association, 281*(14), 1318–1325.

George, T. P., Chawarski, M. C., Pakes, J., Carroll, K. M., Kosten, T. R., & Schottenfeld, R. S. (2000). Disulfiram versus placebo for cocaine dependence in buprenorphine-maintained subjects: A preliminary trial. *Biological Psychiatry, 47*(12), 1080–1086.

Gerstein, D. R., & Harwood, H. J. (1990). *Treating drug problems: A study of the evolution*, effectiveness, and financing of public and private drug treatment systems. Washington, DC: National Academy Press.

Gonzales, D., Bjornson, W., Durcan, M. J., White, J. D., Johnston, J. A., Buist, A. S., Hurt, R. D. (2002). Effects of gender on relapse prevention in smokers treated with bupropion SR. *American Journal of Preventive Medicine, 22*(4), 234–239.

Gonzales, D., Rennard, S. I., Nides, M., Oncken, C., Azoulay, S., Billing, C. B., Reeves, K. R. (2006). Varenicline, an alpha4beta2 nicotinic acetylcholine receptor partial agonist, vs sustained-release bupropion and placebo for smoking cessation: A randomized controlled trial. *Journal of the American Medical Association*, 296(1), 47–55.

Grant, B. F., Hasin, D. S., Blanco, C., Stinson, F. S., Chou, S. P., Goldstein, R. B., Huang, B. (2005). The epidemiology of social anxiety disorder in the United States: Results from the National Epidemiologic Survey on Alcohol and Related Conditions. *Journal of Clinical Psychiatry*, 66(11), 1351–1361.

Griffith, J. D., Rowan-Szal, G. A., Roark, R. R., & Simpson, D. D. (2000). Contingency management in outpatient methadone treatment: A meta-analysis. *Drug and Alcohol Dependency*, 58(1–2), 55–66.

Hameedi, F. A., Rosen, M. I., McCance-Katz, E. F., McMahon, T. J., Price, L. H., Jatlow, P. I., Kosten, T. R. (1995). Behavioral, physiological, and pharmacological interaction of cocaine and disulfiram in humans. *Biological Psychiatry*, 37(8), 560–563.

Haney, M., Hart, C. L., Vosburg, S. K., Comer, S. D., Reed, S. C., & Foltin, R. W. (2008). Effects of THC and lofexidine in a human laboratory model of marijuana withdrawal and relapse. *Psychopharm*, 197(1), 157–168.

Haynes, R. B., Ackloo, E., Sahota, N., McDonald, H. P., & Yao, X. (2008). Interventions for enhancing medication adherence. *Cochrane Database of Systematic Reviews*, 2, CD000011.

Hays, J. T., Hurt, R. D., Rigotti, N. A., Niaura, R., Gonzales, D., Durcan, M. J., White, J. D. (2001). Sustained-release bupropion for pharmacologic relapse prevention after smoking cessation: A randomized, controlled trial. *Annals of Internal Medicine*, 135(6), 423–433.

Hien, D. A., Jiang, H., Campbell, A. N., Hu, M. C., Miele, G. M., Cohen, L. R., Nunes, E. V. (2010). Do treatment improvements in PTSD severity affect substance use outcomes? A secondary analysis from a randomized clinical trial in NIDA's Clinical Trials Network. *American Journal of Psychiatry*, 167(1), 95–101.

Higgins, S. T., Budney, A. J., Bickel, W. K., Foerg, F. E., Donham, R., & Badger, G. J. (1994). Incentives improve outcome in outpatient behavioral treatment of cocaine dependence. *Archives of General Psychiatry*, 51(7), 568–576.

Hubbard, R. L., Craddock, S. G., & Anderson, J. (2003). Overview of 5-year followup outcomes in the drug abuse treatment outcome studies (DATOS). *Journal of Substance Abuse and Treatment*, 25(3), 125–134.

Hughes, J., Stead, L., & Lancaster, T. (2004). Antidepressants for smoking cessation. *Cochrane Database of Systematic Reviews*, 4, CD000031.

Institute of Medicine. (1995). *Development of medications for the treatment of opiate and cocaine addictions: Issues for the government and private sector*. Washington, DC: National Academy Press.

Jason, L. A., Olson, B. D., Ferrari, J. R., Majer, J. M., Alvarez, J., & Stout, J. (2007). An examination of main and interactive effects of substance abuse recovery housing on multiple indicators of adjustment. *Addiction*, 102(7), 1114–1121.

Johnson, B. A. (2008). Update on neuropharmacological treatments for alcoholism: Scientific basis and clinical findings. *Biochemical Pharmacology*, 75(1), 34–56.

Johnson, B. A. (2010). Medication treatment of different types of alcoholism. *American Journal of Psychiatry*, 167(6), 630–639.

Johnson, B. A., Rosenthal, N., Capece, J. A., Wiegand, F., Mao, L., Beyers, K., Swift, R. M. (2007). Topiramate for treating alcohol dependence: A randomized controlled trial. *Journal of the American Medical Association*, 298(14), 1641–1651.

Jorenby, D. E., Hays, J. T., Rigotti, N. A., Azoulay, S., Watsky, E. J., Williams, K. E., Reeves, K. R. (2006). Efficacy of varenicline, an alpha4beta2 nicotinic acetylcholine receptor partial agonist, vs placebo or sustained-release bupropion for smoking cessation: A randomized controlled trial. *Journal of the American Medical Association*, 296(1), 56–63.

Jorenby, D. E., Smith, S. S., Fiore, M. C., Hurt, R. D., Offord, K. P., Croghan, I. T., Baker, T. B. (1995). Varying nicotine patch dose and type of smoking cessation counseling. *Journal of the American Medical Association*, 274(17), 1347–1352.

Kakko, J., Gronbladh, L., Svanborg, K. D., von Wachenfeldt, J., Ruck, C., Rawlings, B., Heilig, M. (2007). A stepped care strategy using buprenorphine and methadone versus conventional methadone maintenance in heroin dependence: A randomized controlled trial. *American Journal of Psychiatry*, 164(5), 797–803.

Kampman, K. M. (2010). What's new in the treatment of cocaine addiction? *Current Psychiatry Report*, 12(5), 441–447.

Kampman, K. M., Pettinati, H., Lynch, K. G., Dackis, C., Sparkman, T., Weigley, C., & O'Brien, C. P. (2004). A pilot trial of topiramate for the treatment of cocaine dependence. *Drug and Alcohol Dependency*, 75(3), 233–240.

Kessler, R. C., Sonnega, A., Bromet, E., Hughes, M., & Nelson, C. B. (1995). Posttraumatic stress disorder in the National Comorbidity Survey. *Archives of General Psychiatry, 52*(12), 1048–1060.

Kranzler, H. R. (1996). Evaluation and treatment of anxiety symptoms and disorders in alcoholics. *Journal of Clinical Psychiatry, 57*(Suppl 7), 15–21; discussion 22–14.

Laken, M. P., & Ager, J. W. (1996). Effects of case management on retention in prenatal substance abuse treatment. *American Journal of Drug and Alcohol Abuse, 22*(3), 439–448.

Levin, F. R., Mariani, J. J., Brooks, D. J., Pavlicova, M., Cheng, W., & Nunes, E. V. (2011). Dronabinol for the treatment of cannabis dependence: A randomized, double-blind, placebo-controlled trial. *Drug and Alcohol Dependency, 116*, 142–150.

Mann, K., Lehert, P., & Morgan, M. Y. (2004). The efficacy of acamprosate in the maintenance of abstinence in alcohol-dependent individuals: Results of a meta-analysis. *Alcoholism: Clinical and Experimental Research, 28*(1), 51–63.

Martell, B. A., Mitchell, E., Poling, J., Gonsai, K., & Kosten, T. R. (2005). Vaccine pharmacotherapy for the treatment of cocaine dependence. *Biological Psychiatry, 58*(2), 158–164.

Martell, B. A., Orson, F. M., Poling, J., Mitchell, E., Rossen, R. D., Gardner, T., & Kosten, T. R. (2009). Cocaine vaccine for the treatment of cocaine dependence in methadone-maintained patients: a randomized, double-blind, placebo-controlled efficacy trial. *Archives of General Psychiatry, 66*(10), 1116–1123.

Mattick, R. P., & Hall, W. (1996). Are detoxification programmes effective? *Lancet, 347*(8994), 97–100.

McLellan, A. T., Arndt, I. O., Metzger, D. S., Woody, G. E., & O'Brien, C. P. (1993). The effects of psychosocial services in substance abuse treatment. *Journal of the American Medical Association, 269*(15), 1953–1959.

McLellan, A. T., Carise, D., & Kleber, H. D. (2003). Can the national addiction treatment infrastructure support the public's demand for quality care? *Journal of Substance Abuse and Treatment, 25*(2), 117–121.

McLellan, A. T., Lewis, D. C., O'Brien, C. P., & Kleber, H. D. (2000). Drug dependence, a chronic medical illness: Implications for treatment, insurance, and outcomes evaluation. *Journal of the American Medical Association, 284*(13), 1689–1695.

McLellan, A. T., & McKay, J. (1998). The treatment of addiction: What can research offer practice? In S. Lamb, M. Greenlick, & D. McCarty (Eds.), *Bridging the gap: Forging new partnerships in community-based drug abuse treatment*. Washington, DC: National Academy Press.

McLellan, A. T., Metzger, D. S., Alterman, A. L., Woody, G. E., Durell, J., & O'Brien, C. P. (1995). Is addiction treatment "worth it"? Public health expectations, policy-based comparisons. In J. S. Fox (Ed.), *Proceedings of Josiah Macy Conference on Medical Education* (pp. 165–212). New York: Josiah Macy Foundation.

Mejta, C. L., Bokos, P. J., Mickenberg, J., Maslar, M. E., & Senay, R. (1997). Improving substance abuse treatment access and retention using a case management approach. *Journal of Drug Issues, 27*(2), 329–340.

Miller, W. R., & Rollnick, S. (1991). *Motivational interviewing: Preparing people to change addictive behavior*. New York: The Guilford Press.

Monterosso, J. R., Flannery, B. A., Pettinati, H. M., Oslin, D. W., Rukstalis, M., O'Brien, C. P., & Volpicelli, J. R. (2001). Predicting treatment response to naltrexone: The influence of craving and family history. *American Journal of Addiction, 10*(3), 258–268.

Moos, R. H., Finney, J. W., Ouimette, P. C., & Suchinsky, R. T. (1999). A comparative evaluation of substance abuse treatment: Treatment orientation, amount of care, and 1-year outcomes. *Alcoholism: Clinical and Experimental Research, 23*(3), 529–536.

Moos, R. H., & King, M. J. (1997). Participation in community residential treatment and substance abuse patients' outcomes at discharge. *Journal of Substance Abuse and Treatment, 14*(1), 71–80.

Moos, R. H., Pettit, B., & Gruber, V. A. (1995). Characteristics and outcomes of three models of community residential care for abuse patients. *Journal of Substance Abuse and Treatment, 7*(1), 99–116.

National Institutes of Health. (1998). Effective medical treatment of opiate addiction. National Consensus Development Panel on Effective Medical Treatment of Opiate Addiction. *Journal of the American Medical Association, 280*(22), 1936–1943.

Nunes, E. V., & Levin, F. R. (2004). Treatment of depression in patients with alcohol or other drug dependence: A meta-analysis. *Journal of the American Medical Association, 291*(15), 1887–1896.

O'Brien, C. P., & McLellan, A. T. (1996). Myths about the treatment of addiction. *Lancet, 347*(8996), 237–240.

O'Connor, P. G., Oliveto, A. H., Shi, J. M., Triffleman, E. G., Carroll, K. M., Kosten, T. R., & Schottenfeld, R. S. (1998). A randomized trial of buprenorphine maintenance for heroin dependence in a primary care clinic for substance users versus a methadone clinic. *American Journal of Medicine, 105*(2), 100–105.

Paoletti, P., Fornai, E., Maggiorelli, F., Puntoni, R., Viegi, G., Carrozzi, L., & Giuntini, C. (1996). Importance of baseline cotinine plasma values in smoking cessation: Results from a double-blind study with nicotine patch. *European Respiratory Journal, 9*(4), 643–651.

Petrakis, I. L., Poling, J., Levinson, C., Nich, C., Carroll, K., & Rounsaville, B. (2005). Naltrexone and disulfiram in patients with alcohol dependence and comorbid psychiatric disorders. *Biological Psychiatry, 57*(10), 1128–1137.

Petry, N. M., Peirce, J. M., Stitzer, M. L., Blaine, J., Roll, J. M., Cohen, A., Li, R. (2005). Effect of prize-based incentives on outcomes in stimulant abusers in outpatient psychosocial treatment programs: A national drug abuse treatment clinical trials network study. *Archives of General Psychiatry, 62*(10), 1148–1156.

Pettinati, H. M., Oslin, D. W., Kampman, K. M., Dundon, W. D., Xie, H., Gallis, T. L., O'Brien, C. P. (2010). A double-blind, placebo-controlled trial combining sertraline and naltrexone for treating co-occurring depression and alcohol dependence. *American Journal of Psychiatry, 167*(6), 668–675.

Piper, M. E., Smith, S. S., Schlam, T. R., Fiore, M. C., Jorenby, D. E., Fraser, D., & Baker, T. B. (2009). A randomized placebo-controlled clinical trial of 5 smoking cessation pharmacotherapies. *Archives of General Psychiatry, 66*(11), 1253–1262.

Pomerleau, O. F., Pomerleau, C. S., Marks, J. L., Snedecor, S. M., Mehringer, A. M., Namenek Brouwer, R. J., & Saules, K. K. (2003). Prolonged nicotine patch use in quitters with past abstinence-induced depressed mood. *Journal of Substance Abuse and Treatment, 24*(1), 13–18.

Prochaska, J. O., & DiClements, C. C. (1992). Stages of change in the modificaiton of problem Behavior. In J. Hersen, R. Eisler, & P. M. Miller (Eds.), *Progress in behavior modification* (pp. 184–214). Sycamore, IL: Sycamore Publishing Company.

Regier, D. A., Farmer, M. E., Rae, D. S., Locke, B. Z., Keith, S. J., Judd, L. L., & Goodwin, F. K. (1990). Comorbidity of mental disorders with alcohol and other drug abuse. Results from the Epidemiologic Catchment Area (ECA) Study. *Journal of the American Medical Association, 264*(19), 2511–2518.

Rice, D. P., Kelman, S., & Miller, L. S. (1991). Estimates of economic costs of alcohol and drug abuse and mental illness, 1985 and 1988. *Public Health Report, 106*(3), 280–292.

Saleh, S. S., Vaughn, T., Hall, J., Levey, S., Fuortes, L., & Uden-Holmen, T. (2002). Effectiveness of case management in substance abuse treatment. *Care Management Journals, 3*(4), 172–177.

Siegal, H. A., Fisher, J. H., Rapp, R. C., Kelliher, C. W., Wagner, J. H., O'Brien, W. F., & Cole, P. A. (1996). Enhancing substance abuse treatment with case management. Its impact on employment. *Journal of Substance Abuse and Treatment, 13*(2), 93–98.

Silverman, K., Higgins, S. T., Brooner, R. K., Montoya, I. D., Cone, E. J., Schuster, C. R., & Preston, K. L. (1996). Sustained cocaine abstinence in methadone maintenance patients through voucher-based reinforcement therapy. *Archives of General Psychiatry, 53*(5), 409–415.

Steinberg, M. B., Foulds, J., Richardson, D. L., Burke, M. V., & Shah, P. (2006). Pharmacotherapy and smoking cessation at a tobacco dependence clinic. *Preventive Medicine, 42*(2), 114–119.

Stitzer, M. L., Bigelow, G. E., & Gross, J. (1989). Behavioral treatment of drug abuse. In T. B. Karasu (Ed.), *Treatments of psychiatric disorders: A task force report of the American Psychiatric Association* (pp. 1430–1447). Washington, DC: American Psychiatric Association.

Strain, E. C., Bigelow, G. E., Liebson, I. A., & Stitzer, M. L. (1999). Moderate- vs high-dose methadone in the treatment of opioid dependence: A randomized trial. *Journal of the American Medical Association, 281*(11), 1000–1005.

Strakowski, S. M., DelBello, M. P., Fleck, D. E., & Arndt, S. (2000). The impact of substance abuse on the course of bipolar disorder. *Biological Psychiatry, 48*(6), 477–485.

Vanderplasschen, W., Rapp, R. C., Wolf, J. R., & Broekaert, E. (2004). The development and implementation of case management for substance use disorders in North America and Europe. *Psychiatric Services, 55*(8), 913–922.

Vanderplasschen, W., Wolf, J., Rapp, R. C., & Broekaert, E. (2007). Effectiveness of different models of case management for substance-abusing populations. *Journal of Psychoactive Drugs, 39*(1), 81–95.

Weisner, C., & Schmidt, L. (1993). Alcohol and drug problems among diverse health and social service populations. *American Journal of Public Health, 83*(6), 824–829.

Treatment Resistance in Personality Disorders

Glen O. Gabbard

Introduction

Personality disorders have always been difficult to treat, so the designation "treatment resistant" could easily be recast as "more difficult than usual." Personality disorders are a complex constellation of genetically based temperamental dispositions and the residuals of environmental experiences early in life that shape who one is (Gabbard, 2005a). Temperamental dispositions include such things as novelty seeking, impulsivity, and proneness to angry outbursts, while the vicissitudes of early interactions with parents and other significant figures lead to internalized object relations that shape what people expect from interpersonal relationships as adults. In addition to the inherent difficulty in trying to treat personality disorders, things are further complicated by the considerable comorbidity with Axis I disorders found in personality disorders (Skodol et al., 2010). Conditions such as major depressive disorder, dysthymia, substance abuse, and posttraumatic stress disorder (PTSD) are all found regularly in association with borderline personality disorder (BPD; Gunderson & Links, 2008). Finally, many patients with personality disorders come to treatment reluctantly or ambivalently because they are reticent to change long-standing adaptations they had made to deal with the fears that haunt them. Although it is a vast overstatement to say that personality disorders are ego syntonic as opposed to Axis I conditions, which are ego dystonic, a significant number of patients with Axis II conditions do not want to undergo the emotional pain and expense of treatment.

Despite the complexity and formidable challenges in treating personality disorders, the prognosis for many personality disorders is surprisingly good. The conventional wisdom on personality disorders had always been that they were more or less stable conditions over time and in many cases became chronic disorders. More recent data suggest that this conceptualization is largely a myth. Two large-scale prospective studies—the Collaborative Longitudinal Personality Disorders Study (Skodol et al., 2010) and the McLean Study of Adult Development (Zanarini et al., 2010)—were funded by the National Institute of

Mental Health in the 1990s and have now accumulated impressive data. In the McLean study that followed 290 patients for a follow-up period of 10 years, 93% of the BPD patients attained remission of symptoms that lasted at least 2 years, while 86% attained a sustained remission lasting at least 4 years. However, 34% of those who achieved recovery ultimately lost it. Investigators concluded that recovery occurs in approximately half of the patients and is relatively stable, with only a third of the recovered patients later losing their recovery. They define true recovery as the combination of a 2-year symptomatic remission and the attainment of good vocational and social functioning. They found that the latter is more difficult to attain than some substantial reduction in symptom severity.

While the McLean study focused on BPD, the Collaborative Longitudinal Personality Disorders Study (CLPS) was a multisite longitudinal study that recruited 668 treatment-seeking or recently treated patients of one of four personality disorder diagnoses—borderline, schizotypal, avoidant, or obsessive-compulsive. The original sample also included patients with major depressive disorder who had no Axis II condition. The results were encouraging in that within the first 2 years of follow-up, between 33% (schizotypal) and 55% (obsessive-compulsive) of patients with personality disorders experienced a period of remission that lasted 2 months. At 2 years' follow-up, between 50% and 60% were below the threshold for a personality disorder diagnosis. Among those patients who continued over the first 6 years of follow-up, three quarters of patients with personality disorders had a 2-month remission and over two thirds had a 12-month remission (Skodol et al., 2010).

The fact that even without systematic outpatient treatment, there can be considerable improvement in the clinical picture of personality disorders is encouraging to those who are mired in impasses and treatment-resistant situations with such patients. There are 10 personality disorders in *DSM-IV-TR* (APA, 2000), and space considerations preclude a thorough discussion of the approach to treatment resistance with each of the 10. Therefore, I will use BPD as a prototype and discuss in detail the treatment-resistant phenomena that clinicians encounter with that entity. Moreover, we have much more data on the treatment of BPD than we do any other Axis II condition; the only possible exception is antisocial personality disorder, which is notoriously refractory to any kind of treatment.

Treatment Resistance as a Construct

The concept of resistance is used in clinical discussions in two primary contexts: (1) to refer to a patient who is unconsciously resisting the treatment because of anxieties about change; and (2) to refer to patients who are motivated to change, are receiving appropriate treatment, but are nevertheless failing to benefit from the treatment. Both of these constructs of resistance may apply to patients with personality disorders.

Freud originated the notion of resistance in 1912, when he stated, "The resistance accompanies the treatment step by step. Every single association, every act of a person under treatment must reckon with the resistance and represent the compromise between the forces that are striving towards recovery and the opposing ones" (1912/1958, p. 103). Resistance to treatment is common in psychotherapeutic practice and may take the form of forgetting appointments, forgetting medication, forgetting the psychiatrist's advice or interpretations, talking about trivia (while concealing important information), or simply becoming silent when one is asked to talk. Unconscious resistance of this nature involves the patient's defenses as they safeguard the patient against unpleasant emotions, such as anxiety and grief. The characteristic defense mechanisms of the patient become resistances when the patient enters treatment (Gabbard, 2010a).

Clinicians must avoid blaming the patient for resisting the treatment. Rather, we understand that the patient has anxieties, fears, and resentments that have long been buried by a set of defenses, and it is difficult to consider giving up that characteristic form of armoring oneself against painful affect states. We allow patients to show us who they are, and we do not exhort them to stop doing whatever it is they are doing. The manner in which the patient resists is likely to be a re-creation of a past relationship that influences a variety of other relationships besides the one with the therapist. Psychodynamic clinicians study the way the patient is resisting as a key to understanding ongoing interpersonal problems outside of therapy.

The other construct or definition of treatment resistance implies that the clinician should be rethinking his or her treatment strategy. Perhaps another medication is needed since the one being prescribed is not working. Perhaps an increase in dosage of the current agent would be sufficient to address the lack of response. A third possibility would be that an augmenting agent is needed. From a psychotherapeutic standpoint, one may consider switching to a different type of therapy if the current modality is not being effective. While for sake of clarity we are differentiating these two types of resistance, they commonly co-occur, and one of the clinician's tasks is to sort out which of the two resistances is relatively more prominent and what interventions are required to deal with the two types of resistance. In the ensuing discussion of BPD, we will touch on both dimensions of treatment resistance as they apply.

Misdiagnosis

BPD is commonly misdiagnosed because of the pleomorphic nature of the disorder. It can mimic a psychotic disorder, depression, bipolar illness, and PTSD. A particularly common problem is differentiating bipolar II disorder from BPD. Both conditions involve affective lability, dysphoria, and impulsive behavior. A useful distinction that has been made between BPD and bipolar II involves duration of the affective episode. Hypomanic episodes in the true bipolar II patient are usually more sustained than the periods of affective lability in BPD patients. In other words, in most cases a hypomanic episode should last at least several days to warrant the diagnosis. On the other hand, in BPD, some periods of increased activity and irritability resembling a hypomanic episode may last no more than a few hours. However, this distinction is not hard and fast as there are cases of ultrarapid cycling in bipolar illness that last only a few hours (Kramlinger & Post, 1996).

Another useful distinction involves the presence or absence of a precipitant before an episode of affective distress. BPD is often accompanied by a form of affective instability that is closely linked to life events; in particular, interpersonal slights or loss. On the other hand, it is common for a hypomanic episode, as part of bipolar II, to have a gradual onset over days, weeks, or even months without a clear stressor that has triggered it. By contrast, the dysphoria or mood lability associated with BPD may appear within minutes of the stressor, particularly if it is an interpersonal injury of some type, such as being jilted by a lover.

Misdiagnosis can have significant treatment implications where one is trying to differentiate between bipolar II and BPD. For example, the first-line psychopharmacologic treatment for the affective and impulsivity symptoms in BPD is often a selective serotonin reuptake inhibitor (SSRI) (American Psychiatric Association, 2001). If such a treatment is administered to a depressed patient with bipolar II, one may precipitate a switch into a hypomanic episode (Altschuler et al., 1995; Coryell et al., 1995). Mood stabilizers and/or a typical antipsychotic may be appropriate and effective in certain cases. However, if the diagnosis of BPD is incorrectly applied, a clinician may discontinue the mood stabilizer or antipsychotic after stabilization, thus depriving the bipolar II patient of prophylaxis and increasing the risk of relapse.

Similar problems or treatment may occur in the psychotherapeutic domain. A variety of psychotherapeutic programs have demonstrated efficacy with BPD, as will be discussed later in this chapter, but none of these have been shown to be efficacious with bipolar II patients. Hence misdiagnosis of the patient may lead to misapplication of a psychotherapeutic technique lacking in demonstrated effectiveness (American Psychiatric Association, 2001). The presence of repeated angry outbursts, acts of deliberate self-harm in response to interpersonal rejection, and a series of suicide attempts are classic for BPD, and it is unlikely that someone with those features will have bipolar II (Gunderson et al., 2006).

Of course, it is also possible for a patient to be accurately diagnosed with both bipolar II and BPD. Gunderson et al (2006) examined rates of co-occurrence in both disorders from a longitudinal prospective database and concluded that there is a modest association of BPD with bipolar II. To be more precise, in a large sample of personality disorder patients, there was a significantly higher co-occurrence rate of bipolar disorder (19.4%) with borderline than with other personality disorders. This co-occurrence leads to another source of diagnostic and treatment difficulty—namely, comorbidity.

Comorbidity

Comorbidity is the rule rather than the exception in BPD. Mood disorders, eating disorders, anxiety disorders, and substance abuse all commonly appear as Axis I conditions in conjunction with BPD (Gunderson & Links, 2008). In the McLean study referred to earlier (Zanarini et al., 2004), Axis I conditions were assessed in 290 patients with BPD. At the beginning of the study, 86.6% of patients were comorbid for Axis I major depression (96.9% if one considered all mood disorders), 62.1% had substance abuse disorders, 89% had anxiety disorders, and 53.8% were comorbid for eating disorders. The investigators reevaluated the subjects at 2-year time intervals. Even at 6-year follow-up, 75% of the patients with BPD met criteria for mood disorder, 60% for an anxiety disorder, 34% for an eating disorder, and 19% for a substance use disorder.

In the 6-year follow-up of 522 patients from the Collaborative Longitudinal Personality Disorders Study (Morey et al., 2010), two thirds of the patients with personality disorders had comorbid depressive episodes on Axis I. Of the patients who were included in this prospective study, only 8% of the depressed patients who did *not* have personality disorders remained depressed at 6-year follow-up. On the other hand, in the group of patients with both depression and a personality disorder, 29% of the group remained depressed.

Traditionally, personality disorder has been viewed as a comorbid factor that interferes with the recovery of depression (Newton-Howes et al., 2006). However, it may also be true that an untreated depression can create a situation where the condition of BPD is more refractory to treatment when one of the standard psychotherapeutic approaches to BPD is the centerpiece of treatment without accompanying pharmacotherapy. Some patients with significant depression may be cognitively slowed in such a way that they find it difficult to do the psychotherapeutic work required of them to make the psychotherapy efficacious.

In the McLean study (Zanarini et al., 2010), the rates of four of the five types of Axis I disorders studied remained relatively constant over time for patients whose BPD did not remit. One of the most important findings involved the role of substance use disorders. Absence of substance use was a stronger predictor of remission from BPD than the absence of any other disorder. The investigators noted that this finding fits with clinical observations that alcohol and drug abuse can exacerbate four core aspects of borderline psychopathology, namely, impulsivity, decreased mood, heightened distrust, and increase relational turbulence. Hence, one sensible clinical implication of this finding is that substance abuse must be aggressively treated as one of the main foci of an integrated treatment of BPD.

Even patients with BPD who appear dysphoric may not receive antidepressant treatment. There is an ongoing controversy regarding whether the depression in BPD is substantively different from major depression (Silk, 2010). Patients with BPD, even if they do not currently meet criteria for major depression, often show similar levels of depression on observer-rated scales such as the HDRS or the SCL. However, as Silk (2010) points out, BPD patients experience their moods at times in different ways from depressed patients without BPD, and they regard them as responsive to problematic interpersonal situations in a way that may be different from the typical patient with major depressive disorder. Moreover, because of the emptiness, dysphoria, loneliness, and fear of abandonment of BPD, the extent to which depression has improved in a patient with BPD is highly difficult to assess.

In any case, there is a strong argument for adding an SSRI to the treatment of a patient with BPD who is not responding to empirically validated psychotherapeutic treatment provided by competent practitioners. A number of double-blind placebo-controlled studies (Coccaro & Kavoussi, 1997; Markovitz, 1995; Rinne et al., 2002; Salzman et al., 1995) have demonstrated some degree of efficacy in patients with borderline and other severe personality disorders. These agents appear to be especially effective in reducing affective lability; anger; impulsive-aggressive behavior, particularly verbal aggression; intense anxiety and a "short fuse," that is, a quick temper. Some studies suggest that higher doses (the equivalent of 80 mg per day of fluoxetine) may be necessary to be maximally effective. Another controversy in the field, however, is that it is unclear whether the medication is treating a true major depressive disorder or personality traits that are an essential part of the temperament of BPD. Recent research suggests that SSRIs may actually result in true personality change when they are being used to treat depression. Tang et al (2009) studied adult patients with moderate-to-severe major depressive disorder randomized to receive cognitive therapy, placebo, or paroxetine. Those who took paroxetine received greater personality change than placebo patients even after controlling for depression improvement. These changes particularly affected the traits of neuroticism and extraversion. Patients taking paroxetine reported 3.5 times as much change on extraversion as placebo patients matched for depression improvement and

6.8 times as much change on neuroticism. The investigators concluded that paroxetine appears to have a specific pharmacological effect on personality that is distinct from its effect on depression.

The available research, preliminary as it is, fits with much clinical experience reported anecdotally. In other words, when a patient receiving psychotherapy for BPD is not improving as one would expect, one should consider the possibility that Axis I disorders, especially mood disorders, may not be receiving the optimal treatment with psychopharmacologic strategies. The resulting improvement may reflect the impact of the antidepressants, especially SSRIs, on the specific personality traits as much as on accompanying Axis I major depression. Similarly, the treatment of eating disorders, anxiety disorders, and other conditions, such as substance abuse, may be equally important in promoting maximum benefit of overcoming treatment resistance.

While substance abuse is widespread among patients with BPD who hope to self-medicate their intense affective states, recent research suggests that an opioid deficit inherent in BPD may contribute to this proclivity (Prossin et al., 2010). This opioid deficit may be managed by many patients through self-cutting, which releases endogenous opioids to counteract the deficit. It is also of interest that patients seeking buprenorphine treatment have a high rate (44.1%) of comorbidity with BPD (Sansone et al., 2008). New and Stanley (2010) point out that BPD patients respond somewhat differently to opiates than others. While patients without BPD tend to report euphoria in response to opiates, BPD patients are more inclined to describe their feeling as simply *euthymic*. Withdrawal of opiates with BPD patients is associated with sustained dysphoria.

Substance abuse goes well beyond the issue of opioid deficits in BPD. Such patients commonly abuse a wide range of different medications and alcohol. Often the substance abuse is concealed from treaters, so that a patient refractory to treatment may be undermining any effective treatment through the use of alcohol or drugs. It is commonplace, for example, for a patient with BPD to use large doses of benzodiazepines during a crisis without checking with the treating psychiatrist. Because some medications in this class, particularly alprazolam, are known to disinhibit patients with BPD (American Psychiatric Association., 2001), the patient may deteriorate further with impulsive behavior and affective outbursts. Treaters may be confused by the clinical picture because the benzodiazepine abuse is hidden from them. Clinicians should have a high index of suspicion in such cases and carefully consider this possibility when patients are not responding as expected.

The comorbidity of substance abuse on Axis I represents a symptom that does not disappear as quickly as others in the treatment of BPD. It carries with it a disconcerting prognosis. Zanarini et al (2004) noted that substance abuse in BPD is associated with a strong tendency for failure of remission in BPD and with suicidality. Hence, this comorbid condition requires careful and persistent attention by clinicians treating the disorder.

Clinicians have long suspected that attention-deficit/hyperactivity disorder (ADHD) occurs at a higher rate in patients with BPD. Fossati et al (2002) noted that the symptom clusters associated with ADHD—impulsivity, mood lability, hyperactivity, inattentiveness, hot temper, irritability, disorganization, and impaired stress tolerance—are also observed in BPD. A recent study confirms the clinical impression of overlap. Ferrer et al (2010) found that 38.1% of patients diagnosed with BPD were comorbid for adult ADHD. The patients with both disorders had more severe symptoms, and the investigators suggest the presence of comorbid ADHD may define a subgroup of BPD patients who are more impulsive. Hence, treatment of both conditions may be necessary for optimal response.

Finally, one must keep in mind that patients may meet criteria for more than one personality disorder. Indeed, one of the chief criticisms of the *DSM-IV* Axis II diagnoses is that if a patient meets criteria for one personality disorder, he or she is likely to be diagnosed with 3–6 other personality disorders by *DSM-IV* criteria (Westen & Muderrisoglu, 2002). BPD is extensively overlapping with antisocial, histrionic, narcissistic, and dependent personality disorders (Skodol, 2005). When BPD patients are treatment resistant, clinicians must entertain the possibility that antisocial personality disorder (ASPD) may be present. In all outcome studies, antisocial features considerably worsen the prognosis of BPD.

Antisocial patients are well known for deceiving and conning clinicians (Gabbard, 2005b). Patients may minimize or leave out criminal activity while focusing on impulsivity, suicidality, and relationship problems. In addition, there tends to be a gender bias to diagnose ASPD in men and BPD in women. Hence, the possibility of ASPD may particularly be overlooked when clinicians are evaluating female patients (Gabbard, 2005b). Women who have been violent or corrupt may be regarded as BPD patients who have problems with impulsivity or victimized women who are defending themselves in the face of abusers. While this characterization may be accurate in some cases, the failure to see the active initiation of aggression in females may result in missing the antisocial features of the patient. As with all patients where the diagnosis of ASPD is being entertained, clinicians should incorporate collateral sources, such as previous medical records, police records, and information from family members when evaluating the patient (Gabbard, 2005b). Even well-trained clinicians are vulnerable to being conned by an antisocial patient in a clinical interview.

Psychotherapeutic Considerations in Treatment Resistance

As noted in the beginning of this chapter, for decades, BPD patients were thought to be refractory to treatment such that there was a pessimism about the value of psychotherapy in their treatment. A common belief was that, regardless of treatment, the patients would continue to be emotionally volatile, impulsive, and interpersonally difficult. We now know that many patients appear to achieve substantial amounts of symptom remission. Moreover, there now is a smorgasbord of structured psychotherapeutic programs from which to choose (see Table 13.1). All have been shown to be efficacious in randomized controlled trials comparing the specific psychotherapy to other empirically validated psychotherapies designed especially for BPD.

These psychotherapies include the following: dialectical behavior therapy (Linehan et al., 2006), mentalization-based therapy (Bateman & Fonagy, 1999), transference-focused psychotherapy (Clarkin et al., 2007), schema-focused therapy (Giesen-Bloo et al., 2006), supportive psychotherapy (Clarkin et al., 2007), systems training for emotional predictability and problem solving (STEPPS) (Blum et al., 2008), and general psychiatric management with dynamically oriented therapy (GPM) (McMain et al., 2009). All of these

TABLE 13.1 Psychotherapies for Borderline Personality Disorder Shown to Be Efficacious in Randomized Controlled Trials

- Dialectical behavior therapy (DBT)
- Mentalization-based therapy (MBT)
- Transference-focused psychotherapy (TFP)
- Schema-focused therapy (SFT)
- Supportive psychotherapy (SP)
- Systems training for emotional predictability and problem solving (STEPPS)
- General psychiatric management with dynamically oriented therapy (GPM)

psychotherapeutic programs are essentially long term, taking many months to over a year to show substantial improvement. They also have in common a built-in supervision/consultation process so that psychotherapists are constantly in dialog with one another regarding the principles of the technique and the potential for therapists to be derailed by countertransference or other considerations.

Certain symptoms of BPD, including impulsive acts like shoplifting and careless sexual encounters, self-mutilation, and suicide attempts/gestures, are more responsive to psychotherapy, medication, or a combination of the two, often showing good results within a year or two (Clarkin et al., 2007). The aspects of BPD that are more related to genetically based temperament, including abandonment concerns, intense anger, irritability, moodiness, and mercuriality, often persist long after the symptoms have been adequately addressed and alleviated (Zanarini et al., 2010). This observation has led many to emphasize that too much attention has been paid to symptom reduction while neglecting the thornier problem of psychosocial rehabilitation (Zanarini et al., 2010).

The fact that there are so many different types of psychotherapy that appear to make significant differences in the symptomatology of BPD have led some to conclude that "all roads lead to Rome" (Gabbard, 2007). There are several possible explanations for why so many treatments, often of different theoretical orientation and diverse technical strategies, are efficacious with patients who suffer from BPD (Gabbard, 2010b). These include the following:

1. All therapeutic approaches, however diverse, nevertheless provide a systematic conceptual framework that organizes the internal chaos of the BPD patient. Hence, any therapeutic strategy that explains the pathogenesis of the illness and has a coherent treatment plan following from that explicit pathogenesis may give patients hope and help them think about their disorder in a different way.

2. BPD patients may respond to different elements of the therapeutic action depending on the specific characteristics of the patient. BPD has a diverse etiology that involves elements such as genetic vulnerability, neuropsychological difficulties, childhood abuse, childhood neglect, confusing and problematic family interactions, and the influence of Axis I disorders. Studies using group mean values for outcome can lead to a "washout effect," as those who benefit cancel out those who do worse (Gabbard & Horowitz, 2009).

3. The therapeutic action may largely be attributed to secondary strategies that are not emphasized by psychotherapists who are advocates of one particular approach. Gabbard and Westen (2003) have identified a number of such strategies that may receive less

attention than transference interpretation and the therapeutic relationship. Various forms of confrontation carry implicit or explicit suggestions for change. For example, therapists frequently confront dysfunctional beliefs in the same way they confront problematic behaviors in patients with BPD. Whereas cognitive therapy emphasizes confrontation, dynamic therapy does not, but few therapists deny that it is of value in the treatment of BPD. Exposure, a central mechanism of change and behavioral treatments, is almost always present in any form of psychotherapy of BPD. Exposure means presenting the patient with a situation that provokes anxiety while assisting the patient in confronting the situation until it no longer creates anxiety because the patient has habituated to it. Transference anxieties diminish over time, which, in part, is related to exposure. As the patient recognizes that the original fears of being criticized or attacked by the therapist are unrealistic, anxiety subsides. Judicious self-disclosure may be yet another mode of action, where a therapist may share a particular feeling with the patient to promote mentalizing. Finally, affirmation may be critically important for patients who have experienced severe trauma (Killingmo, 1989). Such patients may have had parents who invalidated their experiences, and the therapist's affirmative validation of the patient's experience can be highly beneficial.

4. The other possibility is that the nature of the therapeutic alliance is responsible for the improvement of the patient. Norcross (2000) notes that psychotherapy research indicates that the therapeutic relationship accounts for most of the outcome variance: Technique generally accounts for only 12%–15% of the variance across different kinds of therapy. The therapeutic alliance, often defined as the degree to which the patient feels helped by the therapist and is able to collaborate with the therapist in pursuit of common therapeutic goals, has been shown in research to be the most potent predictor of outcome in psychotherapy (Horvath & Symonds, 1991; Martin et al., 2000).

5. From a neuroscience perspective, it may be that all approaches act through similar underlying neurophysiological processes. Amygdalar hyperactivity is probably modified by increased activity in the prefrontal cortex in almost every form of psychotherapy (Gabbard, 2009). The therapeutic relationship is used to sharpen the patient's self-observational capacity for reappraisal of assumptions, presumptions, and "kneejerk" beliefs. In other words, the systematic approach of all these treatments is to use thinking to overcome impulsivity and affective lability and contextualize those aspects.

Returning to the topic of treatment resistance, clinicians have noted for decades that treatment impasses with BPD patients are extremely common in psychotherapy. There are a variety of reasons for these impasses, and this chapter will touch on several of the most common.

Poor Fit Between Type of Therapy and Patient

As noted earlier, BPD is heterogeneous. There are diverse pathways to the condition that involve a variety of pathogenetic and etiological factors. Skilled clinicians attempt to match the patient to the most suitable therapeutic approach, but sometimes a good "fit" is lacking, and adjustments need to be made. We have limited data on how to match patient to therapy, so much of this challenge is based on clinical hunches that do not work out as planned. However, findings of research are emerging that shed light on relevant factors.

Childhood trauma has long been recognized as one of the contributing factors to the etiology and pathogenesis of BPD. Researchers estimate that childhood abuse and neglect are probably relevant in 60%–80% of cases (Gunderson & Links, 2008; Widom et al., 2009). Sexual abuse, physical abuse, verbal abuse, and neglect have all been implicated in the etiology. In a prospective study that matched abused and/or neglected children with nonvictimized children and followed them prospectively into young adulthood (Widom et al., 2009), early trauma clearly elevated the risk of BPD. Five hundred children with documented cases of physical or sexual abuse or neglect were shown to be at greater risk to develop BPD compared with the controls who had no childhood trauma.

Much of the trauma research has shed light on issues relevant to the psychotherapeutic approaches to BPD. In particular, there has been a shift to a more validating, empathic approach that appreciates the role that trauma has played in shaping the patient's personality. However, the impact of trauma is not monolithic. A recent study of PTSD patients (Lanius et al., 2010) investigated two subtypes of PTSD: one subtype, the dissociative variant, was characterized by overmodulation of affect. The more common subtype involved undermodulation of affect with a predominance of hyperarousal and reexperiencing symptoms. Magnetic resonance imaging (MRI) data revealed that the dissociative subtype is a form of emotional dysregulation that involves emotional overmodulation mediated by midline prefrontal inhibition of the limbic regions. By contrast, the subtype involving reexperiencing/hyperarousal involves emotional undermodulation mediated by failure of prefrontal inhibition of limbic regions.

These findings are relevant to a study of inpatient treatment for 57 BPD patients (Kleindienst et al., 2011). These patients were prospectively observed over a 3-month period. They tested the hypothesis that since dialectical behavior therapy relies on emotional learning, dissociation, which generally hinders the learning process, might predict poorer response to dialectical behavior therapy. They confirmed this hypothesis by finding that high levels of dissociation were a negative predictor of outcome in patients with BPD. These results suggest that it is important to assess dissociation before starting exposure-based treatments for BPD. Bypassing the protective function of dissociative defenses may overwhelm patients by confronting them with reliving the trauma and increase PTSD-like symptoms. For these patients a phase-oriented approach that focuses on building better functioning in multiple domains may be better (Chu, 2010). These findings suggest that it may ultimately be possible to predict prospectively which therapy may be most suited to an individual patient. Until then, therapists must use their best clinical judgment when assigning patients to a specific treatment. Unfortunately, in some cities, the choices are very limited, and many BPD patients are simply assigned to whatever treatment is available.

Insufficient Attention to the Therapeutic Alliance

Establishing a therapeutic alliance is the cornerstone of all forms of psychotherapy. As noted earlier, research suggests that the therapeutic alliance is the best predictor of outcome and is more important than any individual technique in studies that compare the relative efficacy of different treatments (Norcross, 2000). The therapeutic alliance is generally defined as having three components: (1) agreement between therapist and patient on the goals for therapy; (2) agreement on the method to reach these goals; and (3) an emotional or relational bond between therapist and patient (Borden, 1979).

Many psychiatric patients readily form a therapeutic alliance in the first meeting, when they feel they are being helped, empathized with, and understood. However, there is a considerable consensus that patients with BPD have greater difficulty in forming a therapeutic alliance (Horwitz et al., 1996). In part, this may be related to a history of having grown up in a household where patients feel they cannot trust parental figures. There is research suggesting that BPD patients show significantly greater left amygdalar activation to facial expressions of emotion compared with normal control subjects (Donegan et al., 2003). Of greater importance is their tendency to attribute negative attributes to neutral faces. They tended to see faces that were without expression as threatening or untrustworthy. Since the therapeutic alliance is based on trust, one can understand why creating a therapeutic alliance with a BPD patient is particularly difficult.

An additional influence may involve the opioid deficit previously described. It is well known that opioids are involved in pathological and normal emotion regulation. Specifically, endogenous opioids facilitate normal social functioning in healthy individuals (Kennedy et al., 2006). Deficits in endogenous opioids have been related to the ubiquitous social dysfunction observed in BPD. In addition, these problems of trusting others and relating to others may well be translated into difficulties forming a therapeutic alliance (New & Stanley, 2010).

Overestimation of Capacity for Insight-Oriented Therapy

When Wallerstein (1986) reviewed the outcome data from the Menninger Foundation Psychotherapy Research Project (PRP), he noted a recurrent theme. He found that in many of the cases (followed over 30 years) that had positive outcomes, therapists had recognized that their initial prediction that the patient would do well with a highly expressive/interpretive approach had to be revised. They realized that they had overestimated the capacity of the patient to use insight and needed to shift to a more supportive-expressive approach. Those who made that shift tended to have positive outcomes. The PRP was started in the 1950s, before the availability of rigorous diagnostic instruments that would confirm the diagnosis of BPD. Neither was there a randomized controlled design used in the study. Nevertheless, psychotherapy researchers agree that most of the patients in that study would now be diagnosed as suffering from BPD. So while we cannot use the data in a definitive way to derive inferences about psychotherapy of BPD, we can resonate with the findings of the study since a familiar reason for treatment resistance is that the therapist is more ambitious than the patient in attempting to apply interpretive techniques. These attempts at insight may be directed at extratransference phenomena or the transference fears and fantasies about the therapist.

In a spin-off study using the PRP data, Colson et al (1985) examined the 11 cases that had negative outcomes. They found a recurrent theme in these cases. The therapists dealt with acting-out behavior by interpreting the unconscious motives rather than by setting limits with the patients. These therapists tended to eschew the use of supportive measures like limit setting and instead counted on highly expressive approaches, such as interpretation, to help the patients reflect on the negative consequences and the underlying motivations that lay behind their behaviors. The therapists assumed that when the patients understood these unconscious phenomena, they would stop the behavior. This hypothesis was not realized. Instead, the patients continued to act out and deteriorate while the therapists offered insight. A capacity to be flexible and depart from a rigidly held view of the "proper" way to conduct psychoanalytic therapy seemed to be characteristic of those therapists who had good outcomes.

The fact that some patients do well with transference-focused psychotherapy suggests that an insight-oriented approach is useful for a subgroup of patients. However, as noted earlier, BPD occurs along a spectrum of patients with different strengths and weaknesses. A significant subgroup may have neuropsychological impairments that make expressive work more difficult. LeGris and van Reekum (2006) reviewed 29 neuropsychological studies of patients with BPD. More than 60% of these studies revealed impairments in attention, verbal memory, and visuospatial functions. Seres et al (2009) compared the neuropsychological performance of 50 patients with BPD to that of patients with other personality disorders ($n = 30$) and to that of healthy controls ($n = 30$). Patients with BPD manifested deficient attention, immediate and delayed memory, and relatively spared visuospatial and language functions compared with controls. They concluded that BPD patients are impaired in neuropsychological domains sensitive for frontal and temporal lobe functioning, and that this deficit is related to impulsivity.

Some of these neuropsychological deficits may not be evident in a clinical interview. Nevertheless, a frequent clinical observation is that a patient with BPD may have difficulty grasping what the therapist is trying to convey through an insight-oriented comment. It may be useful to "check out" with the patient if the gist of the intervention is understood before moving on. Some patients may pretend to grasp what is said because they feel a sense of shame when they cannot comprehend what the therapist is trying to convey. In any case, the key point here is that treatment resistance may relate to the therapist's insistence on using a highly interpretive approach that overestimates the patient's capacity to abstract, reflect, and process what is being said. An adjustment to a more supportive approach may move the therapy forward more effectively.

One challenge for the psychotherapy that results from these difficulties in forming a trusting relationship with the therapist is that the therapeutic alliance cannot be considered a "given" at the beginning of the treatment as it is with many patients who suffer from milder disorders. Rather, a good therapeutic alliance is an achievement of the psychotherapy of BPD that results from careful attention to ruptures in the alliance that may occur as a result of either unempathic comments from the therapist or the perception of malevolence in the therapist, however unwarranted it may be. Ruptures in the alliance may be long lasting in their impact because many BPD patients view a thoughtless comment, an insensitive statement, or a failure to respond in the way that the patient felt the therapist should respond as definitive confirmation that the therapist cannot be trusted.

Similarly, a psychotherapy that is geared to transference interpretation, such as transference-focused psychotherapy (Clarkin et al., 2007), may create difficulties for the patient who is not concentrating on the relationship to the therapist as the primary issue in his or her life. An example will illustrate this phenomenon:

PATIENT: So my boss is sitting there, and I'm trying to explain reasons that I had to leave work in the afternoon. I told him that my mother was upsetting me so much with her phone calls that I could not control my emotions. I told him that if I hadn't left work, I might have caused difficulties for my coworkers, so I was trying to be considerate. I stayed away for only about an hour and a half. The whole time I was telling him this, my boss had this deadpan expression on his face and seemed completely unsympathetic.

THERAPIST: It sounds like you were experiencing your boss in the same way you experience me.

PATIENT: (5-second pause) I can't believe you just said that. This has nothing to do with you. You're always putting yourself into this. Just forget it. (silence)

In this vignette, a poorly timed transference interpretation devastates the alliance and shuts down the patient. Transference interpretation is not necessarily a bad choice of intervention with BPD patients (as the research on transference focused psychotherapy attests). However, when it is introduced outside the context of a good therapeutic alliance, it may have a devastating impact. In a process study involving audiotapes of long-term psychodynamic therapy with three BPD patients, one group of investigators looked at the impact of a therapist's interventions on the therapeutic alliance (Horwitz et al., 1996). A second group collaborated on identifying the interventions used by the therapist. These researchers found the transference interpretation had greater impact on the therapeutic alliance—both positive and negative—than other interventions. They concluded that transference interpretation is a high-risk, high-gain intervention in the psychotherapy of patients with BPD (Horwitz et al., 1996.

When the researchers looked at the interventions made by the therapists leading up to the transference interpretation, they found that the most effective interpretations of transference had something in common. Mainly, the way had been paved for the interpretation by a series of empathic, validating, and supportive interventions that created a strong therapeutic alliance where the patient felt heard, understood, and validated. A surgeon needs anesthesia to operate, and the psychotherapist of a BPD patient needs a solid therapeutic alliance to interpret transference. Hence, the therapeutic alliance and transference interpretation may work synergistically.

It should be clarified that timing is not the only consideration in the use of transference interpretation. In addition, one needs to be judicious in the use of this intervention. There is a time-honored principle in interpreting transference dating back to Freud that suggests the following: Do not interpret the transference until it becomes a resistance (Gabbard, 2010a). Hence, when the transference is facilitating the process, as it was in the vignette described earlier, it is not necessary to interpret the transference, but in addition to the timing issue, most good therapists tend to discourage high-frequency interpretation of the transference in one session. As a general rule, transference interpretation is much more effective when used sparingly (Høglend & Gabbard, 2011).

In any situation where a treatment-resistant patient suffers from BPD, the psychotherapist should be thinking about the possibility that the therapeutic alliance has been ruptured. While BPD patients may be temperamentally irritable, the rupture in the alliance has a specific definition as a strain or breakdown in the collaborative process between therapist and patient or a deterioration of the quality of relatedness between patient and therapist (Safran et al., 2002). In brief, a repair of the alliance simply involves disengaging oneself from what is being enacted with the patient and commenting on the current interaction to invite exploration of how the patient is experiencing the therapist in the here and now. This may help get a process "unstuck." A crucial component of this exploration is the therapist's acknowledgment of his or her participation in the rupture.

Disidentification with the Aggressor

In cases in which childhood trauma is instrumental in shaping the patient with BPD, a set of internal object relations arises from the early trauma. Each child internalizes parent–child interactions as a relational configuration that is embedded in a neural network in the patient's brain (Westen & Gabbard, 2002). Prominent in the internal object relations of these patients are three roles in the internal drama: a victim, an abuser, and a rescuer. These roles are played out in the interaction between patient and therapist such that the patient is in the role of victim while the therapist is in the role of victim or abuser. The unfolding drama may play out in a variety of ways, but a common impasse leading to treatment resistance involves what is known as *disidentification with the aggressor* (Gabbard, 2003). In these instances the therapist is intent on proving to the patient that he or she is not the "bad object" associated with the parent who abused the child. Therapists who defend against the patient's unconscious tendency to re-create the childhood situation may grow more and more saintly in response to patients' verbal attacks. They may clarify again and again how different they are from the "bad" parent and thereby resist the patient's very real need to re-create the parent–child situation in order to work it through in a therapeutic context.

This type of impasse may be particularly true in chronically suicidal BPD patients. In their effort to maintain the position as a "good" object disidentified with the aggressive abuser of childhood, therapists may desperately try to convince the patient that there is no reason to commit suicide since the therapist is giving the patient a reason to live. The message may unwittingly be given to the patient that the therapist may omnipotently and magically keep the patient from committing suicide.

Zealous efforts to eliminate suicidal ideation and save patients from themselves may blur the distinction between suicidality and suicide. In some cases, ruminating about the possibility of suicide may perform valuable psychological functions for the patient. Therapists need to respect that these patients must think about suicide as a way out of an unbearable situation originating in childhood, but that may not mean that they are intent on actually ending their lives.

The therapist who is too intent on saving patients from themselves may become self-sacrificing to a fault and do whatever it takes to prove to the patient that he or she will not repeat the abusive or neglectful situation from childhood. This may provide false hope to the patient, who thinks the therapist really is a parent who will always be available and will ultimately save the patient from suicide. It also colludes with the BPD patient's tendency to assign to others the responsibility for keeping the patient alive (Gabbard & Wilkinson, 1994). Hendin (1982) characterized this assignment as one of the most lethal features of suicidal patients. When therapists place themselves in bondage to the patient, they will soon find that their omnipotent wishes are thwarted and consciously or unconsciously begin to wish the patient would disappear.

An impasse is often reached in which the therapist has become desperate to save the patient and is tormented by the patient's unrelenting demands on the therapist's time. Consultation is often sought at this point, and it may be extremely helpful for a consultant or supervisor to point out to the therapist how desperately the therapist is repudiating his or her own anger, aggression, or hatred of the patient. One of the helpful perspectives in this type of impasse is for therapists to recognize that they must allow themselves to be transformed into the "bad object" for the patient to have the opportunity to work it through (Fonagy, 1998). When therapists resist this transformation, patients may have to escalate the provocativeness and work even harder to re-create the situation of being mistreated by an authority figure in a close relationship with them, namely the therapist. In the worst-case scenario, therapists escalate their efforts to disavow any aggression by crossing boundaries and doing such things as hugging the patient, discontinuing the fee, or taking the patient on trips with the family (Gabbard, 2003). Many ethical transgressions begin with an effort to demonstrate that no aggression toward the patient exists in the therapist.

Negative Therapeutic Reaction

Of the various kinds of treatment resistance encountered in psychotherapy with patients who have BPD, perhaps the most ominous is the negative therapeutic reaction. When Freud (1923/1958) first used the term, he referred to a phenomenon encountered in clinical practice when a patient who received an accurate interpretation got worse in response to the intervention. Freud linked this to the patient's unconscious sense of guilt. Such patients, he suggested, did not feel they deserved to get better because of a profound and often unconscious conviction that they had inflicted grave damage on others, often parents or siblings. Without stating unequivocally that these patients were untreatable, he conveyed a thoroughgoing pessimism about their prognosis in analytic treatment.

Since that time, the term is more broadly used to indicate situations in which a patient gets worse when help is offered to him or her, a variation on "biting the hand that feeds you" (Gabbard, 1989). Some patients with BPD appear to get worse and refuse help even when approached by experienced psychotherapists who are using empirically validated techniques. Rather than blaming the patient in such cases, the wise therapist attempts to investigate the mechanisms at work in the patient. At the core may be a sense of unconscious guilt, commonly found in some patients with childhood sexual abuse, who hold themselves responsible for "seducing" the perpetrator. On the other hand, rage at parents or other caregivers may also be a key factor in the pathogenesis of this form of treatment resistance.

A fundamental psychodynamic principle is that most patients unconsciously re-create their childhood situation or at least their internal version of it (Gabbard, 2010), which is in fact the essence of transference. Patients with BPD who have had particularly traumatic relationships with parents or caregiving figures may be intent on defeating the therapist without really knowing why. Help may be resented for a variety of reasons, but such patients often feel that being a failure in treatment is some form of success (Gabbard, 2000). Parents may have been perceived as using the child for their own sadistic and sexual pleasure. A pathological need to use the child for one's own gratification may infuriate the child, who then deliberately refuses to succeed in life as a way of taking revenge against parents or caregivers.

Other parents may have been perceived by their children as having taken credit for the child's success while blaming the child for failures. Revenge may be a powerful motivator, and the power of revenge fantasies may outweigh the clear advantages of improving one's clinical picture. As the patient gets worse, the therapist may become anxious and try harder and harder to provide a caring and therapeutically useful relationship to the patient. As noted earlier, in working with suicidal patients, any type of *furor therapeutics* may simply gratify the patient even further and intensify the patient's wish to torpedo his or her own treatment in the service of unconsciously defeating parental figures symbolically through the transference re-enactment. Hence, there is considerable value in disengaging from such an intense need to heal the patient and instead enlisting the patient as a collaborator in an exploration of why cutting off one's nose to spite one's face is of particular value to the patient. As with any self-defeating behavior, the therapist's primary question must be this: "What you're doing must be better than something else—can we try to understand what the 'something else' is?"

It's also important to keep in mind that some patients are basically untreatable. A significant percentage of BPD patients, perhaps 9%–10% (Gabbard 2005b), will commit suicide over the course of a lifetime. Those who are relentlessly bent on self-destruction may not be salvageable. Nevertheless, they all deserve our best efforts, and an examination of the dynamics of the self-defeating behavior can sometimes be life-saving.

Family System Issues

The foregoing discussion has been based on individual characteristics of the patient. Another source of treatment resistance is that the patient's pathology is embedded in an entrenched family system. Patients may feel that to improve their situation will somehow betray the family (Choi-Kain & Gunderson, 2009). The family system may in some way unconsciously "need" the patient to be in the sick role so that problems between the parents are triangulated into the child and attention is diverted away from the marital issues of the parents.

Parents may also have deep reservations about psychotherapy of their child who has BPD for fear that horrible things will be said about them in the course of the therapy. They may try to turn the patient against the therapist or may undermine therapy by not paying for it as initially agreed.

In the initial phases of evaluation and treatment, clinicians are well advised to include the family in the process so that they can fully understand the nature of BPD. Educating families about the disorder, its etiology, and its treatment may be of considerable value in heading off disruptions in the treatment and also engaging the family productively in what is generally a long-term process (Gunderson & Hoffman, 2005).

Concluding Comments

While the foregoing discussion has focused on treatment resistance in BPD, many of the sources of treatment resistance identified when one finds oneself at an impasse with BPD patients are applicable to treatment of other personality disorders. Comorbidity with Axis I disorders is a regular finding in the treatment of many personality disorders (Skodol, 2005). Similarly, entrenched re-creations of internal object relationships in the transference-countertransference dimensions of the therapeutic dyad can happen with any of the personality disorders.

Those who attempt long-term psychotherapeutic treatment of personality disorders would be wise to avail themselves of a consultant or supervisor to be sure that they maintain their bearings and do not become blind to a transference-countertransference impasse. The use of a third party helps the therapist take distance from the therapy and benefit from a pair of fresh eyes and ears. It sometimes feels impossible to step outside of treatment impasses, and a new perspective may keep the therapist on course when the way has been lost.

Disclosure Statement

G.O.G. has no conflicts of interest to disclose.

References

Altschuler, LL, RM Post, GS Leverich, K Mikalauskas, A Rosoff, & L Ackerman, (1995). Antidepressant-induced mania and cycle acceleration: a controversy revisited. *American Journal of Psychiatry*, *152*, 1130–1138.

American Psychiatric Association. (2000). Diagnostic and statistical manual of mental disorders (4th ed., text rev.) Washington, DC: Author.

American Psychiatric Association. (2001). Practice guidelines for the treatment of patients with borderline personality disorder. Am J Psychiatry 158 (Suppl 10): 1–52.

Bateman, A, & P Fonagy, (1999). Effectiveness of partial hospitalization in the treatment of borderline personality disorder: a randomized controlled trial. *American Journal of Psychiatry*, *156*, 1563–1569.

Blum, N, D St. John, B Pfohl, S Stuart, B McCormick, J Allen, S Arndt, & DW Black, (2008). Systems training for emotional predictability and problem solving (STEPPS) for outpatients with borderline personality disorder: a randomized controlled trial and 1-year follow-up. *American Journal of Psychiatry*, *165*, 468–478.

Borden, E, (1979). The generalizability of the psychoanalytic concept of the working alliance. *Psychotherapy: Theory, Research, Practice and Training*, *16*(3), 252–260.

Choi-Kain, LW, & JG Gunderson, (2009, August). Borderline personality disorder and resistance to treatment. *Psychiatric Times*, p. 35–36.

Chu, J, (2010). Posttraumatic stress disorder: beyond DSM-IV. *American Journal of Psychiatry*, *167*, 615–617.

Clarkin, JR, KN Levy, MF Lenzenweger, & OF Kernberg, (2007). Evaluating three treatments for borderline personality disorder: a multiwave study. *American Journal of Psychiatry*, *164*, 922–928.

Coccaro, EF, & RJ Kavoussi, (1997). Fluoxetine and impulsive aggressive behavior in personality- disordered subjects. *Archives of General Psychiatry*, *54*, 1081–1088.

Colson, DB, L Lewis, & L Horwitz, (1985). Negative outcome in psychotherapy and psychoanalysis. In DT Mays & CM Frank (Eds.), *Negative Outcome in Psychotherapy and What to Do About It* (pp. 59–75). New York: Springer.

Coryell, W, J Endicott, JD Maser, MB Keller, AC Leon, & HS Akiskal, (1995). Long-term stability of polarity distinctions in the affective disorders. *American Journal of Psychiatry, 152,* 385–390.

Donegan, NH, CA Sanislow, HP Blumberg, RK Fulbright, C Lacadie, P Skudlarski, JC Gore, IR Olson, TH McGlashan, & BE Wexler, (2003). Amygdalar hyperreactivity in borderline personality disorder: implications for emotional dysregulation. *Biological Psychiatry, 54,* 1284–1293.

Ferrer, M, O Andion, J Matali, S Valero, JA Navarro, JA Ramos-Quiroga, R Torrubia, & M Casas, (2010). Comorbid attention-deficit/hyperactivity disorder in borderline patients defines an impulsive subtype of borderline personality disorder. *Journal of Personality Disorders, 24,* 812–822.

Fonagy, P, (1998). An attachment theory approach to treatment of the difficult patient. *Bulletin of the Menninger Clinic, 62,* 147–169.

Fossati, A, L Novella, D Donati, M Donini, & C Maffei, (2002). History of childhood attention deficit/hyperactivity disorder symptoms and borderline personality disorder: a controlled study. *Comprehensive Psychiatry, 43,* 365–377.

Freud, S, (1958). The dynamics of transference. (1912). In T Strachey (Trans. & Ed.), *The Standard Edition of the Complete Psychological Works of Sigmund Freud* (Vol. 12, pp. 97–108). London: Hogarth Press.

Freud, S, (1958). The ego and the id (1923). In T Strachey (Trans. & Ed.), *The Standard Edition of the Complete Psychological Works of Sigmund Freud* (Vol. 19, pp. 3–67). London: Hogarth Press.

Gabbard, GO, (1989). Patients who hate. *Psychiatry, 52*(1), 96–106.

Gabbard, GO, (2000). On gratitude and gratification. *Journal of the American Psychoanalytic Association, 48*(3), 697–718.

Gabbard, GO, (2003). Miscarriages of psychoanalytic treatment with suicidal patients. *International Journal of Psychoanalysis, 84,* 249–261.

Gabbard, GO, (2005a). Mind, brain, and personality disorders. *American Journal of Psychiatry, 162*(4), 648–655.

Gabbard, GO, (2005b). *Psychodynamic Psychiatry in Clinical Practice* (4th edition). Arlington, VA: American Psychiatric Publishing.

Gabbard, GO, (2007). Do all roads lead to Rome? New findings on borderline personality disorder. *American Journal of Psychiatry, 164*(6), 853–855.

Gabbard, GO, (2009). Foreword. In RA Levy & JS Ablon (Eds.), *Handbook of Evidence-Based Psychodynamic Psychotherapy: Bridging the Gap between Science and Practice* (pp. vii–ix), New York: Humana Press.

Gabbard, GO, (2010a). *Long-Term Psychodynamic Psychotherapy: A Basic Text* (2nd edition). Arlington, VA: American Psychiatric Publishing.

Gabbard, GO, (2010b). Therapeutic action in the psychoanalytic psychotherapy of borderline personality disorder. In JF Clarkin, P Fonagy, & GO Gabbard (Eds.), *Psychodynamic Psychotherapy for Personality Disorders: A Clinical Handbook* (pp. 239–256). Arlington, VA: American Psychiatric Association.

Gabbard, GO, & M Horowitz, (2009). Insight, transference interpretation, and therapeutic change in the dynamic psychotherapy of borderline personality disorder. *American Journal of Psychiatry, 166,* 517–521.

Gabbard, GO, & D Westen, D, (2003). Rethinking therapeutic action. *International Journal of Psychoanalysis, 84,* 823–841.

Gabbard, GO, & SM Wilkinson, (1994). *Management of Countertransference with Borderline Patients.* Washington, DC: American Psychiatric Press.

Giesen-Bloo, J, R van Dyck, P Spinhoven, W van Tilburg, C Dirksen, C, T van Affelt, I Kremers, M Nadort, & A Arntz, (2006). Outpatient psychotherapy for borderline personality disorder: randomized trial of schema-focused therapy vs. transference-focused therapy. *Archives of General Psychiatry, 63,* 649–658.

Gunderson, JG, & P Hoffman, (Eds.). (2005). *Understanding and Treating Borderline Personality Disorder: A Guide for Professionals and Families.* Arlington, VA: American Psychiatric Publishing.

Gunderson, JG, & PS Links, (2008). *Borderline Personality Disorder: A Clinical Guide* (2nd edition). Arlington, VA: American Psychiatric Publishing.

Gunderson, JG, I Weinberg, MT Daversa, KD Kueppenbender, MC Zanarini, MT Shea, AE Skodol, CA Sanislow, S Yen, LC Morey, CM Grilo, TH McGlashan, RL Stout, & I Dyck, (2006). Descriptive and longitudinal observations on the relationship of borderline personality disorder and bipolar disorder. *American Journal of Psychiatry, 163,* 1173–1178.

Hendin, H, (1982). *Suicide in America,* New York: W. W. Norton.

Horvath, AD, & BD Symonds, (1991). Relation between working alliance and outcome in psychotherapy: a meta-analysis. *Journal of Counseling Psychology, 38,* 139–149.

Horwitz, L, GO Gabbard, G Allen, SH Frieswyk, DB Colson, GE Newsom, & L Coyne, (1996). *Borderline Personality Disorder: Tailoring the Psychotherapy to the Patient.* Washington, DC: American Psychiatric Press.

Høglend, P, & GO Gabbard, (2011). When is transference work useful in psychodynamic psychotherapy? A review of empirical research. In RA Levy & JS Ablon (Eds.), *Handbook of Evidence-Based Psychodynamic Psychotherapy* (Vol. 2, pp. 449–467). New York: Humana Press.

Kennedy, SE, RA Koeppe, EA Young, & J-K Zubieta, (2006). Dysregulation of endogenous opioid emotion regulation circuitry in major depression in women. *Archives of General Psychiatry*, *63*, 1199–1208.

Killingmo, B, (1989). Conflict and deficits: implications for technique. *International Journal of Psychoanalysis*, *70*, 65–79.

Kleindienst N, MF Limberger, UW Ebner-Priemer, J Mauchnik, A Dyer, M Berger, C Schmahl & M Bohus, (2011). Dissociation predicts poor response to Dialectical Behavior Therapy in female patients with borderline personality disorder. *Journal of Personality Disorders, 25*, 432–437.

Kramlinger, KG, & RM Post, (1996). Ultra-rapid and ultradian cycling in bipolar affective illness. *British Journal of Psychiatry*, *168*, 314–323.

Lanius, RA, E Vermetten, RJ Loewenstein, B Brand, C Schmahl, JD Bremner, & D Spiegel D, (2010). Emotion modulation in PTSD: clinical and neurobiological evidence for a dissociative subtype. *American Journal of Psychiatry*, *167*, 640–647.

LeGris, J, & R van Reekum, (2006). The neuropsychological correlates of borderline personality disorder and suicidal behavior. *Canadian Journal of Psychiatry*, *5*, 131–142.

Linehan, MM, KA Contois, AM Murray, MZ Brown, RJ Gallop, HL Heard, KE Korslund, DA Tutek, FK Reynolds, & N Lindenboim, (2006). Two-year randomized controlled trial on follow-up with dialectical behavior therapy vs. therapy by experts for suicidal behaviors and borderline personality disorder. *Archives of General Psychiatry*, *63*, 757–766.

Markovitz, P, (1995). Pharmacotherapy of impulsivity, aggression, and related disorders. In E Hollander, DJ Stein, & J Zohar (Eds), *Impulsivity and Aggression* (pp. 263–287). New York: Wiley.

Martin, DJ, JP Garske, & MK Davis, (2000). Relation of the therapeutic alliance with outcome and other variables: a meta-analytic review. *Journal of Consulting and Clinical Psychology*, *68*, 438–450.

McMain, SF, PS Links, WH Gnam, T Guimond, RJ Cardish, L Korman, & DL Streiner, (2009). A randomized trial of dialectical behavior therapy versus general psychiatric management for borderline personality disorder. *American Journal of Psychiatry*, *166*, 1365–1374.

Morey, LC, MT Shea, JC Markovitz, RL Stout, TJ Hopwood, JG Gunderson, CM Grilo, TH McLashan, S Yen, CA Sanislow, & AE Skodol. (2010), State effects of major depression on the assessment of personality and personality disorder. *American Journal of Psychiatry*, *167*, 528–535.

New, AS, & B Stanley, (2010). An opioid deficit in borderline personality disorder: self-cutting, substance abuse, and social dysfunction. *American Journal of Psychiatry*, *167*, 883–885.

Newton-Howes, G, T Tyrer, & T Johnson, (2006). Personality disorder and the outcome of depression: meta-analysis of published studies. *British Journal of Psychiatry*, *188*, 13–20.

Norcross, JC, (2000). Toward the delineation of empirically based principles in psychotherapy: commentary on Beutler *Prevention and Treatment*, *3*, 1–5.

Prossin, AR, TM Love, RA Koeppe, J-K Zubieta, & KR Silk, (2010). Dysregulation of regional endogenous opioid function in borderline personality disorder. *American Journal of Psychiatry*, *167*, 925–933.

Rinne, T, W van den Brink, L Wouters & R van Dyck, R, (2002). SSRI treatment of borderline personality disorder: a randomized placebo-controlled clinical trial for female patients with borderline personality disorder. *American Journal of Psychiatry*, *159*, 2048–2054.

Safran, JD, JC Muran, LW Samstag, & C Stevens, (2002). Repairing alliance ruptures. In JC Norcross (Ed.), *Psychotherapy Relationships That Work*. New York: Oxford University Press.

Salzman, C, AN Wolfson, A Schatzberg, J Looper, R Henke, M Albanese, J Schwartz, & E Miyawaki, (1995). Effect of fluoxetine on anger in symptomatic volunteers with borderline personality disorder. *Journal of Clinical Psychopharmacology*, *15*, 23–29.

Sansone, RA, P Whitecar, & MW Wiederman, (2008). The prevalence of borderline personality among buphenorphine patients. *International Journal of Psychiatry in Medicine*, *38*, 217–226.

Seres, I, Z Unoka Z, N Bodi, N Aspan, & S Keri S, (2009). The neuropsychology of borderline personality disorder: relationship with clinical dimensions and comparison with other personality disorders, *Journal of Personality Disorders*, *23*, 555–562.

Silk, KR, (2010). The quality of depression in borderline personality disorder and the diagnostic process. *Journal of Personality Disorders*, *24*, 25–27.

Skodol, AE, (2005). Manifestations, clinical diagnosis, and comorbidity. In JM Oldham, AE Skodol, & DS Bender (Eds.), *The American Psychiatric Publishing Textbook of Personality Disorders* (pp. 57–87). Arlington, VA: American Psychiatric Publishing.

Skodol, AE, MT Shea, S Yen, CN White, & JG Gunderson, (2010). Personality disorders and mood disorders: perspectives on diagnosis and classification from studies of longitudinal course and familial associations. *Journal of Personality Disorders, 24,* 83–108.

Tang, TZ, RJ DeRubeis, SD Hollan, J Amsterdam, R Shelton, & B Schalet, (2009). Personality change during depression treatment: a placebo-controlled trial. *Archives of General Psychiatry, 66,* 1322–1330.

Wallerstein, RW, (1986). *Forty-Two Lives in Treatment.* New York: The Guilford Press.

Westen, D, & GO Gabbard, (2002). Developments in cognitive neuroscience: II. Implications for theories of transference. *Journal of the American Psychoanalytic Association, 50,* 99–134.

Westen, D, & S Muderrisoglu, (2002). Assessing personality disorders using a systematic clinical interview: evaluation of an alternative to structured interviews. *Journal of Personality Disorders, 17,* 351–369.

Zanarini, MC, FR Frankenburg, DB Reich, & G Fitzmaurice, (2010). Time to attainment of recovery from borderline personality disorder and stability of recovery: a 10-year prospective follow-up study. *American Journal of Psychiatry, 167,* 663–667.

Management of Treatment-Resistant Insomnia

Karl Doghramji and Charles F. Reynolds III

Introduction

Insomnia is the complaint of an inability to fall or stay asleep, or unrefreshing sleep. After pain, it represents the second most commonly expressed complaint in clinical settings (Mahowald, Kader, & Schenck, 1997). The past few decades have seen a tremendous increase in the array of treatment modalities for this malady. Nevertheless, these treatments do not confer absolute benefit for insomnia in all patients, as more than one third of insomnia patients remain symptomatic following the application of standard therapies (Mini, Wang-Weigand, & Zhang, 2008). Additionally, insomnia represents a persistent symptom following the management of its comorbidities; for example, nearly half of responders in the pharmacologic management of major depression in one study had persistent sleep disturbances (Nierenberg et al., 1999). The persistence of insomnia represents a treatment complication, as it introduces the possibility of polypharmacy and a wider array of side effects, enhances the risk of daytime cognitive and functional impairment, and is associated with a higher risk of relapse in the case of some disorders. It is fitting, therefore, that insomnia is included in a text on treatment resistance in psychiatric practice.

Prevalence

Studies into the epidemiology of insomnia abound, yet they have been limited by varied definitions of insomnia and inconsistent diagnostic and screening methods. Large community-based surveys suggest, however, that about 35% of the adult population experience insomnia during the course of 1 year (Mellinger, Balter, & Uhlenhuth, 1985). Half experience the problem as severe, and 20.1% of adults are dissatisfied with their sleep or take medication for sleeping difficulties (Ohayon, 1996). Insomnia is also a common complaint in children and adolescents; an estimated 4% of children complain of insomnia at least 3 times per week over the course of a year (Zhang, 2009).

The prevalence of insomnia is greatest in certain populations (Doghramji, Grewal, & Markov, 2009). These include the following:

1. Women—the prevalence of insomnia peaks during pregnancy and the peri- and postmenopausal years
2. Seniors—the prevalence of insomnia increases with advancing age and affects more than one third of the population age 65 and older
3. Individuals who engage in nontraditional occupational schedules, such as shift workers
4. Individuals who fall in the lower socioeconomic range
5. Divorced, widowed, or single individuals
6. Those who live in settings that are not conducive to sound sleep, such as noisy environments
7. Individuals who are affected by poor mental and physical health and those who use and misuse recreational substances

Impact

Clinical experience suggests that a poor night's sleep is generally followed by daytime sleepiness and fatigue. Indeed, compared to individuals without sleep difficulties, insomniacs report a greater rate of difficulty with coping, accomplishing tasks, impaired mood, breaches in interpersonal relationships, psychosocial upheaval, and cognitive deficits (Espie, Inglis, Harvey, & Tessier, 2000; Gallup, 1995; Hauri, 1997). Quality of life impairments are directly related to the severity of insomnia. Insomnia is also associated with work-related impairments and absenteeism (Kupperman et al., 1995) and a greater utilization of health care resources (Chevalier et al., 1999). However, the cross-sectional nature of these studies complicates the interpretation of these data. The effects of insomnia on daytime function appear to be complex, as controlled studies have revealed either no change, or even a greater degree of alertness, in insomniacs compared to normal controls (Stepanski, Zorick, Roehrs, Young, & Roth, 1988), whereas more recent studies have revealed psychomotor performance deficits when responding to challenging reaction time tasks in insomniacs (Espie et al., 2000). There is also emerging evidence linking primary insomnia to cardiovascular abnormalities such as enhanced heart rate (Bonnet & Arand, 1998) and hypertension (Lanfranchi, 2009).

Of possibly greater relevance to the topic of this chapter are observations that persistent insomnia confers a greater risk, than resolved insomnia, for the future development of new psychiatric and medical conditions. The relative contribution of treatment resistance in these studies is unclear, as studies did not divide populations into those who had, and who had not, received prior treatment for their conditions. Nevertheless, the persistence of the complaint of insomnia has been shown to confer an increased risk for the development of new mood, anxiety, and substance use disorders (Breslau, Roth, Rosenthal, & Andreski, 1996; Chang, Ford, Mead, Cooper-Patrick, & Klag, 1997; Ford & Kamerow, 1989; Weissman, Greenwald, Nino-Murcia, & Dement, 1997). Persistent insomnia is also associated with a greater risk of the future development of cardiovascular abnormalities and even predicts mortality (Dew et al., 2003; Mallon, Broman, & Hetta, 2002).

Classification

The three major classification systems used by clinicians and researchers for insomnia are the *Diagnostic and Statistical Manual of Mental Disorders (DSM-IV-TR)*, the International Classification of Sleep Disorders, Second Version (ICSD-2), and the International Classification of Disorders-10 (ICD-10) (American Academy of Sleep Medicine, 2005; American Psychiatric Association [APA], 2000; World Health Organization [WHO], 1992).

The *DSM-IV-TR* broadly organizes sleep disorders into two major categories according to presumed etiology. These include (Mahowald et al., 1997) primary sleep disorders, such as primary insomnia, primary hypersomnia, narcolepsy, and breathing-related sleep disorders, among others, and (Mini et al., 2008) sleep disorders related to other mental disorders, other medical conditions, and those that are substance induced. Diagnostic criteria for primary insomnia appear in Table 14.1.

The *DSM-IV TR* views insomnia, therefore, as a complaint that either stands alone, in which case it is presumed to represent an independent disorder as long as it meets certain duration criteria and is associated with daytime impairment, or one that is secondary to other medical or psychiatric disorders. Inherent in this view is the notion of causality. Recently, however, a National Institutes of Health State of the Science Conference challenged the primary/secondary distinction, noting that the limited understanding of mechanistic pathways in insomnia precludes drawing firm conclusions about the nature of the associations between insomnia and comorbid conditions or the direction of causality (National Institutes of Health [NIH], 2005) and recommended the use of term "comorbid insomnia" for those instances in which insomnia occurs in the context of other medical and psychiatric disorders. This conceptualization, which has been widely accepted in the field of sleep medicine, further emphasizes the potential for the existence of insomnia as an autonomous disorder, either alone or in the context of other disorders, which may warrant independent clinical attention. This movement away from causal attributions is reflected in the proposed *DSM-V* sleep-wake disorders nosology (Table 14.2; Reynolds, 2010).

TABLE 14.1 *DSM-IV TR* Diagnostic Criteria for Primary Insomnia

A. The predominant complaint is difficulty initiating or maintaining sleep, or nonrestorative sleep, for at least 1 month.

B. The sleep disturbance (or associated daytime fatigue) causes clinically significant distress or impairment in social, occupational, or other important areas of functioning.

C. The sleep disturbance does not occur exclusively during the course of Narcolepsy, Breathing-Related Sleep Disorder, Circadian Rhythm Sleep Disorder, or a Parasomnia.

D. The disturbance does not occur exclusively during the course of another mental disorder (e.g., Major Depressive Disorder, Generalized Anxiety Disorder, a delirium).

E. The disturbance is not due to the direct physiological effects of a substance (e.g., a drug of abuse, a medication) or a general medical condition.

Source: From APA (2000).

TABLE 14.2 Proposed *DSM-V* Diagnostic Criteria for Insomnia Disorder

A. The predominant complaint is a global sleep dissatisfaction with one or more of the following symptoms:
   1. Difficulty initiating sleep (*in children*: w/o caregiver intervention)
   2. Difficulty maintaining sleep (i.e., frequent or prolonged awakenings with difficulty returning to sleep) (*in children*: w/o caregiver intervention)
   3. Early morning awakening (i.e., premature awakening with inability to return to sleep)
   4. Nonrestorative sleep (adults)
   5. Resistance to going to bed (children)

B. The sleep complaint is accompanied by significant distress or impairment in social, occupational, or other important areas of functioning as indicated by the presence of at least one of the following:
   1. Fatigue or low energy
   2. Daytime sleepiness
   3. Cognitive impairments (e.g., attention, concentration, memory)
   4. Mood disturbance (e.g., irritability, dysphoria)
   5. Behavioral problems in children (hyperactivity, impulsivity, aggression)
   6. Impaired occupational function
   7. Impaired interpersonal/social function
   8. Impaired academic function (children)
   9. Negative impact on caregiver or family function (children)

C. The sleep difficulty occurs at least 3 nights per week
D. The sleep difficulty is present for at least 3 months
E. The sleep difficulty occurs despite adequate age-appropriate circumstances and opportunity for sleep

Clinically Comorbid Conditions:
1. Mental/psychiatric disorder (specify)
2. Medical disorder (specify)
3. Another disorder (specify)

Duration:
1. Acute insomnia (<1 month)
2. Subacute insomnia (1–3 months)
3. Persistent insomnia (>3 months)

Highlights of the *DSM-V* recommendations with regard to insomnia include the following:

1. The elimination of the diagnosis of "primary insomnia" in favor of "insomnia disorder"
2. The elimination of "sleep disorder related to another mental disorder" and "sleep disorder due to a general medical condition" in favor of "insomnia disorder" with concurrent specification of clinically comorbid medical and psychiatric conditions
3. The elimination of "insomnia" in favor of "sleep dissatisfaction," which is more strongly associated with daytime impairments than insomnia symptoms alone (Ohayon, 2002)
4. The addition of "early morning awakening," which promises to improve specificity of symptoms (Morin, 2006)
5. The provision of specific examples of impairments, which may facilitate the assessment of the impact of insomnia with children and adults (Edinger, 2004)
6. The addition of a minimal insomnia frequency of 3 nights per week and a duration of more than 3 months represent important cut-points for determining the degree of impairment (Buysse et al., 2007; Morin et al., 2009; Ohayon & Reynolds, 2009)

Pathophysiological Models of Primary Insomnia (*DSM-V* "Insomnia Disorder")

The pathophysiology of primary insomnia is poorly understood. Next, we review proposed etiological models.

Neurophysiologic Models

A core neurophysiologic alteration in insomnia is *hyperarousal*, or an overly active arousal system. This is evident during the environment and timing of sleep, and during the waking portions of the 24-hour day. When insomniacs are allowed the opportunity to nap during the course of their typical daytime, they display enhanced alertness, or a decreased ability to fall asleep, compared to normal sleepers (Edinger, Means, Carney, & Krystal, 2008). This is consistent with the complaint of insomniacs that they have difficulty napping during the course of the day, and that even when they are successful in napping, they awaken feeling unrefreshed. Hyperarousal has been described in the following areas:

1. *Sleep electroencephalography*: Reduced low-frequency delta power (typical of deep non-REM sleep) across the night, particularly in the first part of the night, and increased high frequency beta power across the entire night compared to healthy controls (Merica, Blois, & Gaillard, 1998)
2. *Neuroendocrine axis*: Increased cortisol and adrenocorticotropic hormone levels before and during sleep, particularly during the first half of sleep (Vgontzas et al., 2001)
3. *Metabolic brain activity*: Single-photon emission computed tomography (SPECT) and positron emission tomography (PET) scans reveal increased global glucose metabolic rates during both wakefulness and sleep compared with healthy control subjects, and the usual sleep-related decline in metabolism in brainstem arousal centers is attenuated (Nofzinger et al., 2004).
4. *Physiological and metabolic systems*: An increase in heart rate, a decrease in heart beat-to-beat variability (Bonnet & Arand, 1998), and an increase in whole-body metabolic rate (Bonnet & Arand, 1997) during sleep have been noted in patients with insomnia compared with controls.

Circadian Models

These models implicate the importance of the circadian system in the genesis of insomnia, pointing to various circadian rhythm disorders such as delayed sleep phase syndrome and advanced sleep phase syndrome (see later discussion), which are associated with difficulty in falling asleep and early awakening, respectively. In these disorders, the circadian system is deranged, causing sleep/wakefulness, melatonin, cortisol, and presumably other endogenous rhythms to be either delayed or advanced in relationship to the environmental light/dark cycle. Recent findings of a genetic basis for these disorders in at least some individuals (a mutation in a human clock gene (Per2) was shown to produce advanced sleep phase syndrome, and a functional polymorphism in Per3 is associated with delayed sleep phase syndrome) further supports genetic models of insomnia (Hamet & Tremblay, 2006).

Genetic Models

One study noted that the correlation between insomnia was greater with monozygotic than dizygotic twins (0.47 versus 0.15; Watson, Goldberg, Arguelles, & Buchwald, 2006). Other studies have found similar genetic mutations and genotypes in a rare form of insomnia, fatal familial insomnia (Tabernero, 2000).

Psychological Models

Although a variety of *psychoanalytic* models have been proposed throughout the past century, the one most widely recognized is that of Sigmund Freud. This construct proposed, in essence, that insomnia represents a failure of dream work (Freud, 1995). Dreams, according to Freud, are created by a combination of daily events ("residue") and conflictual, anxiety-producing, unconscious wishes. These are, in turn, transformed into dreams through a series of mental processes, including displacement, condensation, symbolic representation, and secondary elaboration, which, are, collectively subsumed under the rubric of "dream work." Freud further hypothesized that successful dream work is necessary for the preservation of sleep. However, in insomnia, "evil, repudiated wishes become active precisely at night and disturb us during sleep" (Freud, 1986). Dream work is unsuccessful because of the intensity of the anxiety caused by the underlying conflict, resulting in the awakening of the dreamer and the complaint of insomnia.

Cognitive/behavioral constructs in the genesis of insomnia rely on the importance of sleep-related thoughts and associated behaviors. Cognitive and emotional arousal due to traumatic events and stressors can *precipitate* insomnia in most individuals. However, insomniacs are theorized to have a *predisposition* for an exaggerated reaction to such stressors, requiring less activation to achieve high levels of arousal, which, in turn leads to disturbed sleep. This predisposition is supported by studies indicating that insomniacs report, more frequently than controls, difficulty relaxing, feeling tense and anxious, being overly preoccupied with a myriad of thoughts, and being worried and depressed (Kales et al., 1984). Other predisposing factors, such as distorted beliefs about sleep itself, including the belief that poor sleep is inevitable, that the lack of a full night of sleep will inevitably lead to disastrous health consequences, and that a minimum of 8 hours of sleep per day is critical to maintain health, can induce further emotional and cognitive arousal. Such catastrophizing is encouraged by many nights of poor sleep, which can foment cognitive rumination and worry about not falling asleep and about the potential for disastrous next-day consequences of sleeplessness. Therefore, such a cycle of apprehension and worry can *perpetuate* insomnia and make future sleep even less likely. Finally, insomniacs are prone to excessive cognitive monitoring at bedtime, which can further perpetuate insomnia; insomniacs carefully monitor mental and body sensations, as well as external cues such as the bedroom clock and environmental noises.

Arousal at bedtime can also be a learned response. The repeated experience of poor sleep promotes an association between sleeplessness and both pre-sleep activities and the sleep setting. Once these connections are established, the bedtime rituals and environment become contextual cues for arousal rather than for sleep (Yang, Spielman, & Glovinsky, 2006). The interaction between predisposing, precipitating, and perpetuating factors in the genesis and progression of insomnia are depicted in Figure 14.1.

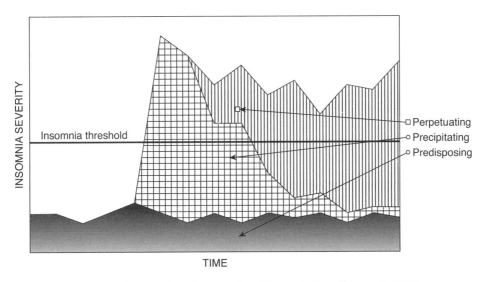

FIGURE 14.1 Factors in the genesis and progression of insomnia (from Yang et al., 2006).

Comorbid Insomnia

As noted earlier, comorbid insomnia refers to insomnia occurring in the context of other medical and psychiatric disorders. Insomnia typically occurs with one or more comorbidities (NIH, 2005), and comorbid insomnia is far more common than insomnia existing in isolation (Ohayon & Partinen, 2002). Some of these disorders are listed in Table 14.3 (Doghramji & Doghramji, 2006). Population studies suggest that 40% to 60% of comorbidities fall within the realm of psychiatric disorders (excluding primary insomnia), the most common of which are mood, anxiety, and substance use disorders (Ford & Kamerow, 1989; Ohayon & Partinen, 2002). Notably, however, a significant proportion of insomniacs suffer from nonpsychiatric comorbidities.

Table 14.4 lists some of the commonly encountered comorbid insomnia disorders and their defining symptoms (American Academy of Sleep Medicine, 2005; Doghramji et al., 2009).

A variety of medications can cause the complaint of insomnia, including anticholinergic agents, antihypertensives, antineoplastics, central nervous system (CNS) stimulants, hormones, antidepressants, antipsychotics, and withdrawal from sedating agents (Doghramji & Doghramji, 2006).

Selected Comorbid Disorders

Mood Disorders

There is a strong association between insomnia and mood disorders. Insomnia is voiced by most patients with major depression. Sleep patterns include difficulty falling asleep, frequent nocturnal awakenings, early morning awakening, nonrestorative sleep, decreased total sleep, and disturbing dreams. Daytime fatigue is also common (Reynolds, 1987). Insomnia is also a common complaint in bipolar patients in the depressed phase, yet hypersomnia is also a frequent complaint, with extended nocturnal sleep periods, difficulty awakening, and excessive daytime sleepiness (Detre, 1972). Hypersomnia is also common in seasonal affective

TABLE 14.3 Selected Conditions Associated with Insomnia

Psychiatric disorders
- Mood disorders (depression, bipolar disorder, dysthymic disorder)
- Anxiety disorders (generalized anxiety disorder, panic disorder, posttraumatic stress disorder)
- Substance use disorders
- Adjustment disorders
- Alzheimer disease
- Schizophrenia

Primary sleep disorders
- Obstructive sleep apnea syndrome
- Restless legs syndrome
- Periodic limb movement disorder
- Circadian rhythm disorders
    Shift work disorder
    Delayed sleep phase disorder
    Advanced sleep phase disorder
    Others

Medical conditions
- Chronic pain
- Cardiovascular disease (congestive heart failure, angina)
- Drug or alcohol intoxication or withdrawal
- Endocrine disorders (thyroid imbalance, dysfunctional uterine bleeding)
- Menopause
- Rheumatic disease (fibromyalgia, arthritis, ankylosing spondylitis, Sjögren syndrome)
- Pulmonary disease (chronic obstructive pulmonary disease, asthma, pneumonia)
- Neurologic disorders (Parkinson disease, Alzheimer disease, multiple sclerosis, uncontrolled migraines, brain tumor, traumatic brain injury)
- Urologic disease (benign prostatic hyperplasia, overactive bladder)
- Gastrointestinal disease (gastroesophageal reflux disease, peptic ulcer disease, irritable bowel syndrome)
- Acquired immunodeficiency syndrome (AIDS)
- Chronic fatigue syndrome
- Lyme disease
- Dermatologic disorders (nocturnal pruritus)
- Systemic cancer

disorder, during episodes of winter depression. During manic periods, however, patients usually report significantly reduced amounts of total sleep, often with a subjective sense of a decreased need for sleep.

Conversely, 14% to 20% of individuals with significant complaints of insomnia show evidence of major depression, whereas rates of depression are less than 1% in those without sleep complaints (Ford & Kamerow, 1989; Mellinger, 1985). Longitudinal studies indicate that insomnia is more likely to emerge prior to, rather than following, the onset of the acute phase of a mood disorder (Ohayon & Roth, 2003). Indeed, the complaint of insomnia also confers an increased risk for the development of new psychiatric disorders over the course of the ensuing year, a risk that diminishes if the insomnia resolves (Ford & Kamerow, 1989). Other studies have noted an enhanced risk for mood disorders for a median of 34 years following the complaint of insomnia (Chang et al., 1997). The occurrence and persistence of insomnia also confers an enhanced future risk for the future occurrence of anxiety and substance use disorders (Breslau et al., 1996; Weissman et al., 1997). There appears, therefore, to be a bidirectional relationship between insomnia and various psychiatric disorders, one which is most robust in the case of depression. From a clinical standpoint, these data suggest that the presence of chronic insomnia should alert the clinician to the possibility of the future

TABLE 14.4 Hallmark Symptoms of Commonly Encountered Comorbid Insomnia Disorders

Disorder	Hallmark Symptoms
Impaired sleep hygiene	Violation of one of the proper sleep hygiene recommendations (see below)
Psychophysiological insomnia	"Trying" to fall asleep Difficulty falling asleep at desired bedtime Frequent nocturnal awakenings Anxiety regarding sleeplessness
Restless legs syndrome (RLS)	Irresistible urge to move the extremities Limb paresthesiae Onset of symptoms during periods of rest and in the evening or at bedtime Relief of symptoms with movement
Periodic limb movement disorder (PLMD)	Repetitive involuntary movements of the extremities during sleep or just prior to falling asleep
Obstructive sleep apnea syndrome (OSAS)	Snoring Breathing pauses during sleep Choking Gasping Morning dry mouth
Chronic obstructive pulmonary disease	Dyspnea
Gastroesophageal reflux	Epigastric pain or burning Laryngospasm Acid taste in mouth Sudden nocturnal awakenings
Prostatic hypertrophy	Frequent nocturia
Nocturnal seizures	Thrashing in bed Loss of bladder or bowel control
Nocturnal panic attacks	Sudden surges of anxiety Tachycardia Diaphoresis Choking Laryngospasm
Posttraumatic stress disorder	Recurring, vivid dreams and nightmares Anxiety and hypervigilance in sleep environment
Delayed sleep phase disorder	Inability to fall asleep at desired time Inability to awaken at desired time
Advanced sleep phase disorder	Inability to stay awake until the desired bedtime Inability to remain asleep until the desired awakening time

emergence of a mood, anxiety, or substance use disorder. In addition, the lack of sufficient response to the treatment of presumed primary insomnia should alert the clinician to the possibility of an underlying, disguised, mood, substance use, or anxiety disorder that may warrant independent management.

Anxiety Disorders

Anxiety disorders represent the most frequent psychiatric comorbidities in individuals with insomnia (Ohayon, 2002). As noted earlier, insomnia often precedes the onset of an anxiety disorder. However, unlike the situation in mood disorders, insomnia is more likely to emerge at the same time (>38%) or after (>34%) the onset of the anxiety disorder (Ohayon & Roth, 2003).

The comorbidity of generalized anxiety disorder (GAD) and insomnia is more frequent than in all other anxiety disorders (Ohayon, Caulet, & Lemoine, 1998). Insomnia is one of the core symptoms of posttraumatic stress disorder (PTSD) and is thought to be a reflection of increased psychological and physiologic arousal associated with the original experience of the traumatic event or its reexperiencing (APA, 2000). Another core symptom of PTSD is that of distressing dreams and nightmares, reflections of the reexperiencing of the traumatic event. As with insomnia, their presence early in the aftermath of trauma is a strong predictor of the later development of PTSD itself (Mellman, David, Kulick-Bell, Hebding, & Nolan, 1995; Mellman & Uhde, 1989). Nightmares may incorporate portions of the actual traumatic event or the entire event, along with affective correlates. However, the latent content of the dream (i.e., the traumatic event and its psychic correlates) may be disguised so that dreams may be affectively charged yet lack the factual recollection of the actual event or may not be remembered at all. In the aftermath of trauma, the latter experience carries a more positive prognosis. Mellman and colleagues (2001) reported that within 6 weeks of traumatic events reports of dreams rated as "highly similar" to the traumatic experience and as distressing were associated with concurrent and subsequent PTSD severity. On the other hand, lack of dream recall or dreams that did not depict actual memories of the traumatic event were more characteristic of the group of individuals exposed to trauma yet who did not subsequently develop PTSD, although their dreams did contain some threatening scenarios. The authors theorized that dreams with highly replicative content represent a failure of adaptive emotional memory processing that is a normal function of REM sleep and dreaming.

Insomnia is not one of the diagnostic symptoms of panic disorder. However, insomnia, characterized by both impaired sleep initiation and maintenance, is more commonly reported by those with panic disorder than by normal individuals (Stein, Chartier, & Walker, 1993). Insomnia can be related to episodes of panic, which can arise during sleep and result in the complaint of insomnia. The first awareness of panic in most people with this disorder is a somatic symptom such as racing heart or shortness of breath (Shapiro & Sloan, 1998), which results in sudden awakening with a feeling of physical intensity. Taylor and colleagues (1986) noted that major spontaneous panic attacks clustered during the sleep period between 1:30 and 3:30 a.m. Contrary to popular belief, they generally do not occur in REM sleep. They have been observed to occur in slow-wave sleep and during the transition from stage 2 to slow-wave sleep (Mellman & Uhde, 1989). Dreams are not commonly reported preceding panic episodes. Not all patients with panic disorder experience panic episodes during sleep.

Insomnia can also arise from recurrent sleep panic attacks, which, in turn, can create a state of anticipatory anxiety and apprehension over the prospect of yet another night of sleeplessness followed by another day of fatigue. A vicious cycle can then ensue where excessive focus on sleep and trying to sleep causes greater tension and even greater impairment in sleep initiation and maintenance, thereby resulting in a second comorbid condition, that is, psychophysiological (or conditioned) insomnia (see earlier).

From the earlier discussion, it is evident that the complaint of insomnia can be associated with a host of sleep disorders and medical and psychiatric comorbidities. The complaint of insomnia warrants, therefore, a systematic and comprehensive evaluation process prior to proceeding to direct management of insomnia itself in clinical settings. Such an evaluation seems even more important when insomnia persists despite management. Although studies have not directly examined the causes of incomplete resolution of insomnia after direct management, it is likely that, at least in some cases, the presence of comorbid disorders is an important contributory factor. Once all of the related disorders are established, treatment can be conducted with greater accuracy and confidence (Doghramji & Choufani, in press; Sateia, Doghramji, Hauri, & Morin, 2000).

Evaluation

History

Essential elements of the history are outlined in Table 14.5 (Doghramji et al., 2009).

TABLE 14.5 Essential Elements of the Sleep/Wake History in the Evaluation of Insomnia

1. Nature of the complaint of insomnia
    a. Nocturnal pattern (initial, middle, terminal)
    b. Duration (acute, long term)
    c. Frequency (nightly, weekly, monthly, etc.)
    d. Precipitants (illnesses, shift work, medications, substances, etc.)
    e. Perpetuating factors (learned/conditioned response, hyperarousal, sleep hygiene habits, etc.)

2. Daytime symptoms
    a. Fatigue
    b. Irritability
    c. Anergia
    d. Memory impairment
    e. Mental slowing

3. Habits and behaviors related to sleep and the sleep environment that aggravate insomnia
    a. Caffeine and alcohol prior to bedtime
    b. Nicotine (both smoking and cessation)
    c. Large meals or excessive fluid intake within 3 hours of bedtime
    d. Exercising within 3 hours of bedtime
    e. Utilizing the bed for nonsleep activities (work, telephone, Internet)
    f. Staying in bed while awake for extended periods of time
    g. Activating behaviors up to the point of bedtime
    h. Excessive worrying at bedtime
    i. Clock-watching prior to sleep onset or during nocturnal awakenings
    j. Exposure to bright light prior to bedtime or during awakenings
    k. Keeping the bedroom too hot or too cold
    l. Noise
    m. Behaviors of a bed partner (e.g., snoring, leg movements)

4. Daytime habits and behaviors that aggravate insomnia
    a. Prolonged bed rest, inactivity, and excessive napping
    b. Insufficient light exposure
    c. Frequent travel and shift work

5. Patterns of sleep and wakefulness
    a. Bedtime
    b. Sleep latency (time to fall asleep after lights out)
    c. Nocturnal awakenings; number and duration
    d. Time of final morning awakening
    e. Rising time (i.e., time out of bed)
    f. Number, time, and duration of daytime naps
    g. Daytime symptoms, including levels of sleepiness and fatigue over the course of the day

1. The *nocturnal pattern* of insomnia can distinguish between various diagnostic possibilities; for example, delayed sleep phase syndrome is characterized by difficulty falling asleep, whereas advanced sleep phase syndrome is characterized by early bedtimes and early morning awakening. This can also be useful in determining treatment choice, as longer acting hypnotic agents may be better suited for midnocturnal awakenings and early morning insomnia.

2. The *duration and frequency* of symptoms are important in identifying degree of impairment. Insomnias of long duration and greater frequency are thought to have greater impact on daytime functioning, and they may require earlier and more aggressive management. Inventories can assist in the dimensional assessment or quantification of the severity of insomnia; although many are available, the Insomnia Severity Index (ISI; Fig. 14.2) is one of the few that have been subjected to empirical validation (Bastien, Vallieres, & Morin, 2001). The ISI takes into account subjective symptoms and consequences of insomnia and the degree of concern or distress caused by the disturbance. It is a useful clinical and research tool for measuring treatment outcome.

3. *Precipitants* of the insomnia complaint can identify etiology and guide management. Common precipitants include job loss, engaging in shift work or travel across time zones, breaches in relationships or loss of relatives through bereavement, onset of medical and psychiatric illness, and introduction of new medications or changes in dosages and times of administration of existing medications, among others. As noted earlier, following the onset of insomnia, *perpetuating factors* can transform insomnia into a chronic disorder. They include the development of poor sleep hygiene practices and of anticipatory anxiety with the approach of bedtime. Similarly, the patient's attitude toward his or her insomnia can itself have an important influence on the ability to sleep. In particular, the extent of dysfunctional beliefs and attitudes as well as sleep-related anxiety as bedtime approaches and during the bedtime hours provides the clinician with important insights into to the role these processes play in perpetuating or exacerbating the insomnia. Therefore, information about the dysfunctional cognitions of the insomniac such as catastrophic attributions of the effects of insomnia, the time of day that the insomniac begins to worry about sleep, and the state of mind of the insomniac during time awake during the night should all be solicited (Yang et al., 2006).

4. An assessment of *daytime symptoms* is useful in understanding the impact of insomnia on an individual's functioning. Additionally, the correction of daytime impairment is an important measure of treatment efficacy.

5. *Sleep-related habits and behaviors* in which the patient engages during the few hours prior to bedtime, during bedtime hours, and just after morning awakening can cause or significantly intensify existing insomnia. Although these factors are seldom the lone cause of an insomnia complaint, a lack of awareness of them can lead to a failure in other treatment modalities.

6. *Daytime habits and behaviors* that can adversely affect nocturnal sleep include intense exercise too close to bedtime (Stepanski & Wyatt, 2003). Long periods of bed rest, inactivity, and excessive napping can foment circadian rhythm disturbances and

Insomnia Severity Index (ISI)

Subject ID: _____   **Date:** _____

For each question below, please circle the number corresponding most accurately to your sleep patterns in the **LAST MONTH.**

For the first three questions, please rate the **SEVERITY** of your sleep difficulties.

1. Difficulty falling asleep:

None	Mild	Moderate	Severe	Very Severe
0	1	2	3	4

2. Difficulty staying asleep:

None	Mild	Moderate	Severe	Very Severe
0	1	2	3	4

3. Problem waking up too early in the morning:

None	Mild	Moderate	Severe	Very Severe
0	1	2	3	4

4. How **SATISFIED**/dissatisfied are you with your current sleep pattern?

Very Satisfied	Satisfied	Neutral	Dissatisfied	Very Dissatisfied
0	1	2	3	4

5. To what extent do you consider your sleep problem to **INTERFERE** with your daily functioning (e.g., daytime fatigue, ability to function at work/daily chores, concentration, memory, mood).

Not at all Interfering	**A Little** Interfering	**Somewhat** Interfering	**Much** Interfering	**Very Much** Interfering
0	1	2	3	4

6. How **NOTICEABLE** to others do you think your sleeping problem is in terms of impairing the quality of your life?

Not at all Noticeable	**A Little** Noticeable	**Somewhat** Noticeable	**Much** Noticeable	**Very Much** Noticeable
0	1	2	3	4

7. How **WORRIED**/distressed are you about your current sleep problem?

Not at all	**A Little**	**Somewhat**	**Much**	**Very Much**
0	1	2	3	4

Guidelines for Scoring/Interpretation:

Add scores for all seven items = _____
Total score ranges from 0–28

   0–7 = No clinically significant insomnia
   8–14 = Subthreshold insomnia
   15–21 = Clinical insomnia (moderate severity)
   22–28 = Clinical insomnia (severe)

FIGURE 14.2 The Insomnia Severity Index (printed with permission).

aggravate insomnia. Exposure to bright light can be helpful in establishing circadian cycling and, conversely, lack of sufficient light exposure during the morning hours can disrupt sleep timing. Frequent travel and shift work can also disrupt sleep and contribute to both insomnia and daytime sleepiness. It is useful to understand the patient's preferred social and occupational activities as this information can be helpful in devising a daily structure that promotes consistent sleep scheduling.

7. *Patterns of sleep and wakefulness* should be clarified during initial and follow-up visits. These patterns can also be assessed by utilizing patient-completed sleep logs or diaries that track sleep-wake patterns over time (Fig. 14.3). Importantly and of great clinical relevance, sleep logs and diaries may be more useful than subjective summaries since insomniacs tend to underestimate total sleep time and overestimate sleep latency, possibly resulting from a preferential recall bias for particularly bad nights of sleep that do not reflect the longitudinal course of their complaints (Carskadon et al., 1976).

Ideally, individuals retire and emerge from bed at consistent times day to day, including weekends. The time spent in bed between retiring and falling asleep would preferably be less than 20 minutes, and individuals would emerge from bed soon after awakening in the morning. Additionally, awakenings in good sleepers are typically limited to one or two, and time spent in bed following awakenings kept to a minimum (i.e., less than 15 minutes). These variables are affected by age (Cooke & Ancoli-Israel, 2006). Patients with insomnia can have large discrepancies from these norms, and patterns may emerge that suggest specific underlying causes of insomnia and/or help guide treatment. It is also useful to ascertain each of these parameters not only for the "average" day but also for a sequence of days, as such a temporal record can demonstrate variability in sleep patterns over time that can, in turn, contribute to poor sleep. The assessment of variability between workdays/schooldays, weekends, and vacations can also be useful. Insomniacs characteristically do not maintain rigorous sleep/wake schedules, and introducing such regularity into their lives is one of the primary elements of sleep hygiene education and other cognitive-behavioral techniques (see later discussion).

8. *Hallmark symptoms* of the various disorders described earlier should be inquired about (Table 14.4). In the case of obstructive sleep apnea syndrome (OSAS), The STOP-Bang Scoring Model is a validated inventory that succinctly summarizes the essential symptoms and historical findings, and predicts individuals who are at high risk for the disorder (Fig. 14.4; Chung et al., 2008). "Yes" answers to three or more questions identify the patient at high risk for OSA. Collateral information from bed partners can be useful in obtaining information that the patient may not be aware of, such as snoring, breathing pauses during sleep, limb movements, and the extent and frequency of naps. The history should also include the past medical history, history of medications, and substance use history. Family history is relevant since certain sleep disorders can have a hereditary component; for example, 50% of primary restless legs syndrome (RLS) cases have a positive family history (Montplaisir, Allen, Walters, & Ferini-Strambi, 2005). Social and occupational history can also contribute to irregular sleep/wake habits.

TWO WEEK SLEEP DIARY

INSTRUCTIONS:

1. Write the date, day of the week, and type of day: Work, School, Day Off, or Vacation.
2. Put the letter "C" in the box when you have coffee, cola or tea. Put "M" when you take any medicine. Put "A" when you drink alcohol. Put "E" when you exercise.
3. Put a line (I) to show when you go to bed. Shade in the box that shows when you think you fell asleep.
4. Shade in all the boxes that show when you are asleep at night or when you take a nap during the day.
5. Leave boxes unshaded to show when you wake up at night and when you are awake during the day.

SAMPLE ENTRY BELOW: On a Monday when I worked, I jogged on my lunch break at 1 PM, had a glass of wine with dinner at 6 PM, fell asleep watching TV from 7 to 8 PM, went to bed at 10:30 PM, fell asleep around Midnight, woke up and couldn't got back to sleep at about 4 AM, went back to sleep from 5 to 7 AM, and had coffee and medicine at 7:00 in the morning.

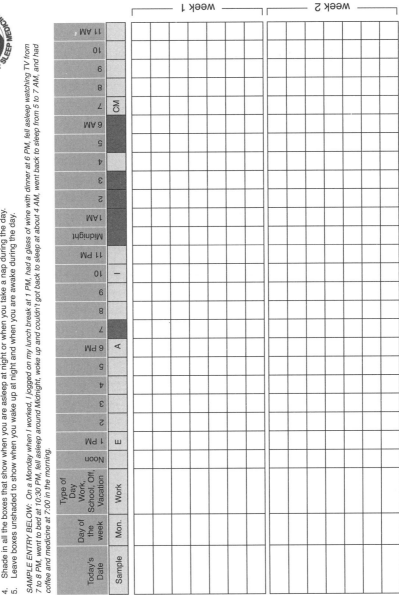

FIGURE 14.3 Sleep log.

1. *Snoring*
   Do you snore loudly (louder than talking or loud enough to be heard through closed doors)?
      Yes   No
2. *Tired*
   Do you often feel *tired*, fatigued, or sleepy during daytime?
      Yes   No
3. *Observed*
   Has anyone *observed* you stop breathing during your sleep?
      Yes   No
4. Blood *pressure*
   Do you have or are you being treated for high blood *pressure*?
      Yes   No
5. *BMI*
   BMI more than 30 kg/m^2?
      Yes   No
6. *Age*
   Age over 50 yr old?
      Yes   No
7. *Neck* circumference
   Neck circumference greater than 40 cm?
      Yes   No
8. *Gender*
   Gender male?
      Yes   No

High risk of OSA: answering yes to three or more items
Low risk of OSA: answering yes to less than three items

FIGURE 14.4 The STOP-Bang Scoring Model.

Physical and Mental Status Examinations

Although a *physical examination* is not routinely performed in psychiatric practice, it is essential in the evaluation of insomnia; for example, a neck circumference of 16 inches or greater in women and 17 inches or greater in men, is associated with an increased risk for sleep-related breathing disorders (Millman, Carlisle, McGarvey, Eveloff, & Levinson, 1995). Obesity with fat distribution around the neck or midriff suggests the diagnosis of OSA. Other contributors to sleep-related breathing disorders include nasal obstruction, mandibular hypoplasia, and retrognathia. Oropharyngeal abnormalities can also be involved, including enlarged tonsils and tongue, an elongated uvula and soft palate, diminished pharyngeal patency, and redundant pharyngeal mucosa (American Academy of Sleep Medicine, 2005). The Mallampati Airway Classification score should be determined (Fig. 14.5), which is useful in assessing the risk for OSA. On average, for every 1-point increase in the Mallampati score, the odds of having OSA increases more than twofold (Nuckton, Glidden, Browner, & Claman, 2006).

    The chest examination should be scrutinized for expiratory wheezes and kyphoscoliosis, indicative of, among others, asthma and restrictive lung disease, respectively, which, in turn, can be associated with the complaint of insomnia. Signs of right heart failure should be noted; heart failure can cause abnormalities of breathing during sleep, which, in turn, can be associated with the complaint of frequent nocturnal awakenings and unrefreshing sleep.

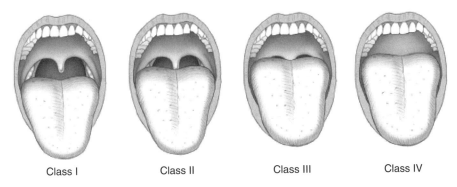

Class I   Class II   Class III   Class IV

FIGURE 14.5 Mallampati Airway Classification.

A basic neurological examination can clarify the presence of neurological disorders; for example, the presence of increased resting muscle tone, cogwheel rigidity, and tremor can indicate the presence of Parkinson disease. The *mental status examination* should include an evaluation of affect, anxiety, psychomotor agitation or slowing, cognition, the possibility of reduced alertness and slurred speech, and perceptual disturbances (Vaughn & O'Neill, 2005).

Diagnostic Testing

Potentially useful scales and inventories have been described earlier. The utility of *serum laboratory tests* has not been systematically explored in the evaluation of insomnia, yet it seems reasonable that general serum laboratory tests, including thyroid function studies, be considered if they have not been performed in the past 6 months to 1 year. RLS is more common in iron deficiency states and conditions associated with iron deficiency such as pregnancy and anemia (Sun, Chen, Ho, Earley, & Allen, 1998). The level of serum ferritin, an important indicator of iron deficiency, is inversely correlated with severity of RLS symptoms, and iron supplementation has been shown to reduce RLS symptoms. Therefore, serum ferritin should be obtained in patients presenting with insomnia or ES and associated RLS symptoms, and a level of 50 µg/l is considered significant.

Actigraphy utilizes small, wristwatch-like devices to record movement. It assumes that lack of movement is equivalent to sleep and is not, therefore, useful to measure exact sleep times. It can be useful for the assessment of sleep-wake patterns when such information is not reliably available by other means such as sleep logs. It can be appropriate for the documentation of changes in sleep patterns over prolonged diagnosis and treatment periods and for the assessment of whether an insomniac follows certain sleep hygiene advice (e.g., to curtail time in bed or to regularize wake-up times) and of improvement in sleep following behavioral treatment.

Polysomnography (PSG) is the technique of monitoring multiple physiologic measures during sleep, including brain waves, eye movements, heart rate, respirations, oxyhemoglobin saturation, and muscle tone and activity. Video recording identify abnormal movements during sleep. This test is typically performed in a sleep laboratory, although home testing is gradually gaining popularity. In the evaluation of insomnia, it is appropriate if the evaluation raises the suspicion of OSAS or PLMD (periodic limb movement disorder), if the patient reports violent or potentially injurious nocturnal behaviors, and for the diagnosis of paroxysmal arousals or other sleep disruptions thought to be seizure related. *Sleep medicine consultations* may be helpful if the office-based evaluation is not fruitful, or if the patient does not respond appropriately to treatment of the presumed disorder (Kushida et al., 2005).

Management of Comorbid Disorders

A systematic evaluation is the first step in the identification of conditions that are comorbid with insomnia. Once these have been identified, clinical wisdom suggests that they should be managed, or their existing management modalities should be optimized, in an effort to achieve resolution of the insomnia complaint. While this practice has not been well explored in the vast majority of comorbid disorders, the available data certainly support it. In this section, we will review therapeutic modalities specifically targeting comorbid conditions and their effects on insomnia.

Psychiatric Disorders

In general, effective management of these comorbid psychiatric disorders results in a decrement in insomnia complaints (van Mill, Hoogendijk, Vogelzangs, van Dyck, & Penninx, 2010). In the case of anxiety disorders, for example, GAD-specific cognitive-behavioral therapy (CBT) can ameliorate insomnia when used for the treatment of GAD (Belanger, Morin, Langlois, & Ladouceur, 2004) and imagery rehearsal with dream rescripting for the nightmares of patients with PTSD can improve sleep continuity, presumably as a secondary consequence of diminished nightmares (Krakow et al., 2001). Nonpharmacologic treatments directed primarily at the mood disorder can also diminish sleep disturbances, yet their effects may be more modest than those of antidepressants.

Pharmacologic therapies directed at comorbid psychiatric disorders can also diminish insomnia complaints, yet 25% to 45% of those treated with pharmacologic agents for mood or anxiety disorders continue to complain of insomnia following remission (Nierenberg et al., 1999; van Mill et al., 2010). In the case of major depressive disorder, one prospective study noted that sleep complaints were the most common residual symptoms following the achievement of remission with fluoxetine, followed by fatigue and loss of interest. This finding was irrespective of baseline severity of depression, length of the episode, age, gender, or marital status (Nierenberg et al., 1999). Residual depressive symptoms are associated with higher rates, and earlier occurrence, of relapse and recurrence, as compared to asymptomatic recovery, in major depression (Judd et al., 1998). However, the association between the persistence of insomnia and depression recurrence is independent of other depressive symptoms, chronic medical disease, and antidepressant medication use (Cho et al., 2008).

The causes of persistent sleep abnormalities following remission of psychiatric disorders are varied. In the case of major depression, these abnormalities may represent trait markers of depression; certain sleep electroencephalogram (EEG) alterations predict the future onset of depression (Modell, Ising, Holsboer, & Lauer, 2005) and persist following its remission (Kupfer, 1995). However, other studies have suggested that they may be state specific (Leistedt et al., 2007), raising the possibility that the persistence of sleep abnormalities represents incomplete treatment despite the achievement of conventionally established remission criteria. In addition, as is implicit from the discussion in prior sections, the persistence of subjective complaints such as insomnia following the achievement of remission can represent the effects of comorbid medical and other psychiatric disorders and medications, which have been reviewed earlier. With respect to medications, iatrogenic causes related to the medications used to treat the comorbid psychiatric disturbance must also be considered.

Although medications used to treat psychiatric disorders generally lead to a reduction of sleep-related complaints in parallel with other disease-specific symptoms, they may also produce additional sleep-related effects due to their direct pharmacologic effects on the processes governing sleep and wakefulness. These effects have been the subject of extensive exploration over the past few decades, yet these studies are limited by a number of shortcomings. They do not entirely represent prospective studies specifically examining sleep-related effects. Many are derived from the examination of side effects in studies with individuals with various psychiatric and neurological conditions. In some, distinctions between medication effects and the effects of the underlying conditions are blurred and few studies have examined the effects of these agents on normal subjects. Many studies, especially those utilizing antipsychotic and antiepileptic medications, have employed a small number of subjects of various disease types and have utilized inconsistent methodologies. Despite these shortcomings, the findings described generally have consistency across multiple studies. With the exception of low-dose doxepin, none of the antidepressants and antipsychotics is approved by the US Food and Drug Administration (FDA) for the treatment of insomnia.

Effects of antidepressants on sleep can be partially attributed to their unique receptor profiles. These are listed in Table 14.6 (Espana & Scammell, 2004). The positive effects on sleep continuity and latency appear to be largely mediated by these agents' blockade of histaminic, alpha-1 adrenergic, and 5HT2 receptors, whereas enhanced activity at these receptors confers a greater degree of sleep continuity disturbance. However, these same agents have a greater potential for the production of undesirable daytime sedation.

The effects of psychotropic medications used to treat anxiety and mood disorders on subjective and objective measures of sleep continuity are listed in Table 14.7 (Winokur et al., 2001).

The effects of antipsychotic drugs on sleep continuity are likely mediated through inhibitory effects at alpha-1 adrenergic, 5-HT-2, and histamine H-1 receptors. Their effects are summarized in Table 14.8 (Krystal, Goforth, & Roth, 2008). As is evident, all are likely to diminish awakenings and improve continuity of sleep following sleep onset, yet some may be more efficacious for sleep latency reduction.

In addition to receptor profile, pharmacokinetic considerations are likely involved in their effects on sleep. The lower effect on sleep latency with certain agents such as clozapine, olanzapine, and ziprasidone may be a product of their relatively slow absorption.

TABLE 14.6 Impact of Receptor Systems on Sleep Continuity

Increased Sleep Continuity	Decreased Sleep Continuity
Antihistaminic	5HT1A binding
5HT2 blockade	5HT2 binding
Alpha-1 norepinephrine blockade	Dopamine binding
	Norepinephrine binding

TABLE 14.7 Effects of Antidepressants on Sleep Continuity

Antidepressant	Receptor Profile	Impact on Sleep Continuity
MAOI	↑ 5HT1A, 5HT2; NE, and DA	↓
TCA	↑ 5HT1A,5HT2, NE, DA (weak); ↓ HA, NE, Ach	→ To ↑
SSRI	↑ 5HT1A,5HT2 binding	→ To ↓
Venlafaxine	↑ 5HT1A,5HT2; NE and DA (weak) binding	↓
Bupropion	↑ NE, and DA	→ To ↓
Nefazodone	↓ 5HT2	↑
Trazodone	↓ HA, 5HT2, NE; weak ↑ 5HT1A,5HT2	↑
Mirtazapine	↓ HA, 5HT2; ↑ NE, 5HT1A,5HT2	↑

MAOI, monoamine oxidase inhibitors; SSRI, selective serotonin re-uptake inhibitors; TCA, tricyclic antidepressant.

Sleep Disorders
Obstructive Sleep Apnea Syndrome

The effective management of various sleep disorders appears to be helpful in diminishing insomnia complaints and improving sleep latency and continuity. Approximately 39%–55% of OSAS patients report insomnia symptoms, primarily a difficulty in staying asleep (Luyster, Buysse, & Strollo, 2010). Established treatment modalities for OSAS include lifestyle changes such as the avoidance of CNS depressants and weight loss, body positioning devices, dental (oral) appliances, upper airway surgery, and positive airway devices that are utilized during sleep such as continuous positive airway pressure (CPAP). A few studies have documented the improvement in insomnia severity following the treatment of sleep disordered breathing in patients with insomnia and comorbid OSAS. Treatments that have been examined in this regard include nasal-dilator-strips (Krakow et al., 2006), surgery (Guilleminault, Davis, & Huynh, 2008), and a combination of treatments, including CPAP, oral appliances, or bilateral turbinectomy (Krakow et al., 2004). In the latter study, the addition of CBT provided additional benefit for insomnia symptoms. It should be noted, however, that insomnia can also complicate the course of treatment with CPAP in certain OSAS patients and possibly diminish compliance with CPAP, in which case direct management of insomnia may be beneficial, a practice that will be discussed in the next section (Luyster et al., 2010).

TABLE 14.8 Effects of Antipsychotics on Sleep Continuity

Antipsychotic	Shorten Sleep Latency	Decrease Awakenings and/or WASO
Clozapine	+	+++
Quetiapine	+++	+++
Ziprasidone	+	+++
Olanzapine	+	+++
Resperidone	+	++
Thiothixene	+++	+++
Haloperidol	+++	+++

WASO, wake after sleep onset. 0, no effect; +, mild effect; + +, moderate effect; + + +, strong effect.

Restless Legs Syndrome

Ninety percent of RLS sufferers report insomnia (Montplaisir et al., 1997), which is associated with motor restlessness and an irresistible urge to move the extremities. These symptoms peak in severity around bedtime and shortly thereafter, and they interfere with the ability to fall asleep or awaken sleepers following sleep onset. Insomnia is the single most troubling symptom for the RLS patient, and insomnia and daytime fatigue are the most common reasons for consulting a physician (Hening et al., 2004). Treatments for the condition include various behavioral measures, iron supplementation, dopamine agonists, benzodiazepines, opioids, and antiepileptic compounds, yet only the dopamine agonists pramipexole and ropinorole are indicated by the FDA for the condition and seem to provide specific therapy directed at the presumed etiology and have, therefore, received the most extensive studies (Littner et al., 2004). In general, these studies reveal a reduction in sleep-related complaints, both at sleep onset and following sleep onset, following effective management of RLS paresthesiae, motor disturbances, and periodic limb movements in sleep (Erichsen, Ferri, & Gozal, 2010).

Circadian Rhythm Disorders

Insomnia is a hallmark symptom of all of the circadian rhythm sleep disorders. It results from a mismatch between the ambient light-dark cycle and endogenous rhythms, so that the circadian alerting signal occurs during the desired (or required) time for sleep. Management of the sleep component of these conditions includes behavioral measures such as sleep schedule adjustment and proper sleep hygiene practices, timed bright light administration, melatonin, and hypnotic agents. Studies have shown that correction of the underlying sleep phase misalignment can result in improved sleep continuity, diminished sleep latency, and a lessening of insomnia severity (Sack et al., 2007a, 2007b). Although melatonin has not been widely accepted as a consistently effective treatment modality for undifferentiated insomnia complaints, it has been shown to be effective in advancing the sleep-wake rhythm and endogenous melatonin rhythm in delayed sleep phase disorder, leading to a decrease in sleep latency in that disorder (van Geijlswijk, Korzilius, & Smits, 2010). It has also been shown to hold promise in the treatment of shift work disorder, where results have been inconsistent, with some studies revealing a shift in circadian phase in parallel with improved sleep quality and duration (Morgenthaler et al., 2007).

Miscellaneous Medical Conditions

A wide variety of medical and neurological conditions are associated with the complaint of insomnia. The extent of this complaint in each condition, and its response to treatment targeting the comorbid condition, has not been well explored. Next, we discuss two medical disorders in which data are available and refer the reader to reviews published elsewhere (Culpepper, 2006; McCrae & Lichstein, 2001; Stepanski & Rybarczyk, 2006).

Gastroesophageal Reflux Disease

Heartburn that is associated with nocturnal awakening affects approximately 25% of the general US population >40 years of age. In a recent national survey, 79% of individuals suffering from heartburn reported having these symptoms at night (Locke, Talley, Fett,

Zinsmeister, & Melton, 1997). Of those, 63% reported that their symptoms affected their ability to get a good night's sleep, 75% reported that symptoms kept them from falling asleep or woke them up during sleep, and 40% indicated that heartburn had some effect on their ability to function well at work the next day. Diminished esophageal acid clearance during sleep, which occurs under normal conditions, is thought to be responsible for the high rate of sleep-related reflux symptoms in gastroesophageal reflux disease (GERD) sufferers, which, in turn, is due to a variety of factors, including the loss of gravitational drainage, diminished swallowing, and slower gastric emptying. The severity of GERD symptoms is related to the severity of the sleep disturbance (Dickman et al., 2007). Disturbed sleep in the form of arousals and awakenings is, in turn, thought to serve a protective function for the esophagus, as it facilitates esophageal acid clearance. However, it is also associated with insomnia and daytime fatigue (Dickman et al., 2007). Enhanced esophageal acid exposure is also related to the development of esophagitis, Barrett's esophagus, and adenocarcinoma (Rubenstein, Scheiman, Sadeghi, Whiteman, & Inadomi, 2010).

Treatment of GERD with proton pump inhibitor medications reduces esophageal acid exposure and restores sleep continuity by diminishing their associated arousals and awakenings (Dimarino et al., 2005). Conversely, symptomatic treatment of insomnia with hypnotic agents, although it results in an improvement of sleep quality, can also lead to an increase in esophageal acid exposure by reducing the protective arousal response to nocturnal acid exposure, raising the possibility of an increased risk of future complications (Gagliardi et al., 2009).

Chronic Obstructive Pulmonary Disease

Sleep disturbances are the third most commonly reported symptoms, after dyspnea and fatigue, in chronic obstructive pulmonary disease (COPD) and 53% of patients with chronic bronchitis complain of insomnia characterized by difficulty in falling asleep and maintaining sleep (Kinsman et al., 1983; Klink & Quan, 1987). Insomnia is thought to be related to a variety of disease-specific factors (George & Bayliff, 2003), such as excessive mucus production and cough and the increased work of breathing associated with airflow limitation, and hypoxemia and/or hypercapnia during sleep, resulting in an increase in ventilation and respiratory effort, which, in turn, leads to sleep-related arousals and awakenings.

Studies into the effects of disease-specific treatments and their effects on sleep are scant. The beta-2 agonist albutamol (albuterol) does not appear to affect sleep quality adversely in patients with asthma and COPD (Veale, Cooper, Griffiths, Corris, & Gibson, 1994) and the anticholinergic medication ipratropium resulted in improved subjective sleep quality and an increase in REM sleep time in patients with moderate to severe COPD (Martin et al., 1999). No data are available on the effects of inhaled steroids on sleep in patients with COPD, and the methylxanthine theophylline is known to have negative effects on sleep continuity variables and subjective sleep quality in normal volunteers. In patients with COPD, it was reported to impair sleep quality in one study (Mulloy & McNicholas, 1993) and had no effect on sleep in two others (Brander & Salmi, 1992; Martin & Pak, 1992). The effects of oxygen supplementation on sleep in COPD have been variable, with some studies revealing improvement and others revealing no change (Stege et al., 2008).

The limited data that are available regarding disease-specific treatments for comorbid insomnia disorders suggest, therefore, that treatment of the comorbid disorder can produce a diminution of insomnia severity. Furthermore, they send a note of caution regarding the management of insomnia directly, without first addressing the comorbid disorder. Finally, they suggest that in many cases insomnia complaints remain even after effective management of comorbid disorders. The direct management of insomnia will be the subject of the next section.

Management of Insomnia

Nonpharmacologic Methods

The various established options in this category, and levels of evidence supporting the use of each method, are listed in Table 14.9 (Morgenthaler et al., 2006). A majority of insomniacs respond to nonpharmacologic methods. When compared with pharmacologic methods, they are at least as efficacious and have the advantage of longer duration of benefit (Morin, 2006).

Sleep hygiene education attempts to correct habits and behaviors that may be counterproductive to good sleep. Although evidence supporting sleep hygiene education as a stand-alone therapeutic modality is lacking, this modality is considered to be a necessary component of any nonpharmacologic strategy since poor sleep hygiene habits may impair the efficacy of other techniques. Many versions of sleep hygiene instructions have been described. A composite of the various recommendations appears in Table 14.10 (Hauri, 1997; Stepanski & Wyatt, 2003).

Stimulus control therapy (SCT) is based on the premise that insomnia is caused by the conditioned arousal that occurs in response to the stimulus of repeated wakefulness and the bedroom environment; this is further elaborated upon in the section on "Pathophysiological

TABLE 14.9 Psychological and Behavioral Therapies for Insomnia

Technique	Goal	Method
Sleep hygiene education	Promote habits that help sleep; eliminate habits that interfere with sleep	Promote habits that help sleep; eliminate habits that interfere with sleep
Stimulus control therapy*	Strengthen bed and bedroom as sleep stimuli	If unable to fall asleep within 20 minutes, get out of bed and repeat as necessary
Restriction of time in bed (sleep restriction)	Improve sleep continuity by limiting time spent in bed	Decrease time in bed to equal time actually asleep and increase as sleep efficiency improves
Cognitive therapy	Dispel faulty beliefs that may perpetuate insomnia	Talk therapy to dispel unrealistic and exaggerated notions about sleep
Relaxation therapies*	Reduce arousal and decrease anxiety	Biofeedback, progressive muscle relaxation
Paradoxical intention	Relieve performance anxiety	Patient is instructed to try to stay awake
Cognitive-behavioral therapy*	Combines sleep restriction, stimulus control, and sleep hygiene education with cognitive therapy	Combines sleep restriction, stimulus control, and sleep hygiene education with cognitive therapy

*Standard therapy (high clinical certainty).

TABLE 14.10 Elements of Sleep Hygiene Education

Do the following:
- Awaken at the same time every morning
- Increase exposure to bright light during the day
- Establish a daily activity routine
- Exercise regularly in the morning and/or afternoon
- Set aside a worry time
- Establish a comfortable sleep environment
- Do something relaxing prior to bedtime
- Try a warm bath

Avoid the following:
- Napping, unless a shift worker
- Alcohol
- Caffeine, nicotine, and other stimulants
- Exposure to bright light during the night
- Exercise within 3 hours of bedtime
- Heavy meals or drinking within 3 hours of bedtime
- Noise
- Excessive heat/cold in room
- Using your bed for things other than sleep (or sex)
- Watching the clock
- Trying to sleep

Models of Primary Insomnia." The assumption is that spending time awake in bed while eating, talking, watching television, or worrying strengthens the association between the bedroom cues and sleeplessness, perpetuating insomnia. The goal of SCT is to break the association between bedroom cues and conditioned arousal that occurs with repeated wakefulness, to imprint bed as sleep stimulus, and to associate the bedroom environment with falling asleep. Specific instructions are listed in Table 14.11 (Yang et al., 2006).

Sleep restriction therapy strives to improve sleep continuity by curtailing time spent in bed. This results in some sleep curtailment, which, in turn, results in greater sleep continuity as long as naps are avoided. It also leads to enhanced sleep efficiency, which, in turn, may result in the perception of improved sleep quality. Principles of this approach are summarized in Table 14.12.

Cognitive therapy attempts to address the dysfunctional cognitions, catastrophic thinking, and preoccupation with sleeplessness that accompany insomnia and ultimately contribute to poor sleep. These are described earlier in this chapter. In the course of the therapy, insomniacs' dysfunctional beliefs and attitudes toward sleep need to be challenged, their unrealistic expectations about sleep need to be corrected, and their perceptions of the consequences of insomnia need to be reappraised (Yang et al., 2006).

TABLE 14.11 Rules of Stimulus Control Therapy

- Go to bed only when sleepy
- Use bed for sleep and sex only; avoid watching television, reading, or eating in bed
- If not able to fall asleep in 15 minutes, then leave the bedroom as soon as start to feel anxious or irritable and go to another room. Do not watch the clock
- Return to bed only when sleepy
- Repeat above tactic as often as needed
- Regardless of total sleep time, always wake up at the same time
- Avoid daytime naps

TABLE 14.12 Sleep Restriction Therapy

- Determine average time spent asleep from 1–2 week sleep diary
- Set time in bed to equal time spent asleep, never less than 5 hours
- Determine mean sleep efficiency (time spent asleep ÷ time in bed × 100 = %) over 5-day period
  - If efficiency ≥90%, increase time in bed by 15–20 minutes
  - If efficiency <85%, decrease time in bed by 15–20 minutes
- Regular wake time
- No napping

Relaxation therapy was developed around the theory that hyperarousal leads to insomnia. The goal of the relaxation therapy is not to induce sleep; the goal is to reduce arousal and induce a relaxed state (relaxation), thus allowing sleep to occur. Progressive muscle relaxation, autogenic training, guided imagery, and biofeedback are among the many techniques that have been used to reduce arousal and induce relaxation. Before applying relaxation therapy at bedtime, the patients are trained and instructed to practice relaxation techniques during the day (Yang et al., 2006).

Paradoxical intention is intended for patients with sleep onset insomnia. Patients are instructed to try to stay awake for as long as possible. Its effectiveness may be a result of redefining the task, thus removing the performance anxiety associated with the urgency of falling asleep (Ascher & Efran, 1978).

Cognitive-behavioral therapy (CBT) combines various nonpharmacologic strategies, as noted in the table. Individual treatment sessions are typically conducted once per week over the course of 6 to 8 weeks. It has been shown to have consistent short-term (average 5 weeks) efficacy, and durability of benefit of up to 6 months following the termination of treatment (Morin et al., 2006). It enjoys greater patient acceptance than pharmacotherapy and has few, if any, adverse effects, although these have not been systematically explored (Morin, Gaulier, Barry, & Kowatch, 1992). Its major drawback lies in the limited availability of trained therapists, inconvenience, time commitment, and cost. It also necessitates active patient participation. Attempts have recently been made to address some of these drawbacks through the provision of treatment in groups, training primary care nurse practitioners to provide CBT, and even devising telephone, videotape, and Internet treatment modalities; a recent study demonstrated both short-term efficacy and long-term durability of benefit with internet CBT (Ritterband et al., 2009). Attempts have also been made to provide CBT with an abbreviated number of sessions; a recent study of Brief Behavioral Treatment of Insomnia (BBTI) demonstrated the efficacy of individualized behavioral instructions delivered in two intervention sessions and two telephone calls over the course of 4 weeks; improvements were maintained over the course of 6 months (Buysse et al., 2011).

Pharmacologic Agents

FDA-Approved Hypnotic Medications

These are summarized in Table 14.13 (Curry, Eisenstein, & Walsh, 2006; Markov & Doghramji, 2010; Neubauer, 2012).

They include benzodiazepine and nonbenzodiazepine agents, both of which are also agonists at the benzodiazepine receptor site on the GABA-A receptor complex (BzRAs), the melatonin receptor agonist ramelteon, and the H-1 receptor antagonist doxepin. With the

TABLE 14.13 FDA-Approved Hypnotic Agents

Class	Hypnotic	Doses (mg)	Elimination Half-Life (hr)	Indications	DEA Class
Benzodiazepine receptor agonist benzodiazepines	Flurazepam	15, 30	48–120	treatment of insomnia characterized by difficulty in falling asleep, frequent nocturnal awakenings, and/or early morning awakening	IV
	Temazepam	7.5, 15, 22.5, 30	8–20	short-term treatment of insomnia	IV
	Triazolam	0.125, 0.25	2–4	short-term treatment of insomnia	IV
	Quazepam	7.5, 15	48–120	treatment of insomnia characterized by difficulty in falling asleep, frequent nocturnal awakenings, and/or early morning awakenings	IV
	Estazolam	1, 2	8–24	short-term management of insomnia characterized by difficulty in falling asleep, frequent nocturnal awakenings, and/or early morning awakenings; administered at bedtime improved sleep induction and sleep maintenance	IV
Benzodiazepine receptor agonist nonbenzodiazepines	Zolpidem	5, 10	1.5–2.4	short-term treatment of insomnia characterized by difficulties with sleep initiation	IV
	Zaleplon	5, 10	1	short-term treatment of insomnia; has been shown to decrease the time to sleep onset	IV
	Eszopiclone	1, 2, 3	5–7	treatment of insomnia; administered at bedtime decreased sleep latency and improved sleep maintenance	IV
	Zolpidem ER	6.25, 12.5	2.8–2.9	treatment of insomnia characterized by difficulties with sleep onset and/or sleep maintenance as measured by wake time after sleep onset	IV
	Zolpidem Oral spray	5, 10	~2.5	short-term treatment of insomnia characterized by difficulties with sleep initiation	IV
	Zolpidem Sublingual	5, 10	~2.5	short-term treatment of insomnia characterized by difficulties with sleep initiation	IV
Melatonin receptor agonist	Ramelteon	8	1–2.6	treatment of insomnia characterized by difficulty with sleep onset	None
H-1 receptor antagonist	Doxepin	3, 6	15.3	treatment of insomnia characterized by difficulties with sleep maintenance	None

exception of doxepin, all of these agents have established efficacy for difficulties in falling asleep and some for difficulties in maintaining sleep. One of the most relevant distinctions between these agents is elimination half-life. Although other factors are also involved in the determination of clinical efficacy, in general agents with longer half-lives have a longer duration of action and are beneficial for sleep maintenance insomnia, yet they may produce residual daytime sedation and cognitive impairment. In the case of zolpidem ER, the efficacy for sleep maintenance insomnia is achieved by its extended-release feature. Agents with shorter half-lives are better suited for sleep initiation difficulties and have less of a likelihood of daytime sedation. Zaleplon, an ultrashort half-life agent, has also been evaluated for administration in the middle of the night following nocturnal awakenings (Zammit et al., 2006), a practice that should not be utilized unless the patient has the opportunity to be in bed for at least 4 hours after administration, although no hypnotic agents are FDA approved for this specific use.

The main adverse effects of the BzRAs are daytime sedation and psychomotor and cognitive impairment, whose likelihood is greater with the longer half-life hypnotics and in the case of hypnotics with active metabolites. Therefore, the clinical challenge in using this class of compounds is the identification of a particular medication along the half-life continuum that produces maximum efficacy across the night and minimum daytime residual effects. BzRA hypnotics should be used with caution in individuals with respiratory depression (e.g., COPD and OSAS), in the elderly, in those with hepatic disease, those with multiple medical conditions, and those who are taking other medications that have CNS-depressant properties. Individuals who must awaken during the course of the drug's active period should not take these medications. All of the BzRAs are DEA Schedule IV agents carry a risk of abuse liability (Doghramji & Doghramji, 2006).

The most common adverse effects that are associated with ramelteon include somnolence, fatigue, and dizziness. It is not recommended for use with fluvoxamine due to a CYP 1A2 interaction. A mild elevation in prolactin levels has been noted in a small number of females and a mild decrease in testosterone values has been noted in elderly males, yet the clinical relevance of these changes remains unclear. Ramelteon does not demonstrate respiratory depression in mild to moderate OSAS or in mild to moderate COPD. It is DEA nonscheduled and does not carry the risk of abuse liability (Zammit et al., 2007).

The most common adverse effects associated with low-dose doxepin are somnolence/sedation, nausea, and upper respiratory tract infection. At higher, antidepressant, doses, it is associated with anticholinergic side effects, including sedation, confusion, urinary retention, constipation, blurred vision, and dry mouth, and other effects such as hypotension and dose-dependent cardiotoxicity; nevertheless, these effects have not been observed at hypnotic doses. Antidepressants are associated with an increased risk, when compared to placebo, of suicidal thinking and behavior in children, adolescents, and young adults in short-term studies of major depressive disorder and other psychiatric disorders. The risk for suicide from the lower dose of doxepin cannot be excluded. Doxepin is contraindicated in patients with severe urinary retention, narrow angle glaucoma, and who have used monoamine oxidase inhibitors (MAOIs) within the previous 2 weeks (Markov & Doghramji, 2010).

Tolerance, a decrement in clinical efficacy following repeated use, and rebound insomnia, an escalation of insomnia beyond baseline severity levels following abrupt discontinuation, can occur even after a few weeks of administration. They appear to be more pronounced following the administration of higher doses of hypnotics and of the older, benzodiazepine, agents that have a short elimination half-life, such as triazolam, than the longer elimination half-life benzodiazepines and some of the newer nonbenzodiazpine BzRAs (Soldatos, Dikeos, & Whitehead, 1999). Eszopiclone (Krystal et al., 2003), zolpidem ER (Krystal et al., 2008), and ramelteon (Mayer et al., 2009) have been evaluated for up to 6 months in controlled studies, and they have demonstrated a low proclivity for the production of these effects. Nevertheless, clinical wisdom suggests that all hypnotics should be utilized for short periods of time as much as possible. Patients utilizing these medications for longer periods of time should be evaluated periodically for tolerance and carefully monitored for withdrawal symptoms following abrupt discontinuation. The risk of rebound insomnia and withdrawal symptoms can be minimized by utilizing the lowest effective dose and by gradually tapering the dose over the course of a few nights.

Hypnotics carry the potential for severe allergic reactions and complex sleep-related behaviors, which include sleep driving. The latter may be associated with concomitant ingestion of alcohol and other sedating substances (Southworth, Kortepeter, & Hughes, 2008). It may be prudent, therefore, to advise patients to limit the use of such substances whenever possible.

Hypnotics should be utilized at reduced dosages in the elderly, and, whenever possible those with the shortest half-lives should be considered. The BzRAs should also not be offered to patients with a history of drug and alcohol dependence without close monitoring. The addition of alcohol and other sedating agents may lead to potentiation of sedative effects and decreased margin of safety.

Medications Not FDA Approved as Hypnotics

A recent NIH state-of-the-science conference concluded that "evidence supports the efficacy of cognitive-behavioral therapy and benzodiazepine receptor agonists in the treatment of this disorder. Very little evidence supports the efficacy of other treatments, despite their widespread use" (NIH, 2005). These agents consist mainly of the sedating antidepressants and antipsychotic agents, typically utilized at low doses that are subtherapeutic from the standpoint of their intended applications. The effects of these agents on sleep and insomnia have been reviewed in Tables 14.6, 14.7, and 14.8. Trazodone and mirtazapine are the most commonly utilized agents; there are no published studies on the latter, and the former has received little scientific attention, in primary insomnia (Ford & Kamerow, 1989). Although trazodone does increase total sleep time in patients with major depressive disorder, there are virtually no dose–response data for trazodone vis-à-vis sleep and, similarly, no available data on tolerance to its possible hypnotic effects. Concerns have been raised regarding daytime somnolence, the significant dropout rates in clinical studies, and the induction of cardiac arrhythmias, primarily in patients with histories of cardiac disease, as well as the development of priapism. Sedating antipsychotic agents have also received little scientific attention for the management of insomnia, and their spectrum of potential side effects includes sedation and metabolic disturbances; their use in primary insomnia cannot, therefore, be wholeheartedly supported.

Over-the-Counter Agents

Over-the-counter agents marketed for insomnia contain the antihistamines diphenhydramine or doxylamine. Although the evidence supporting their efficacy in insomnia is scant, antihistamines may produce mild to moderate sedation and may improve sleep latency and continuity for some individuals. However, tolerance to their sedating effects can develop rapidly (Richardson, Roehrs, Rosenthal, Koshorek, & Roth, 2002). They are also associated with morning grogginess, daytime sleepiness possibly leading to impairment of driving ability, delirium, urinary retention, constipation, dry mouth, blurry vision, and psychomotor impairment (Basu, Dodge, Stoehr, & Ganguli, 2003).

Although their use is not regulated by the FDA, dietary supplements and herbal remedies also enjoy extensive usage, owing to a variety of factors, including their widespread availability, lack of prescription requirements, relatively low cost, and the widespread belief that they are safe and have a relatively low abuse risk. These include, among others, valerian, kava-kava (Piper methysticum), melatonin, chamomilla, passiflora, avena sativa, and humulus lupulus. Most of these have not been well studied for safety and efficacy; melatonin, which has received the widest evaluations, may be effective in the treatment of delayed sleep phase disorder and shift work disorder, but it does not appear to be consistently effective in treating most primary or comorbid sleep disorders with short-term use (Buscemi et al., 2004).

Conclusions

Insomnia is a common complaint in the community and in clinical settings. Its persistence following management may reflect the existence of comorbid sleep, psychiatric, and medical disorders. Therefore, a systematic evaluation, which strives to uncover these disorders, may offer inroads into more specific treatment modalities, which, in turn, can diminish insomnia complaints.

Disclosure Statement

K.D. is a consultant for UCB, Inc. and holds stock in Merck.

C.F.R. has received pharmaceutical supplies for NIH-sponsored research from BMS, Lilly, Pfizer, and Forest Laboratories.

References

American Academy of Sleep Medicine. International Classification of Sleep Disorders. 2nd ed. Westchester, IL: American Academy of Sleep Medicine; 2005.

American Psychiatric Association. Diagnostic and Statistical Manual of Mental Disorders. 4th ed., text rev. Arlington, VA: American Psychiatric Association; 2000.

Ascher LM, Efran JS. Use of paradoxical intention in a behavioral program for sleep onset insomnia. *J Consult Clin Psychol* 1978;46(3):547–550.

Bastien CH, Vallieres A, Morin CM. Validation of the Insomnia Severity Index as an outcome measure for insomnia research. *Sleep Med* 2001;2(4):297–307.

Basu R, Dodge H, Stoehr GP, Ganguli M. Sedative-hypnotic use of diphenhydramine in a rural, older adult, community-based cohort: effects on cognition. *Am J Geriatr Psychiatry* 2003;11(2):205–213.

Belanger L, Morin CM, Langlois F, Ladouceur R. Insomnia and generalized anxiety disorder: effects of cognitive behavior therapy for gad on insomnia symptoms. *J Anxiety Disord* 2004;18(4):561–571.

Bonnet MH, Arand DL. Physiological activation in patients with sleep state misperception. *Psychosom Med* 1997;59(5):533–540.

Bonnet MH, Arand DL. Heart rate variability in insomniacs and matched normal sleepers. *Psychosom Med* 1998;60(5):610–615.

Brander PE, Salmi T. Nocturnal oxygen saturation and sleep quality in patients with advanced chronic obstructive pulmonary disease during treatment with moderate dose CR-theophylline. *Eur J Clin Pharmacol* 1992;43(2):125–129.

Breslau N, Roth T, Rosenthal L, Andreski P. Sleep disturbance and psychiatric disorders: a longitudinal epidemiological study of young adults. *Biol Psychiatry* 1996;39(6):411–418.

Buscemi N, Vandermeer B, Pandya R, Hooton N, Tjosvold L, Hartling L, et al. Melatonin for treatment of sleep disorders. *Evid Rep Technol Assess (Summ)* 2004;108:1–7.

Buysse DJ, Germain A, Moul DE, Franzen PL, Brar LK, Fletcher ME, et al. Efficacy of brief behavioral treatment for chronic insomnia in older adults. *Arch Intern Med* 2011;171:887–895.

Buysse DJ, Thompson W, Scott J, Franzen PL, Germain A, Hall M, et al. Daytime symptoms in primary insomnia: a prospective analysis using ecological momentary assessment. *Sleep Med* 2007;8(3):198–208.

Carskadon MA, Dement WC, Mitler MM, Guilleminault C, Zarcone VP, Spiegel R. Self-reports versus sleep laboratory findings in 122 drug-free subjects with complaints of chronic insomnia. *Am J Psychiatry* 1976;133(12):1382–1388.

Chang PP, Ford DE, Mead LA, Cooper-Patrick L, Klag MJ. Insomnia in young men and subsequent depression. The Johns Hopkins Precursors Study. *Am J Epidemiol* 1997;146(2):105–114.

Chevalier H, Los F, Boichut D, Bianchi M, Nutt DJ, Hajak G, et al. Evaluation of severe insomnia in the general population: results of a European multinational survey. *J Psychopharmacol* 1999;13(4 Suppl 1):S21–24.

Cho HJ, Lavretsky H, Olmstead R, Levin MJ, Oxman MN, Irwin MR. Sleep disturbance and depression recurrence in community-dwelling older adults: a prospective study. *Am J Psychiatry* 2008;165(12):1543–1550.

Chung F, Yegneswaran B, Liao P, Chung SA, Vairavanathan S, Islam S, et al. STOP questionnaire: a tool to screen patients for obstructive sleep apnea. *Anesthesiology* 2008;108(5):812–821.

Cooke JR, Ancoli-Israel S. Sleep and its disorders in older adults. *Psychiatr Clin North Am* 2006;29(4):1077–93; abstract x–xi.

Culpepper L. Secondary insomnia in the primary care setting: review of diagnosis, treatment, and management. *Curr Med Res Opin* 2006;22(7):1257–1268.

Curry DT, Eisenstein RD, Walsh JK. Pharmacologic management of insomnia: past, present, and future. *Psychiatr Clin North Am* 2006;29(4):871–93; abstract vii–viii.

Detre T, Himmelhoch J, Swartzburg M, Anderson CM, Byck R, Kupfer DJ. Hypersomnia and manic-depressive disease. *Am J Psychiatry* 1972;128(10):1303–1305.

Dew MA, Hoch CC, Buysse DJ, Monk TH, Begley AE, Houck PR, et al. Healthy older adults' sleep predicts all-cause mortality at 4 to 19 years of follow-up. *Psychosom Med* 2003;65(1):63–73.

Dickman R, Green C, Fass SS, Quan SF, Dekel R, Risner-Adler S, et al. Relationships between sleep quality and pH monitoring findings in persons with gastroesophageal reflux disease. *J Clin Sleep Med* 2007;3(5):505–513.

Dimarino Jr AJ, Banwait KS, Eschinger E, Greenberg A, Dimarino M, Doghramji K, et al. The effect of gastro-oesophageal reflux and omeprazole on key sleep parameters. *Aliment Pharmacol Ther* 2005;22(4):325–329.

Doghramji K, Choufani D. Taking a sleep history. In: Winkelman J, Plante D, editors. Foundations of Psychiatric Sleep Medicine Cambridge, MA: Cambridge University Press;Cambridge, 2010, pp. 95–110.

Doghramji K, Doghramji P. Clinical Management of Insomnia. 1st ed. West Islip, NY: Professional Communications; 2006.

Doghramji K, Grewal R, Markov D. Evaluation and management of insomnia in the psychiatric setting. *Focus: The Journal of Lifelong Learning in Psychiatry* 2009;VII(4):441–454.

Edinger JD, Bonnet MH, Bootzin RR, Doghramji K, Dorsey CM, Espie CA, et al. Derivation of research diagnostic criteria for insomnia: report of an American Academy of Sleep Medicine Work Group. *Sleep* 2004;27(8):1567–1596.

Edinger JD, Means MK, Carney CE, Krystal AD. Psychomotor performance deficits and their relation to prior nights' sleep among individuals with primary insomnia. *Sleep* 2008;31(5):599–607.

Erichsen D, Ferri R, Gozal D. Ropinirole in restless legs syndrome and periodic limb movement disorder. *Ther Clin Risk Manag* 2010;6:173–182.

Espana RA, Scammell TE. Sleep neurobiology for the clinician. *Sleep* 2004;27(4):811–820.

Espie CA, Inglis SJ, Harvey L, Tessier S. Insomniacs' attributions. psychometric properties of the Dysfunctional Beliefs and Attitudes about Sleep Scale and the Sleep Disturbance Questionnaire. *J Psychosom Res* 2000; 48(2):141–148.

Ford DE, Kamerow DB. Epidemiologic study of sleep disturbances and psychiatric disorders. An opportunity for prevention? *JAMA* 1989;262(11):1479–1484.

Freud S. The Interpretation of Dreams. 2nd ed. London: Hogarth Press; 1955.

Freud S. Dreams. In: Strachey J, editor. The Standard Edition of the Complete Psychological Works of Sigmund Freud. London: Hogarth Press;, volume 15, page 218; 1953/1986: 83–239.

Gagliardi GS, Shah AP, Goldstein M, Denua-Rivera S, Doghramji K, Cohen S, et al. Effect of zolpidem on the sleep arousal response to nocturnal esophageal acid exposure. *Clin Gastroenterol Hepatol* 2009;7(9):948–952.

Gallup. Sleep in America. 1995. http://www.stanford.edu/~dement/95poll.html, accessed 2/6/12

George CF, Bayliff CD. Management of insomnia in patients with chronic obstructive pulmonary disease. *Drugs* 2003;63(4):379–387.

Guilleminault C, Davis K, Huynh NT. Prospective randomized study of patients with insomnia and mild sleep disordered breathing. *Sleep* 2008;31(11):1527–1533.

Hamet P, Tremblay J. Genetics of the sleep-wake cycle and its disorders. *Metabolism* 2006;55(10 Suppl 2): S7–S12.

Hauri PJ. Cognitive deficits in insomnia patients. *Acta Neurol Belg* 1997;97(2):113–117.

Hening W, Walters AS, Allen RP, Montplaisir J, Myers A, Ferini-Strambi L. Impact, diagnosis and treatment of restless legs syndrome (RLS) in a primary care population: the REST (RLS epidemiology, symptoms, and treatment) primary care study. *Sleep Med* 2004;5(3):237–246.

Judd LL, Akiskal HS, Maser JD, Zeller PJ, Endicott J, Coryell W, et al. Major depressive disorder: a prospective study of residual subthreshold depressive symptoms as predictor of rapid relapse. *J Affect Disord* 1998;50 (2–3):97–108.

Kales JD, Kales A, Bixler EO, Soldatos CR, Cadieux RJ, Kashurba GJ, et al. Biopsychobehavioral correlates of insomnia, V: clinical characteristics and behavioral correlates. *Am J Psychiatry* 1984;141(11):1371–1376.

Kinsman RA, Yaroush RA, Fernandez E, Dirks JF, Schocket M, Fukuhara J. Symptoms and experiences in chronic bronchitis and emphysema. *Chest* 1983;83(5):755–761.

Klink M, Quan SF. Prevalence of reported sleep disturbances in a general adult population and their relationship to obstructive airways diseases. *Chest* 1987;91(4):540–546.

Krakow B, Hollifield M, Johnston L, Koss M, Schrader R, Warner TD, et al. Imagery rehearsal therapy for chronic nightmares in sexual assault survivors with posttraumatic stress disorder: a randomized controlled trial. *JAMA* 2001;286(5):537–545.

Krakow B, Melendrez D, Lee SA, Warner TD, Clark JO, Sklar D. Refractory insomnia and sleep-disordered breathing: a pilot study. *Sleep Breath* 2004;8(1):15–29.

Krakow B, Melendrez D, Sisley B, Warner TD, Krakow J, Leahigh L, et al. Nasal dilator strip therapy for chronic sleep-maintenance insomnia and symptoms of sleep-disordered breathing: a randomized controlled trial. *Sleep Breath* 2006;10(1):16–28.

Krystal AD, Erman M, Zammit GK, Soubrane C, Roth T, ZOLONG Study Group. Long-term efficacy and safety of zolpidem extended-release 12.5 mg, administered 3 to 7 nights per week for 24 weeks, in patients with chronic primary insomnia: a 6-month, randomized, double-blind, placebo-controlled, parallel-group, multicenter study. *Sleep* 2008;31(1):79–90.

Krystal AD, Goforth HW, Roth T. Effects of antipsychotic medications on sleep in schizophrenia. *Int Clin Psychopharmacol* 2008;23(3):150–160.

Krystal AD, Walsh JK, Laska E, Caron J, Amato DA, Wessel TC, et al. Sustained efficacy of eszopiclone over 6 months of nightly treatment: results of a randomized, double-blind, placebo-controlled study in adults with chronic insomnia. *Sleep* 2003;26(7):793–799.

Kupfer DJ. Sleep research in depressive illness: clinical implications—a tasting menu. *Biol Psychiatry* 1995; 38(6):391–403.

Kuppermann M, Lubeck DP, Mazonson PD, Patrick DL, Stewart AL, Buesching DP, et al. Sleep problems and their correlates in a working population. *J Gen Intern Med* 1995;10(1):25–32.

Kushida CA, Littner MR, Morgenthaler T, Alessi CA, Bailey D, Coleman J, Jr, et al. Practice parameters for the indications for polysomnography and related procedures: an update for 2005. *Sleep* 2005;28(4):499–521.

Lanfranchi PA, Pennestri MH, Fradette L, Dumont M, Morin CM, Montplaisir J. Nighttime blood pressure in normotensive subjects with chronic insomnia: implications for cardiovascular risk. *Sleep* 2009;32(6): 760–766.

Leistedt S, Dumont M, Coumans N, Lanquart JP, Jurysta F, Linkowski P. The modifications of the long-range temporal correlations of the sleep EEG due to major depressive episode disappear with the status of remission. *Neuroscience* 2007;148(3):782–793.

Littner MR, Kushida C, Anderson WM, Bailey D, Berry RB, Hirshkowitz M, et al. Practice parameters for the dopaminergic treatment of restless legs syndrome and periodic limb movement disorder. *Sleep* 2004;27(3): 557–559.

Locke GR, 3rd, Talley NJ, Fett SL, Zinsmeister AR, Melton LJ, 3rd. Prevalence and clinical spectrum of gastroesophageal reflux: a population-based study in Olmsted County, Minnesota. *Gastroenterology* 1997;112(5): 1448–1456.

Luyster FS, Buysse DJ, Strollo PJ, Jr. Comorbid insomnia and obstructive sleep apnea: challenges for clinical practice and research. *J Clin Sleep Med* 2010;6(2):196–204.

Mahowald MW, Kader G, Schenck CH. Clinical categories of sleep disorders I. *Continuum* 1997;3(4):35–65.

Mallon L, Broman JE, Hetta J. Sleep complaints predict coronary artery disease mortality in males: a 12-year follow-up study of a middle-aged Swedish population. *J Intern Med* 2002;251(3):207–216.

Markov D, Doghramji K. Doxepin for insomnia. *Current Psychiatry* 2010;9(10):67–77.

Martin RJ, Bartelson BL, Smith P, Hudgel DW, Lewis D, Pohl G, et al. Effect of ipratropium bromide treatment on oxygen saturation and sleep quality in COPD. *Chest* 1999;115(5):1338–1345.

Martin RJ, Pak J. Overnight theophylline concentrations and effects on sleep and lung function in chronic obstructive pulmonary disease. *Am Rev Respir Dis* 1992;145(3):540–544.

Mayer G, Wang-Weigand S, Roth-Schechter B, Lehmann R, Staner C, Partinen M. Efficacy and safety of 6-month nightly ramelteon administration in adults with chronic primary insomnia. *Sleep* 2009;32(3):351–360.

McCrae CS, Lichstein KL. Secondary insomnia: diagnostic challenges and intervention opportunities. *Sleep Med Rev* 2001;5(1):47–61.

Mellinger GD, Balter MB, Uhlenhuth EH. Insomnia and its treatment. Prevalence and correlates. *Arch Gen Psychiatry* 1985;42(3):225–232.

Mellman TA, David D, Bustamante V, Torres J, Fins A. Dreams in the acute aftermath of trauma and their relationship to PTSD. *J Trauma Stress* 2001;14:241–247.

Mellman TA, David D, Kulick-Bell R, Hebding J, Nolan B. Sleep disturbance and its relationship to psychiatric morbidity after Hurricane Andrew. *Am J Psychiatry* 1995;152(11):1659–1663.

Mellman TA, Uhde TW. Electroencephalographic sleep in panic disorder. A focus on sleep-related panic attacks. *Arch Gen Psychiatry* 1989;46(2):178–184.

Merica H, Blois R, Gaillard JM. Spectral characteristics of sleep EEG in chronic insomnia. *Eur J Neurosci* 1998;10(5):1826–1834.

Millman RP, Carlisle CC, McGarvey ST, Eveloff SE, Levinson PD. Body fat distribution and sleep apnea severity in women. *Chest* 1995;107(2):362–366.

Mini L, Wang-Weigand S, Zhang J. Ramelteon 8 mg/d versus placebo in patients with chronic insomnia: post hoc analysis of a 5-week trial using 50% or greater reduction in latency to persistent sleep as a measure of treatment effect. *Clin Ther* 2008;30(7):1316–1323.

Modell S, Ising M, Holsboer F, Lauer CJ. The Munich vulnerability study on affective disorders: premorbid polysomnographic profile of affected high-risk probands. *Biol Psychiatry* 2005;58(9):694–699.

Montplaisir J, Allen R, Walters A, Ferini-Strambi L. Restless legs syndrome and periodic limb movements in sleep. In: Kryger M, Roth T, Dement W, editors. Principles and Practice of Sleep Medicine, 4th ed. Philadelphia: Elsevier; 2005: 839–852.

Montplaisir J, Boucher S, Poirier G, Lavigne G, Lapierre O, Lesperance P. Clinical, polysomnographic, and genetic characteristics of restless legs syndrome: a study of 133 patients diagnosed with new standard criteria. *Mov Disord* 1997;12(1):61–65.

Morgenthaler T, Kramer M, Alessi C, Friedman L, Boehlecke B, Brown T, et al. Practice parameters for the psychological and behavioral treatment of insomnia: an update. An American Academy of Sleep Medicine report. *Sleep* 2006;29(11):1415–1419.

Morgenthaler TI, Lee-Chiong T, Alessi C, Friedman L, Aurora RN, Boehlecke B, et al. Practice parameters for the clinical evaluation and treatment of circadian rhythm sleep disorders. An American Academy of Sleep Medicine report. *Sleep* 2007;30(11):1445–1459.

Morin CM. Combined therapeutics for insomnia: should our first approach be behavioral or pharmacological? *Sleep Med* 2006;7(Suppl 1):S15–19.

Morin CM, Belanger L, LeBlanc M, Ivers H, Savard J, Espie CA, et al. The natural history of insomnia: a population-based 3-year longitudinal study. *Arch Intern Med* 2009;169(5):447–453.

Morin CM, Bootzin RR, Buysse DJ, Edinger JD, Espie CA, Lichstein KL. Psychological and behavioral treatment of insomnia:update of the recent evidence (1998–2004). *Sleep* 2006;29(11):1398–1414.

Morin CM, Gaulier B, Barry T, Kowatch RA. Patients' acceptance of psychological and pharmacological therapies for insomnia. *Sleep* 1992;15(4):302–305.

Mulloy E, McNicholas WT. Theophylline improves gas exchange during rest, exercise, and sleep in severe chronic obstructive pulmonary disease. *Am Rev Respir Dis* 1993;148(4 Pt 1):1030–1036.

National Institutes of Health. National Institutes of Health State of the Science Conference Statement on Manifestations and Management of Chronic Insomnia in Adults, June 13–15, 2005. *Sleep* 2005;28(9):1049–1057.

Neubauer, DN. Pharmacotherapeutic approach to insomnia in adults. In: Barkoukis TJ, Matheson JK, Ferber R, Doghramji K. Therapy in Sleep Medicine. Elsevier Saunders, Philadelphia, 2012. pp. 172–180.

Nierenberg AA, Keefe BR, Leslie VC, Alpert JE, Pava JA, Worthington JJ, 3rd et al. Residual symptoms in depressed patients who respond acutely to fluoxetine. *J Clin Psychiatry* 1999;60(4):221–225.

Nofzinger EA, Buysse DJ, Germain A, Price JC, Miewald JM, Kupfer DJ. Functional neuroimaging evidence for hyperarousal in insomnia. *Am J Psychiatry* 2004;161(11):2126–2128.

Nuckton TJ, Glidden DV, Browner WS, Claman DM. Physical examination: Mallampati score as an independent predictor of obstructive sleep apnea. *Sleep* 2006;29(7):903–908.

Ohayon M. Epidemiological study on insomnia in the general population. *Sleep* 1996;19(Suppl 3):S7–15.

Ohayon MM. Epidemiology of insomnia: what we know and what we still need to learn. *Sleep Med Rev* 2002;6(2):97–111.

Ohayon MM, Caulet M, Lemoine P. Comorbidity of mental and insomnia disorders in the general population. *Compr Psychiatry* 1998;39(4):185–197.

Ohayon MM, Partinen M. Insomnia and global sleep dissatisfaction in Finland. *J Sleep Res* 2002;11(4):339–346.

Ohayon MM, Reynolds CF, 3rd. Epidemiological and clinical relevance of insomnia diagnosis algorithms according to the DSM-IV and the International Classification of Sleep Disorders (ICSD). *Sleep Med* 2009;10(9):952–960.

Ohayon MM, Roth T. Place of chronic insomnia in the course of depressive and anxiety disorders. *J Psychiatr Res* 2003;37(1):9–15.

Reynolds CF, 3rd, Kupfer DJ. Sleep research in affective illness: state of the art circa 1987. *Sleep* 1987;10(3):199–215.

Reynolds CF, 3rd, Redline S, DSM-V Sleep-Wake Disorders Workgroup and Advisors. The DSM-v sleep-wake disorders nosology: an update and an invitation to the sleep community. *J Clin Sleep Med* 2010;6(1):9–10.

Richardson GS, Roehrs TA, Rosenthal L, Koshorek G, Roth T. Tolerance to daytime sedative effects of H1 antihistamines. *J Clin Psychopharmacol* 2002;22(5):511–515.

Ritterband LM, Thorndike FP, Gonder-Frederick LA, Magee JC, Bailey ET, Saylor DK, et al. Efficacy of an Internet-based behavioral intervention for adults with insomnia. *Arch Gen Psychiatry* 2009;66(7):692–698.

Rubenstein JH, Scheiman JM, Sadeghi S, Whiteman D, Inadomi JM. Esophageal adenocarcinoma incidence in individuals with gastroesophageal reflux: synthesis and estimates from population studies. *Am J Gastroenterol* 2010;106(2):254–260.

Sack RL, Auckley D, Auger RR, Carskadon MA, Wright KP, Jr, Vitiello MV, et al. Circadian rhythm sleep disorders: part II, advanced sleep phase disorder, delayed sleep phase disorder, free-running disorder, and irregular sleep-wake rhythm. An American Academy of Sleep Medicine review. *Sleep* 2007a;30(11):1484–1501.

Sack RL, Auckley D, Auger RR, Carskadon MA, Wright KP, Jr, Vitiello MV, et al. Circadian rhythm sleep disorders: part I, basic principles, shift work and jet lag disorders. An American Academy of Sleep Medicine review. *Sleep* 2007b;30(11):1460–1483.

Sateia MJ, Doghramji K, Hauri PJ, Morin CM. Evaluation of chronic insomnia. An American Academy of Sleep Medicine review. *Sleep* 2000;23(2):243–308.

Shapiro CM, Sloan EP. Nocturnal panic—an underrecognized entity. *J Psychosom Res* 1998;44(1):21–23.

Soldatos CR, Dikeos DG, Whitehead A. Tolerance and rebound insomnia with rapidly eliminated hypnotics: a meta-analysis of sleep laboratory studies. *Int Clin Psychopharmacol* 1999;14(5):287–303.

Southworth MR, Kortepeter C, Hughes A. Nonbenzodiazepine hypnotic use and cases of "sleep driving". *Ann Intern Med* 2008;148(6):486–487.

Stege G, Vos PJ, van den Elshout FJ, Richard Dekhuijzen PN, van de Ven MJ, Heijdra YF. Sleep, hypnotics and chronic obstructive pulmonary disease. *Respir Med* 2008;102(6):801–814.

Stein MB, Chartier M, Walker JR. Sleep in nondepressed patients with panic disorder: I. Systematic assessment of subjective sleep quality and sleep disturbance. *Sleep* 1993;16(8):724–726.

Stepanski EJ, Rybarczyk B. Emerging research on the treatment and etiology of secondary or comorbid insomnia. *Sleep Med Rev* 2006;10(1):7–18.

Stepanski EJ, Wyatt JK. Use of sleep hygiene in the treatment of insomnia. *Sleep Med Rev* 2003;7(3):215–225.

Stepanski E, Zorick F, Roehrs T, Young D, Roth T. Daytime alertness in patients with chronic insomnia compared with asymptomatic control subjects. *Sleep* 1988;11(1):54–60.

Sun ER, Chen CA, Ho G, Earley CJ, Allen RP. Iron and the restless legs syndrome. *Sleep* 1998;21(4):371–377.

Tabernero C, Polo JM, Sevillano MD, Munoz R, Berciano J, Cabello A, et al. Fatal familial insomnia: clinical, neuropathological, and genetic description of a Spanish family. *J Neurol Neurosurg Psychiatry* 2000;68(6): 774–777.

Taylor CB, Sheikh J, Agras WS, Roth WT, Margraf J, Ehlers A, et al. Ambulatory heart rate changes in patients with panic attacks. *Am J Psychiatry* 1986;143(4):478–482.

van Geijlswijk IM, Korzilius HP, Smits MG. The use of exogenous melatonin in delayed sleep phase disorder: a meta-analysis. *Sleep* 2010;33(12):1605–1614.

van Mill JG, Hoogendijk WJ, Vogelzangs N, van Dyck R, Penninx BW. Insomnia and sleep duration in a large cohort of patients with major depressive disorder and anxiety disorders. *J Clin Psychiatry* 2010;71(3):239–246.

Vaughn BV, O'Neill DF. Cardinal manifestations of sleep disorders. In: Kryger M, Roth T, Dement WC, editors. Principles and Practice of Sleep Medicine, 4th ed. Philadelphia: Elsevier; 2005:589.

Veale D, Cooper BG, Griffiths CJ, Corris PA, Gibson GJ. The effect of controlled-release salbutamol on sleep and nocturnal oxygenation in patients with asthma and chronic obstructive pulmonary disease. *Respir Med* 1994;88(2):121–124.

Vgontzas AN, Bixler EO, Lin HM, Prolo P, Mastorakos G, Vela-Bueno A, et al. Chronic insomnia is associated with nyctohemeral activation of the hypothalamic-pituitary-adrenal axis: clinical implications. *J Clin Endocrinol Metab* 2001;86(8):3787–3794.

Watson NF, Goldberg J, Arguelles L, Buchwald D. Genetic and environmental influences on insomnia, daytime sleepiness, and obesity in twins. *Sleep* 2006;29(5):645–649.

Weissman MM, Greenwald S, Nino-Murcia G, Dement WC. The morbidity of insomnia uncomplicated by psychiatric disorders. *Gen Hosp Psychiatry* 1997;19(4):245–250.

Winokur A, Gary KA, Rodner S, Rae-Red C, Fernando AT, Szuba MP. Depression, sleep physiology, and antidepressant drugs. *Depress Anxiety* 2001;14(1):19–28.

World Health Organization. International Statistical Classification of Diseases and Related Health Problems. 10th rev. ed. Geneva, Switzerland: World Health Organization; 1992.

Yang CM, Spielman AJ, Glovinsky P. Nonpharmacologic strategies in the management of insomnia. *Psychiatr Clin North Am* 2006;29(4):895–919; abstract viii.

Zammit GK, Corser B, Doghramji K, Fry JM, James S, Krystal A, et al. Sleep and residual sedation after administration of zaleplon, zolpidem, and placebo during experimental middle-of-the-night awakening. *J Clin Sleep Med* 2006;2(4):417–423.

Zammit G, Erman M, Wang-Weigand S, Sainati S, Zhang J, Roth T. Evaluation of the efficacy and safety of ramelteon in subjects with chronic insomnia. *J Clin Sleep Med* 2007;3(5):495–504.

Zhang J, Li AM, Kong AP, Lai KY, Tang NL, Wing YK. A community-based study of insomnia in Hong Kong Chinese children: prevalence, risk factors and familial aggregation. *Sleep Med* 2009;10(9):1040–1046.

Management of Treatment-Resistant Childhood Mood and Anxiety Disorders

Karen Dineen Wagner

The focus of this chapter will be on the management of treatment-resistant childhood mood and anxiety disorders. The theme throughout the chapter is the importance of using evidence-based treatments in the acute management of mood and anxiety disorders in children and adolescents. This strategy may reduce the likelihood of treatment-resistant disorders.

Clinical issues may affect response to treatment and should be assessed if a child does not have a positive response to evidence-based treatment. These issues include diagnostic accuracy, comorbid disorders, psychosocial factors, and treatment compliance (Wagner & Pliszka, 2009). Since there may be symptom overlap among disorders, the diagnosis should be reassessed. For example, irritability and sleep disturbance may be present for children with major depression, bipolar disorder, and anxiety disorders. Unrecognized comorbid disorders may adversely affect the outcome of treatment. As an example, comorbid attention-deficit/hyperactivity disorder has been found to lower response rates in the treatment of bipolar disorder (Masi et al., 2004; Pavuluri, Henry, Carbray et al., 2006). Psychosocial factors such as child abuse, family conflict, parental psychopathology, and bullying by peers may exacerbate symptoms. Lack of compliance with medication treatment will adversely affect treatment response. Similarly, failure to complete cognitive-behavioral therapy homework assignments may impact negatively on treatment outcomes.

Major Depressive Disorder

The prevalence of major depression is estimated to be 2% in children and up to 8% in adolescents (Birmaher et al., 1996). The mean length of an episode of major depression ranges from 8 to 13 months. Relapse is common, with rates ranging from 30% to 70% (Birmaher, Arbelaez, & Brent, 2002; Birmaher et al., 2004; Rao, Hammen, & Poland, 2010).

Pharmacotherapy

Acute Treatment

There are only two medications that have Food and Drug Administration (FDA) approval for the acute treatment of major depression in youth: fluoxetine for ages 8 years and older and escitalopram for ages 12 years and older.

There have been three positive controlled trials of fluoxetine treatment of major depression in children and adolescents. In one study, 96 children and adolescents with major depression were randomized to fluoxetine 20 mg per day or placebo for an 8-week trial (Emslie et al., 1997). Fifty-six percent of youths who received fluoxetine were much or very much improved (Clinical Global Impression-Improvement (CGI-I ≤2) compared to 33% for placebo-treated youth. A similar response rate to fluoxetine was found in a double-blind, placebo-controlled multicenter study in which 219 children and adolescents with major depression were randomly assigned to fluoxetine 20 mg per day or placebo for an 8-week trial (Emslie et al., 2002). Fifty-two percent of youths treated with fluoxetine were much or very much improved compared to 37% of youths treated with placebo. In the Treatment for Adolescents with Depression Study (TADS) (2004), the response rate (CGI-I < 2) for adolescents randomized to fluoxetine (10–40 mg/day) for 12 weeks was 61% compared to 35% in the placebo group.

In the positive study of escitalopram, response rates (CGI ≤ 2) were similar to those found in the fluoxetine studies. In this study, 157 adolescents with major depression were randomly assigned to escitalopram 10–20 mg per day or placebo in an 8-week double-blind controlled trial (Emslie, Ventura, Korotzer, & Tourkodimitris, 2009). Sixty-four percent of the adolescents who received escitalopram were much or very improved compared to 53% of placebo-treated youths.

The efficacy of other selective serotonin reuptake inhibitors (SSRIs) in the acute treatment of children and adolescents with major depression has shown mixed results in double-blind placebo-controlled trials. Citalopram has one positive study in children and adolescents (Wagner, Robb et al., 2004) and one negative study in adolescents (von Knorring, Olsson, Thomsen, Lemming, & Hultén, 2006). In an a priori defined pooled analysis of two identical multicenter studies, sertraline was superior to placebo (Wagner, Ambrosini et al., 2003); however, the individual trials were negative. Other negative trials include three studies of paroxetine (Berard, Fong, Carpenter, Thomason, & Wilkinson, 2006; Emslie et al., 2006; Keller et al., 2001) and one study of escitalopram that included children and adolescents (Wagner, Jonas, Findling, Ventura, & Saikali, 2006).

Other classes of antidepressants have failed to demonstrate superiority of medication to placebo in randomized controlled trials for the treatment of children and adolescents with major depression, including mirtazapine (US Food and Drug Administration, 2004), nefazodone (Rynn et al., 2002; US Food and Drug Administration, 2004), and venlafaxine (Emslie, Findling, Yeung, Kunz, & Li, 2007).

There are no published reports of randomized controlled studies of bupropion or duloxetine for the treatment of children and adolescents with major depressive disorder.

Efficacy of Acute Pharmacotherapy

In a meta-analysis of published and unpublished randomized placebo-controlled antidepressant trials in youth with major depression, the pooled absolute rates of response were 61% for youth treated with antidepressants and 50% for youth treated with placebo. The number needed to treat (NNT) to benefit was 10 (Bridge et al., 2007). In another meta-analysis of randomized controlled trials of antidepressants in youth, a modest pooled drug/placebo response ratio of 1.22 was found (Tsapakis, Soldani, Tondo, & Baldessarini, 2008). The NNT for SSRIs was 9. The NNT decreased with increasing age: children (NNT = 21) and adolescents (NNT = 8). Another meta-analysis of controlled antidepressants trials in children and adolescents showed greater improvement in the medication groups compared to the placebo groups with an odds ratio of 1.52 (Papanikolaou, Richardson, Pehlivanidis, & Papadopoulou-Daifoti, 2006).

Remission rates in acute treatment antidepressant treatment trials for youth are substantially lower than response rates. Remission (defined as a Children's Depression Rating Scale Revised (CDRS-R: Poznanski, Freman, & Mokros, 1985) score ≤28 have ranged from 23% to 39% in fluoxetine-treated youth (Emslie et al., 1997, 2002; TADS Team, 2004). Similarly, in the positive escitalopram study, the remission rate was 42% (Emslie et al., 2009). In the meta-analysis of published and unpublished randomized placebo-controlled antidepressant trials of youth with major depression, the rate of remission ranged from 30% to 40% (Bridge et al., 2007).

The evidence base supports the use of SSRIs as first-line treatment for major depression in children and adolescents (Hughes et al., 2007). Approximately 60% of youth will have a positive response to acute treatment. Remission rates are approximately 30%–40% for acute pharmacotherapy.

Continuation Treatment

Consensus guidelines recommend that antidepressants be continued for 6–12 months after symptom remission (Birmaher et al., 2007; Hughes et al., 2007).

The effectiveness of continuation of escitalopram treatment for adolescent depression was evaluated in a 24-week controlled trial. Three hundred eleven adolescents with major depression participated in a double-blind placebo-controlled trial with an 8-week acute phase and 16-week continuation phase (Emslie et al., 2009; Findling, Boseet et al., 2009). The most reduction in depressive symptoms occurred in the first 6 weeks of treatment; however, this improvement was maintained during the 16-week continuation phase.

The long-term effectiveness of venlafaxine extended-release (ER) was evaluated in children and adolescents with major depressive disorder. Eight-six youth participated in an open-label study of venlafaxine ER for 6 weeks of acute treatment, which was followed by continuation treatment for up to 6 months (Emslie, Yeung, & Kunz, 2007). The greatest improvement in depressive symptoms occurred during the first 6 weeks (acute phase) of treatment. However, after continuing treatment for 6 months, an additional 10% of youth met response criteria.

In the TADS study the response (CGI-I ≤ 2) was 62% at week 12. With continuation of treatment, response rates were 81% at 36 weeks (Kennard et al., 2009; TADS Team, 2007).

Continuation of treatment beyond 12 weeks also resulted in higher remission rates. In the TADS study, the remission rate (CDRS-R ≤ 28) with fluoxetine treatment was 24% at 12 weeks. With continued treatment, remission rates were 55% at 36 weeks (Kennard et al., 2009). In the Treatment of Resistant Depression in Adolescents (TORDIA) trial (Brent et al., 2008), remission rates were 17.7% after 12 weeks of treatment, 38.9% after 24 weeks of treatment, 64.8% after 48 weeks of treatment, and 78.8% after 72 weeks of treatment (Emslie et al., 2010; Vitiello et al., 2011).

Continuing treatment beyond acute response also helps to prevent relapse. In a randomized placebo-controlled discontinuation trial, 102 children and adolescents who had an adequate response after 12 weeks of treatment with fluoxetine were randomly assigned to continue treatment with fluoxetine or placebo for an additional 6 months (Emslie et al., 2008). Forty-two percent of the fluoxetine group relapsed compared with 69.2% of the placebo group. The odds of relapse in the placebo group were 3.2 times more likely than for the fluoxetine group. The median time to relapse was shorter in the placebo group than fluoxetine group (8 weeks vs. greater than 24 weeks, respectively). At the end of acute treatment, those youths with no residual symptoms were much less likely to relapse during continuation treatment than those with residual symptoms. Importantly, youths with no residual symptoms at the end of acute treatment who were switched to placebo for continuation treatment were six times as likely to relapse than those youths who remained on fluoxetine.

Maintenance Treatment

Two medications, escitalopram and fluoxetine, have FDA approval for maintenance treatment for major depression in children and adolescents. Escitalopram is indicated for maintenance treatment for major depression in adolescents 12 years and older. This indication was based upon extrapolation from adult data along with comparisons of escitalopram pharmacokinetic parameters in adult and adolescent patients (FDA approved Lexapro prescribing label, 03–19-2009). Fluoxetine has approval for maintenance treatment of major depression in children and adolescents 8 years and older. This indication was based upon extrapolation from adult data (FDA approved Prozac prescribing label).

There is a paucity of data regarding maintenance treatment for major depressive disorder in youth. In a maintenance study of sertraline for the treatment of adolescents with depression, 93 adolescents with major depression received sertraline for 12 weeks (Cheung et al., 2008). Of these, 51 adolescents were responders and were enrolled in a 24-week continuation study. At the end of the continuation phase, responders were randomized to a sertraline ($n = 13$) or a placebo ($n = 9$) for a 52-week maintenance phase. At the end of 52 weeks, 38% of the adolescents treated with sertraline maintained response (i.e., no recurrence) compared to 0% of the placebo-treated patients. This study provides preliminary support for maintenance treatment of depression in adolescents for a minimum of 1 year following 9 months of adequate treatment response.

It is clinical consensus that the longer the recovery period and the higher the number of recurrences, the longer should be the maintenance period (Birmaher et al., 2007). For adolescents with at least two episodes of depression or one severe episode or chronic episodes of depression, it is recommended that maintenance treatment be for longer than 1 year.

Predictors of Treatment Response

More severe depression, baseline suicidality, comorbid psychiatric disorders (especially anxiety and substance abuse), hopelessness, and family conflict are predictors of poorer treatment outcome for depressed youth (Asarnow et al., 2009; Emslie, Kennard, & Mayes, 2011; Goldstein, Axelson, Birmaher, & Brent, 2007).

Clinical response by week 12 of treatment has been shown to increase the likelihood of clinical remission. In the TORDIA study, remission rates were 61.6% for those adolescents with clinical response at week 12 compared to 18.3% for those adolescents who had not responded by week 12 (Emslie et al., 2010). In the TADS study, recovery by 2 years was more likely for acute treatment responders (96.2%) than for partial responders (79.1%) (Curry et al., 2011). In a 12-week open-label study of fluoxetine treatment for 168 youths with major depression, a reduction in depressive symptoms of approximately 50% by week 4 was most predictive of remission at the end of the 12 weeks of acute treatment (Tao et al., 2009).

Similarly, more residual symptoms following acute treatment increase the likelihood of relapse. In the TADS study, the greater the number of residual symptoms after 12 weeks of acute treatment, the less likely remission was achieved at weeks 18 and 36 (Kennard et al., 2009).

Psychotherapy

Acute Treatment

Cognitive-behavioral therapy (CBT) has the most evidence to support its efficacy as a psychotherapy treatment for major depression in children and adolescents. In a randomized trial, 175 adolescents with major depressive disorder were randomized to individual CBT, systemic behavior family therapy, or individual nondirective supportive therapy for 12–16 sessions (Brent et al., 1997). At the end of treatment, those adolescents who received CBT had a higher rate of remission: CBT, 64.7%; systemic behavior family therapy, 37.9%, and nondirective supportive therapy, 39.4%. Other studies support the efficacy of CBT for the treatment of adolescent depression (Clarke, Rohde, Lewinsohn, Hops, & Seeley, 1999; Lewinsohn, Clarke, Hops, & Andrews, 1990; Roselló & Bernal, 1999; Wood, Harrington, & Moore, 1996).

However, in the National Institute of Mental Health (NIMH)–funded Treatment of Adolescents with Depression Study (TADS) (TADS Team, 2004), CBT was not shown to be significantly superior to placebo. Four hundred thirty-nine adolescents with major depression were randomized to CBT, fluoxetine, CBT plus fluoxetine, or placebo for a 12-week period. Response rates (CGI-I < 2) were 43% for CBT and 35% for placebo, which was not a statistically significant difference.

Interpersonal psychotherapy has shown some efficacy for the treatment of adolescents with major depression. Interpersonal psychotherapy modified for depressed adolescents (IPT-A) was compared to treatment as usual in school-based mental health clinics in a 16-week randomized clinical trial for 63 depressed adolescents (Mufson et al., 2004). The adolescents who were treated with IPT-A showed a greater reduction in depression symptoms compared to the treatment-as-usual group. Other controlled trials of interpersonal psychotherapy have also shown efficacy for IPT-A for depressed adolescents (Mufson, Wiessman,

Moreau, & Garfinkel, 1999; Rosselló & Bernal, 1999; Tang, Jou, Ko, Huang, & Yen, 2009; Young, Mufson, & Gallop, 2010;).

Continuation Treatment

Continuation of psychotherapy beyond acute treatment may increase response and remission rates. In the TADS study, the response rate (CGI-I ≤ 2) for CBT was 48% at 12 weeks treatment. With continued treatment, the response rate for CBT at week 18 was 65% and at week 36 was 81%. (TADS Team, 2007). Similarly, remission rates increased with continuation of CBT beyond acute treatment. After 12 weeks of CBT treatment, the remission rate (CDRS-R ≤ 28) was 19%. At week 18 the remission rate was 27%, and at week 36 the remission rate increased to 64% (Kennard et al., 2009).

Efficacy of Psychotherapy

A meta-analysis of 35 randomized psychotherapy trials for the treatment of depression in children and adolescents was conducted to determine the effectiveness of psychotherapy, the comparative efficacy of cognitive versus noncognitive psychotherapies, and long-term effects of psychotherapy (Weisz, McCarty, & Valeri, 2006). A modest effect of psychotherapy was found for the treatment of children and adolescents with depression (effect size 0.34). No specific advantage was found for cognitive therapy over other noncognitive therapies for the treatment of depressed youth. One-year follow-up studies showed no treatment effect.

To increase the long-term effectiveness of psychotherapy, booster sessions may be needed to maintain treatment effect (Clarke et al., 1999).

Treatment-Resistant Depression

In the NIMH-funded multisite Treatment of SSRI-Resistant Depression in Adolescents (TORDIA) trial (Brent et al., 2008), treatment-resistant depression was defined as clinically significant depression despite treatment with an SSRI for at least 8 weeks, with the last 4 weeks at dosages of fluoxetine 40 mg, or its equivalent (citalopram 40 mg, escitalopram 40 mg, paroxetine 40 mg, or sertraline 150 mg).

In this trial, 334 adolescents with SSRI-resistant depression were randomized to one of four treatments for 12 weeks: switch to an alternate SSRI; switch to an alternate SSRI plus CBT; switch to venlafaxine; or switch to venlafaxine plus CBT. The highest rate of response (54.8%) was for CBT plus switch to either medication. Response rates (CGI-I ≤ 2 and CDRS-R ≥ 50% reduction from baseline) were similar for a switch to an alternate SSRI (47%) or to venlafaxine (48.2%). Adverse events of increase in diastolic blood pressure and pulse and skin problems occurred more frequently with venlafaxine than SSRI treatment.

Based on the findings from the TORDIA study, approximately 50% of adolescents who fail to respond to treatment with an initial SSRI will respond to treatment with another antidepressant. Since adverse events were lower in the SSRI-treated patients, a switch to an alternate SSRI would be a reasonable medication strategy for depressed youth who do not have an adequate clinical response to an initial SSRI.

For adolescents with SSRI treatment-resistant depression, the addition of CBT to a medication switch increased response rates from 41% to 55%. Those adolescents who had more than nine CBT sessions were 2.5 times more likely to have a positive clinical response than those with fewer than nine sessions (Kennard et al., 2008). The addition of CBT to medication was more effective for those adolescents with a greater number of comorbidities, no abuse history, and lower hopelessness (Asarnow et al., 2009).

Strategies for Treatment-Resistant Depression

A medication algorithm has been developed for the treatment of major depression in children and adolescents (Hughes et al., 2007). The medication stages are as follows:

> Stage 1: Monotherapy with an SSRI. If the youth does not respond to an SSRI, then move to next stage.
> Stage 2: Switch to an alternate SSRI. If the youth has a partial response to alternate SSRI treatment, then augment with another medication. If there is no response to treatment, then move to the next stage.
> Stage 3: Monotherapy with an alternate class of medication. If the youth has a partial or nonresponse, then move to the next stage.
> Stage 4: Reassess, treatment guidance.

Since the development of this medication treatment algorithm, there have been additional studies (as described in this chapter) to guide treatment decisions. Fluoxetine has the most evidence to support its use as the initial SSRI treatment for children and adolescents with depression. Escitalopram has evidence of efficacy for adolescents with major depression. Approximately 60% of youth will respond to initial treatment with an SSRI.

Based upon the findings from the TORDIA study, approximately 50% of those youths with SSRI treatment-resistant depression will respond to a switch to an alternate SSRI or an alternate class of medication. Switch to an alternate SSRI is recommended because of the lower side-effect profile than venlafaxine. Approximately 20% of youths will not respond to treatment after two different medication trials. For depressed youth who are treatment resistant to two antidepressant medications, a number of strategies may be utilized as discussed in the following sections.

Switch to an Alternate Antidepressant

To date, only the SSRIs have demonstrated efficacy in double-blind placebo-controlled trials for the treatment of major depression in children and adolescents. If a depressed youth fails to respond to two SSRI trials, then a switch to an alternate medication would be indicated. Although venlafaxine was not demonstrated to be superior to placebo in controlled trials for the treatment of major depression, in children and adolescents, approximately 50% of adolescents with SSRI treatment-resistant depression had a positive response to venlafaxine in the TORDIA trial. Other antidepressant options include bupropion, duloxetine, and mirtazapine.

Combination Medication

Atypical antipsychotics have been utilized to augment antidepressant treatment response. However, there are no controlled data for this augmentation strategy in depressed children and adolescents. In a case series of 10 adolescents with SSRI-resistant depression, 70% of adolescents responded (CGI-I ≤ 2) to augmentation with quetiapine (dose range 150–800 mg per day; median dose 200 mg) (Pathak, Johns, & Kowatch, 2005).

Based upon extrapolation from adult data, other augmentation agents for SSRI-resistant depression include lithium, bupropion, and mirtazapine (Hughes et al., 2007).

Combination Medication and Psychotherapy

The results have been mixed regarding the relative efficacy of medication plus CBT compared to medication alone for the treatment of adolescent depression.

In the TADS study (TADS Team, 2004), 439 adolescent outpatients with major depression were randomized to combination CBT plus fluoxetine, fluoxetine alone, CBT alone, or placebo for 12 weeks. Medication plus CBT was the most effective treatment. Response rates (CGI-I ≤ 2) were as follows: combination fluoxetine plus CBT, 73%; fluoxetine alone, 62%; CBT, 48%; and placebo, 35%. There was a greater decrease in suicidal ideation with combination treatment than with fluoxetine monotherapy.

In the Adolescent Depression and Psychotherapy Trial (ADAPT) (Goodyer et al., 2008), 208 adolescents with major depression who had not responded to a brief psychotherapy were randomly assigned to an SSRI or an SSRI plus CBT for 12 weeks. At 12 weeks, 44% of the SSRI alone group and 42% of the SSRI plus CBT group were much or very much improved on the CGI-I. Suicidality decreased in both groups and there was no added advantage of CBT in the reduction of suicidality. At the end of 28 weeks of treatment, there was no significant difference in treatment response between the groups; 61% of the youth in the SSRI alone group and 53% of the youth in the SSRI plus CBT group were much or very much improved.

The efficacy of CBT, sertraline, and combined CBT plus sertraline was assessed in a randomized 12-week trial for the treatment of 73 adolescents with depressive disorders (Melvin et al., 2006). All treatment groups showed a significant improvement on depression outcome measures. The combination of CBT and sertraline was not superior to CBT alone or sertraline alone. At 6-month follow-up, improvement was maintained for all of the treatments.

The addition of fluoxetine to CBT compared to CBT plus placebo was evaluated in a 16-week randomized controlled trial for 126 adolescents with major depressive disorder, substance use disorder, and conduct disorder (Riggs et al., 2007). The combination of fluoxetine with CBT showed greater efficacy than CBT plus placebo on changes in CDRS-R scores but not on CGI-I treatment response (76% versus 67%).

The addition of CBT to SSRI treatment was evaluated in a 1-year study of 152 depressed adolescents in a pediatric primary care setting (Clarke et al., 2005). No significant reduction in depressive symptoms was found for those adolescents who received CBT in addition to as-usual treatment with an SSRI.

The combination of medication plus CBT may result in quicker time to response than either treatment alone for depression in youth. In the TADS study, the combination of fluoxetine plus CBT accelerated response time compared to CBT alone (Kratochvil et al., 2006). There was also a 1.5-fold greater probability of sustained early response for combination treatment than fluoxetine alone. Combined treatment was also demonstrated to be more effective than fluoxetine for those adolescents with mild to moderate depression and who had high levels of cognitive distortion (Curry et al., 2006). However, combined treatment was not more effective than medication alone for adolescents with severe depression or those adolescents who had low levels of cognitive distortion.

CBT has been shown to prevent relapse in children and adolescents with major depression who responded to acute pharmacotherapy. In one study, 46 youths who responded to 12 weeks of treatment with fluoxetine were randomized to either continued antidepressant medication management or antidepressant medication management plus CBT for 6 months (Kennard et al., 2008). Relapse rates were significantly higher in the fluoxetine group (37%) compared to the fluoxetine plus CBT group (15%). The addition of CBT during the continuation phase of treatment reduced the risk of relapse by eightfold compared to antidepressant medication alone.

Omega-3 Fatty Acids

In a small randomized study, 28 children with major depression were randomized to omega-3 (1,000 mg/day; contained 400 mg EPA and 200 mg DHA) or placebo for 16 weeks (Nemets, Nemets, Apter, Bracha, & Belmaker, 2006). The response rate (> 50% reduction in CDRS-R) was 70% for the omega-3–treated children and 0% for the placebo-treated children. Remission rate (CDRS-R ≤ 28) was 40% for the omega-3–treated children and 0% for the placebo-treated children.

Large controlled trials are needed to further assess the efficacy of omega-3 fatty acids in the treatment of depressed youth.

Electroconvulsive Therapy

There are no controlled data on the use of electroconvulsive therapy (ECT) for treatment-resistant depression in children and adolescents. In a retrospective study of adolescents with treatment-resistant depression, one third of the adolescents who received ECT had a 60% improvement in depressive symptoms (Hegeman et al., 2008). The American Academy of Child and Adolescent Psychiatry Practice Parameters on Use of ECT (Ghaziuddin et al., 2004) recommends that ECT could be considered for severe, persistent, and significantly disabling depression if an adolescent has failed at least two adequate trials of appropriate psychopharmacological agents along with other appropriate treatment modalities. Similarly, the Texas Children's Medication Algorithm Project recommends consideration of ECT if an adolescent has severe and nonresponsive depression (Hughes et al., 2007).

Repetitive Transcranial Magnetic Stimulation

There is recent interest in the role of repetitive transcranial magnetic stimulation (rTMS) for treatment-resistant depression in youths. In an open-label study of rTMS, nine adolescents with treatment-resistant depression received twenty 10-Hz, 2-second trains given over 20 min per day for 14 days (Bloch et al., 2008). Three (30%) adolescents were responders (≥30% reduction in CDRS-R). In a case series of adolescents with treatment-resistant depression, two of four adolescents responded to rTMS (Walter, Tormos, Israel, & Pascual-Leone, 2001).

Although the data are scant for rTMS in adolescent depression, Croarkin and colleagues (2010) suggest that rTMS may be a clinically useful treatment for depressed adolescents.

Bipolar Disorder

The prevalence of bipolar disorder in children and adolescents is estimated to be 1%–2.9% (Lewinsohn, Klein, & Seeley, 1995; Merikangas et al., 2010). Bipolar disorder is a chronic disorder in youth. Recovery rates of 87% and relapse rates of 64% have been reported (Geller, Tillman, Craney, & Bolhofner, 2004). In an 8-year follow-up of children with bipolar disorder, the relapse rate was 73% (Geller, Tillman, Bolhofner, & Zimerman, 2008).

Pharmacotherapy

Acute Treatment

Five medications have FDA approval for the acute treatment of bipolar I disorder, mixed or manic in youth. These medications are aripiprazole (≥10 years old), risperidone (≥10 years old), quetiapine (≥10 years old), olanzapine (≥13 years old), and lithium (≥12 years old).

In a 3-week multicenter controlled trial, 161 adolescents with bipolar 1 disorder, manic or mixed, were randomized to treatment with olanzapine (mean modal dose 10.7 mg/day) (Tohen et al., 2007). The olanzapine group had a significantly greater reduction in Young Mania Rating Scale scores (YMRS; Young, Biggs, Ziegler, & Meyer, 1978) than the placebo-treated youth. Response rates (≥50% reduction in baseline YMRS scores) were 48.6% for the olanzapine group and 22% for the placebo group.

The efficacy of risperidone was evaluated in a 3-week double-blind placebo-controlled trial that included 169 youths with bipolar I disorder, manic or mixed (Haas et al., 2009). Low-dose risperidone (0.5–2.5 mg/day) and high-dose risperidone (3.0–6 mg/day) were assessed in this study. Both dose ranges of risperidone showed significant superiority to placebo in reduction of YMRS scores. The response rate (≥50% reduction in baseline YMRS) was 59% for risperidone 0.5–2.5 mg/day and 63% for risperidone 3–6 mg/day, whereas the placebo response rate was 26%. However, adverse events, particularly extrapyramidal symptoms, were more frequent in the high-dose risperidone group.

In a 4-week multicenter controlled trial of aripiprazole, 296 youths with bipolar I disorder, manic or mixed, were randomized to treatment with aripiprazole or placebo (Findling, Nyilas et al., 2009). Low-dose aripiprazole (10 mg) and high-dose aripiprazole (30 mg) were evaluated in this study. Both dose ranges of aripiprazole were significantly superior to placebo in reduction of YMRS scores. The response rate (≥0% reduction in YMRS) was 44.8% for aripiprazole 10 mg, 63.6% for aripiprazole 30 mg, and 26.1% for placebo. Adverse events, including somnolence and extrapyramidal side effects, had higher rates for the aripiprazole 30 mg compared to aripiprazole 10 mg groups.

The efficacy of quetiapine was assessed in a 3-week double-blind placebo-controlled trial that included 277 youths with bipolar I disorder, manic or mixed (DelBello et al., 2007). Lower dose quetiapine (400 mg/day) and higher dose quetiapine (600 mg/day) were assessed in this study. Both dose ranges of quetiapine showed significant superiority to placebo in reduction of YMRS scores. The response rate (≥50% reduction in baseline YMRS) was 64% for quetiapine 400 mg, 58% for quetiapine 600 mg, and 37% for placebo.

In a 4-week multicenter controlled trial of ziprasidone, 150 youths with bipolar I disorder, manic or mixed, were randomized to ziprasidone 80–160 mg/day or placebo (DelBello et al., 2008). Ziprasidone was significantly superior to placebo in reduction of YMRS scores.

The response rates (≥50% reduction in YMRS) were 62% for ziprasidone and 35% for placebo.

Remission rates in these acute 3–4 week trials of the atypical antipsychotics are substantially lower than response rates. Remission rates (YMRS ≤ 12) ranged from 25% to 54%.

Although lithium has FDA approval for acute mania in youths ages 12 and older, this approval was based on efficacy in adults. Data regarding the efficacy of lithium in youth are limited. In an NIMH-funded study, 153 children and adolescents with bipolar I disorder, mixed or manic, were randomized in an 8-week double-blind trial to treatment with lithium, divalproex, or placebo (Kowatch, Findling, Scheffer, & Stanford, 2007). Target serum levels for lithium were 0.8–1.2 mEq/l. Lithium was not significantly superior to placebo. In a 4-week open lithium trial of 100 adolescents with mania, response rate (≥ 50% reduction in baseline YMRS) was 55% (Kafantaris, Coletti, Dicker, Padula, & Kane, 2003).

Most anticonvulsants have not demonstrated superiority to placebo in controlled trials for youth with bipolar I disorder, mixed or manic state.

The efficacy of oxcarbazepine was assessed in a 6-week double-blind placebo-controlled trial for 116 children and adolescents with bipolar I disorder, mixed or manic. No significant difference was found in YMRS scores at endpoint between the oxcarbazepine and placebo groups (Wagner, Kowatch et al., 2006). Response rates (≥50% reduction in YMRS) were 42% for oxcarbazepine and 16% for placebo.

The efficacy of topiramate was assessed in a 4-week double-blind placebo-controlled trial for 56 children with bipolar I disorder, mixed or manic (DelBello et al., 2005). The mean topiramate dose was 278 mg/day. No significant difference was found on reduction in YMRS scores between the topiramate and placebo groups. Response rates (CGI-I ≤ 2) were 34.5% for topiramate and 22.2% for placebo.

In a 4-week double-blind placebo-controlled trial of divalproex ER, which included 150 youth, there was no significant difference in reduction in YMRS scores from baseline to endpoint between divalproex ER and placebo (Wagner et al., 2009). Response rates (≥50% reduction in YMRS) were 24% for divalproex ER group and 23% for the placebo group.

In the previously cited NIMH trial comparing lithium, divalproex, and placebo (Kowatch et al., 2007), the response rate (≥50% reduction in YMRS) for divalproex was 56%, which was significantly greater than for placebo (30%). Similarly, response rates based on CGI-I ≤ 2 were significantly greater for divalproex (54%) than for placebo (29%). The target serum level for divalproex was 85–110 μg/mL.

The efficacy of lamotrigine was assessed in a 12-week open-label trial for 30 children and adolescents with bipolar spectrum disorders (Biederman et al., 2010). Mean endpoint lamotrigine dose was 160.7mg/day. Approximately half of the youth completed the trial and seven subjects discontinued because of rash. Significant improvement in mean YMRS scores was reported.

Comparator Medication Studies

In a 6-week open-label comparator study of divalproex, carbamazepine, and lithium, response rates (≥50% reduction in baseline YMRS) were similar among these medications, divalproex 53%, carbamazepine 38%, and lithium 38% (Kowatch et al., 2000).

The efficacy of risperidone compared to divalproex was assessed in an 8-week double-blind randomized trial (Pavaluri et al., 2010). Sixty-six youth with bipolar disorder were randomized to risperidone or divalproex. Response rates (≥50% reduction in baseline YMRS) were significantly higher for risperidone (78.1%) compared to divalproex (45.5%). Improvement was more rapid for the risperidone group than for the divalproex group. Remission rates (YMRS ≤ 12 and CDRS ≤ 28) were significantly higher for risperidone (62.5%) than for divalproex (33.3%).

Quetiapine and divalproex efficacy was compared in 50 adolescents with bipolar I disorder, manic or mixed in a 4-week double-blind placebo-controlled trial (DelBello et al., 2006). There was no significant group difference in YMRS scores during the trial. Response rates (CGI-BP-I ≤ 2) and remission rates (YMRS ≤2) were significantly greater in the quetiapine-treated youth (72% and 60%, respectively) compared to the divalproex-treated youth (40% and 28%, respectively). Improvement also occurred more rapidly in the quetiapine group.

Olanzapine and risperidone were compared in an open-label 8-week trial for the treatment of preschool-age children with bipolar disorder (Biederman et al., 2005). Response rates (CGI ≤ 2 or ≥30% reduction in YMRS) were 69% for risperidone and 53% for olanzapine, which were not significantly different.

Efficacy of Acute Pharmacotherapy

A comparative analysis of the efficacy of antipsychotics and mood stabilizers for the treatment of pediatric bipolar disorder was conducted by Correll and colleagues (2010). Nine double-blind, placebo-controlled trials in youth, of which five evaluated second-generation antipsychotics and four evaluated mood stabilizers, were included in the analysis. A significantly greater improvement in YMRS scale scores was shown with antipsychotics compared to mood stabilizers in youth. Effect size for the antipsychotics was 0.65 and for mood stabilizers was 0.24. Using a definition of response of ≥50% reduction in the YMRS, the NNT was 4. However, antipsychotics caused more weight gain and somnolence than mood stabilizers in youth.

Based upon available evidence, atypical antipsychotics or lithium is a first-line treatment for bipolar I disorder, mixed or manic in youth. Approximately 50%–60% of youth will respond to acute treatment. Response rates are approximately 25% to 50% for acute pharmacotherapy.

Continuation Treatment

There are no data to guide the duration of continuation treatment for bipolar disorder in youth. Clinical recommendations are to continue the medication for at least 12 to 24 months following sustained remission (Kowatch et al., 2005).

Maintenance Treatment

There are limited data about maintenance treatment for bipolar disorder in youth. Lithium has a maintenance indication for acute mania in youth ages 12 and older; however, this indication is based on adult data.

The effectiveness of lamotrigine in maintenance of manic and depressive symptom control was assessed in a 14-week open trial (Pavuluri et al., 2009). Forty-six children and adolescents with bipolar I disorder, mixed or manic, or bipolar II disorder were titrated to a therapeutic dose of lamotrigine over 8 weeks while receiving an atypical antipsychotic for mood stabilization. This acute phase was followed by a 6-week lamotrigine monotherapy phase. Mean endpoint lamotrigine dose was 1.8 mg/lb. At 14-week endpoint, response rate on mania symptoms (YMRS ≤ 12) was 72% and on depressive symptoms (CDRS-R ≤ 40) was 82%. Approximately half of the subjects were in remission at week 8, but 23% relapsed by week 14.

Sixty youth who responded to treatment with a combination of divalproex and lithium were randomized in a double-blind trial to either divalproex or lithium for 18 months (Findling et al., 2005). The time to relapse was not significantly different between the divalproex and lithium groups (median days: divalproex, 112; lithium, 114).

Predictors of Treatment Response

Comorbid attention-deficit/hyperactivity disorder, conduct disorder, more severe bipolar disorder, earlier age of onset, and history of sexual abuse are predictors of poorer outcome for youth with bipolar disorder (Masi et al., 2004; Pavuluri, Henry, Carbray et al., 2006).

Treatment-Resistant Bipolar Disorder

To date, there are no large controlled studies for treatment-resistant pediatric bipolar disorder. Moreover, there is not a standard definition of treatment-resistant pediatric bipolar disorder. For the purpose of this chapter, treatment resistance will be defined as inadequate response to treatment with an atypical antipsychotic or lithium at adequate dose for a minimum 6-week duration.

Strategies for Treatment-Resistant Bipolar Disorder

A medication algorithm was developed for the treatment of bipolar I disorder, manic or mixed (Kowatch et al., 2005). This algorithm was based on expert consensus and a review of the treatment literature.

> Stage 1: Monotherapy with mood stabilizer or atypical antipsychotic.
> > If partial response, then monotherapy plus augmentation with different class of agent.
> > If no response, move to next stage.
> Stage 2: Alternate monotherapy.
> > If partial response, then alternate monotherapy plus augmentation with an agent that was not used in Stage 1.
> > If no response, then move to next stage.
> Stage 3: Switch monotherapy agent or combination of two mood stabilizers.
> > If no response, move to next stage.
> Stage 4: Combination of two mood stabilizers or combination of three mood stabilizers (if the youth had a partial or no response to combination of two mood stabilizers in Stage 3).
> > If no response, move to next stage.
> Stage 5: Alternate monotherapy.
> > If no response, move to next stage.
> Stage 6: Electroconvulsive therapy for adolescents or clozapine.

Since the development of this medication treatment algorithm, there have been additional studies to guide treatment decisions as described in this chapter. The atypical antipsychotics have the most evidence to support use as an initial treatment for children and adolescents with bipolar disorder. Lithium also has FDA approval for treatment of adolescents with acute mania. Approximately 50% of youth will respond to initial treatment with an antimanic agent. For youths with bipolar disorder who fail to respond to an atypical antipsychotic or lithium, a number of strategies may be utilized as discussed next.

Combination Medication

If a child does not respond to monotherapy treatment, combination treatment may be needed. Kowatch et al (2000) found that 20 of 35 (38%) youths with bipolar disorder required additional psychotropic medication after 6 weeks of treatment with one mood stabilizer.

The efficacy of combination divalproex and lithium was assessed in a 20-week open trial for 90 youths with bipolar I or II disorder (Findling et al., 2003). The remission rate (defined as contiguous weekly ratings of YMRS ≤ 12.5, CDRS-R≤40, Children's Global Assessment Scale [CGAS] ≥ 51; no mood cycling and clinical stability) was 42%. Significant improvement on all outcome measures was found by week 8.

In a 6-month open-label trial, the efficacy of risperidone plus lithium was compared to risperidone plus divalproex sodium for 37 youths with bipolar I disorder, mixed or manic (Pavuluri et al., 2004). Similar response rates (≥50% reduction in baseline YMRS scores) were found for risperidone plus lithium (82.4%) and risperidone plus divalproex sodium (80%).

Medication Augmentation

Aripiprazole and quetiapine have FDA approval as an adjunct to lithium or valproate for children ages 10 and older with bipolar I disorder, mixed or manic. FDA approval of aripiprazole was based upon extrapolation from adult data along with comparison of aripiprazole pharmacokinetics in adults and pediatric patients (Abilify prescribing information, 2009). FDA approval of quetiapine was based on a 3-week monotherapy trial (Seroquel prescribing information, 2010).

The efficacy of divalproex and adjunctive quetiapine has been assessed in a small controlled study. Thirty adolescents with bipolar disorder who received divalproex were randomly assigned to adjunctive quetiapine or placebo in a 6-week trial (DelBello, Schwiers, Rosenberg, & Strakowski, 2002). The divalproex and quetiapine group showed a significantly greater reduction in YMRS scores than the divalproex and placebo group. Response rates (≥50% reduction in baseline YMRS) were significantly higher in the divalproex and quetiapine group (87%) compared to the divalproex and placebo group (53%).

Risperidone has been used as augmentation for lithium nonresponders (Pavuluri, Henry et al., 2006). Twenty-one youths who did not respond to lithium monotherapy received risperidone for up to 11 months in an open-label trial. Response rates (≥50% reduction in YMRS) were 85.7% for the combination of lithium and risperidone.

Overall, although the data are limited, a combination of two antimanic medications increases response rates from approximately 50% to 80%.

Switch to an Alternate Mood Stabilizer

If a child with bipolar disorder fails to respond to a second-generation antipsychotic or lithium, other mood stabilizers may be considered, including divalproex, oxcarbazepine, and carbamazepine, although controlled data have shown minimal efficacy compared to placebo.

In a retrospective chart review, clozapine demonstrated efficacy for 10 adolescents with treatment refractory bipolar disorder (Masi, Mucci, & Millepiedi, 2002). The mean dose of clozapine was 142.5 mg. All patients were responders (CGI-I ≤ 2).

Adjunctive Psychotherapy

The addition of psychotherapy to medication may improve treatment response for youth with bipolar disorder. To date, there are no published studies of psychotherapy as monotherapy treatment for pediatric bipolar disorder.

Multifamily psychoeducational psychotherapy has been examined as an adjunctive treatment for children with bipolar disorder (Fristad, Verducci, Walters, & Young, 2009). Components of the treatment included psychoeducation, family systems, and cognitive-behavioral techniques. One hundred sixty-five children with mood disorders (70% bipolar spectrum disorders) were randomized to multifamily psychoeducational psychotherapy plus treatment as usual or a wait-list control plus treatment as usual. The group that received multifamily psychoeducational psychotherapy had significantly greater improvement in mood symptoms than the wait-list control group over a 1-year follow-up period.

Child and family focused cognitive-behavioral therapy (CFF-CBT) has been shown to improve manic symptoms in children when used as an adjunctive treatment to pharmacotherapy (West et al., 2009). Twenty-six families with a child with bipolar spectrum disorders participated in this 12-session weekly therapy.

Dialectic behavior therapy has shown potential as an adjunctive treatment for adolescent bipolar disorder. In an open pilot study of 10 adolescents with bipolar disorder, adjunctive dialectical behavior therapy resulted in significant improvement in emotional dysregulation, suicidality, and depressive symptoms (Goldstein et al., 2007).

Electroconvulsive Therapy

There are no controlled data for the use of ECT in children and adolescents with bipolar disorder. Case reports of the use of ECT for adolescents with bipolar mania have reported response rates based upon clinical impression ranging from 75% to 100% (Cohen, Paillere-Martinot, & Basquin, 1997; Rey & Walter, 1997; Walter & Rey, 1997). The American Academy of Child and Adolescent Psychiatry Practice Parameter for the Assessment and Treatment of Children with Bipolar Disorder recommends that ECT should only be considered for adolescents with well-defined bipolar I disorder who have severe episodes of mania or depression and are unresponsive to standard medication therapies (McClellan, Kowatch, & Findling, 2007).

Obsessive-Compulsive Disorder

The prevalence rate of obsessive-compulsive disorder (OCD) in children and adolescents is 2% to 4% (Douglass, Moffitt, Dar, McGee, & Silva, 1995; Zohar, 1999). OCD has a chronic course in youth. A meta-analysis of longitudinal studies of children with OCD revealed a persistence of 60% for full or subthreshold OCD (Stewart et al., 2004).

Pharmacotherapy

Acute Treatment

Four medications have FDA approval for the treatment of OCD in youth. These medications are sertraline (6 years and older), fluoxetine (7 years and older), fluvoxamine (7 years and older), and clomipramine (10 years and older).

Sertraline was shown to be significantly superior to placebo in an 8-week double-blind placebo-controlled trial that included 187 children and adolescents with OCD (March et al., 1998). The mean dose of sertraline was 167 mg/day at endpoint. Forty-two percent of the sertraline-treated patients compared to 26% of the placebo-treated patients were rated as much or very much improved.

A 13-week double-blind placebo-controlled trial that included 103 children and adolescents with OCD showed significant reduction in OCD severity in the group treated with fluoxetine compared to placebo (Geller et al., 2001). The mean daily fluoxetine dose was 24.6 mg/day. Fluoxetine was significantly superior to placebo in reduction of OCD symptoms. Response rates (>40% reduction in Children's Yale-Brown Obsessive-Compulsive Scale (CY-BOCS) were 49% in the fluoxetine group and 25% in the placebo group. Fluoxetine was also shown to be efficacious in two small controlled trials (Liebowitz et al., 2002; Riddle et al., 1992).

Fluvoxamine efficacy was demonstrated in a 10-week double-blind placebo-controlled trial that included 120 children and adolescents with OCD (Riddle et al., 2001). The mean daily dose of fluvoxamine was 165 mg/day. Response rates (>25% reduction in CY-BOCS) were 42% for the fluvoxamine group and 25% for the placebo group.

In two double-blind placebo-controlled trials, clomipramine was effective for the treatment of pediatric OCD. One small study included 19 children and adolescents with OCD who were randomly assigned to clomipramine (mean daily dose 141 mg) or placebo for 5 weeks. Improvement in obsessions and compulsions were found (Flament et al., 1985). In an 8-week double-blind placebo-controlled trial that included 60 children with OCD, the mean reduction in CY-BOCS scores was 37% in the clomipramine group and 8% in the placebo group (DeVeaugh-Geiss et al., 1992).

Although not FDA approved for the treatment of OCD in children and adolescents, paroxetine efficacy was shown in one 10-week double-blind placebo-controlled trial that included 203 children and adolescents with OCD (Geller, Wagner et al., 2004). The mean daily dose of paroxetine was 23 mg. There was significantly greater reduction in CY-BOCS scores from baseline to endpoint in the paroxetine group compared to the placebo group. Response rates (>25% reduction in CY-BOCS scores) were 64.9% in the paroxetine group and 41.2% in the placebo group. However, another study of paroxetine did not demonstrate efficacy for OCD treatment in 335 youth who received 16 weeks open-label paroxetine followed by randomization of responders to placebo or paroxetine for an additional 6 weeks. There was no significant difference in response rates between the paroxetine and placebo group (Emslie et al., 2000).

There are no large-scale double-blind placebo-controlled trials of citalopram for the treatment of pediatric OCD. In a small double-blind trial, 29 children and adolescents with OCD were randomized to citalopram or fluoxetine for 6 weeks (Alaghband-Rad & Hakimshooshtary, 2009). Both groups showed a significant improvement in CY-BOCS scores with no significant difference between either medication. An open-label 10-week trial that included 23 children with OCD who received citalopram (mean daily dose 37 mg) showed significant improvement in CY-BOCS scores (Thomsen, 1997). Fourteen of 15 youths with OCD showed significant improvement in CY-BOCS scores in an 8-week open-label study of citalopram (Mukaddes & Abali, 2003).

Efficacy of Acute Pharmacotherapy

Medium effect sizes have been reported for the SSRIs in the treatment of pediatric OCD. In one meta-analysis of 12 randomized controlled trials of pediatric OCD, the overall effect size for four SSRIs (paroxetine, fluoxetine, fluvoxamine, and sertraline) was 0.46 (Geller et al., 2003). Effect sizes for the individual medications were as follows: paroxetine, 0.41; fluoxetine, 0.55; fluvoxamine, 0.38; sertraline, 0.33; and clomipramine, 0.69. In another meta-analysis of 10 randomized controlled trials of SSRIs for pediatric OCD, the pooled effect size for medication was 0.48 (Watson & Rees, 2008). The effect sizes for the individual medications were as follows: fluoxetine, 0.51; fluvoxamine, 0.31; paroxetine, 0.44; sertraline, 0.47; and clomipramine, 0.85. Although clomipramine has been shown to have the largest effect size compared to SSRIs, its side-effect profile limits its use as a first-line agent in children. In a meta-analysis of six randomized controlled trials of SSRIs for the treatment of OCD in children and adolescents, the pooled rate of response was 52% in the SSRI treatment patients and 32% in the placebo-treated patients. The NNT was 6 (Bridge et al., 2007).

Continuation Treatment

The long-term effectiveness of sertraline for children and adolescents with OCD was assessed in a 52-week extension study (Cook et al., 2001) following the 12-week double-blind placebo-controlled study (March et al., 1998). Significant improvement of OCD symptoms was found during this 1 year follow-up. Rates of responses (>25% decrease in CY-BOCS and a CGI-I score of ≤2) were 72% for children and 61% for adolescents. Forty-seven percent of patients achieved full remission (CY-BOCS score < 8) and an additional 25% achieved partial remission (CY-BOCS score <15 but >8) (Wagner, Cook, Chung, & Messig, 2003).

A 1-year open-label extension study (Walkup et al., 1998) of an acute double-blind placebo-controlled fluvoxamine study of 99 youth with OCD (Riddle et al., 2001) showed that improvement plateaued at about 6 months of treatment.

The long-term use of citalopram was assessed in an open study of 30 adolescents who received citalopram for 1–2 years (Thomsen, Ebbesen, & Persson, 2001). A significant reduction in CY-BOCS scores was found from baseline to assessment at 2 years.

Clomipramine was shown to remain effective in a 1-year open-label extension trial for 47 patients following an 8-week randomized controlled trial (DeVeaugh-Geiss et al., 1992).

Maintenance

There are no large maintenance studies of medication treatment for pediatric OCD. In a small study, 26 children and adolescents with OCD received clomipramine maintenance treatment for 4 to 32 months (mean duration 17.1 months) followed by an 8-month double-blind desipramine substitution trial (Leonard et al., 1991). Eighteen percent of the patients in the clomipramine group relapsed compared to 89% in the desipramine group.

Predictors of Treatment Response

Predictors of low response rates to SSRI treatment in children and adolescents with OCD include comorbid disorders of attention-deficit/hyperactivity disorder, oppositional defiant disorder, and tic disorder (Geller, Biederman, Wagner et al., 2001). Without comorbid disorders, response rate to SSRI treatment was 75%, but comorbidity reduced response rates to as low as 39%.

Psychotherapy

The American Academy of Child and Adolescent Psychiatry Practice Parameters recommends that CBT should be first-line treatment for mild to moderate OCD in children and adolescents (King, Leonard, March, & The Work Group on Quality Issues, 1998).

CBT with exposure and response prevention had been shown in randomized controlled trials to be an efficacious treatment for children and adolescents with OCD (Asbahr, Castillo, Ito, Moreira, & Lotufo-Neto, 2005; Barrett, Healy-Farrell, & March, 2004; deHaan, Hoodgum, Buitelaar, & Keijsers, 1998; POTS, 2004; Storch et al., 2007). Therapy generally occurs over a 12–14 week period of time. CBT may be delivered on an individual basis (Piacentini, Bergman, Jacobs, McCracken, & Kretchman 2002), in a group (Asbahr et al., 2005), and with family (Barrett et al., 2004). Intensive (daily psychotherapy for 3 weeks) was compared to 14 weekly sessions of CBT for children and adolescents with OCD, and both were found to be efficacious (Storch et al., 2007).

Efficacy of Acute Psychotherapy

In a meta-analysis that included 12 open and randomized controlled trials, the effect size for CBT in the treatment of pediatric OCD was 1.55 (Freeman et al., 2006). In another meta-analysis of five randomized controlled treatment trials for pediatric OCD, the mean pooled effect size was 1.45 (Watson & Rees, 2008). Barrett et al (2008) evaluated CBT trials for children and adolescents with OCD and reported that results have been consistent across studies with remission rates ranging from 40% to 85%. Individual exposure-based CBT for pediatric OCD was considered to be a probably efficacious treatment, whereas CBT delivered in a group or family-focused individual format was considered as a possibly efficacious treatment. The NICE guideline (2005) supports the use of CBT that includes exposure and response prevention in the treatment of OCD for children and adolescents. Inclusion of parents in the treatment results in better outcomes for the children. Based on a review of OCD studies (O'Kearney, 2007), it was concluded that following CBT treatment there is a 37% reduction in the risk of continued OCD.

There is some evidence to support the stability of acute treatment gains made with CBT. The long-term effects of family-focused individual CBT and group CBT for 48 youths with OCD was assessed at 12 and 18 months following treatment (Barrett, Farrell, Dadds, & Boulter, 2005). Seventy percent of youth in individual therapy and 84% in group therapy did not meet diagnostic criteria for OCD at follow-up. No differences were found between the different delivery formats of CBT. Thirty-eight youths who had participated in a randomized controlled trial of individual or group cognitive-behavioral family-based therapy (CBFT) for OCD were evaluated 7 years post treatment (O'Leary, Barrett, & Fjermestad, 2009). Ninety-five percent from group CBFT and 79% of youth from individual CBFT had no diagnosis of OCD at 7-year follow-up.

Predictors of Treatment Response

Predictors of poor response to CBT treatment for pediatric OCD include higher baseline OCD symptoms, family dysfunction, family accommodations to rituals, comorbid attention-deficit/hyperactivity disorder, disruptive behavior disorders, and major depression (Ginsburg et al., 2008; Storch, Merlo, et al., 2008, Storch, Björgvinsson, et al., 2010).

Combination Medication and Psychotherapy

The efficacy of CBT, SSRI, and CBT plus an SSRI was compared in a large NIMH-funded multicenter study (POTS, 2004). One hundred twelve children and adolescents with OCD were randomly assigned to sertraline, CBT, sertraline plus CBT, or placebo for 12 weeks. Combined treatment was more efficacious than CBT alone or sertraline alone. CBT, sertraline, and combination treatment were superior to placebo. Sertraline alone and CBT alone did not significantly differ in response. Effect size for combined treatment was 1.4, for CBT 0.97, and for sertraline 0.67. The rate of remission (CY-BOCS score ≤10) was 53.6% for combined treatment, 39.3% for CBT, 21.4% for sertraline, and 3.6% for placebo.

In a study of 30 youth with OCD who were partial responders or nonresponders to two or more medication trials, the addition of 14 sessions of intensive family-based CBT improved response (Storch, Lehmkuhl, et al., 2010). At the end of treatment, 80% of the youth were considered improved (a CY-BOCS reduction of ≥30% and at 3-month follow-up). Fifty-seven percent of youth were in remission (CY-BOCS ≤ 10 or ADIS-IV-P ≤ 3) at post treatment, and 53% were in remission at follow-up.

Treatment-Resistant Obsessive-Compulsive Disorder

The SSRIs (sertraline, fluvoxamine, and fluoxetine) have shown efficacy in controlled trials and are first-line medication treatments for children and adolescents with OCD. Clomipramine is also an efficacious treatment for pediatric OCD. Approximately 50% of youth will respond to initial treatment with SSRIs. In a critical review of studies that included CBT for pediatric OCD, CBT was demonstrated to be equally effective to SSRIs for first-line treatment of youth with OCD (O'Kearney, 2007).

Treatment-resistant OCD as defined by expert consensus is persistent and substantial OCD symptomatology despite having received adequate treatment that is known to be effective in treating pediatric OCD (Geller, 2010). A CY-BOCS score of ≥16 or CGI-S of marked or severe impairment has been recommended as a guideline for defining persistent symptoms of at least moderate severity. An adequate trial of medication is defined as a minimum of 10 weeks of each SSRI or clomipramine at maximum recommended or tolerated doses, with no change in that dose for the preceding 3 weeks. An adequate trial of CBT dose is 8–10 total sessions or 5–6 sessions of exposure. Therefore, treatment resistance is defined as the failure of adequate trials of at least two SSRIs or one SSRI and a clomipramine trial in addition to failure of adequately delivered CBT.

Strategies for Treatment-Resistant Obsessive-Compulsive Disorder

If a child fails to respond to treatment with two SSRIs or one SSRI and clomipramine as well as CBT, a number of strategies may be utilized as described next.

Medication Augmentation

Atypical antipsychotic medications have been used as an augmentation strategy to SRIs for treatment-resistant OCD.

In a naturalistic sample of 220 children and adolescents with OCD, 89 (40.5%) were treated with SSRI alone and 131 (59.5%) required polypharmacy (Masi et al., 2009). Patient characteristics related to receiving augmentation medication were higher rates of comorbid bipolar disorder, tic disorder, and disruptive behavior disorders. Forty-three children were treated with an atypical antipsychotic as an augmenting agent. Twenty-five of these youths (58.1%) responded to treatment. Those youths who responded to treatment had less severe impairment at baseline.

In a large case series in a naturalistic study, the efficacy of aripiprazole augmentation to an SRI was assessed in 39 adolescents with OCD who had not responded to two initial trials with SRI monotherapy (Masi, Pfanner, Millepiedi, & Berloffa, 2010). The mean endpoint aripirazole dose was 12.2 mg/day. Fifty-nine percent of youths responded to treatment (CGI-I ≤ 2 and CGI-S ≤ 3 during 3 consecutive months).

Risperidone as augmentation to an SSRI was evaluated in a 12-week open-label trial for 17 adolescents who had failed two SSRI monotherapy trials (Thomsen, 2004). Risperidone dosages ranged from 1 to 2 mg. Four adolescents had >25% reduction in CY-BOCS scores and 10 adolescents had a reduction of 10%–25% in CY-BOCS scores. In a case series of four youths who had failed SSRI monotherapy, risperidone augmentation of an SRI resulted in improvement of OCD symptoms (Fitzgerald, Stewart, Tawile, & Rosenberg, 1999). Risperidone (0.5 mg/day) augmentation to sertraline was shown to be effective for two preschool children with OCD (Oner & Oner, 2008). One child was symptom free after 8 weeks and the other symptom free after 6 months of treatment.

The addition of clomipramine to an SSRI may increase treatment response based on the combination of serotonergic effects (Geller, 2010), although there are no published trials of this augmentation strategy in youth.

There are two case reports of the use of benzodiazepines for treatment-resistant OCD in adolescents. One adolescent received clonazepam up to 2 mg/day over an 11-week period and had a substantial decrease in obsessive-compulsive symptoms (Ross & Pigott, 1993). In another case, clonazepam augmentation (4 mg/day) to fluoxetine resulted in a 75% improvement in an adolescent's OCD symptoms (Leonard et al., 1994).

Buspirone augmentation (30 mg/day) of fluoxetine produced significant improvement in OCD symptoms for a child whose symptoms had not responded to fluoxetine alone (Alessi & Bos, 1991).

Cognitive-Behavioral Therapy Augmentation

The addition of motivational interviewing to CBT for the treatment of pediatric OCD was assessed in a small randomized trial of 16 youth (Merlo et al., 2010). At posttreatment, there was no significant difference between youth randomized to intensive family-based CBT plus extra psychoeducation compared to CBT plus motivational interviewing. Mean reduction of CY-BOCS scores ranged from 46% to 70%. However, the motivational interviewing group showed more rapid improvement.

Aripiprazole augmentation of CBT was shown to be effective for an adolescent who had a partial response to sertraline plus CBT (Storch, Lehmkuhl et al., 2008).

Riluzole

Riluzole, a glutamate antagonist, has been evaluated in an open-label trial for pediatric treatment-resistant OCD (Grant, Lougee, Hirschtritt, & Swedo, 2007). Six children and adolescents participated in a 12-week open-label trial of riluzole. The mean dose of riluzole was 101 mg/day at the end of 12 weeks. Four of 6 youths had a reduction of more than 46% on the CY-BOCS and a CGI-I ≤ 2 at the end of 12 weeks. One participant who continued treatment with riluzole experienced improvement in symptoms after the trial.

Non–Obsessive-Compulsive Disorder Anxiety Disorders

Estimates in children and adolescents of the prevalence of generalized anxiety disorder (GAD) are 2.9% to 7.3%; social anxiety disorder, 0.9%–7%; and separation anxiety disorder, 3.5% (Anderson, Williams, McGee, & Silva, 1987; Kashani & Orvaschel, 1988; Stein et al., 2001). The course of GAD and social anxiety disorder in youth tends to be chronic (Keller et al., 1992; Stein et al., 2001).

Most treatment studies of pediatric non-OCD anxiety disorders include GAD, separation anxiety disorder, and social anxiety disorder, rather than examining treatment response for the individual disorders.

Pharmacotherapy

Acute Treatment

There are no FDA-approved medications for the treatment of GAD, social anxiety disorder, or separation anxiety disorder in children and adolescents.

The efficacy of fluvoxamine was investigated in a multicenter trial for the treatment of GAD, social anxiety disorder, or separation anxiety disorder (Research Units on Pediatric Psychopharmacology Anxiety Study Group, 2001). One hundred twenty-eight children and adolescents who were nonresponders to 3 weeks of psychoeducational therapy were randomized to fluvoxamine (up to 300 mg/day) or placebo for an 8-week trial. The fluvoxamine group had a significantly greater reduction in scores on the Pediatric Anxiety Rating Scale (PARS) (Research Units on Pediatric Psychopharmacology Anxiety Study Group, 2002) compared to the placebo group. The response rate (CGI-I ≤ 2) was 76% for the fluvoxamine-treated patients and 29% for the placebo-treated patients.

Fluoxetine efficacy for the treatment of GAD, separation anxiety disorder, and/or social anxiety disorder was evaluated in a randomized 12-week controlled trial that included 74 children and adolescents (Birmaher et al., 2003). Flouxetine was significantly superior to placebo in reduction of anxiety symptoms on the PARS and Screen for Child Anxiety Disorders (SCARED). Response rates (CGI-I ≤ 2) were significantly greater for the fluoxetine-treated patients (61%) than for the placebo-treated patients (35%).

In a 9-week double-blind placebo-controlled trial of sertraline for the treatment of GAD, 22 children and adolescents were randomly assigned to sertraline (maximum dose 50 mg/day) or placebo (Rynn, Siqueland, & Rickels, 2001). Sertraline was significantly superior to placebo in reduction of Hamilton Anxiety Scale scores. The CGI-I ≤ 2 was 90% for sertraline-treated patients and 10% for placebo-treated patients. An open-label study of sertraline for the treatment of 14 children and adolescents with social anxiety disorder showed that 36% of the patients were much or very much improved and 29% had a partial response by the end of 8 weeks (Compton et al., 2001).

The efficacy of paroxetine was evaluated in a 16-week double-blind placebo-controlled trial for 322 children and adolescents with social anxiety disorder (Wagner, Berard et al., 2004). The mean daily dose of paroxetine was 32.6 mg/day. Paroxetine was significantly superior to placebo. Response rates (CGI-I ≤ 2) were 77.6% for paroxetine treated patients and 38.3% for placebo treated patients.

In a 12-week open-label study of escitalopram for the treatment of 20 children with social anxiety disorder, 65% of participants responded (CGI-I ≤ 2) to treatment (Isolan et al., 2007). The mean daily dosage of escitalopram at end point was 13 mg.

The efficacy of venlafaxine ER for the treatment of pediatric social anxiety disorder was evaluated in a randomized controlled 16-week trial (March, Entusah, Rynn, Albano, & Tourian, 2007). Two hundred ninety-three children and adolescents with social anxiety disorder were randomized to venlafaxine ER (dose range, 37.5 mg to 222 mg; mean daily dose range, 2.6 mg/kg to 3.0 mg/kg) or placebo. Venlafaxine ER was significantly superior to placebo on the reduction in The Society Anxiety Scale, Child and Adolescent Version (SAS-CA) scores. Response rates (CGI-I ≤ 2) were 56% for venlafaxine ER-treated patients and 37% for placebo-treated patients.

Venlafaxine ER was also evaluated for the treatment of GAD in children and adolescents in two double-blind placebo-controlled trials (Rynn, Riddle, Yeung, & Kunz, 2007). Three hundred twenty youth were randomized to venlafaxine ER or placebo for 8 weeks. Venlafaxine was flexibly dosed up to 225 mg/day. In one study, venlafaxine ER was superior on primary and secondary efficacy measures, but in the other study venlafaxine ER was not significantly superior to placebo on the primary outcome measure (baseline to endpoint change in a composite measure of GAD symptoms). In a pooled analysis, the response rate (CGI-I ≤ 2) was significantly greater for venlafaxine ER (69%) compared to placebo (48%).

Other than the SSRIs and venlafaxine ER, there are no limited controlled data regarding medications for the treatment of children with non-OCD anxiety disorders.

Mirtazapine was evaluated in an 8-week open-label study for the treatment of 18 children and adolescents with social anxiety disorder (Mrakotsky et al., 2008). Response rate

(CGI-I ≤ 2) was 56%, and 17% of youth achieved full remission. The mean endpoint daily dose of mirtazapine was 28.75 mg/day.

Buspirone (up to 30 mg/day) efficacy was evaluated in two small open studies for the treatment of pediatric GAD (Kutcher, Reiter, Gardner, & Klein, 1992; Simeon, 1993) and demonstrated reduction in anxiety clinical ratings after 4–6 weeks.

Alprazolam efficacy was evaluated for anxiety disorders in children and adolescents. In a double-blind placebo-controlled trial, 30 children with *DSM-III-R* diagnoses of overanxious disorder or avoidance disorder were randomized to alprazolam (mean daily dose 1.57 mg) or placebo for a 4-week trial (Simeon et al., 1992). No statistically significant difference was found on global ratings of improvement between the alprazolam group and the placebo group. Alprazolam was not found to be significantly superior to placebo in a double-blind crossover trial of 4 weeks of clonazepam and 4 weeks of placebo in 15 children with anxiety disorders, predominantly separation anxiety disorder (Graae, Milner, Rizzotto, & Klein, 1994).

Imipramine has been studied in small controlled trials for separation anxiety disorder, and the results have been mixed (Bernstein, Garfinkel, & Borchardt, 1990; Gittelman-Klein & Klein, 1971; Klein, Koplewicz, & Kanner, 1992). The side-effect profile of imipramine limits its use in children.

Efficacy of Acute Pharmacotherapy

A meta-analysis was conducted of six randomized controlled trials for non-OCD anxiety that included 1,136 children and adolescents who had been treated with antidepressants (Bridge et al., 2007). The pooled rates of response were 69% in the antidepressant treated youth and 39% in the youth who received placebo. The NNT was 3.

An analysis of two studies of pharmacologic treatment for children and adolescents with generalized anxiety disorder found an effect size of 1.38 (Hidalgo, Tupler, & Davidson, 2007).

Continuation Treatment

The long-term efficacy of fluoxetine treatment for childhood anxiety disorders (GAD, separation anxiety disorder, and/or social phobia) was assessed in a 1-year open-label long-term extension (Clark et al., 2005) of the randomized controlled trial comparing fluoxetine and placebo (Birmaher et al., 2003). Forty-two youth took fluoxetine and 10 youth took no medication during the 1 year follow-up. Those youths who took fluoxetine had significantly superior outcomes on most anxiety measures, including clinician, parent, and child ratings.

A 6-month open-label extension (Walkup et al., 2002) followed the 8-week placebo-controlled study of fluvoxamine (RUPP, 2001) in the treatment of pediatric GAD, separation disorder, or social anxiety disorder. Thirty-three of 35 (94%) youths who had initially responded to fluvoxamine continued to maintain their response. Fourteen fluvoxamine nonresponders were switched to fluoxetine, and anxiety symptoms significantly improved in 10 (71%) of these youth. For the 48 placebo nonresponders, 27 (56%) had clinically significant improvement in anxiety on fluvoxamine.

Psychotherapy

Acute Treatment

CBT is the major treatment modality for children with non-OCD anxiety disorders. The efficacy of CBT for the treatment of these disorders has been demonstrated in randomized controlled trials (Barrett, 1998; Flannery-Schroeder & Kendall, 2000; Gallagher, Rabian, & McCloskey, 2003; Hayward et al., 2000; Herbert et al., 2009; Kendall, 1994; Kendall et al., 1997; Liber et al., 2008; Manassis et al., 2002; Rapee, Abbott, & Lyneham, 2006; Silverman et al., 1999; Spence, Donovan, & Brechman-Toussaint, 2000; Spence, Holmes, March, & Lipp, 2006).

Social effectiveness training for children with social anxiety disorder has also demonstrated efficacy in controlled trials (Beidel, Turner, et al., 2000).

Efficacy of Acute Pharmacotherapy

A review of evidence-based psychosocial treatments for anxiety disorders in children and adolescents found that individual CBT, group CBT, group CBT with parents, group CBT for social anxiety disorders, and social effectiveness training for children with social anxiety disorder met criteria for probably efficacious (Silverman, Pina, & Viswesvaran, 2008). Treatment effects ranged from 46% to 79%. Ninety-six percent of treatments showed at least a 46% improvement in diagnostic recovery. No significant differences in response rates were found between CBT that was delivered in an individual format compared to a group format (59% vs. 62%). No differences in response rates were found whether parents participated in treatment or did not participate in treatment (68% vs. 64%).

A 1-year follow-up was conducted of 161 children and adolescents who had participated in a randomized clinical trial of individual CBT, family-based CBT, and family-based education, support, and attention treatment for separation anxiety disorder, social phobia, and/or GAD (Kendall, Hudson, Gosch, Flannery-Schroeder, & Suveg, 2008). Treatment gains were maintained at 1 year follow-up. Other follow-up studies (Barrett, Duffy, & Rapee, 2001; Kendall, Stafford, Flannery-Schroeder, & Webb, 2004) found similar positive long-term effects of short-term CBT for anxiety disorders in children and adolescents.

A 5-year follow-up study of adolescents who had received social effectiveness training for social anxiety disorder showed maintenance of treatment gains with diagnostic recovery rates of 43% (Garcia-Lopez et al., 2006).

The long-term effects of CBT for childhood anxiety disorders on adult outcomes was assessed (Saavedra, Silverman, Morgan-Lopez, & Kurtines, 2010). Sixty-seven participants with a mean age of 19 years old were followed 8–13 years post CBT for an anxiety disorder. Of the participants, 92.5% did not meet diagnostic criteria for an anxiety disorder, and 82.1% did not meet diagnostic criteria for any new disorders.

Treatment-Resistant Non–Obsessive-Compulsive Disorder Anxiety Disorders

The SSRIs have shown efficacy in controlled trials and are first-line medication treatment for children and adolescents with non-OCD anxiety disorders. Approximately 60% of youth will respond to initial treatment with SSRIs. CBT has also shown efficacy as a first-line psychotherapy treatment for non-OCD anxiety disorders in youth. Data are extremely limited with regard to alternate treatments for children and adolescents with non-OCD anxiety disorders who do not respond to treatment with an SSRI or CBT.

Strategies for Treatment Resistant Non–Obsessive-Compulsive Disorder Anxiety Disorders

If a child fails to respond to treatment with an SSRI or with CBT, some strategies that may be utilized are described in the sections that follow.

Combination Medication and Cognitive-Behavioral Therapy

The combination of an SSRI plus CBT has been shown to improve treatment response compared to either modality alone.

The Child-Adolescent Anxiety Multimodal Study (CAMS) evaluated the relative efficacy of sertraline, CBT, sertraline plus CBT, and placebo in a 12-week randomized controlled trial (Walkup et al., 2008). Four hundred eighty-eight children and adolescents who had a diagnosis of GAD, separation anxiety disorder, or social phobia were randomized to one of the four treatments. Sertraline dosing was titrated upward to 200 mg/day by week 8. Response rates (CGI-I ≤ 2) were 80.7% for combination treatment, 59.7% for CBT, and 54.9% for sertraline; all of these treatments were significantly superior to placebo (23.7%). Combination treatment was significantly superior to both CBT alone and sertraline alone. Effect size was 0.86 for combination treatment, 0.45 for sertraline, and 0.31 for CBT. The NNT was 1.7 for combination treatment, 3.2 for sertraline, and 2.8 for CBT.

The efficacy of fluoxetine, social effectiveness therapy for children (SET-C), and placebo was evaluated in a 12-week trial for the treatment of 122 children and adolescents with social anxiety disorder (Biedel et al., 2007). SET-C and fluoxetine were significantly superior to placebo in reducing social distress and behavioral avoidance and increasing general functioning, but SET-C was more efficacious on these measures than fluoxetine. SET-C was the only treatment superior to placebo in improving social skills, decreasing anxiety in specific social interactions, and improving social competence.

The effectiveness of combined psychoeducation and citalopram was evaluated in a 12-week open-label trial for 12 children and adolescents with social anxiety disorder (Chavira & Stein, 2002). As a result, 41.7% of youths were very much improved, and 41.7% of youths were much improved on clinical global ratings.

Alternate Medications

Venlafaxine is the only non-SRRI medication that has demonstrated some efficacy in the treatment of non-OCD anxiety disorders and is a treatment option for children who fail to respond to treatment with SSRIs. Buspirone is another option, although data are limited regarding its efficacy. Benzodiazepines may be used briefly (1–3 weeks) to reduce debilitating anxiety; however, long-term use with children and adolescents is not recommended.

Parent–Child and Family Interventions

In some cases, parents and families foster the development and maintenance of anxiety in children. Psychotherapeutic interventions that improve parent–child relationships, increase family problem solving, reduce parental anxiety, and facilitate parenting skills that reinforce adaptive coping and appropriate autonomy in the child may be helpful for anxious children (Connolly, Bernstein, & Work Group on Quality Issues, 2007). Models for family treatment with anxious children have been proposed (Dadds & Roth, 2001); however, controlled trials of family therapy are needed to determine the efficacy of this treatment modality for children with anxiety disorders.

Disclosure Statement

K.D.W. has received honoraria from American Psychiatric Association, Physicians Post-graduate Press, CMP Medica, American Academy of Child and Adolescent Psychiatry, NIH, Mexican Psychiatric Association, Contemporary Forums, Doctors Hospital at Renaissance, UBM Medica, Quantia Communications, CME LLC, Nevada Psychiatric Association, Slack Inc., Mercy, and Hospital Universitario Ramón y Cajal.

References

Alaghband-Rad, J., & Hakimshooshtary, M. (2009). A randomized controlled clinical trial of citalopram versus fluoxetine in children and adolescents with obsessive-compulsive disorder (OCD). *European Child and Adolescent Psychiatry, 18*, 131–135.

Alessi, N., & Bos, T. (1991). Buspirone augmentation of fluoxetine in a depressed child with obsessive-compulsive disorder. *American Journal of Psychiatry, 148*, 1605–1606.

Anderson, J. C., Williams, S., McGee, R., & Silva, P. A. (1987). DSM-III disorders in preadolescent children. Prevalence in a large sample from the generation population. *Archives of General Psychiatry, 44*, 69–76.

Asarnow, J. R., Emslie, G., Clarke, G., Wagner, K. D., Spirito, A., Vitiello, B., et al. (2009). Treatment of selective serotonin reuptake inhibitor-resistant depression in adolescents: Predictors and moderators of treatment response. *Journal of the American Academy of Child and Adolescent Psychiatry, 48*, 330–339.

Asbahr, F., Castillo, R., Ito, L., Moreira, L. M., & Lotufo-Neto, F. (2005). Group cognitive-behavioural therapy versus sertraline for the treatment of children and adolescents with obsessive-compulsive disorder. *Journal of the American Academy of Child and Adolescent Psychiatry, 44*, 1128–1136.

Barrett, P. M. (1998). Evaluation of cognitive-behavioral group treatments for childhood anxiety disorders. *Journal of Clinical Child Psychology, 27*, 459–468.

Barrett, P. M., Duffy, A. L., & Rapee, R. M. (2001). Cognitive-behavioral treatment of anxiety disorders in children: Long-term (6-year) follow-up. *Journal of Consulting and Clinical Psychology, 69*, 135–141.

Barrett, P. M., Farrell, L. J., Dadds, M., & Boulter, N. (2005). Cognitive-behavioral family treatment of childhood obsessive-compulsive disorder: Long-term follow-up and predictors of outcomes. *Journal of the American Academy of Child and Adolescent Psychiatry, 44*, 1005–1014.

Barrett, P. M., Farrell, L., Pina, A. A., Peris, T. S., & Piacentini, T. S. (2008). Evidence-based psychosocial treatment for child and adolescent obsessive-compulsive disorder. *Journal of Clinical Child and Adolescent Psychopharmacology, 37*, 131–155.

Barrett, P. M., Healy-Farrell, L. J., & March, J. S. (2004). Cognitive-behavioral family treatment of childhood obsessive-compulsive disorder: A controlled trial. *Journal of the American Academy of Child and Adolescent Psychiatry, 43*, 46–62.

Beidel, D. C., Turner, S. M., & Morris, T. L. (2000). Behavioral treatment of childhood social phobia. *Journal of Consulting and Clinical Psychology, 68*, 1072–1080.

Beidel, D. C., Turner, S. M., Sallee, F. R., Ammerman, R. T., Crosby, L. A., & Pathak, S. (2007). SET-C versus fluoxetine in the treatment of childhood social phobia. *Journal of the American Academy of Child and Adolescent Psychiatry, 46*, 1622–1632.

Berard, R., Fong, R., Carpenter, D. J., Thomason, C., & Wilkinson, C. (2006). An international, multicenter, placebo-controlled trial of paroxetine in adolescents with major depressive disorder. *Journal of Child and Adolescent Psychopharmacology, 16*, 59–75.

Bernstein, G. A., Garfinkel, B. D., & Borchardt, C. M. (1990). Comparative studies of pharmacotherapy for school refusal. *Journal of the American Academy of Child and Adolescent Psychiatry, 29*, 773–781.

Biederman, J., Joshi, G., Mick, E., Doyle, R., Georgiopoulos, A., Hammerness, P., et al. (2010). A prospective open-label trial of lamotrigine monotherapy in children and adolescents with bipolar disorder. *CNS Neuroscience and Therapuetics, 16,* 91–102.

Biederman, J., Mick, E., Hammerness, P., Harpold, T., Aleardi, M., Dougherty, M., et al. (2005). Open-label, 8-week trial of olanzapine and risperidone for the treatment of bipolar disorder in preschool-age children. *Biological Psychiatry, 58,* 589–594.

Birmaher, B., Arbelaez, C., & Brent, D. (2002). Course and outcome of child and adolescent major depressive disorder. *Child and Adolescent Psychiatric Clinics of North America, 11,* 619–637.

Birmaher, B., Axelson, D. A., Monk, K., Kalas, C., Clark, D. B., Ehmann, M., et al. (2003). Fluoxetine for the treatment of childhood anxiety disorders. *Journal of the American Academy of Child and Adolescent Psychiatry, 42,* 415–423.

Birmaher, B., Ryan, N. D., Williamson, D. E., Brent, D. A., Kaufman, J., Dahl, R. E., et al. (1996). Childhood and adolescent depression: a review of the past ten years, Part I. *Journal of the American Academy of Child and Adolescent Psychiatry, 35,* 1427–1439.

Birmaher, B., Williamson, D. E., Dahl, R. E., Axelson, D. A., Kaufman, J., Dorn, L. D., & Ryan, N. D. (2004) Clinical presentation and course of depression in youth: Does onset in childhood differ from onset in adolescence? *Journal of the American Academy of Child and Adolescent Psychiatry, 43,* 63–70.

Birmaher, B., Brent, D., AACAP Work Group on Quality Issues, Bernet, W., Bukstein, O., Walter, H., et al. (2007). Practice parameter for the assessment and treatment of children and adolescents with depressive disorders. *Journal of the American Academy of Child and Adolescent Psychiatry, 46,* 1503–1526.

Bloch, Y., Grisaru, N., Harel, E. V., Beitler, G., Faivel, N., Ratzoni G., et al. (2008). Repetitive transcranial magnetic stimulation in the treatment of depression in adolescents: An open-label study. *Journal of the ECT, 24,* 156–159.

Brent, D. A., Holder, D., Kolko, D., Birmaher, B., Baugher, M., Roth, C., et al. (1997). A clinical psychotherapy trial for adolescent depression comparing cognitive, family, and supportive therapy. *Archives of General Psychiatry, 54,* 877–885.

Brent, D., Emslie, G., Clarke, G., Wagner, K. D., Asarnow, J. R., Keller, M., et al. (2008) Switching to another SSRI or to venlafaxine with or without cognitive behavioral therapy for adolescents with SSRI-resistant depression: The TORDIA randomized controlled trial. *Journal of the American Medical Association, 299,* 901–913.

Bridge, J. A., Iyengar, S., Salary, C. B., Barbe, R. P., Birmaher, B., Pincus, H. A., et al. (2007). Clinical response and risk for reported suicidal ideation and suicide attempts in pediatric antidepressant treatment: A meta-analysis of randomized controlled trials. *Journal of the American Medical Association, 297,* 1683–1696.

Chavira, D. A., & Stein, M. B. (2002). Combined psychoeducation and treatment with selective serotonin reuptake inhibitors for youth with generalized anxiety disorder. *Journal of Child and Adolescent Psychopharmacology, 12,* 47–54.

Cheung, A., Kusumakar, V., Kutcher, S., Dubo, E., Garland, J., Weiss, M., et al. (2008). Maintenance study for adolescent depression. *Journal of Child and Adolescent Psychopharmacology, 18,* 389–394.

Clark, D. B., Birmaher, B., Axelson, D., Monk, K., Kalas, C., Ehmann, M., et al. (2005). Fluoxetine for the treatment of childhood anxiety disorders: Open-label, long-term extension to a controlled trial. *Journal of the American Academy of Child and Adolescent Psychiatry, 44,* 1263–1270.

Clarke, G. N., Rohde, P., Lewinsohn, P. M., Hops, H., & Seeley, J. R. (1999). Cognitive-behavioral treatment of adolescent depression. *Journal of the American Academy of Child and Adolescent Psychiatry, 38,* 272–279.

Clarke, G., DeBar, L., Lynch, F., Powell, J., Gale, J., O'Connor, E., et al. (2005). A randomized effectiveness trial of brief cognitive-behavioral therapy for depressed adolescents receiving antidepressant medication. *Journal of the American Academy of Child and Adolescent Psychiatry, 44,* 888–898.

Cohen, D., Paillere-Martinot, M. L., & Basquin, M. (1997). Use of electroconvulsive therapy in adolescents. *Convulsive Therapy, 13,* 25–31.

Compton, S. N., Grant, P. J., Chrisman, A. K., Gammon, P. J., Brown, V. L., & March, J. S. (2001). Sertraline in children and adolescents with social anxiety disorder: An open trial. *Journal of the American Academy of Child and Adolescent Psychiatry, 40,* 564–571.

Connolly, S. D., Bernstein, G. A., & Work Group on Quality Issues. (2007). Practice parameter for the assessment and treatment of children and adolescents with anxiety disorders. *Journal of the American Academy of Child and Adolescent Psychiatry, 46,* 267–283.

Cook, E. H., Wagner, K. D., March, J. S., Biederman, J., Landau, P., Wolkow, R., et al. (2001). Long-term sertraline treatment of children and adolescents with obsessive-compulsive disorder. *Journal of the American Academy of Child and Adolescent Psychiatry, 40,* 1175–1181.

Correll, C. U., Sheridan, E. M., & DelBello, M. P. (2010). Antipsychotic and mood stabilizer efficacy and tolerability in pediatric and adult patients with bipolar I mania: A comparative analysis of acute, randomized, placebo-controlled trials. *Bipolar Disorders, 12*, 116–141.

Croarkin, P. E., Wall, C. A., McClintock, S. M., Kozel, F. A., Husain, M. M., & Sampson, S. M. (2010). The emerging role for repetitive transcranial magnetic stimulation in optimizing the treatment of adolescent depression. *Journal of ECT, 26*, 323–329.

Curry, J., Rohde, P., Simons, A., Silva, S., Vitiello, B., Kratochvil, C., et al. (2006). Predictors and moderators of acute outcome in the treatment of adolescents with depression study (TADS). *Journal of the American Academy of Child and Adolescent Psychiatry, 45*, 1427–1439.

Curry, J., Silva, S., Rohde, P., Ginsburg, G., Kratochvil C., Simons, A., et al. (2011). Recovery and recurrence following treatment for adolescent major depression. *Archives of General Psychiatry, 68*, 263–270.

Dadds, M. R., & Roth, J. H. (2001). Family process in the development of anxiety problems. In M. W. Vasey & M. R. Dadds (Eds.), *The developmental psychopathology of anxiety* (pp. 278–303). New York: Oxford University Press.

De Haan, E., Hoodgum, K. A. L, Buitelaar, J. K., & Keijsers, G. (1998). Behavior therapy versus clomipramine in obsessive-compulsive disorders in children and adolescents. *Journal of the American Academy of Child and Adolescent Psychiatry, 37*, 1022–1029.

DelBello, M. P., Kowatch, R. A., Adler, C. M., Stanford, K. E., Welge, J. A., Barzman, D. H., et al. (2006) A double-blind randomized pilot study comparing quetiapine and divalproex for adolescent mania. *Journal of the American Academy of Child and Adolescent Psychiatry, 45*, 305–313.

DelBello, M. P., Findling, R. L., Kushner, S., Wang, D., Olson, W. H., Capece, J. A., et al. (2005). A pilot controlled trial of topiramate for mania in children and adolescents with bipolar disorder. *Journal of the American Academy of Child and Adolescent Psychiatry, 44*, 539–547.

DelBello, M. P., Findling, R. L., Earley, W. R., Acevedo, l., Stankowski, J.l. (2007, December 9–13). *Efficacy of quetiapine in children and adolescents with bipolar mania: A 3-week, double blind, randomized, placebo-controlled trial.* Poster presented at the 46th Annual Meeting of the American College of Neuropsychopharmacology (ACNP), Boca Raton, FL.

DelBello, M. P., Findling, R. L., Wang, P. P., Gundapaneni, B., Versavel, M. (2008, May 1-3). *Safety and efficacy of ziprasidone in pediatric bipolar disorder.* Poster presented at the 63rd Annual Meeting of the Society of Biological Psychiatry, Washington, DC.

DelBello, M. P., Schwiers, M. L., Rosenberg, H. L., & Strakowski, S. M. (2002). A double-blind, randomized, placebo-controlled study of quetiapine as adjunctive treatment for adolescent mania. *Journal of the American Academy of Child and Adolescent Psychiatry, 41*, 1216–1223.

DeVeaugh-Geiss, J, Moroz, G., Biederman, J., Cantwell, D., Fontaine, R., Greist, J. H., et al. (1992). Clomipramine hydrochloride in childhood and adolescent obsessive-compulsive disorder—a multicenter trial. *Journal of the American Academy of Child and Adolescent Psychiatry, 31*, 45–49.

Douglass, H. M., Moffitt, T. E., Dar, R., McGee, R., & Silva, P. (1995). Obsessive-compulsive disorder in a birth cohort of 18-year-olds: Prevalence and predictors. *Journal of the American Academy of Child and Adolescent Psychiatry, 34*, 1424–1431.

Emslie, G. J., Findling, R. L., Yeung, P. P., Kunz, N. R., & Li, Y. (2007). Venlafaxine ER for the treatment of pediatric subjects with depression: Results of two placebo-controlled trials. *Journal of the American Academy of Child and Adolescent Psychiatry, 46*, 479–488.

Emslie, G. J., Heiligenstein, J. H., Wagner, K. D., Hoog, S. L., Ernest, D. E., Brown, E., et al. (2002). Fluoxetine for acute treatment of depression in children and adolescents: A placebo-controlled, randomized clinical trial. *Journal of the American Academy of Child and Adolescent Psychiatry, 41*, 1205–1215.

Emslie, G. J., Kennard, B. D., & Mayes, T. L. (2011). Predictors of treatment response. *Psychiatric Annals, 41*, 223–229.

Emslie, G. J., Kennard, B. D., Mayes, T. L., Nightingale-Teresi, J., Carmody, T., Hughes, C. W., et al. (2008). Fluoxetine versus placebo in preventing relapse of major depression in children and adolescents. *American Journal of Psychiatry, 165*, 459–467.

Emslie, G. J., Mayes, T., Porta, G., Vitiello, B., Clarke, G., Wagner, K. D., et al. (2010). Treatment of resistant depression in adolescents (TORDIA): Week 24 outcomes. *American Journal of Psychiatry, 167*, 782–791.

Emslie, G. J., Rush, A. J., Weinberg, W. A., Kowatch, R. A., Hughes, C. W., Carmody, T., et al.(1997). A double-blind, randomized, placebo-controlled trial of fluoxetine in children and adolescents with depression. *Archives of General Psychiatry, 54*, 1031–1037.

Emslie, G. J., Ventura, D., Korotzer, A., & Tourkodimitris, S. (2009). Escitalopram in the treatment of adolescent depression: A randomized placebo-controlled multisite trial. *Journal of the American Academy of Child and Adolescent Psychiatry, 48*, 721–729.

Emslie, G. J., Wagner, K. D., Kutcher, S., Krulewicz, S., Fong, R., Carpenter, D. J., et al. (2006). Paroxetine treatment in children and adolescents with major depressive disorder: A randomized, multicenter, double-blind, placebo-controlled trial. *Journal of the American Academy of Child and Adolescent Psychiatry, 45*, 709–719.

Emslie, G. J., Wagner, K. D., Riddle, M., Lawrinson, S., Carpenter, J. C. (2000, May 13–18). Safety and Efficacy of Paroxetine in the Treatment of Children and Adolescents with OCD Poster presented at the 153rd Annual Meeting of the American Psychiatric Association, Chicago, IL.

Emslie, G. J., Yeung, P. P., & Kunz, N. R. (2007). Long-term, open-label venlafaxine extended-release treatment in children and adolescents with major depressive disorder. *CNS Spectrums, 12*, 223–233.

Findling, R. L., McNamara, N. K., Gracious, B. L., Youngstrom, E. A., Stansbrey, R. J., Reed, M. D., et al. (2003). Combination lithium and divalproex sodium in pediatric bipolarity. *Journal of the American Academy of Child and Adolescent Psychiatry, 42*, 895–901.

Findling, R. L., McNamara, N. K., Youngstrom, E. A., Stansbrey, R., Gracious, B. L., Reed, M. D., et al. (2005). Double-blind 18-month trial of lithium versus divalproex maintenance treatment in pediatric bipolar disorder. *Journal of the American Academy of Child and Adolescent Psychiatry, 44*, 409–417.

Findling, R. L., Bose, A., Aquino, D., Tourkodimitris, (2009, June 29-July 2). *24 week controlled trial of escitalopram for adolescent depression.* Poster presentation at the 49th New Clinical Drug Evaluation Unit Annual Meeting, Hollywood, FL.

Findling, R. L., Nyilas, M., Forbes, R. A., McQuade, R. D., Jin, N., Iwamoto, T., et al. (2009). Acute treatment of pediatric bipolar I disorder, manic or mixed episode, with aripiprazole: A randomized, double-blind, placebo-controlled study. *Journal of Clinical Psychiatry, 70*, 1441–1451.

Fitzgerald, K. D., Stewart, C. M., Tawile, V., & Rosenberg, D. (1999). Risperidone augmentation of serotonin reuptake inhibitor treatment of pediatric obsessive compulsive disorder. *Journal of Child and Adolescent Psychopharmacology, 9*, 115–123.

Flament, M. F., Rapoport, J. L., Berg, C. J., Sceery, W., Kilts, C., Mellström, B., et al. (1985). Clomipramine treatment of childhood obsessive-compulsive disorder. A double-blind controlled study. *Archives of General Psychiatry, 42*, 977–983.

Flannery-Schroeder, E. C., & Kendall, P. C. (2000). Group and individual cognitive-behavioral treatments for youth with anxiety disorders: A randomized clinical trial. *Cognitive Therapy and Research, 24*, 251–278.

Freeman, J. B., Garcia, A. B., Swedo, S. E., Rapoport, J. L., Ng, J. S., & Leonard, H. D. (2006). Obsessive-compulsive disorder. In M. K. Dulcan & J. M. Wiener (Eds.), *Essentials of child and adolescent psychiatry* (pp. 441–454). Washington, DC: American Psychiatric Publishing.

Fristad, M. A., Verducci, J. S., Walters, K., & Young, M. E. (2009). Impact of multifamily psychoeducational psychotherapy in treating children aged 8 to 12 years with mood disorders. *Archives of General Psychiatry, 66*, 1013–1021.

Gallagher, H. M., Rabian, B. A., & McCloskey, M. S. (2003). A brief group cognitive behavioral intervention for social phobia in childhood. *Journal of Anxiety Disorders, 18*, 459–479.

Garcia-Lopez, L., Olivares, J., Beidel, D. C., Albano, A. M., Turner, S. M., & Rosa, A. I. (2006). Efficacy of three treatment protocols for adolescents with social anxiety disorder: A 5-year follow-up assessment. *Journal of Anxiety Disorders, 20*, 459–479.

Geller, D. (2010). Obsessive-compulsive disorder. In *Dulcan's textbook of child and adolescent psychiatry* (pp. 349–366). M. K. Dulcan (Ed.), Washington, DC: American Psychiatric Publishing.

Geller, D. A., Biederman, J., Stewart, S. E., Mullin, B., Martin, A., Spencer, T., et al. (2003). Which SSRI? A meta-analysis of pharmacotherapy trials in pediatric obsessive-compulsive disorder. *American Journal of Psychiatry, 160*, 1919–1928.

Geller, D., Biederman, J., Wagner, K.D., Emslie, G. J., Gallagher, D., Wetherhold, E., Carpenter, D.J.,l. (2001, May 28–31). *Comorbid psychiatric illness and response to treatments, relapse rates, and behavioral adverse event incidents in pediatric OCD.* Abstracts of the Child and Adolescent Program of the 41st Annual Institute of Mental Health (NIMH) New Clinical Evaluation Unit (NCDEU) Meeting, Phoenix, Arizona. Z.

Geller, D. A., Hoog, S. L., Heiligenstein, J. H., Ricardi, R. K., Tamura, R., Kluszynski, S., et al. (2001). Fluoxetine treatment for obsessive-compulsive disorder in children and adolescents: a placebo-controlled clinical trial. *Journal of the American Academy of Child and Adolescent Psychiatry, 40*, 773–779.

Geller, B., Tillman, R., Craney, J. L., & Bolhofner, K. (2004). Four-year prospective outcome and natural history of mania in children with a prepubertal and early adolescent bipolar disorder phenotype. *Archives of General Psychiatry*, 61, 459–467.

Geller, B., Tillman, R., Bolhofner, K., & Zimerman, B. (2008). Child bipolar I disorder: Prospective continuity with adult bipolar I disorder; characteristics of second and third episodes; predictors of 8-year outcome. *Archives of General Psychiatry*, 65, 1125–1133.

Geller, D. A., Wagner, K. D., Emslie, G., Murphy, T., Carpenter, D. J., Wetherhold, E., et al. (2004). Paroxetine treatment in children and adolescents with obsessive-compulsive disorder: A randomized, multicenter, double-blind, placebo-controlled trial. *Journal of the American Academy of Child and Adolescent Psychiatry*, 43, 1387–1396.

Ghaziuddin, N., Kutcher, S.P., Knapp, P., Bernet, W., Arnold, V., Beitchman, J., Benson, R.S., Bukstein, O., Kinlan, J., McClellan, J., Rue, D., Shaw, J.A., Stock, S., Kroeger Ptakowski, K.; Work Group on Quality Issues; AACAP (2004). Practice parameter for use of electroconvulsive therapy with adolescents. *Journal of the American Academy of Child and Adolescent Psychiatry*, 43, 1521–1539.

Ginsburg, G.S., Kingery, J.N., Drake, K.L., Grados, M.A. (2008). Predictors of treatment response in pediatric obsessive-compulsive disorder. *Journal of the American Academy of Child and Adolescent Psychiatry*, 47, 868–878.

Gittelman-Klein, R., & Klein, D. F. (1971) Controlled Imipramine treatment of school phobia. *Archives of General Psychiatry*, 25, 204–207.

Goldstein, T. R., Axelson, D. A., Birmaher, B., & Brent, D. A. (2007). Dialectical behavior therapy for adolescents with bipolar disorder: A 1-year open trial. *Journal of the American Academy of Child and Adolescent Psychiatry*, 46, 820–830.

Goodyer, I. M., Dubicka, B., Wilkinson, P., Kelvin, R., Roberts, C., Byford, S., et al. (2008). A randomized controlled trial of cognitive behaviour therapy in adolescents with major depression treated by selective serotonin reuptake inhibitors. The ADAPT trial. *Health Technology Assessment*, 12(14), iii–iv.

Graae, F., Milner, J., Rizzotto, L., & Klein, R. G. (1994). Clonazepam in childhood anxiety disorders. *Journal of the American Academy of Child and Adolescent Psychiatry*, 33, 372–376.

Grant, P., Lougee, L., Hirschtritt, M., & Swedo, S. E. (2007). An open-label trial of riluzole, a glutamate antagonist, in children with treatment-resistant obsessive-compulsive disorder. *Journal of Child and Adolescent Psychopharmacology*, 17, 761–767.

Haas, M., DelBello, M. P., Pandina, G., Kushner, S., Van Hove, I., Augustyns, I., et al. (2009). Risperidone for the treatment of acute mania in children and adolescents with bipolar disorder: A randomized, double-blind, placebo-controlled study. *Bipolar Disorders*, 11, 687–700.

Hayward, C., Vardy, S., Albano, A. M., Thienemann, M., Henderson, L., & Schatzberg, A. F. (2000). Cognitive-behavioral group therapy for social phobia in female adolescents: Results of a pilot study. *Journal of the American Academy of Child and Adolescent Psychiatry*, 39, 721–726.

Hegeman, J. M., Doesborgh, S. J., van Niel, M. C., & van Megen, H. J. (2008). The efficacy of electroconvulsive therapy in adolescents. A retrospective study. *Tijdschrift voor Psychiatrie*, 50, 23–31.

Herbert, J. D, Gaudiano, B. A., Rheingold, A. A., Moitra, E., Myers, V. H., Dalrymple, K. L., et al. (2009). Cognitive behavior therapy for generalized anxiety disorder in adolescents: A randomized controlled trial. *Journal of Anxiety Disorders*, 23, 167–177.

Hidaldo, R. S., Tupler, L. A., & Davidson, J. R. T. (2007). An effect-size analysis of pharmacologic treatments for generalized anxiety disorder. *Journal of Psychopharmacology*, 21, 864–872.

Hughes, C. W., Emslie, G. J., Crismon, M. L., Posner, K., Birmaher, B., Ryan, N., et al. (2007). Texas Children's Medication Algorithm Project: update from Texas Consensus Conference Panel on Medication Treatment of Childhood Major Depressive Disorder. *Journal of the American Academy of Child and Adolescent Psychiatry*, 46, 667–686.

Isolan, L., Pheula, G., Salum, G. A., Oswald, S., Rohde, L. A., & Manfro, G. G. (2007). An open-label trial of escitalopram in children and adolescents with social anxiety disorder. *Journal of Child and Adolescent Psychopharmacology*, 17, 751–759.

Kafantaris, V., Coletti, D. J., Dicker, R., Padula, G., & Kane, J. M. (2003). Lithium treatment of acute mania in adolescents: A large open trial. *Journal of the American Academy of Child and Adolescent Psychiatry*, 42, 1038–1045.

Kashani, J. J., & Orvaschel, H. (1988). Anxiety disorders in mid-adolescence: A community sample. *American Journal of Psychiatry*, 145, 960–964.

Keller, M. B., Lavori, P. W., Wunder, J., Beardslee, W. R., Schwartz, C. E., & Roth, J. (1992). Chronic course of anxiety disorders in children and adolescents. *Journal of the American Academy of Child and Adolescent Psychiatry*, 31, 595–599.

Keller, M. B., Ryan, N. D., Strober, M., Klein, R. G., Kutcher, S. P., Birmaher, B., et al. (2001). Efficacy of paroxetine in the treatment of adolescent major depression: A randomized, controlled trial. *Journal of the American Academy of Child and Adolescent Psychiatry, 40*, 762–772.

Kendall, P. C. (1994). Treating anxiety disorders in children: Results of a randomized clinical trial. *Journal of Consulting and Clinical Psychology, 62*, 200–210.

Kendall, P. C., Hudson, J. L., Gosch, E., Flannery-Schroeder, E., & Suveg, C. (2008) Cognitive-behavioral therapy for anxiety disordered youth: A randomized clinical trial evaluating child and family modalities. *Journal of Consulting and Clinical Psychology, 76*, 282–297.

Kendall, P. C., Flannery-Schroeder, E., Panichelli-Mindal, S. M., Southam-Gerow, M., Henin, A., et al. (1997). Therapy for youth with anxiety disorders: A second randomized clinical trial. *Journal of Consulting and Clinical Psychology, 65*, 366–380.

Kendall, P. C., Stafford, S. Flannery-Schroeder, E., & Webb, A. (2004). Child anxiety treatment: Outcomes in adolescence and impact on substance use and depression at 7.4 year follow-up. *Journal of Consulting and Clinical Psychology, 72*, 276–287.

Kennard, B. D., Emslie, G. J., Mayes, T. L., Nightingale-Teresi, J., Nakonezny, P. A., Hughes, J. L., et al. (2008). Cognitive-behavioral therapy to prevent relapse in pediatric responders to pharmacotherapy for major depressive disorder. *Journal of the American Academy of Child and Adolescent Psychiatry, 47*, 1395–1404.

Kennard, B. D., Silva, S. G., Tonev, S., Rohde, P., Hughes, J. L., Vitiello, B., et al. (2009). Remission and recovery in the treatment for adolescents with depression study (TADS): Acute and long-term outcomes. *Journal of the American Academy of Child and Adolescent Psychiatry, 48*, 186–195.

King, R., Leonard, H., March, J., & the Work Group on Quality Issues. (1998). *Practice parameters for the assessment and treatment of children and adolescents with obsessive-compulsive disorder.* Retrieved January 2012, from http://aacap.browsermedia.com/galleries/PracticeParameters/Ocd.pdf

Klein, R. G., Koplewicz, H. S., & Kanner, A. (1992). Impiramine treatment of children with separation anxiety disorder. *Journal of the American Academy of Child and Adolescent Psychiatry, 31*, 21–28.

Kowatch, R. A., Findling, R. L., Scheffer, R. E., & Stanford, K. (2007, October 23–28). Pediatric bipolar collaborative mood stabilizer trial. Poster presented at the 54th Annual Meeting of the American Academy of Child and Adolescent Psychiatry, Boston, MA.

Kowatch, R. A., Fristad, M., Birmaher, B., Wagner, K. D., Findling, R. L., Hellander, M., et al. (2005). Treatment guidelines for children and adolescents with bipolar disorder. *Journal of the American Academy of Child and Adolescent Psychiatry, 44*, 213–235.

Kowatch, R. A., Suppes, T., Carmody, T. J., Bucci, J. P., Hume, J. H., Kromelis, M., et al. (2000). Effect size of lithium, divalproex sodium, and carbamazepine in children and adolescents with bipolar disorder. *Journal of the American Academy of Child and Adolescent Psychiatry, 39*, 713–720.

Kratochvil, C., Emslie, G., Silva, S., McNulty, S., Walkup, J., Curry, J., et al. (2006). Acute time to response in the treatment for adolescents with depression study (TADS). *Journal of the American Academy of Child and Adolescent Psychiatry, 45*, 1412–1418.

Kutcher, S. P., Reiter, S., Gardner, D. M., & Klein, R. G. (1992). The pharmacotherapy of social anxiety disorders in children and adolescents. *Psychiatric Clinics of North America, 15*, 41–67.

Leonard, H. L., Swedo, S. E., Lenane, M. C., Rettew, D. C., Cheslow, D. L., Hamburger, S. D., et al. (1991). A double-blind desipramine substitution during long-term clomipramine treatment in children and adolescents with obsessive-compulsive disorder. *Archives of General Psychiatry, 48*, 922–927.

Leonard, H. L., Topol, D., Bukstein, O., Hindmarsh, D., Allen, A. J., & Swedo, S. E. (1994). Clonazepam as an augmenting agent in the treatment of childhood-onset obsessive-compulsive disorder. *Journal of the American Academy of Child and Adolescent Psychiatry, 33*, 792–794.

Lewinsohn, P. M., Clarke, G. N., Hops, H., & Andrews, J. (1990). Cognitive-behavioral treatment for depressed adolescents. *Behavioral Therapy, 21*, 385–401.

Lewinsohn, P. M., Klein, D. N., & Seeley, J. R. (1995). Bipolar disorders in a community sample of older adolescents: Prevalence, phenomenology, comorbidity, and course. *Journal of the American Academy of Child and Adolescent Psychiatry, 34*, 454–463.

Liber, J. M., Van Widenfelt, B. M., Utens, E. M. W. J., Ferdinand, R. F., Van der Leeden, A. J. M., Van Gastel, W., et al. (2008). No differences between group versus individual treatment of childhood anxiety disorders in a randomized clinical trial. *Journal of Child Psychology and Psychiatry, 49*, 886–893.

Liebowitz, M. R., Turner, S. M., Piacentini, J., Beidel, D. C., Clarvit, S. R., Davies, S. O., et al. (2002). Fluoxetine in children and adolescents with OCD: A placebo-controlled trial. *Journal of the American Academy of Child and Adolescent Psychiatry, 41*, 1431–1438.

Manassis, K., Mendlowitz, S. L., Scapillato, D., Avery, D., Fiksenbaum, L., Freire, M., et al. (2002). Group and individual cognitive behavioral therapy for childhood anxiety disorders. A randomized trial. *Journal of the American Academy of Child and Adolescent Psychiatry, 41*, 1423–1430.

March, J. S., Biederman, J., Wolkow, R., Safferman, A., Mardekian, J., Cook, E. H., et al. (1998). Sertraline in children and adolescents with obsessive-compulsive disorder: A multicenter randomized controlled trial. *Journal of the American Medical Association, 280*, 1752–1756.

March, J. S., Entusah, R., Rynn, M., Albano, A. M., & Tourian, K. A. (2007). A randomized controlled trial of venlafaxine ER versus placebo in pediatric social anxiety disorder. *Biological Psychiatry, 62*, 1149–1154.

Masi, G., Mucci, M., & Millepiedi, S. (2002). Clozapine in adolescent inpatients with acute mania. *Journal of Child and Adolescent Psychopharmacology, 12*, 93–99.

Masi, G., Millepiedi, S., Perugi, G., Pfanner, C., Berloffa, S., Pari, C., et al. (2009). Pharmacotherapy in paediatric obsessive-compulsive disorder: A naturalistic, retrospective study. *CNS Drugs, 23*, 241–252.

Masi, G., Perugi, G., Toni, C., Millepiedi, S., Mucci, M., Bertini, N., et al. (2004). Predictors of treatment nonresponse in bipolar children and adolescents with manic or mixed episodes. *Journal of Child and Adolescent Psychopharmacology, 14*, 395–404.

Masi, G., Pfanner, C., Millepiedi, S., & Berloffa, S. (2010). Aripiprazole augmentation in 39 adolescents with medication-resistant obsessive-compulsive disorder. *Journal of Clinical Psychopharmacology, 30*, 688–693.

McClellan, J., Kowatch, R., & Findling, R. L. (2007). Practice parameter for the assessment and treatment of children and adolescents with bipolar disorder. *Journal of the American Academy of Child and Adolescent Psychiatry, 46*, 107–125.

Melvin, G. A., Tonge, B. J., King, N. J., Heyne, D., Gordon, M. S., & Klimkeit, E. (2006). A comparison of cognitive-behavioral therapy, sertraline, and their combination for adolescent depression. *Journal of the American Academy of Child and Adolescent Psychiatry, 45*, 1151–1161.

Merikangas, K. R., He, J. P., Burstein, M., Swanson, S. A., Avenevoli, S., Cui, L., et al. (2010). Lifetime prevalence of mental disorders in U.S. adolescents: Results from the National Comorbidity Survey Replication—Adolescent Supplement (NCS-A). *Journal of the American Academy of Child and Adolescent Psychiatry, 49*, 980–989.

Merlo, L. J., Storch, E. A., Lehmkuhl, H. D., Jacob, M. L., Murphy, T. K., Goodman, W. K., et al. (2010). Cognitive behavioral therapy plus motivational interviewing improves outcomes for pediatric obsessive-compulsive disorder: a preliminary study. *Cognitive Behavior Therapy, 39*, 24–27.

Mrakotsky, C., Masek, B., Biederman, J., Raches, D., Hsin, O., Forbes, P., et al. (2008) Prospective open-label pilot trial of mirtazapine in children and adolescents with social phobia. *Journal of Anxiety Disorders, 22*, 88–97.

Mufson, L., Weissman, M. M., Moreau, D., & Garfinkel, R. (1999). Efficacy of interpersonal psychotherapy for depressed adolescents. *Archives of General Psychiatry, 56*, 573–579.

Mufson, L., Dorta, K. P., Wickramaratne, P., Nomura, Y., Olfson, M., & Weissman, M. M. (2004). A randomized effectiveness trial of interpersonal psychotherapy for depressed adolescents. *Archives of General Psychiatry, 61*, 577–584.

Mukaddes, N. M., & Abali, O. (2003). Quetiapine treatment for children and adolescents with Tourette's Disorder. *Journal of Child and Adolescent Psychopharmacology, 13*, 295–299.

Nemets, H., Nemets, B., Apter, A., Bracha, Z., & Belmaker, R. H. (2006). Omega-3 treatment of childhood depression: A controlled, double-blind study. *American Journal of Psychiatry, 163*, 1098–1100.

O'Kearney, R. (2007). Benefits of cognitive-behavioural therapy for children and youth with obsessive-compulsive disorder: Re-examination of the evidence. *Australian and New Zealand Journal of Psychiatry, 41*, 199–212.

O'Leary, E. M., Barrett, P., & Fjermestad, K. W. (2009). Cognitive-behavioral family treatment for childhood obsessive-compulsive disorder: A 7-year follow-up study. *Journal of Anxiety Disorders, 23*, 973–978.

Oner, O., & Oner, P. (2008). Psychopharmacology of pediatric obsessive-compulsive disorder: Three case reports. *Journal of Psychopharmacology, 22*, 809–811.

Papanikolaou, C., Richardson, C., Pehlivanidis, A., & Papadopoulou-Daifoti, Z. (2006). Efficacy of antidepressants in child and adolescent depression: A meta-analytic study. *Journal of Neural Transmission, 113*, 399–415.

Pathak, S., Johns, E. S., & Kowatch, R. A. (2005). Adjunctive quetiapine for treatment-resistant adolescent major depressive disorder: a case series. *Journal of Child and Adolescent Psychopharmacology, 15*, 696–702.

Pavuluri, M. N., Henry, D. B., Carbray, J. A., Sampson, G., Naylor, M. W., & Janicak, P. G. (2004). Open-label prospective trial of risperidone in combination with lithium or divalproex sodium in pediatric mania. *Journal of Affective Disorders, 82*(Suppl 1), S103–S111.

Pavuluri, M. N., Henry, D. B., Carbray, J. A., Sampson, G. A., Naylor, M. W., & Janicak, P.G. (2006). A one-year open-label trial of risperidone augmentation in lithium nonresponder youth with preschool-onset bipolar disorder. *Journal of Child and Adolescent Psychopharmacology, 16*, 336–350.

Pavuluri, M. N., Henry, D. B., Devineni, B., Carbray, J. A., & Birmaher, B. (2006). Child mania rating scale: Development, reliability, and validity. *Journal of the American Academy of Child and Adolescent Psychiatry*, *45*, 550–560.

Pavuluri, M. N., Henry, D. B., Findling, R. L., Parnes, S., Carbray, J. A., Mohammed, T., et al. (2010). Double-blind randomized trial of risperidone versus divalproex in pediatric bipolar disorder. *Bipolar Disorders*, *12*, 593–605.

Pavuluri, M. N., Henry, D. B., Moss, M., Mohammed, T., Carbray, J. A., & Sweeney, J. A. (2009). Effectiveness of lamotrigine in maintaining symptom control in pediatric bipolar disorder. *Journal of Child and Adolescent Psychopharmacology*, *19*, 75–82.

The Pediatric OCD Treatment Study (POTS) Team. (2004). Cognitive-behavior therapy, sertraline, and their combination for children and adolescents with obsessive-compulsive disorder. The pediatric OCD treatment study (POTS) randomized controlled trial. *Journal of the American Medical Association*, *292*, 1969–1976.

Piacentini, J., Bergman, R. L., Jacobs, C. McCracken, J., & Kretchman, J. (2002). Cognitive-behavior therapy for childhood obsessive-compulsive disorder: Efficacy and predictors of treatment response. *Journal of Anxiety Disorders*, *16*, 207–219.

Poznanski, E. O., Freman, L. N., & Mokros, H. B. (1985). Children's Depression Rating Scale-revised. *Psychopharmacology Bulletin*, *21*, 979–989.

Rao, U., Hammen, C. L., & Poland, R. E. (2010). Longitudinal course of adolescent depression: Neuroendocrine and psychosocial predictors. *Journal of the American Academy of Child and Adolescent Psychiatry*, *49*, 141–151.

Rapee, R. M., Abbott, M. J., & Lyneham, H. J. (2006). Bibliotherapy for children with anxiety disorders using written materials for parents: A randomized controlled trial. *Journal of Consulting and Clinical Psychology*, *74*, 436–444.

Research Units on Pediatric Psychopharmacology Anxiety Study Group. (2001). Fluvoxamine for the treatment of anxiety disorders in children and adolescents. *New England Journal of Medicine*, *344*, 1279–1285.

Research Units on Pediatric Psychopharmacology Anxiety Study Group. (2002). The pediatric anxiety rating scale (PARS): Development and psychometric properties. *Journal of the American Academy of Child and Adolescent Psychiatry*, *41*, 1061–1069.

Rey, J. M., & Walter, G. (1997). Half a century of ECT use in young people. *American Journal of Psychiatry*, *154*, 595–602.

Riddle, M. A., Reeve, E. A., Yaryura-Tobias, J. A., Yang, H. M., Claghorn, J. L., Greist, J. H., et al. (2001). Fluvoxamine for children and adolescents with obsessive-compulsive disorder: A randomized, controlled, multicenter trial. *Journal of the American Academy of Child and Adolescent Psychiatry*, *40*, 222–229.

Riddle, M. A., Scahill, L., King, R. A., Hardin, M. T., Anderson, G. M., Ort, S. I., et al. (1992). Double-blind, crossover trial of fluoxetine and placebo in children and adolescents with obsessive-compulsive disorder. *Journal of the American Academy of Child and Adolescent Psychiatry*, *31*, 1062–1069.

Riggs, P. D., Mikulich-Gilbertson, S. K., Davies, R. D., Lohman, M., Klein, C., & Stover, S. K. (2007). A randomized controlled trial of fluoxetine and cognitive behavioral therapy in adolescents with major depression, behavior problems, and substance use disorders. *Archives of Pediatric Adolescent Medicine*, *161*, 1026–1034.

Roselló, J., & Bernal, G. (1999). The efficacy of cognitive-behavioral and interpersonal treatments for depression in Puerto Rican adolescents. *Journal of Consulting and Clinical Psychology*, *67*, 734–745.

Ross, D. C., & Piggott, L. R. (1993). Clonazepam for OCD. *Journal of the American Academy of Child and Adolescent Psychiatry*, *32*, 470–471.

Rynn, M. A., Findling, R. L., Emslie, G. J., Marcus, R.N., Fernandes, L.A., D'Amico, M.F., Hardy, S.A., (2002, May 18–23). *Efficacy and safety of nefazodone in adolescents with MDD*. Poster presented at the 155th Annual Meeting of the American Psychiatric Association, Philadelphia, PA.

Rynn, M. A., Riddle, M., Yeung, P. P., & Kunz, N. R. (2007). Efficacy and safety of extended-release venlafaxine in the treatment of generalized anxiety disorder in children and adolescents: Two placebo-controlled trials. *American Journal of Psychiatry*, *164*, 290–300.

Rynn, M. A., Siqueland, L., & Rickels, K. (2001). Placebo-controlled trial of sertraline in the treatment of children with generalized anxiety disorder. *American Journal of Psychiatry*, *158*, 2008–2014.

Saavedra, L. M., Silverman, W. K., Morgan-Lopez, A. A., & Kurtines, W. M. (2010). Cognitive behavioral treatment for childhood anxiety disorders: Long-term effects on anxiety and secondary disorders in young adulthood. *Journal of Child Psychology and Psychiatry*, *51*, 924–934.

Silverman, W. K., Kurtines, W. M., Ginsburg, G. S., Weems, C. F., Lumpkin, P. W., & Carmichael, D. H. (1999). Treating anxiety disorders in children with group cognitive-behavioural therapy: A randomized clinical trial. *Journal of Consulting and Clinical Psychology*, *67*, 995–1003.

Silverman, W. K., Pina, A. A., & Viswesvaran, C. (2008). Evidence-based psychosocial treatments for phobic and anxiety disorders in children and adolescents. *Journal of Clinical Child and Adolescent Psychiatry Psychology, 37*, 105–130.

Simeon, J. G. (1993). Use of anxiolytics in children. *Encephale, 19*, 71–74.

Simeon, J. G., Ferguson, H. B., Knott, V., Roberts, N., Gauthier, B., Dubois, C., et al. (1992). Clinical, cognitive, and neurophysiological effects of alprazolam in children and adolescents with overanxious and avoidant disorders. *Journal of the American Academy of Child and Adolescent Psychiatry, 31*, 29–33.

Spence, S. H., Donovan, C., & Brechman-Toussaint, M. (2000). The treatment of childhood social phobia: The effectiveness of a social skills training-based, cognitive-behavioral intervention with and without parental involvement. *Journal of Child Psychology and Psychiatry, 41*, 713–726.

Spence, S. H., Holmes, J. M., March, S., & Lipp, O. V. (2006). The feasibility and outcome of clinic plus internet delivery of cognitive behavior therapy for childhood anxiety. *Journal of Consulting and Clinical Psychology, 74*, 614–621.

Stein, M. B., Fuetsch, M., Müeller, N., Höfler, M., Lieb, R., & Wittchen, H. U. (2001). Social anxiety disorder and the risk of depression: A prospective community study of adolescents and young adults. *Archives of General Anxiety, 58*, 251–256.

Stewart, S. E., Geller, D. A., Jenike, M., Pauls, D., Shaw, D., Mullin, B., et al. (2004). Long-term outcome of pediatric obsessive-compulsive disorder: A meta-analysis and qualitative review of the literature. *Acta Psychiatrica Scandinavica, 110*, 4–13.

Storch, E. A., Björgvinsson, T., Riemann, B., Lewin, A. B., Morales, M. J., & Murphy, T. J. (2010). Factors associated with poor response in cognitive-behavioral therapy for pediatric obsessive-compulsive disorder. *Bulletin of the Menninger Clinic, 74*, 167–185.

Storch, E. A., Geffken, G. R., Merlo, L. J., Mann, G., Duke, D., Munson, M., et al. (2007). Family-based cognitive behavioral therapy for pediatric obsessive-compulsive disorder: Comparison of intensive and weekly approaches. *Journal of the American Academy of Child and Adolescent Psychiatry, 46*, 469–478.

Storch, E. A., Lehmkuhl, H., Geffken, G. R., Touchton, A., & Murphy, T. K. (2008). Aripiprazole augmentation of incomplete treatment response in an adolescent male with obsessive-compulsive disorder. *Depression and Anxiety, 25*, 172–174.

Storch, E. A., Lehmkuhl, H. D., Ricketts, E., Geffken, G. R., Marien, W., & Murphy, T. K. (2010). An open-label trial of intensive family based cognitive-behavioral therapy in youth with obsessive-compulsive disorder who are medication partial responders or nonresponders. *Journal of Clinical Child and Adolescent Psychology, 39*, 260–268.

Storch, E. A., Merlo, L. J., Larson, M. J., Geffken, G. R., Lehmkuhl, H. D., Jacob, M. L., et al. (2008). Impact of comorbidity on cognitive-behavioral therapy response in pediatric obsessive-compulsive disorder. *Journal of the American Academy of Child and Adolescent Psychiatry, 47*, 583–592.

Tang, T., Jou, S., Ko, C., Huang, S., & Yen, C. (2009). Randomized study of school-based intensive interpersonal psychotherapy for depressed adolescents with suicidal risk and parasuicide behaviors. *Psychiatry and Clinical Neurosciences, 63*, 463–470.

Tao, R., Emslie, G., Mayes, T., Nakonezny, P., Kennard, B., & Hughest, C. (2009). Early prediction of acute antidepressant treatment response and remission in pediatric major depressive disorder. *Journal of the American Academy of Child and Adolescent Psychiatry, 48*(1), 71.

The Pediatric OCD Treatment Study (POTS) Team. (2004). Cognitive-behavior therapy, sertraline, and their combination for children and adolescents with obsessive-compulsive disorder. The pediatric OCD treatment study (POTS) randomized controlled trial. *Journal of the American Medical Association, 292*, 1969–1976.

The TADS Team. (2007). The treatment for adolescents with depression study (TADS). *Archives of General Psychiatry, 64*, 1132–1144.

Thomsen, P. H. (1997). Child and adolescent obsessive-compulsive disorder treated with citalopram: Findings from an open trial of 23 cases. *Journal of Child and Adolescent Psychopharmacology, 7*, 157–166.

Thomsen, P. H. (2004). Risperidone augmentation in the treatment of severe adolescent OCD in SSRI-refractory cases: A case-series. *Annals of Clinical Psychiatry, 16*, 201–207.

Thomsen, P. H., Ebbesen, C., & Persson, C. (2001). Long-term experience with citalopram in the treatment of adolescent OCD. *Journal of the American Academy of Child and Adolescent Psychiatry, 40*, 895–902.

Tohen, M., Kryzhanovskaya, L., Carlson, G., Delbello, M., Wozniak, J., Kowatch, R., et al. (2007). Olanzapine versus placebo in the treatment of adolescents with bipolar mania. *American Journal of Psychiatry, 164*, 1547–1556.

Treatment for Adolescents With Depression Study (TADS) Team. (2004). Fluoxetine, cognitive-behavioral therapy, and their combination for adolescents with depression: Treatment for Adolescents With Depression Study (TADS) randomized controlled trial. *Journal of the American Medical Association, 292,* 807–820.

Tsapakis, E. M., Soldani, F., Tondo, L., & Baldessarini, R. J. (2008). Efficacy of antidepressants in juvenile depression: Meta-analysis. *British Journal of Psychiatry, 193,* 10–17.

US Food and Drug Administration. (2004, September 13–14). Joint Meeting of the Psychopharmacologic Drugs Advisory Committee and Pediatric Advisory Committee. Available at: http:www.fda.gov/ohrms/dockets/as/04/briefing/2004-4065b1.htm. Assessed January 2011.

Vitiello, B., Emslie, G., Clarke, G., Wagner, K. D., Asarnow, J. R., Keller, M. B., et al. (2011). Long-term outcome of adolescent depression initially resistant to selective serotonin reuptake inhibitor treatment: A follow-up study of the TORDIA sample. *Journal of Clinical Psychiatry, 71,* 388–396.

von Knorring, A. L., Olsson, G. I., Thomsen, P. H., Lemming, O. M., & Hultén, A. (2006). A randomized, double-blind, placebo-controlled study of citalopram in adolescents with major depressive disorder. *Journal of Clinical Psychopharmacology, 26,* 311–315.

Wagner, K. D., Ambrosini, P., Rynn, M., Wohlberg, C., Yang, R., Greenbaum, M. S., et al. (2003). Efficacy of sertraline in the treatment of children and adolescents with major depressive disorder: Two randomized controlled trials. *Journal of the American Medical Association, 290,* 1033–1041.

Wagner, K. D., Berard, R., Stein, M. D., Wetherhold, E., Carpenter, D. J., Perera, P., et al. (2004). A multicenter, randomized, double-blind placebo-controlled trial of paroxetine in children and adolescents with social anxiety disorder. *Archives of General Psychiatry, 61,* 1153–1162.

Wagner, K. D., Cook, E. H., Chung, H., & Messig, M. (2003). Remission status after long-term sertraline treatment of pediatric obsessive-compulsive disorder. *Journal of Child and Adolescent Psychopharmacology, 13*(Suppl 1): S53–S60.

Wagner, K. D., Jonas, J., Findling, R. L., Ventura, D., & Saikali, K. (2006). A double-blind, randomized, placebo-controlled trial of escitalopram in the treatment of pediatric depression. *Journal of the American Academy of Child and Adolescent Psychiatry, 45,* 280–288.

Wagner, K. D., Kowatch, R. A., Emslie, G. J., Findling, R. L., Wilens, T. E., McCague, K., et al. (2006). A double-blind, randomized, placebo-controlled trial of oxcarbazepine in the treatment of bipolar disorder in children and adolescents. *American Journal of Psychiatry, 163,* 1179–1186.

Wagner, K. D., & Pliszka, S. R. (2009). Treatment of child and adolescent disorders. In *Textbook of psychopharmacology* (4th ed., pp. 1309–1366). (Schatzberg, A.F., Nemeroff, C.B. Eds). Washington, DC: American Psychiatric Publishing.

Wagner, K. D., Redden, L., Kowatch, R. A., Wilens, T. E., Segal, S., Chang, K., et al. (2009). A double-blind, randomized, placebo-controlled trial of divalproex extended-release in the treatment of bipolar disorder in children and adolescents. *Journal of the American Academy of Child and Adolescent Psychiatry, 48,* 519–532.

Wagner, K. D., Robb, A. S., Findling, R. L., Jin, J., Gutierrez, M. M., & Heydorn, W. E. (2004). A randomized, placebo-controlled trial of citalopram for the treatment of major depression in children and adolescents. *American Journal of Psychiatry, 161,* 1079–1083.

Walkup, J. T., Albano, A. M., Piacentini, J., Birmaher, B., Compton, S. N., Sherrill, J. R., et al. (2008). Cognitive behavioral therapy, sertraline, or a combination in childhood anxiety. *New England Journal of Medicine, 359,* 2753–2766.

Walkup, J., Labellarte, M., Riddle, M. A., Pine, D. S., Greenhill, L., Fairbanks, J., et al. (2002). Treatment of pediatric anxiety disorders: An open-label extension of the research units on pediatric psychopharmacology anxiety study. *Journal of Child and Adolescent Psychopharmacology, 12,* 175–188.

Walkup, J. T., Reeve, E., Yaryura-Tobias, J., Wong, J., Claghorn, G., Gaffney, J., Greist, D., Holland, B. McConville, T. Pibott, M. Pravetz, L. Scahill, M. Riddle et al. (1998, October 27–November 1). *Fluvoxamine for childhood OCD: Long-term treatment.* Poster presented at the 45th Annual Meeting of the American Academy of Child and Adolescent Psychiatry, Anahiem, CA (abstract Also published in *Eur Neuropsychopharmacol.* 1999; 9 (Suppl 5) 307.

Walter, G., & Rey, J. M. (1997). An epidemiological study of the use of ECT in adolescents. *Journal of the American Academy of Child and Adolescent Psychiatry, 36,* 809–815.

Walter, G., Tormos, J. M., Israel, J. A., & Pascual-Leone, A. (2001). Transcranial magnetic stimulation in young persons: A review of known cases. *Journal of Child and Adolescent Psychopharmacology, 11,* 69–75.

Watson, H. J., & Rees, C. S. (2008). Meta-analysis of randomized, controlled treatment trials for pediatric obsessive-compulsive disorder. *Journal of Child Psychology and Psychiatry, 49,* 489–498.

Weisz, J. R., McCarty, C. A., & Valeri, S. M. (2006). Effects of psychotherapy for depression in children and adolescents: A meta-analysis. *Psychological Bulletin, 132,* 132–149.

West, A. E., Jacobs, R. H., Westerholm, R., Lee, A., Carbray, J., Heidenreich, J., et al. (2009). Child and family-focused cognitive-behavioral therapy for pediatric bipolar disorder: Pilot study of group treatment format. *Journal of the Canadian Academy of Child and Adolescent Psychiatry, 18,* 239–246.

Wood, A., Harrington, R., & Moore, A. (1996). A controlled trial of a brief cognitive-behavioural intervention in adolescent patients with depressive disorders. *Journal of Child Psychology and Psychiatry, 37,* 737–746.

Young, J. F., Mufson, L., & Gallop, R. (2010). Preventing depression: A randomized trial of interpersonal psychotherapy-adolescent skills training. *Depression and Anxiety, 27,* 426–433.

Young, R. C., Biggs, J. T., Ziegler, V. E., & Meyer, D. A.(1978). A rating scale for mania: Reliability, validity and sensitivity. *British Journal of Psychiatry, 133,* 429–435.

Zohar, A. H. (1999). The epidemiology of obsessive-compulsive disorder in children and adolescents. *Child and Adolescent Psychiatric Clinics North America, 8,* 445–460.

Index

Note: Page numbers followed by *f* or *t* indicate figures or tables, respectively.